PRACTICAL MANUAL IN CLINICAL MEDICINE

PRACTICAL MANUAL IN CLINICAL MEDICINE

ABM Abdullah
MRCP (UK) FRCP (Edin)
Dean, Faculty of Medicine
Professor, Department of Medicine
Bangabandhu Sheikh Mujib Medical University
Dhaka, Bangladesh

Foreword
Kamrul Hasan Khan

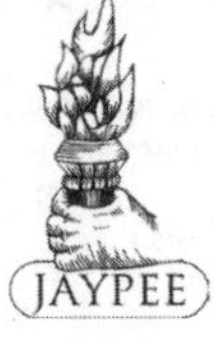

The Health Sciences Publisher
New Delhi | London | Philadelphia | Panama

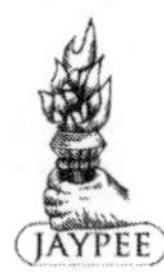

Jaypee Brothers Medical Publishers (P) Ltd

Headquarters

Jaypee Brothers Medical Publishers (P) Ltd
4838/24, Ansari Road, Daryaganj
New Delhi 110 002, India
Phone: +91-11-43574357
Fax: +91-11-43574314
Email: jaypee@jaypeebrothers.com

Overseas Offices

J.P. Medical Ltd
83 Victoria Street, London
SW1H 0HW (UK)
Phone: +44 20 3170 8910
Fax: +44 (0)20 3008 6180
Email: info@jpmedpub.com

Jaypee-Highlights Medical Publishers Inc
City of Knowledge, Bld. 235, 2nd Floor, Clayton
Panama City, Panama
Phone: +1 507-301-0496
Fax: +1 507-301-0499
Email: cservice@jphmedical.com

Jaypee Medical Inc
325, Chestnut Street
Suite 412, Philadelphia, PA 19106, USA
Phone: +1 267-519-9789
Email: support@jpmedus.com

Jaypee Brothers Medical Publishers (P) Ltd
17/1-B Babar Road, Block-B, Shaymali
Mohammadpur, Dhaka-1207
Bangladesh
Mobile: +08801912003485
Email: jaypeedhaka@gmail.com

Jaypee Brothers Medical Publishers (P) Ltd
Bhotahity, Kathmandu, Nepal
Phone: +977-9741283608
Email: kathmandu@jaypeebrothers.com

Website: www.jaypeebrothers.com
Website: www.jaypeedigital.com

Inquiries for bulk sales may be solicited at: jaypee@jaypeebrothers.com

Practical Manual in Clinical Medicine

First Edition: **2017**

ISBN 978-93-85999-71-0

Printed at Nutech Print Services - India

Dedicated to

The memory of

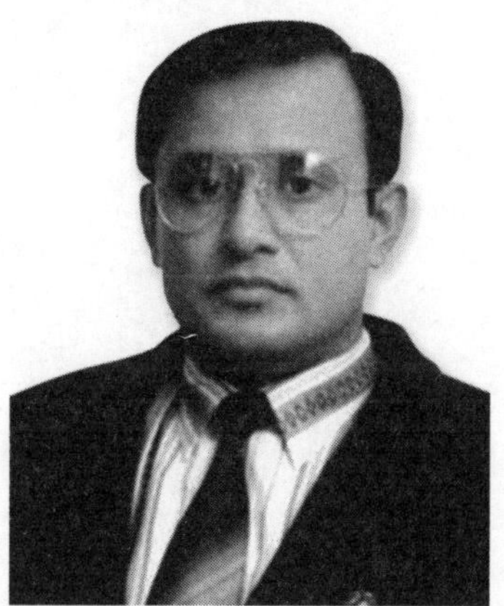

Professor AKM Khorshed Alam

My closest friend, colleague, a well-wisher and source of continued love, affection and inspiration

Foreword

It is my profound delight and pleasure to write a few words about *Practical Manual in Clinical Medicine* by Professor ABM Abdullah. This book sheds light on the important aspects of different diseases covering all the branches of clinical medicine. While going through the manuscript of the book, I keenly observed that all the chapters in this book are arranged in an excellent form. The book is the first of its kind in the country enlightening the crucial facts of different diseases, which will help both undergraduate and postgraduate students of different specialities. Even the busy practicing specialists and general practitioners will be greatly benefitted from the concise and rational format of the book. Dr Abdullah has written this book in such a methodical way that I firmly believe it will become a powerful tool for doctors from all quarters to enhance their knowledge, which will positively impact the standard of medical care throughout the world.

Kamrul Hasan Khan
Vice-Chancellor
Bangabandhu Sheikh Mujib Medical University
Dhaka, Bangladesh

Preface

By the grace of Almighty and persistent support from my family and well-wishers, I am pleased to present the first edition of *Practical Manual in Clinical Medicine.*

There is no doubt that medicine is a vast discipline. Advances are taking place in different branches of this field of science every day. It is a crucial duty of every health professional to keep track with these advances, so that they can come up with the best services possible. For that purpose, one needs to know what he or she must know about a disease and which information are trivial. During the preparation of this book, I solely focused on the information, a physician must memorize during his/her day-to-day practice.

On the other hand, as the syllabus of medicine is overwhelming for the students, they often find it very difficult to retain the necessary knowledge from the large textbooks. This book will also serve to that cause. Medical students, junior doctors, general practitioners, specialist physicians and all other health professionals can use this book as an important tool to quickly brush up on their knowledge. This book can be used by practicing doctors from different specialities to equip themselves with updated knowledge of modern medicine.

I am enthusiastic about *Practical Manual in Clinical Medicine* and all it offers to the readers. I wholeheartedly invite constructive criticism from readers, so that any error can be corrected in future edition.

ABM Abdullah

Acknowledgements

My sincere gratitude to Professor Kamrul Hasan Khan, Vice-Chancellor, Bangabandhu Sheikh Mujib Medical University, Bangladesh, for his inspiration and valuable suggestions regarding this book.

I am deeply indebted to the contributions of my colleagues, fellow doctors and students during the preparation of this book.

- Dr Masuda Begum FCPS, Chairman and Professor, Department of Haematology
- Dr Tahmida Hassan MBBS DDV MD (Dermatol)
- Dr Sanjana Zaman Diploma in Child Psychology PhD (Paed Haematol and Oncol)
- Dr Md Rafiquzzaman Khan FCPS, Associate Professor, Department of Haematology
- Dr Mohammad Abul Kalam Azad FCPS (Med) MD (Rheumat)
- Dr Tazin Afrose Shah FCPS
- Dr Shahnoor Sarmin MCPS FCPS MD (Cardiol)
- Dr Sadi Abdullah MBBS DTCD
- Dr Abhijit Chowdhury PhD Student (University of Newcastle, Australia)
- Dr Ahmed-Al-Muntasir-Niloy MBBS MD (USA)
- Dr Samprity Islam MBBS
- Dr Khaled Mahbub Murshed MBBS
- Dr Nazma Ahmed MBBS DDV
- Dr Shamin Fatema Islam MPH MD (Residency Student)
- Dr Naila Akhter MBBS MD (Residency Student)
- Dr Shailesh Shah MBBS MD (Residency Student)
- Dr Mohona Zaman MBBS MD (Residency Student)
- Dr Sadia Sabah MBBS
- Dr Imtiaz Ahmed MBBS
- Dr Shakhawat Hossain (Rokan) MBBS
- Dr Saiful Islam Alin MBBS MD (Student)
- Dr Omar Serajul Hasan MD (USA)
- Dr Tanjim Sultana MD (USA)

My special thanks to Shri Jitendar P Vij (Group Chairman), Mr Ankit Vij (Group President) and Mr Tarun Duneja (Director–Publishing) of M/s Jaypee Brothers Medical Publishers (P) Ltd, New Delhi, India, for their effort and relentless help which made this book possible to come into light.

Lastly, I am grateful to my wife and children, whose untiring support had been the driving force behind writing this book.

Contents

CHAPTER

1

General Examination

CHAPTER CONTENTS

- Face in different diseases
- Xanthelasma
- Xanthoma
- Hands in different diseases
- Claw hand
- Clubbing
- Koilonychia
- Leuconychia
- Nail changes in different dieases
- Cyanosis
- Fever
- Neuroleptic malignant syndrome
- Malignant hyperthermia
- Pyrexia of unknown origin
- Generalized lymphadenopathy
- Cervical lymphadenopathy
- Oedema
- Pigmentation
- Hirsutism
- Hypertrichosis
- Gynaecomastia
- Hyperhydrosis
- Pyoderma gangrenosum

FACE IN DIFFERENT DISEASES

By looking at the patient's face, many clinical diagnoses are possible. Some examples are given below—

- Myxoedematous face—patient looks apathetic, face is puffy with periorbital swelling, baggy eyelids with loss of outer 1/3rd of the eyebrows. There may be malar flash.
- Cretinism—idiotic look, coarse face with thick lips, large ears.
- Thyrotoxic face or Graves' disease—bilateral or unilateral exophthalmos, the patient looks anxious, restless and fidgety. Thyroid gland is diffusely enlarged.
- Cushingoid face—rounded, plethoric face giving rise to moon face appearance, also hirsutism and acne.
- Acromegalic face—coarse facies, prominent supraorbital ridges, increased wrinkling of the forehead. Mandible, nose, lips and ears are large.
- Mongoloid face (Down's syndrome)—flat nasal bridge, low set small ears, mouth appears small and tends to remain open. Tongue appears protruding with large, horizontal fissure.
- Haemolytic face—frontal and parietal bossing with prominent malar bones.
- Puffy face—see below.
- Leonine face (in lepromatous leprosy)—skin of the face and forehead is thick and corrugated. Multiple nodules of variable sizes and shapes involving ear lobule, face and nose.
- Bell's palsy (see in the Chapter Neurological Bell's Palsy).
- Parkinsonian face—mask like, expressionless face with less blinking of the eyes, staring look and dribbling of saliva.
- Marfanoid face—face is long, lean, elongated and narrow.
- Mitral facies—malar flush.
- Myopathic face—frontal baldness, long, lean, triangular, sad and expressionless face with wasting of temporalis and masseter.
- Nephrotic face—puffy with periorbital swelling.
- Achondroplasia—skull appears enlarged.
- Superior vena caval (SVC) obstruction—puffy, oedematous, plethoric face with congested conjunctival vessels (blood shot eyes) and engorged nonpulsatile neck vein.
- Sturge-Weber's syndrome—port wine stain.
- Hepatic facies—muddy or pigmented discolouration, pinched face and sunken eyes, prominent malar bones.
- Hippocratic face (in advanced peritonitis)—pinched nose, sunken eyes, collapsed temples, with crust on lips and clammy forehead.
- Psychiatric disorders—depressed or anxious face.
- Butterfly rash—photosensitive rash over both cheeks and bridge of the nose.
- Systemic sclerosis—smooth, shiny, tight with hypopigmented and hyperpigmented areas. Nose is pinched up and tapered (beaking of nose, bird beak), loss of wrinkling of forehead. Lips are thin, pursed with puckering of the skin around mouth. Orifice of mouth is small (microstomia).
- Myasthenic face—ptosis, usually bilateral, may be unilateral with frontalis over activity.
- Turner's face—short and webbed neck, low hairline and redundant skinfold on the back of neck. Small lower jaw (micrognathia), small and fish-like mouth with low set, deformed ears.
- Bilateral parotid enlargement.
- Virile (virilization in female).

- Tabetic face—pseudoptosis (due to paralysis of tarsal muscles) with compensatory wrinkling of forehead.
- Paget's disease—large cranium or mandible or forehead.
- Facial asymmetry—hemiplegia and hemiatrophy.
- Lupus perniopigmentation of the tip of the nose in sarcoidosis.

Loss of Lateral One Third of Eyebrow

- Physiological.
- Hypothyroidism.
- Leprosy.

Butterfly Rash

Rash on the cheeks and bridge of the nose sparing the nasolabial fold.
Causes are—

- Systemic lupus erythematosus or discoid lupus erythematosus (DLE).
- Dermatomyositis.
- Mixed connective tissue disease (MCTD).
- Sarcoidosis.
- Drug rash.
- Acne rosacea (characterized by red patch with telangiectasia on the face with papules and pustules, which are absent in systemic lupus erythematosus (SLE)).
- Lepromatous leprosy.
- Post-kala-azar dermal leishmaniasis (PKDL).

Depressed Nasal Bridge

Causes are—

- Trauma.
- Tuberculosis (TB)(lupus vulgaris).
- Leprosy.
- Sarcoidosis.
- Congenital syphilis (also tertiary).
- Wegener's granulomatosis.
- Fungal infection (deep).
- Idiopathic midline granuloma.
- Cutaneous leishmaniasis.

Puffy Face

Causes are—

- Nephrotic syndrome.
- Acute glomerulonephritis (AGN).
- Myxoedema.
- SVC obstruction.
- Acromegaly.
- Angioneurotic oedema.
- Cushing's syndrome.

- Chronic alcoholism.
- Severe congestive cardiac failure.
- Hereditary angio-oedema.

Chloasma or Melasma

It is the discrete pigmentation in the face of females, due to imbalance between oestrogen and progesterone. Melanocyte-stimulating hormone is normal. Causes are—

- Pregnancy.
- Sunlight exposure.
- Drugs (oral contraceptive and phenytoin).
- Others—ovarian tumour (rare).

Malar Flush

Causes are—

- Normal person.
- Mitral stenosis.
- Hypothyroidism.
- Polycythaemia due to any cause.

Plethoric Face

Causes are—

- Normal physiological.
- Polycythaemia (due to any cause).
- Cushing's syndrome.
- Alcoholism.
- SVC obstruction.

Bilateral Parotid Enlargement

Causes are—

- Sarcoidosis.
- Alcoholic liver disease or chronic alcoholism.
- Bilateral mumps (usually it is painful).
- Sjögren's syndrome.
- Malnutrition.
- Diabetes mellitus.
- Lymphoma.
- Leukaemia.
- Mikulicz syndrome.

Cachexia or Emaciation

Causes are—

- Tuberculosis.
- Diabetes mellitus.
- Thyrotoxicosis.
- Malignancy.

- Malabsorption.
- Malnutrition.
- Anorexia nervosa.
- Addison's disease.

Tall Stature

Causes are—

- Familial or constitutional.
- Marfan's syndrome.
- Homocystinuria.
- Gigantism.
- Klinefelter's syndrome.
- Kallmann's syndrome.
- Hypogonadism.
- Thyrotoxicosis before fusion of epiphysis.

Short Stature

Causes are—

- Familial or constitutional.
- Genetic disease—Turner's syndrome, Down's syndrome, achondroplasia.
- Endocrine—juvenile hypothyroidism, hypopituitarism.
- Cardiac—cyanotic congenital heart disease.
- Alimentary—malabsorption syndrome, cystic fibrosis, Coeliac disease, Crohn's disease.
- Nutritional—protein energy malnutrition, ricket.
- Renal—CKD.

Large Skull

- Hydrocephalus in early childhood.
- Acromegaly.
- Hereditary haemolytic anaemia (beta thalassemia major).
- Paget's disease.
- Achondroplasia.

XANTHELASMA

Definition

These are yellowish plaque in subcutaneous or intracutaneous tissues around the eyelids due to deposition of cholesterol or lipids.

Causes

- Familial.
- Primary biliary cirrhosis.
- Hyperlipidaemia (types II and III).
- Hypothyroidism.
- Diabetes mellitus.

- Nephrotic syndrome.
- Alcoholism.
- Drugs—thiazide diuretic, ciclosporin, steroid, androgen, oral contraceptive pill.

Xanthelasma is associated with corneal arcus, xanthoma in other parts (patella, Achilles' tendon and dorsum of the hand) and evidence of primary disease.

Diseases associated with hypercholesterolaemia:
- Tendon xanthoma.
- Tuberous xanthoma.
- Xanthelasma.
- Corneal arcus.
- Atherosclerosis and ischaemic heart disease (IHD).

Diseases associated with hypertriglyceridaemia:
- Acute pancreatitis.
- Lipaemia retinalis.
- Retinal vein thrombosis
- Eruptive xanthoma.

NB: Hypertriglyceridaemia alone is not associated with atherosclerosis and IHD.

Diseases associated with mixed hyperlipidaemia: Tuberous, tendon and palmar xanthoma.

XANTHOMA

Definition

These are deposits of fatty material in the skin, subcutaneous tissue and tendons due to primary or secondary hyperlipidaemia.

Types: Four Types

1. Eruptive xanthoma (multiple, yellow or brown papule on trunk and buttock).
2. Tendon xanthoma (subcutaneous nodules attached to tendons over dorsum of fingers and Achilles' tendon).
3. Tuberous xanthoma (elbow and knee).
4. Palmar xanthoma.

Treatment of Xanthelasma and Xanthoma

General measures
- If obese—weight reduction, exercise, diet control (avoid cholesterol containing diet, animal fat).
- Smoking and alcohol should be avoided.
- Treatment of primary disease.
- If hyperlipidaemia—lipid lowering drugs.

Lipid lowering drugs are
- HMG Co-A reductase inhibitors (simvastatin, pravastatin and lovastatin) are used in treating hypercholesterolaemia.

- Fibrates (fenofibrate, bezafibrate, gemfibrozil)are used in treating hypertriglyceridaemia.
- Others—nicotinic acid, probucol and fish oil (omega-3 triglyceride).

NB: Tendon xanthoma may be confused with—

- Rheumatoid nodule.
- Tophi of gout.
- Neurofibroma.
- Lipoma.

HANDS IN DIFFERENT DISEASES

By looking at the hands, obvious findings may be—
- Rheumatoid arthritis.
- Systemic sclerosis.
- Tophaceous gout.
- Bouchard's nodes, Heberden's node (in osteoarthritis).
- Skin rash and Gottron's patch (dermatomyositis).
- Large hand (acromegaly).
- Claw hand.
- Wrist drop.
- Myotonic dystrophy (diagnosed by handshake or asking the patient to close and open the hands).
- Raynaud's disease or phenomenon.
- Polydactyly.
- Syndactyly.
- Arachnodactyly.
- Short 4th metacarpal.
- Palmar erythema.
- Nail and nail bed change.
- Dupuytren's contracture.
- Carpopedal spasm due to tetany.
- Trophic change (gangrene, ulceration).
- Wasting—thenar, hypothenar or generalized.
- Tremor due to any cause.
- Palm—warm and sweaty palm (thyrotoxicosis), cold and sweaty palms (anxiety).
- Single palmar crease (in Down's syndrome).
- Hyperkeratosis of palm with pigmentation (arsenicosis).

Polydactyly

It means presence of extra fingers and toes. Causes are—
- Congenital.
- Laurence-Moon-Biedl syndrome.

Syndactyly

It means fusion of two fingers. Usually congenital.

Arachnodactyly

It means long slender spider leg-like fingers. Causes—
- Constitutional or congenital.
- Marfan's syndrome.
- Homocystinuria.
- Ehler's-Danlos syndrome.
- Pseudoxanthoma elasticum.

Causes of Short 4th or 5th Metacarpal

- Congenital.
- Pseudohypoparathyroidism.
- Pseudo-pseudohypoparathyroidism.
- Turner's syndrome.

Wasting of Hand Muscles

- Thenar wasting—indicates median nerve lesion.
- Hypothenar and other muscles wasting (except thenar)— indicates ulnar nerve lesion.
- On the dorsum—wasting with dorsal guttering (interossei) indicates ulnar nerve lesion.
- Generalized wasting—indicates C8 and T1 lesion.

Findings in Hand in Infective Endocarditis

- Osler's nodes (small painful violaceous raised nodule, 0.5–1.5 cm, present on the tip of the fingers and toes, also palmar aspect, probably due to development of vasculitis or septic emboli).
- Splinter haemorrhage.
- Clubbing.
- Janeway lesion (large painless erythematous macule containing bacteria on palm, pulp of the fingers. It may be found in the sole).
- Petechial haemorrhage.
- Infarction on the tip of the fingers.

Hands in Chronic Liver Disease

- Palmar erythema.
- Dupuytren's contracture.
- Clubbing.
- Leuconychia.
- Flapping tremor.
- Spider angioma.
- Pigmentation.
- Jaundice.
- Scratch mark.
- Xanthoma.
- Cyanosis.

CLAW HAND

Definition

It is a deformity of hand characterized by flexion of interphalangeal (IP) joints and hyperextension of metacarpophalyngeal joints (MCP) joints.

It is due to weakness of the lumbricals and interossei with unopposed action of long extensors of finger.

Only LMN lesions of C8 and T1 nerves, C8 and T1 nerve root lesion and brachial plexus lesion will produce localized wasting of lumbricals and interossei causing claw hand.

Combined ulnar and median nerve lesion will produce true claw hand. Ulnar claw hand involves 4th and 5th fingers, because 1st and 2nd lumbricals are supplied by median nerve.

Causes of Claw Hand

- Combined ulnar and median nerve lesion—trauma, leprosy.
- Brachial plexus lesion (C8 and T1)—cervical rib, thoracic inlet syndrome, Klumke's paralysis.
- Neurological disease—MND, Charcot-Marie-Tooth disease, syringomyelia, intramedullary tumour and polio.

CLUBBING

Definition

In this condition, there is bulbous swelling of the terminal end of fingers and toes, where nail becomes thick and convex. In advanced stage, nail looks drumstick and parrot beak appearance.

Causes of Clubbing

1. **Respiratory—**
   - Bronchial carcinoma (common in squamous cell type).
   - Suppurative lung disease—bronchiectasis, lung abscess, empyema thoracis.
   - Interstitial lung disease (ILD) or diffuse parenchymal lung disease (DPLD).
   - Cystic fibrosis.
   - Pulmonary TB (in advanced stage with fibrosis).
   - Pleural mesothelioma.
2. **Cardiac—**
   - Infective endocarditis.
   - Cyanotic congenital heart disease (e.g. Fallot's tetralogy).
3. **Others—**
   - Cirrhosis of liver.
   - Inflammatory bowel disease.
   - Familial.
   - Idiopathic.

NB: Commonest cause is bronchial carcinoma in elderly and bronchiectasis in young.

Differential Clubbing

It means clubbing in the toes, but not in the fingers.
Causes are—

- PDA with reversal shunt (also there is cyanosis in toes, not in finger called differential cyanosis).
- Infected abdominal aortic aneurysm.
- Coarctation of abdominal aorta.

Causes of Unilateral Clubbing

- Axillary artery aneurysm.
- Bronchial arteriovenous aneurysm.
- Others—aneurysm of ascending aorta, subclavian or innominate artery.

Causes of Clubbing in a Single Finger

- Trauma (commonest cause).
- Chronic tophaceous gout.
- Sarcoidosis.

Causes of Clubbing with Cyanosis

- Fibrosing alveolitis.
- Cyanotic heart disease (Fallot's tetralogy).
- Cystic fibrosis.
- Bilateral extensive bronchiectasis.

Investigations in Clubbing

- Full blood count.
- Chest X-ray.
- Ultrasonography of whole abdomen.
- Echocardiography.
- Other—according to suspicion of cause (barium enema, follow through, colonoscopy for inflammatory bowel disease, liver function test).

Hypertrophic Osteoarthropathy

- Hypertrophic osteoarthropathy (HOA) is the **triad** of clubbing, arthritis and subperiosteal new bone formation (periosteal inflammation at the distal ends of long bones in radius, ulna, tibia, fibula, although any bone may be involved).
- There is swelling and tenderness at the lower ends of forearm and leg.
- Hypertrophic osteoarthropathy may be primary or secondary to any cause of clubbing. Commonest causes are bronchial carcinoma (squamous cell type) and pleural mesothelioma.

KOILONYCHIA

Definition

It is a disorder in which nail is concave or spoon shaped.

Causes

1. Iron deficiency anaemia (commonest cause).
2. Others (rare)—
   - Trauma (rarely in garage mechanics, who regularly fit tyres).
   - Thyrotoxicosis.
   - Fungal infection.
   - Raynaud's disease.

Mechanism of Koilonychia

Unknown, probably results from slow growth of nail plate.

Stages of Koilonychia

- Dryness, brittleness and ridging (first stage).
- Flattening and thinning (second stage).
- Spooning or concavity (third stage).

Plummer-Vinson Syndrome

It is the combination of—

- Iron deficiency anaemia.
- Dysphagia (due to postcricoid web secondary to epithelial degeneration).
- Glossitis.

It is also called Paterson-Brown-Kelly syndrome, common in women. Cause unknown. There is constriction in the upper oesophageal sphincter in the postcricoid region, which appears radiologically as a web. This web may be asymptomatic or may produce dysphagia. It may be difficult to see endoscopically. Rarely, there is increased risk of squamous cell carcinoma.

Treatment of Plummer-Vinson Syndrome

- Iron therapy.
- If severe anaemia—blood transfusion.
- Rarely, endoscopic dilatation may be required.

LEUCONYCHIA

Definition

It means white nail. It may be diffuse, punctate, linear or striate (white transverse flecks—a normal finding). Leuconychia indicates hypoalbuminaemia.

Causes

- Renal—nephrotic syndrome, chronic renal failure.
- Liver diseases—chronic liver disease (CLD), cirrhosis of liver.

- Malnutrition—malabsorption, less intake.
- May be normal finding.
- Others - rare (lymphoma, fungal infection, congenital).

Investigations

According to the suspicion of cause—
- Liver function tests.
- Renal function tests.
- GIT—endoscopy, colonoscopy, barium follow through.

NAIL CHANGES IN DIFFERENT DISEASES

Nail abnormality may occur in many local, systemic and dermatological diseases. A good visual impression is very essential and a spot diagnosis can be done easily.

Clubbing, koilonychia, leuconychia—Already described.

Pale nail: found in anaemia.

Nail Fold Infarction

Causes are (usually vasculitis due to any cause)—
- SLE.
- Dermatomyositis.
- Systemic sclerosis.
- Rheumatoid arthritis.
- Polyarteritis nodosa.

Splinter Haemorrhage

Bleeding under nail. Causes are—
- Trauma (commonest).
- Infective endocarditis.
- Septicaemia.
- Vasculitis—SLE, RA and polyarteritis nodosa.
- Others—haematological malignancy, severe anaemia, psoriasis. Rarely, in trichinosis (usually transverse haemorrhage).

Half and Half Nail

Proximal part of nail is white and distal part is brown. Causes are—
- Chronic renal failure (commonest).
- Cirrhosis of liver.
- Occasionally, in normal person.

Nail Fold Telangiectasia

New vessels at the base of nail. Causes are—
- SLE.
- Systemic sclerosis.
- Dermatomyositis.
- Mixed connective tissue disease (MCTD).
- Raynaud's phenomenon.

Beau's Line

Nonpigmented transverse line or groove in nail due to transient arrest of nail growth, few weeks after acute illness. Causes are—
- Chronic illness (chronic infection, malignancy, collagen disease).
- Prolonged fever.
- Pneumonia.

- Coronary artery disease.
- Others—cachexia, malnutrition, psychiatric illness, cytotoxic drugs.

Onycholysis

Separation of distal nail plate from the nail bed (free edge looks white). Causes are—

- Psoriasis (commonest).
- Fungal infection.
- Thyrotoxicosis (Plummer's sign).
- Idiopathic.
- Occasionally drugs (tetracycline, psoralen).
- Porphyria.
- Trauma or faulty manicure.

Mees' Line

Single transverse white band in nail. Causes are—

- Chronic arsenic poisoning.
- CRF.
- Also, after chemotherapy and severe illness.

Yellow Nail

Found in yellow nail syndrome, an inherited disease in which the nails are thick, yellow or pigmented with separation of distal part of nail bed due to hypoplasia of lymphatic system.Yellow nail syndrome is associated with lymphoedema of legs, bronchiectasis and pleural effusion.

Loss of Nail (or Dystrophy)

Causes are—

- Severe lichen planus.
- Epidermolysis bullosa.
- Trauma (tooth biting).

Nail Pitting (Depression in Nail)

Causes are—

- Psoriasis.
- Alopecia areata.
- Atopic eczema (when involves proximal nail bed).
- Pityriasis rosacea.

Brittle Nail (Easily Broken)

Causes are—

- Iron deficiency anaemia.
- Peripheral vascular disease.
- Fungal infection.
- Hypocalcaemia.
- Psoriasis.
- Injury (nail biting).
- Idiopathic.

Blue Nail

Normal white lunulae become blue, found in Wilson's disease due to deposition of copper. Also found in cyanosis and ochronosis.

Red Nail

May be normal finding. Also in polycythaemia, carbon monoxide poisoning (cherry red).

Brown Nail

Usually present in CKD.

Periungual or Subungual Fibroma

Found in tuberous sclerosis (epiloia).

Fungal Nail

Nail is white, green, black, thick with discolouration and crust formation.

Absent or Small, Dysplastic Nail

Causes are—

- Nail patella syndrome (AD, associated with no or hypoplastic patella and glomerulonephritis, abnormalities in eye).
- Others—congenital, traumatic and vasculitis.

Nail Hyperpigmentation

May occur due to some drugs (such as zidovudine, doxorubicin, bleomycin, cyclophosphamide, 5-fluorouracil, melphalan and nitrosoureas).

Terry's Nail

Proximal part is white or pink but nail tip is red or brown. Causes are—

- Old age (normally present in elderly).
- Cirrhosis of liver.
- Congestive cardiac failure.
- Hyperthyroidism.
- Malnutrition.
- Renal failure.

Dark Nail

May be a normal finding, mostly in black people. Sometimes may be due to subungual melanoma.

CYANOSIS

Definition

It is the bluish discolouration of the skin and mucous membrane due to increased amount of deoxygenated haemoglobin in blood. Cyanosis is not seen until the **amount** of deoxygenated haemoglobin is >5 g/dl.

- In severe anaemia, haemoglobin is low and fully saturated. So, there is no cyanosis.
- Tongue is always warm, so it is not involved in peripheral cyanosis.

Types of Cyanosis: 2 Types

Two types of cyanosis are discussed below and differentiated in Table 1.

Peripheral cyanosis: Due to localized reduction of blood flow on exposure to cold causing capillary vasoconstriction (lip is blue in cold weather). Also, occurs in reduced cardiac output (heart failure or shock). Tongue is spared in peripheral cyanosis. Causes of peripheral cyanosis—

- Exposure to cold.
- Raynaud's phenomenon.
- Heart failure.

Central cyanosis: Either due to imperfect oxygenation of blood in lung or admixture of venous and arterial blood. It is seen when O_2 saturation falls below 80–85%. Best site is tongue.

Causes of central cyanosis:

1. Respiratory—There is defect in oxygenation of blood in the lungs—
   - Chronic obstructive pulmonary disease (COPD).
   - Severe pneumonia.
   - Acute severe bronchial asthma.
   - Massive pulmonary embolism.
   - Pulmonary infarction.
   - Diffuse parenchymal lung disease (DPLD).

Table 1
Differences between central and peripheral cyanosis

Points	Central cyanosis	Peripheral cyanosis
Mechanism	Imperfect oxygenation of blood in lung or admixture of venous and arterial blood in heart disease	Local vasoconstriction or reduction of arterial flow
Area involved	Generalized	Localized
Affected part	Warm	Cold
Application of warmth	Does not disappear	Disappears
Oxygen	Cyanosis may disappear in pulmonary case (except in right-to-left shunt)	Disappears
Tongue	Always involved	Never involved

2. Cardiac—
   - Cyanotic congenital heart disease—Fallot's tetralogy, transposition of great vessels.
   - Shunt anomaly (right-to-left shunt called Eisenmenger syndrome due to ASD, VSD, PDA).
   - Heart failure.
   - Cardiogenic shock.
3. Others—
   - High altitude (physiological).
   - Polycythaemia.

FEVER

Definition

Rise of body temperature above the normal range.

Normal body temperature is 36.8°C (mouth), 36.4°C (axilla), 37.3°C (rectum). A morning temperature >37.3°C in mouth or 37.7°C in rectum is considered as fever.

Hyperpyrexia

Temperature above 41.1°C is called hyperthermia or hyperpyrexia. Causes are—

- Severe infection (septicaemia, bacteraemia).
- Pontine haemorrhage.
- Heat stroke.
- Malignant hyperthermia.
- Neuroleptic malignant syndrome.
- Thyroid crisis.
- Lobar pneumonia.
- Datura poisoning.

Hyperpyrexia is a serious condition. May cause brain damage, multiorgan failure, rhabdomyolysis, renal failure.

Treatment of Hyperpyrexia

- Removal of clothing.
- Sponging with tepid water.
- Fanning.
- Antipyretic—paracetamol (oral or suppository).

Hypothermia

It means temperature less than 35°C (or 95°F). Causes are—

- Exposure to cold.
- Drug—high dose antipyretic, opium poisoning, ethanol, phenol thiazine, benzodiazepine.
- Shock.
- Hypothyroidism (myxoedema coma).
- Adrenal insufficiency.
- Hypoglycaemia.
- Prolonged postoperative period.
- Infusion of refrigerated blood products without rewarming.

Treatment of Hypothermia

- Covering the body.
- Rewarming.
- IV fluid.
- Treatment of primary cause.

Types of Fever

- Usually 3 types—intermittent, remittent and continued.
- Other types—hyperpyrexia, hectic, Pel-Ebstein fever.

Intermittent

Fever that persists for several hours in a day and always touches the baseline between attack is called intermittent fever. It is of 3 types—

- Quotidian—characterized by paroxysm of fever that occurs daily (daily rise and fall). This type of fever may be found in kala-azar.
- Tertian—characterized by paroxysm of fever that occurs on alternate days. Found in benign tertian malaria (due to *Plasmodium vivax*, rarely *P. ovale*).
- Quartan—characterized by paroxysm of fever that occurs in two days interval between consecutive attacks. This is found in quartan malaria due to *Plasmodium malariae* (rare).

Remittent

If the fluctuation of fever is > 2°C (3°F), but does not touch the baseline, it is called remittent. Found in pyogenic infection (pyogenic liver abscess, acute bronchopneumonia, acute tonsillitis, septicaemia, acute pyelonephritis), miliary TB, lymphoma.

Continued

If the fluctuation of fever is not > 1°C (1.5°F) and does not touch the baseline, it is called continued fever. Found in typhoid, typhus, miliary TB, meningococcal meningitis, rheumatic fever, drug fever.

Pel–Ebstein Fever

Recurrent bouts of pyrexia followed by apyrexial period is called Pel-Ebstein fever. It is found in Hodgkin's disease (in 10% cases). This type of fever may be found in brucellosis (called undulant fever).

Drugs causing fever: Many drugs can cause drug fever. Common drugs are—

- MAO inhibitor.
- Tricyclic antidepressant.
- Alphamethyldopa.
- Betalactam antibiotics.
- Salicylate poisoning.
- LSD.
- Ecstacy.
- Procainamide.
- Anticonvulsant.
- Sulphonamide.
- Neuroleptic malignant syndrome may be caused by phenothiazine, butyrophenon, etc.

Saddleback Fever

Fever that persists for few days, then no fever for one or two days, followed by reappearance of fever. It occurs in dengue fever, Colorado tick fever, borreliosis, leptospira, yellow fever and influenza.

Hectic Fever

It means sudden rise of very high temperature usually associated with chill and rigor, persist for few hours and then fall with profuse sweating. This may be found in pus in anywhere in the body, e.g. lung abscess, pyogenic liver abscess, empyema thoracis, subphrenic abscess, empyema of gallbladder, perinephric abscess. Sometimes in septicaemia or pyaemia.

Aseptic (noninfectious) Fever

It means the fever without infection. May be found in SLE, lymphoma, leukaemia, malignancy (such as hepatoma, renal cell carcinoma), pontine haemorrhage, drug fever, early stage of acute myocardial infarction, heat stroke, thyrotoxic crisis, acute gout, excessive use of atropine injection (in OPC poisoning).

Factitious Fever

Sometimes patient purposefully show false rise of temperature. Usually found in young woman, sometimes due to deliberate intake of thyroxine.

Temperature Fall by Crisis and Lysis

- When temperature subsides quickly to subnormal level, it is called fall by crisis. Causes are lobar pneumonia, septicaemic shock, enteric fever associated with perforation or bleeding.
- When temperature falls gradually over several days, it is called fall by lysis. Causes are enteric fever, rheumatic fever, acute bronchopneumonia.

Pattern of Fever in Different Diseases

- Low grade fever with evening rise—TB.
- Fever with chill and rigor—acute pyelonephritis, acute cholangitis, infective endocarditis, subphrenic abscess, pyogenic lung abscess, septicaemia, lobar pneumonia, pyrogenic reaction after infusion or transfusion.
- Fever with chill and rigor that subsides with sweating— malaria.
- Fever with unconsciousness—cerebral malaria, meningitis, encephalitis, pontine haemorrhage.
- Fever with neck rigidity—meningitis, encephalitis.
- Fever with drenching night sweat—lymphoma, TB.
- Feverish with excessive sweating—thyrotoxicosis.
- Pel-Ebstein fever (undulant fever)—Hodgkin's lymphoma.
- Fever with double rise (or triple rise)—Kala-azar.
- Step ladder pattern of fever—enteric fever.
- Relapsing fever—malaria, borreliosis, occasionally lymphoma (HD).
- Fever with myalgia—viral infection (e.g. like influenza, dengue).

Causes of Fever with Skin Rash with Days

Remember: "Very Sick Person Must Take Double Eggs."

- 1st day - Varicella (chickenpox).
- 2nd day - Scarlet fever.
- 3rd day - Pox (smallpox).
- 4th day - Measles, german measles (rubella).

- 5th day - Typhus.
- 6th day - Dengue.
- 7th day - Enteric fever (rose spot).
- Drug rash may appear anytime.

Other Causes of Skin Rash with Fever

- Still's disease.
- Erythema nodosum.
- Erythema multiforme.
- Toxic shock syndrome.
- Staphylococcal scalded skin syndrome.
- Sweet's syndrome.
- Anthrax.

Fever with Relative Bradycardia

Normally, if temperature rises 1°F, pulse rate increases 10 beats. If rise of pulse rate is less than that, it is called relative bradycardia. Causes are—

- Viral fever.
- First week of enteric fever.
- Brucellosis.
- Psittacosis.
- Weil's disease.

Fever with Relative Tachycardia

If rise in pulse rate is more than that, it is called relative tachycardia. Causes are—

- Acute rheumatic carditis.
- Diphtheric myocarditis.
- Severe TB.
- Polyarteritis nodosa.

Other Points in Fever

- High temperature with pink maculopapular skin rash, which disappears with the fall of temperature is found in Still's disease (this rash is called Salmon rash).
- Hyperpyrexia and rigidity of the body in patient who is taking antipsychotic drug is suggestive of neuroleptic malignant syndrome.

NEUROLEPTIC MALIGNANT SYNDROME

Definition

Unexplained high fever in a psychiatric patient who is on antipsychotic drug is called neuroleptic malignant syndrome. It is rare, but serious complication of any neuroleptic drug therapy, such as phenothiazine, butyrophenones (commonly haloperidol), irrespective of dose. It occurs in 0.2% of cases, usually after days or weeks of neuroleptic drug therapy.

It is characterized by high fever, stiffness or rigidity of the body, fluctuating consciousness, autonomic dysfunction (tachycardia, labile BP, pallor).

There may be leucocytosis and abnormal liver function tests. High CPK (due to myonecrosis) is highly suggestive of the diagnosis. Sometimes, metabolic acidosis, respiratory failure, cardiac failure, rhabdomyolysis and even renal failure may occur.

Mortality is 20% in untreated cases and 5% in treated cases.

Treatment

- Offending drug should be stopped.
- Measures to reduce the temperature—tepid sponging, fanning or air-conditioning, antipyretic (oral or suppository).
- Dopamine receptor agonist—bromocriptine 2.5–7.5 mg orally.
- Antispastic agent—dantrolene IV may be helpful.
- Supportive therapy (hydration).

MALIGNANT HYPERTHERMIA

Definition

It is a rare disorder, develops 30 minutes to several hours after inhalational anaesthesia or to succinylcholine.

It is characterized by high temperature, muscle rigidity, rhabdomyolysis, hypotension and electrolytes abnormality.

Treatment

- Aggressive cooling.
- Dantrolene 2–5 mg/kg should be given IV.

PYREXIA OF UNKNOWN ORIGIN

Definiton

Pyrexia of unknown origin (PUO) is defined as fever higher than 38.3°C (101°F) persisting for more than three weeks despite initial investigation during 3 days of inpatient care or after more than two outpatient visits.

Causes

Infections

- Tuberculosis (commonest cause).
- Abscess (amoebic or pyogenic liver abscess, subphrenic or at any site).
- Infective endocarditis.
- Urinary tract infection, especially prostatitis.
- Dental infection.
- Sinusitis.
- Cholecystitis or cholangitis.
- Bone and joint infections.
- Malaria, brucellosis, toxoplasmosis
- Viral infections (cytomegalovirus (CMV), HIV).
- Fungal infections.

Connective Tissue Disorders

- Systemic lupus erythematosus, rheumatoid arthritis, polymyositis.

Malignancy

- Lymphoma.
- Myeloma.
- Leukaemia.
- Carcinoma of kidney, liver, colon, stomach, pancreas.

Vasculitis

- Giant cell arteritis.
- Vasculitic disorders, e.g. PAN and rheumatoid disease with vasculitis.

Miscellaneous

- Polymyalgia rheumatica.
- Adult Still's disease.
- Drug fever.
- Atrial myxoma.
- Thyrotoxicosis.
- IBD.
- Liver disease (cirrhosis and granulomatous hepatitis).
- Sarcoidosis.
- Familial Mediterranean fever.
- Factitious fever.

Undiagnosed

In 5% cases, diagnosis may not be possible even after postmortem examination.

History to be Taken in PUO

1. For TB—low-grade fever with evening rise, weight loss, night sweat, H/O of contact with TB patient.
2. For other infections—
   - Cough, fever, sputum, chest pain.
   - Diarrhoea, abdominal pain.
   - Dysuria, frequency, urgency, burning micturition.
   - Place of residence and overseas travel (malaria, kala-azar, amoebiasis).
   - History of sexual exposure (HIV, venereal disease, PID).
   - Contact with domestic or wild animals (psittacosis, brucellosis, Q-fever, leptospirosis).
3. For collagen diseases—
   - Skin rash.
   - Mouth ulcer.
   - Joint pain.
   - Alopecia.
4. Unilateral headache, arthralgia, myalgia (giant cell arteritis, polymyalgia rheumatica).
5. Occupation (farming, veterinary surgeon, etc.).
6. Drug history to exclude drug fever.
7. History of any intervention, e.g. catheterization, A-V fistula, prosthetic valve, colonoscopy.

Physical Findings in PUO

- Pattern of temperature.
- In skin—rash, erythema nodosum, erythema multiforme, vasculitic rash.
- Hand—stigmata of infective endocarditis, rheumatoid arthritis, dermatomyositis, clubbing, puncture marks (I/V drug abuse, HIV, HBV, etc.).
- Lymph node—epitrochlear, axillary, cervical, inguinal.
- Eye—iritis, conjunctivitis to exclude seronegative arthritis, collagen disease, sarcoidosis.
- Face—butterfly rash to exclude SLE, heliotrope rash for dermatomyositis, lupus pernio and bilateral parotid enlargement for sarcoidosis.
- Mouth—ulcer, gum disease, teeth, tonsil.
- Thyroid gland to exclude subacute thyroiditis.
- Chest—bony tenderness, murmur (SBE, myxoma), prosthetic valve.
- Abdomen—tenderness over the liver (liver abscess, sub-diaphragmatic abscess), spleen, per rectal examination to exclude prostatic abscess, carcinoma prostate.
- Nervous system—look for signs of meningism, focal neurological signs.
- Fundus—Roth's spot (SBE), retinal haemorrhage or infarction (leukaemia).

Investigations

- CBC with ESR, PBF,
- Malarial parasite (MP).
- Blood culture.

- Blood sugar (to exclude DM).
- Urine R/E and culture.
- Chest X-ray P/A view.
- MT.
- USG of whole abdomen.
- If a lymph node or a palpable mass is found- FNAC and/ or biopsy.
- Serum ferritin (high in adult Still's disease).
- Echocardiography.
- Autoimmune screen - ANA, ENA, anti ds-DNA, CRP, rheumatoid factor, c-ANCA, p-ANCA.
- HIV screen.
- Bone marrow examination.
- Renal function test.
- Liver function test.
- Other investigation according to suspicion of cause—CT scan, MRI, PET scan, bronchoscopy, colonoscopy.

Treatment

According to the cause.

Causes of Absent Radial Pulse:

- Anatomical aberration (may be congenital)
- Atherosclerosis
- Coarctation of aorta (before origin of the left subclavian artery).
- Takayasu's arteritis
- Iatrogenic—Blalock Taussig shunt (done in TOF), A-V fistula for haemodialysis
- Occlusion by thrombosis
- Occlusion of subclavian artery by cervical rib or neoplasm
- Dissecting aneurysm.

GENERALIZED LYMPHADENOPATHY

Definition

Usually three or more areas of lymph node involvement, such as cervical, axillary, inguinal, abdominal, etc.

Causes

1. Hematological malignancy—
   - Lymphoma.
   - Acute lymphoblastic leukaemia (ALL).
   - Chronic lymphocytic leukaemia (CLL).
2. Viral—
   - Infectious mononucleosis.
   - Cytomegalovirus infection.
   - HIV.
3. Collagen disease—SLE
4. Others—
   - Disseminated tuberculosis.
   - Sarcoidosis.
   - Brucellosis.
   - Toxoplasmosis.
   - Secondary syphilis.
5. Drugs—phenytoin or diphenylhydantoin (called pseudolymphoma).

Causes of Lymphadenopathy with Splenomegaly (and/or hepatomegaly)

- Lymphoma.
- ALL.
- CLL.
- Infectious mononucleosis.
- SLE.
- Kala-azar—mainly African and Chinese kala-azar.
- Others—sarcoidosis, brucellosis and toxoplasmosis, HIV.

Causes of Generalized Lymphadenopathy with Fever

- Lymphoma.
- ALL.
- CLL.
- Viral infections (e.g. infectious mononucleosis, CMV infection).
- Disseminated TB.
- Brucellosis.
- Sarcoidosis.
- Toxoplasmosis.

Investigations in Generalized Lymphadenopathy

1. CBC, ESR and PBF (to exclude leukaemia, increased eosinophil in Hodgkin's lymphoma, atypical lymphocyte in infectious mononucleosis, high ESR in TB).
2. Chest X-ray (to see TB, bilateral hilar lymphadenopathy in sarcoidosis, lymphoma, lymphatic leukaemia).
3. USG or CT scan of abdomen (to see hepatomegaly, splenomegaly, para-aortic and other lymphadenopathy).
4. Other investigations—according to the suspicion of cause—
   - If lymphoma is suspected—FNAC or biopsy of lymph nodes (biopsy is preferable).
   - If leukaemia is suspected—Bone marrow study.
   - If disseminated tuberculosis—MT, lymph node FNAC or biopsy.
   - If HIV is suspected—HIV screening test.
   - If SLE is suspected—ANA, anti-ds DNA.

   NB: Following points are important—

   - Normal LN may be palpable in axilla, groin, usually up to 0.5 cm, which are soft, rubbery. Submandibular LN < 1 cm is normal in children and inguinal LN < 2 cm is normal in adult.
   - Reactive LN expand rapidly and may be painful.
   - Localized lymphadenopathy means single anatomical area of LN involvement.
   - Generalized lymphadenopathy means three or more anatomical noncontiguous areas of LN involvement.
   - Enlargement of supraclavicular and scalene LN are always pathological.

CERVICAL LYMPHADENOPATHY

Causes

According to the characteristics of lymph nodes, causes are—

If Matted Cervical Lymphadenopathy

- Tuberculous lymphadenitis (commonest).
- Infection by atypical mycobacteria.
- Actinomycosis.

If Lymphadenopathy with Sinus

- Tuberculous lymphadenitis.
- Actinomycosis.

If Lymphadenopathy with Biopsy Marking

- Tuberculosis.
- Lymphoma.
- Secondaries.

If Hard Lymphadenopathy

- Metastatic malignancy (e.g. from bronchial carcinoma).

If Tender Lymphadenopathy

- Acute inflammation (may be secondary to dental sepsis, tonsillitis and mastoiditis).
- Infection of LN itself.

If Lymphadenopathy is Discrete

- Lymphoma.
- Infectious mononucleosis.
- Reactive hyperplasia.

If Lymphadenopathy with Goitre

- Papillary carcinoma of thyroid with metastasis.

If Lymphadenopathy is Soft, Fleshy, Rubbery and Discrete

- Lymphoma

If Lymphadenopathy is Immobile, Fixed to Skin

- Metastatic malignancy.

Investigations in Tuberculous Lymphadenitis

- CBC and ESR (high).
- Chest X-ray PA view (to see TB in chest).
- Tuberculin test.
- For confirmation—FNAC or biopsy (shows casseating granuloma).

Treatment of Tuberculous Lymphadenitis

- Standard anti-Koch's therapy for 9 months to 1 year.
- Prednisolone may be added.

NB With anti-TB drug therapy, lymph nodes may be enlarged. It is due to hypersensitivity reaction to tuberculoprotein released from dead mycobacteria.

OEDEMA

Definition

It may be defined as excessive accumulation of fluid in the interstitial space. It may be pitting and nonpitting.

Causes of Pitting Oedema

- CCF.
- Nephrotic syndrome
- Hypoproteinaemia due to any other cause (protein loosing enteropathy or less protein intake).
- Deep venous thrombosis.
- Compression of large veins by tumour or lymph nodes.
- Chronic venous insufficiency (varicose vein).
- Drugs—calcium channel blockers (e.g. nifedipine, amlodipine), some NSAIDs (e.g. etoricoxib).
- Idiopathic (called 'fluid retention syndrome', common in women).

Causes of Nonpitting Oedema

- Myxoedema.
- Chronic lymphatic obstruction or lymphoedema due to any cause (see below).

Causes of Unilateral Leg Oedema

- Lymphoedema.
- DVT.
- Cellulitis.
- Ruptured Baker's cyst.
- Chronic venous insufficiency.

Causes of Bilateral Leg Odema

- CCF.
- Hypoproteinaemia due to any cause.
- Cirrhosis of liver in advanced stage.
- Myxoedema.
- Drugs—calcium channel blocker (nifedipine, amlodipine), some NSAIDs (e.g. etoricoxib).
- Lymphoedema.
- Fluid retention syndrome.

Causes of Lymphoedema

1. Primary—
   - Secondary to agenesis or hypoplasia.
   - Hereditary (Milroy's disease).
   - Associated with Turner's syndrome, Noonan's syndrome and yellow nail syndrome.
2. Secondary—
   - Recurrent lymphangitis or cellulitis.
   - Filariasis.

- Trauma.
- Tuberculosis.
- Neoplasm.
- Surgery (in the arm, it may be due to mastectomy).
- Radiation.
- Burn.

Causes of Periorbital oedema

- Nephrotic syndrome.
- AGN.
- Myxoedema.
- Angioneurotic oedema.
- Surgical emphysema.
- Orbital cellulitis.
- Malignant exophthalmos (in Graves' disease).
- Dermatomyositis.

Investigation in Generalized Oedema: According to the Cause

- Nephrotic syndrome—Urine R/E, blood for total protein, 24-hour urinary protein.
- CCF—chest X-ray, ECG, echocardiogram.
- Cirrhosis of liver—LFT (total protein, A:G ratio, prothrombin time, ultrasonogram).
- Hypoproteinaemia—serum total protein, other investigations according to the history to find out cause.
- Hypothyroidism—FT3, FT4, TSH.

Characteristics of Oedema in Different Diseases

- Nephrotic syndrome—oedema is generalized. It starts in face and then involves whole body. May be ascites, bilateral pleural effusion, pericardial effusion due to hypoalbuminaemia.
- Congestive cardiac failure—oedema starts in leg (dependent oedema). In severe advanced case, there may be ascites, swelling of face.
- Cirrhosis of liver—first there is ascites, then may be oedema in leg.
- Malnutrition or hypoproteinaemia—oedema of the feet and face, later may be ascites or even generalized.

PIGMENTATION

Pigmentation may be generalized or localized.

Causes

Physiological

- Familial.
- Racial.
- Pregnancy.
- Sun bath.

Pathological

1. Infections—kala-azar (visceral leishmaniasis).
2. Endocrine causes—
   - Addison's disease.
   - Nelson's syndrome (in bilateral adrenalectomy).
   - Ectopic ACTH syndrome.
   - Acromegaly.
1. Liver disease—
   - Haemochromatosis (greenish or bronze).
   - Cirrhosis of liver (common in primary biliary cirrhosis).
2. GIT—malabsorption syndrome (Whipple's disease, Peutz-Jeghers syndrome).
3. Chronic debilitating illness—
   - Internal malignancy (commonly ectopic ACTH syndrome).
   - CKD.
   - Any chronic illness.
4. Drugs—
   - Busulphan.
   - Bleomycin.
   - Amiodarone (violaceous or brown or blue or slaty grey, in exposed parts).
   - Phenothiazine (slaty grey).
   - Phenytoin (melasmalike pigmentation).
   - Oral contraceptive pill.
   - Chloroquine (blue grey).
   - Clofazimine (red or pinkish).
   - Psoralen (brown).
   - Minocycline.
   - Other cytotoxic drugs.
5. Others—
   - Chronic arsenic poisoning.
   - Pellagra (necklace area and exposed part).
   - Systemic sclerosis.
   - Ochronosis (mainly in the joint, nose, ear and face).
   - Argyria (slaty grey hue due to silver deposition).
   - Porphyria cutaneatarda.
   - Acanthosisnigricans.

Evaluation of Pigmentation

By history, clinical examination and investigations.

1. History of fever (e.g. kala-azar).
2. History of drugs.
3. History suggestive of chronic disease (e.g. CLD, CKD) and Addison's disease or other diseases.
4. Physical examinations—
   - BP (low in Addison's disease).
   - Hepatosplenomegaly (kala-azar).
   - Signs of CLD or haemochromatosis or PBC.
   - Abdomen (scar of bilateral adrenalectomy in Nelson's syndrome).
   - Evidence of other chronic illness.
5. Laboratory investigations—according to the history and suspicion of causes (kala-azar, Addison's disease and haemochromatosis).

HIRSUTISM

Definition

It is the male pattern of hair growth in women due to excess of androgen.

Sites

Hair growth involves chin, moustache. Also in breast, chest, axilla, abdominal midline, pubic and thigh area.

Causes

- Hirsutism without virilization.
- Hirsutism with virilization.

Hirsutism without Virilization

- Idiopathic (commonest cause).
- Familial.
- Drugs—steroid, phenytoin, ciclosporin, androgen, minoxidil, progesterone.
- Others—PCOS (in mild cases, hirsutism is more and virilisation is less), acromegaly and porphyria cutaneatarda.

Hirsutism with Virilization

- Ovarian causes—PCOS (severe case), androgen-secreting ovarian tumour, arrhenoblastoma.
- Adrenal causes—late onset congenital adrenal hyperplasia, Cushing's syndrome, adrenal carcinoma or androgen secreting adrenal tumour.
  Signs of virilization:
- Frontal baldness.
- Male body habitus.
- Deepening of voice.
- Others—clitoromegaly, atrophy of breast, male pattern of pubic hair, acne, greasy skin.

Evaluation and Investigations

- History.
- Drug history.
- Family history.
- Blood for testosterone, LH, FSH and prolactin. If testosterone is high (twice the normal), low LH and FSH, it is likely to be idiopathic hirsutism rather than PCOS.

After exclusion of these, causes may be in ovarian or adrenal. Then USG of abdomen should be done to see ovarian or adrenal abnormality.

1. If **ovarian origin,** following tests should be done—
   - LH and FSH—if LH is high and FSH is normal or high (ratio of LH:FSH is 2 or 3)—it is likely to be PCOS.
   - Sex hormone binding globulin (SHBG)—high.
   - Androgens—high, but testosterone is normal or low.
   - Other tests—CT scan, MRI and laparoscopy may be done.

2. If **adrenal origin,** following tests should be done—
   - If adrenal carcinoma or adenoma—urinary 17- ketosteroid is high.
   - Dexamethasone suppression test may be done—shows failure of suppression.
   - In congenital adrenal hyperplasia—serum 17- hydroxyprogesterone is high, also high pregnanetriol and ACTH.
   - Other tests—CT scan, MRI and laparoscopy may be done.

   NB: A good history regarding hirsutism is essential—
   - If the onset is shortly after menarche, tumour is unlikely.
   - If it occurs in childhood, more chance of underlying disease.
   - If menstruation is regular, more likely to be constitutional rather than tumour or other pathology.
   - Greater the menstrual abnormality (irregular or cessation), more likely there is a serious disease (ovarian or adrenal).
   - Rapid onset, prepubertal or late-onset is suggestive of underlying disease (ovarian or adrenal).
   - Increased libido and signs of virilization indicates increased androgen.

Treatment of Hirsutism

1. Treatment of primary cause. If due to drug, it should be stopped.
2. Local therapy—
   - Plucking, bleaching, depilatory cream, shaving, electrolysis, epilation.
   - Topical eflornithine cream applied locally for 6 months.
3. Systemic therapy (in severe cases)—
   - Cyproterone acetate (antiandrogen), 50–100 mg daily for 1–14 days of each cycle. In women of child bearing age, contraception is essential.

- Oestrogen (in oral contraceptive) is helpful in idiopathic or PCOS. It reduces free androgens by increasing SHBG, when it is low.
- Other antiandrogens—spironolactone, flutamide, fenesteride are also helpful.

HYPERTRICHOSIS

Definition

It is the generalized excess hair growth in any sex which is nonandrogenic in origin. Causes are—

- Familial.
- Sexual precocity.
- Hypothyroidism.
- Adrenal hyperplasia or neoplasm.
- Virilising ovarian tumour.
- Drugs—minoxidil, ciclosporin, androgen.

Causes of decreased body hair:

- Cirrhosis of liver.
- Klinefelter's syndrome.
- Hypopituitarism.
- Bilateral testicular atrophy due to any cause (e.g. leprosy).

GYNAECOMASTIA

Definition

Enlargement of male breast due to proliferation of glandular components.

It is due to disturbance of normal ratio of active androgen to oestrogen in plasma or breast (normal ratio of testosterone:oestrogen is 100:1 and normal ratio of these in blood is 300:1).

Imbalance occurs either due to less testosterone production or action or increased oestrogen synthesis or both.

Causes

Physiological

- Pubertal, may be unilateral due to transient increase in oestradiol level. Resolves spontaneously in 6–18 months.
- Senile, due to increased conversion of oestrogen from androgen (also less Leydig cell in testis).
- Newborn (due to transplacental transfer of maternal oestrogen).

Pathological

1. Chronic liver disease (common in alcoholic liver disease), HCC (hCG secreting).
2. Bronchial carcinoma (5% case, hCG-secreting).
3. Hypogonadism—
   - Primary testicular disease (testicular tumour, teratoma, Leydig cell tumour).
   - Testicular failure (trauma, orchidectomy, radiation, leprosy, TB, mumps orchitis, haemochromatosis, Klinefelter's syndrome).
   - Secondary testicular failure (hypopituitarism, hyperprolactinaemia, Kallman's syndrome).
4. Endocrine disease (acromegaly, thyrotoxicosis, hypothyroidism, adrenal carcinoma, Addison's disease).
5. Drugs—spironolactone, digoxin, INH, oestrogen therapy for prostate carcinoma, alcohol, alkylating agent, methyldopa, marijuana, amiodarone.
6. Chromosomal abnormalities—Klinefelter's syndrome, Kallman's syndrome.
7. Others—testicular feminisation syndrome, starvation, idiopathic.

Difference between Gynaecomastia from Lipomastia

- Lipomastia is due to deposition of fat in the breast. So it is soft.
- Gynaecomastia is the enlargement of male breast due to glandular tissue proliferation.So it is firm, hard or rubbery.

NB: Following points are important—

- Unilateral gynaecomastia in the elderly is highly suspicious of malignancy (hard, fixed to underlying tissue, associated with skin tethering and nipple discharge).
- Carcinoma of breast is 16 times common in Klinefelter's syndrome.

Causes of Painful Gynaecomastia

- Puberty.
- Drugs—spironolactone.
- Chronic liver disease.

Mechanism of Gynaecomastia in CLD

- Excess oestrogen due to increased conversion from androgens and altered oestrogen metabolism by liver.
- Drug (spironolactone therapy for ascites).

Mechanism of Gynaecomastia in Alcoholism

- By causing CLD.
- By damaging Leydig cells of testis without CLD.

Investigations in Gynaecomastia

If the patient is young, it may be due to puberty. No need of further investigation. Other investigations according to suspicion of cause—

1. History of drug intake.
2. Chest x-ray (to exclude bronchial carcinoma).
3. Liver function tests (in CLD).
4. Endocrine evaluation—
   - In hypogonadism—serum testosterone, LH, FSH, oestradiol, prolactin and HCG.
   - If LH and FSH are high, but testosterone is low—cause is primary testicular failure.
   - If both LH and testosterone are low—cause is increased oestrogen production from tumour of testis.
   - If both LH and testosterone are high—cause is androgen resistant state or gonadotrophin secreting tumour.
   - 24 hours urinary 17-ketosteroid or serum androstenedione should be done.
   - If plasma β-HCG is high—indicates testicular tumour. It is also increased in bronchial carcinoma.
5. Chromosomal analysis in Klinefelter's syndrome.

Treatment

- Explanation and reassurance, especially in younger age. Usually improve or disappears spontaneously.
- Treatment of primary cause. If any offending drug is responsible, it should be stopped.
- If severe and progressive or suspicion of malignancy— mastectomy.

HYPERHYDROSIS

Definition

It is defined as excessive sweating.

Causes

- Exposure to hot environment.
- Exercise.
- Anxiety.
- Any pyogenic infection.
- Drugs—antipyretic, alcohol, pilocarpine.
- Endrocrine—thyrotoxicosis, acromegaly, phaeochromocytoma, hyperpituitarism.

- Hypoglycaemia.
- Dumping syndrome.
- Carcinoid syndrome.
- Tylosis.
- Ricket.
- Infantile scurvy.
- Rarely, gustatory sweating, lymphoma, malignancy.

PYODERMA GANGRENOSUM

Definition

It is a noninfective, necrotising ulceration with clear bluish-red overhanging edge. The lesion starts as a blister or pustule, breaks down centrally, expands rapidly to an ulcer with indurated or undermined purplish or pustular edge.

Occurs commonly in legs, but may be anywhere in the body, may be single or multiple. It is common in adults (25–54 years).

Types: 4 types

1. Ulcerative.
2. Pustular.
3. Bullous.
4. Vegetative.

Causes of Pyoderma Gangrenosum

- Inflammatory bowel disease—ulcerative colitis (common), less in Crohn's disease.
- Rheumatoid arthritis.
- Polycythaemia rubravera.
- Chronic myeloid leukaemia (also in acute myeloid leukaemia).
- Multiple myeloma and other paraproteinaemias (especially IgA type).
- Myelofibrosis.
- Wegener's granulomatosis.
- Chronic active hepatitis.
- HIV infection.
- Idiopathic in >20% cases.

Investigations

Diagnosis is usually clinical. Investigations are done to find out the cause—

1. CBC, ESR.
2. Blood sugar.
3. Biopsy from the lesion.
4. Other investigations according to suspicion of cause—
   - For IBD—barium enema, colonoscopy.
   - For collagen disease—ANA, anti-dsDNA, antiphospholipid antibody.
   - For vasculitis—c-ANCA, p-ANCA.
   - For myeloma—protein electrophoresis, bone marrow.

Treatment

1. Treatment of underlying diseases.
2. General measures—
   - Control of infection.
   - Local dressing
   - Analgesic for relief of pain.

3. Topical—
   - Corticosteroid. Triamcinolone may be injected into the ulcer edge (alone or with systemic treatment).
   - Tacrolimus may be given.
4. Systemic—
   - Oral prednisolone in high dose. Methylprednisolone 1 g IV for 3 days may be given.
   - Minocycline 100 mg/day may help reduce the dose of steroid.
   - Immunosuppressive agents—ciclosporin, tacrolimus, azathioprine may be used to reduce steroid dependence or in resistant cases.
   - Anti-TNF a (infliximab, etenercept) may be used if others fail.
   - Dapsone, in milder case.
   - Other drug therapy—colchicine, clofazimine, cyclophosphamide, mycophenolatemofetil.

CHAPTER

2 Cardiovascular System

CHAPTER CONTENTS

- Common symptoms of CVS
- Valvular heart diseases
  - Mitral stenosis (MS)
  - Myxoma of heart
  - Mitral regurgitation (MR)
  - Mitral valve prolapse (MVP)
  - Tricuspid regurgitation (TR)
  - Pulmonary stenosis (PS)
  - Pulmonary regurgitation (PR)
  - Aortic stenosis (AS)
  - Aortic regurgitation (AR)
- Heart Failure
  - Acute left ventricular failure (LVF)
  - Congestive cardiac failure (CCF)
- Hypertension
- Rheumatic fever
- Congenital heart diseases
  - Ventricular septal defect (VSD)
  - Atrial septal defect (ASD)
  - Patent ductus arteriosus (PDA)
  - Eisenmenger's syndrome
  - Tetralogy of Fallot (TOF)
  - Coarctation of aorta (COA)
- Ischaemic heart disease (IHD)
  - Angina pectoris
  - Myocardial infarction (MI)
- Acute pericarditis
- Pericardial effusion
- Chronic constrictive pericarditis
- Myocarditis
- Endocarditis
  - Acute endocarditis
  - Subacute bacterial endocarditis (SBE)
- Cardiomyopathy
  - Hypertrophic cardiomyopathy (HCM)
  - Dilated cardiomyopathy (DCM)
  - Restrictive cardiomyopathy (RCM)
  - Postpartum cardiomyopathy
- Arrhythmia
  - Sinus arrhythmia
  - Sinus tachycardia
  - Sinus bradycardia
  - Sick sinus syndrome
  - Supraventricular tachycardia (SVT)
  - WPW syndrome

- Nodal rhythm or junctional rhythm
- Atrial fibrillation (AF)
- Atrial flutter
- Ectopics
- Atrial ectopics
- Ventricular ectopics
- Ventricular tachycardia (VT)
- Ventricular fibrillation (VF)
- Heart block
- SA block (Sino atrial block)
- First degree AV block
- Second degree AV block
- Complete heart block
- Right bundle brunch block (RBBB)
- Fascicular block (Hemiblock)
- Left bundle brunch block (LBBB)

❖ Takayasu's disease
❖ Pacemaker
❖ Pulmonary hypertension
❖ Cardiac arrest
❖ Marfan's syndrome

COMMON SYMPTOMS OF CVS

- Chest pain (usually central, retrosternal).
- Palpitation.
- Breathlessness or dyspnoea.
- Others—leg swelling (in CCF), syncopal attack (in aortic stenosis, HOCM, arrhythmia, hypotension), cough (in pulmonary oedema), haemoptysis (in pulmonary hypertension).

Causes of Central or Retrosternal Chest Pain

- Cardiac—
  - Acute myocardial infarction.
  - Angina pectoris.
  - Pericarditis
  - Myocarditis.
  - Dissecting aortic aneurysm.
- Others—
  - Spontaneous pneumothorax.
  - Pulmonary embolism.
  - Reflux oesophagitis.
  - Oesophageal tear (Mallory Weis syndrome).
  - Mediastinitis.
  - Tracheitis.
  - Functional.

Palpitation

It is the feeling of rapid heartbeat. Any cause of tachycardia is associated with palpitation (see in arrhythmia).

Dyspnoea

It means difficulty in breathing or subjective awareness of breathing. Cardiac causes of dyspnoea—
- Acute left ventricular failure.
- Any vulvular heart disease like MS, MR, AS, AR, etc.
- CCF.

Types of Dyspnoea

- Dyspnoea on exertion—mild, moderate, severe.
- Paroxysomal nocturnal dyspnea (PND)—it is the difficulty in breathing in which patient wakes up from sleep at late hours of night, relieved by sitting on bed or standing, taking air by going near the windows. It indicates pulmonary oedema (in LVF, mitral stenosis).
- Orthopnoea—It means dyspnoea during lying flat or recumbent position. It indicates pulmonary oedema (LVF, Mitral stenosis).

VALVULAR HEART DISEASES

Any valve narrowing called stenosis or unable to close called regurtitation. The most common cause of valvular heart disease is rheumatic heart disease.

MITRAL STENOSIS (MS)

Normal area of mitral valve is 4–6 cm^2.

Cause

The most common cause is chronic rheumatic heart disease. Rarely congenital.

Symptoms

- Breathlessness, usually on exertion.
- Palpitation.
- Cough, may be haemoptysis.
- Weakness.

Signs

- Pulse—low volume (in severe stenosis).
- JVP—normal but raised in pulmonary hypertension.

Precordium

- Inspection: Visible cardiac impulse in mitral area.
- Palpation:
  - Tapping apex beat.
  - Diastolic apical thrill.
- Auscultation:
  - 1st heart sound—loud in all the areas, more in mitral area.
  - 2nd heart sound—normal in all the areas.
  - Mid-diastolic murmur (MDM) in mitral area, which is low-pitched, localized, rough, rumbling (LLRR), best heard with the bell of stethoscope, in left lateral position with breathing hold after expiration, with presystolic accentuation.
  - Opening snap, just medial to the mitral area.
- Investigations
  - X-ray chest P/A view—shows straightening of left border of heart, double border on the right side.
  - ECG—'P' is bifid called P mitrale. Later on, there may be right ventricular hypertrophy(RVH), right atrial hypertrophy (RAH), atrial fibrillation(AF).
  - Echocardiogram (preferably colour Doppler).
  - Cardiac catheter may be done in some cases.

Complications

- Atrial fibrillation.
- Pulmonary oedema.

- Pulmonary hypertension leading to CCF.
- Left atrial thrombus with systemic embolism.
- Pulmonary congestion, embolism, infarction.
- Ortner's syndrome (enlarged left atrium gives pressure on left recurrent laryngeal nerve, causing hoarseness of voice).
- Dysphagia due to enlarged left atrium.
- Recurrent bronchopulmonary infection.
- Very rarely—infective endocarditis.

Signs of Pulmonary Hypertension (PHTN)

- Palpable P2.
- Prominent 'a' wave in JVP.
- Left parasternal heave (indicates RVH).
- Epigastric pulsation (indicates RVH).
- Loud P2 on auscultation.
- Early diastolic murmur (Graham Steel murmur due to pulmonary regurgitation).
- Signs of Severe MS.

Severe when Mitral Valve Area is <1 cm^2

- Pulse—low volume.
- 1st heart sound—soft.
- Opening snap—nearer to the 2nd sound.
- MDM—prolonged.
- Evidence of pulmonary hypertension and pulmonary oedema.

Treatment

- Medical
  - Restriction of activity.
  - Low dose diuretic—thiazide or frusemide.
  - Anticoagulant (e.g. warfarin) to reduce the risk of embolism.
  - If atrial fibrillation—digoxin, beta-blocker, rate limiting calcium antagonist (e.g. verapamil, diltiazem).
  - If there is CCF—diuretic, digoxin.
- Surgical—when indicated.

Surgical Options

- Valvotomy (CMC—closed mitral commissurotomy, OMC—open mitral commissurotomy).
- Valvuloplasty (percutaneous balloon mitral valvuloplasty)- treatment of choice.
- Valve replacement.

Indications of Surgery

- Symptomatic moderate or severe MS.
- Moderate or severe MS with moderate or severe MR.
- Recurrent thromboembolism.

- Episodes of pulmonary oedema without precipitating cause.
- Associated atrial fibrillation which does not respond to medical therapy.
- Pulmonary hypertension or recurrent haemoptysis.
- Occasionally in pregnancy, with pulmonary oedema (surgery may be done in second trimester as blood volume increases significantly with increased pulmonary pressure).

Indications of Valve Replacement

- Associated MR.
- If the valve is calcified and rigid.
- Thrombus in left atrium despite anticoagulation.

MYXOMA OF HEART

Definition

It is the common primary tumour of heart, usually benign, may be pedunculated, polypoid, gelatinous, attached by a pedicle to the atrial septum. It may be sporadic and familial. It occurs in any age (third to sixth decade), and any sex (more in females).

Sites of Origin

- Left atrium (75%), near the fossa ovalis or its margin.
- Right atrium, rarely from ventricles.

Clinical Features

There are 3 groups of manifestations—

- Obstructive features like MS, signs vary with posture. Occasionally, there is a low-pitched sound called tumour plop. There may be syncope or vertigo.
- Embolic features either systemic or pulmonary embolism.
- Constitutional features like fever, malaise, weakness, loss of weight, myalgia, arthralgia, clubbing, skin rash, Raynaud's phenomenon.

Investigations

- CBC—anaemia, leucocytosis, polycythaemia, high ESR, thrombocytopaenia or thrombocytosis.
- Hypergammaglobulinaemia.
- Chest X-ray (may be similar to MS).
- Echocardiogram—2D or transoesophageal.
- CT scan or MRI may be done.

Treatment

Surgical excision. Recurrence may occur.

MITRAL REGURGITATION (MR)

Causes

- Chronic rheumatic heart disease.
- Mitral valve prolapse.
- Papillary muscle dysfunction.
- Infective endocarditis.
- Trauma or mitral valvotomy.
- Connective tissue diseases (rheumatoid arthritis, SLE, Marfan's syndrome, Ehler-Danlos syndrome).
- Ankylosing spondylitis.
- Cardiomyopathy.
- Secondary to left ventricular dilatation (hypertension, aortic valve disease).

Symptoms

- Breathlessness on exertion.
- Palpitation.
- Cough.
- Weakness.

Signs

Precordium

- Inspection:
  - Visible cardiac impulse in mitral area.
- Palpation:
  - Apex beat is shifted, diffuse, thrusting in character.
  - Systolic thrill in mitral area.
- Auscultation:
  - 1st heart sound—soft in mitral area, normal in other areas.
  - 2nd sound—normal in all the areas.
- Pansystolic murmur in mitral area, which radiates to the left axilla.

Investigations

- X-ray chest P/A view (cardiomegaly may be found).
- ECG (LVH, LAH).
- Echocardiogram, preferably colour doppler.
- Cardiac catheterization may be needed in some cases.

Complications

- Acute LVF.
- Infective endocarditis.
- Embolism.
- Arrhythmia (atrial fibrillation, ectopics).
- CCF.

Treatment

- In mild to moderate case—
  - Diuretic—frusemide or thiazide.
  - Vasodilator—ACE inhibitor.
  - If fast AF—digoxin.
  - Anticoagulant if associated AF or history of pulmonary embolism.
  - Prophylactic penicillin to prevent endocarditis.
  - Follow-up every 6 months by echocardiogram.
  - If ejection fraction falls to 55% and left ventricular dilatation > 60 mm, valve replacement may be considered.
- In severe MR—replacement of valve.

Indications of Surgery in MR

- Symptomatic MR.
- Asymptomatic patient with severe MR with mild to moderate LV dysfunction or pulmonary hypertension.

MITRAL VALVE PROLAPSE (MVP)

Also called Barlow's syndrome or floppy mitral valve. In this condition, a mitral valve leaflet, commonly the posterior leaflet prolapses into the left atrium during ventricular systole. It is one of the most common causes of MR. It may be congenital or due to degenerative myxomatous change.

Symptoms

- More common in thin, young women, may be familial.
- The most common symptom is atypical chest pain, usually in left submammary region, stabbing in quality, may be confused with anginal pain.
- There may be palpitation, dyspnoea, fatigue.

Signs

- Midsystolic click followed by late systolic murmur (cardinal sign).
- Later, signs of MR arc found.

Investigation

- Echocardiogram.

Treatment

- If asymptomatic—reassurance, periodic echocardiography.
- Atypical chest pain and palpitation—beta-blocker.
- Significant MR or AF—anticoagulation to prevent thromboembolism (aspirin may be given).
- In severe MR—mitral valve repair or replacement.
- Prophylactic penicillin to prevent infective endocarditis.

TRICUSPID REGURGITATION (TR)

Causes

- Functional—secondary to pulmonary hypertension, cor pulmonale, right heart failure (commonest cause).
- Chronic rheumatic heart disease.
- Infective endocarditis (commonly involved in drug addicts).
- Congenital heart disease (e.g. Ebstein's anomaly).
- Carcinoid syndrome.
- Right ventricular papillary muscle infarction, trauma or steering wheel injury in chest.

Symptoms

- May be asymptomatic. Symptoms of primary disease.

Signs

- Pulse—normal in volume, rhythm and character.
- JVP—raised, giant 'V' wave, oscillating upto ear lobule.

Precordium

- On palpation:
  - Left parasternal lift and epigastric pulsation (due to RVH).
- On auscultation:
  - First heart sound—soft in tricuspid area, normal in other areas.
  - Second sound—normal in all the areas.
  - Pan systolic murmur (PSM) in left lower parasternal area with no radiation, louder with inspiration.
- Others:
  - Liver—enlarged, tender and pulsatile.
  - Occasionally ascites, oedema and pleural effusion may occur in TR.

Cardinal Findings in TR

- Prominent 'V' wave in JVP.
- Pansystolic murmur (PSM) in left lower parasternal area, louder with inspiration and reduced on expiration.
- Liver—enlarged, tender and pulsatile (Table 1).

Table 1
Differences between MR and TR

MR	TR
1. PSM in mitral area	PSM in left lower parasternal area
2. PSM radiate to left axilla	No radiation
3. Murmur increases with expiration	Murmur increases with inspiration
4. No pulsatile liver	Pulsatile liver
5. No V-wave in JVP	V-wave in JVP

Investigations

- Chest X-ray—heart may be enlarged.
- ECG.
- Echocardiogram, preferably colour Doppler.

Complications

- Right-sided heart failure.
- Infective endocarditis.

Treatment

- Treatment of primary cause.
- In severe organic TR—operative repair. Occasionally, valve replacement is needed.
- Ebstein's anomaly: It is a congenital heart disease associated with downward displacement of tricuspid valve into the right ventricle. Hence, right atrium is large and right ventricle is small. Characteristically, multiple clicks occur due to asynchronous closure of tricuspid valve. ASD is commonly associated with this anomaly.

PULMONARY STENOSIS (PS)

Causes

- Congenital (most common).
- Associated with Carcinoid syndrome, Noonan's syndrome, Fallot's tetralogy.
- May occur, if there is rubella in pregnancy.

Symptoms

- May be asymptomatic.
- Symptoms, such as fatigue, weakness and effort syncope may occur.

Signs

Precordium

- On palpation:
  - Left parasternal lift and epigastric pulsation (due to RVH).
  - Systolic thrill—Present in pulmonary area.
- On auscultation:
  - First heart sound—normal in all the areas.
  - Second heart sound—P2 is soft in pulmonary area and A2 is normal (wide splitting of the second sound may be present).
  - Ejection systolic murmur (ESM) in pulmonary area, which radiates to the neck (more on inspiration).
  - Fourth heart sound may be present (due to right atrial contraction).

Investigations

- ECG—shows RVH and RAH.
- Chest X-ray—shows enlarged pulmonary conus, oligaemic lung fields, poststenotic dilatation of pulmonary artery.
- Echocardiogram.

Types of PS

There are three of PS:

- Valvular.
- Subvalvular.
- Supravalvular.

Complications

- Right heart failure.
- Pulmonary embolism.

Treatment

- In mild case, compatible with normal life (no specific treatment).
- In severe symptomatic case, when the pressure gradient is >50 mm Hg, balloon valvuloplasty is the treatment of choice.
  NB: Infective endocarditis is unusual in PS. Prophylactic antibiotic is unnecessary.

PULMONARY REGURGITATION (PR)

Causes

- Dilatation of pulmonary valve secondary to pulmonary hypertension.
- Secondary to mitral stenosis producing an early diastolic murmur (Graham Steel murmur).
- Rheumatic fever.
- Carcinoid syndrome.

Symptoms

- May be asymptomatic or symptoms of primary disease.
- Features of right-sided heart failure.

Signs

- Left parasternal lift.
- P2 may be soft.
- Early diastolic murmur in 3rd or 4th left intercostal space.

Investigations

- Chest X-ray.
- ECG.
- Echocardiogram.

Treatment

- Teatment of underlying cause.
- In severe regurgitation—valve replacement.

AORTIC STENOSIS (AS)

Normal area of aortic valve is 1.5–2 cm^2. It is severe, if the area is < 1 cm^2. If the valve area is < 0.7 cm^2, it is called critical aortic stenosis.

Causes

- Chronic rheumatic heart disease.
- Congenital bicuspid aortic valve (common in male).
- Calcification in old age.
- Congenital (in early age).

Symptoms

- Breathlessness, mainly on exertion.
- Palpitation.
- Anginal chest pain.
- Syncope (transient loss of consciousness) during effort.
- Sudden death (probably due to ventricular fibrillation).

Signs

- Pulse—low volume, slow rising.
- BP—low systolic, normal diastolic, narrow pulse pressure.

Precordium

- Inspection:
  - Visible cardiac impulse in mitral area.
- Palpation:
  - Palpable apex beat, heaving in nature.
  - Systolic thrill in aortic area.
- Auscultation:
  - 1st heart sound—normal in all the areas.
  - 2nd heart sound—A2 is soft in all the areas, P2 is normal.May be reversed splitting of S2.
  - Ejection systolic murmur in aortic area, radiates to the neck.

Investigations

- X-ray of chest—shows enlarged heart.
- ECG shows left ventriculay hypertrophy (LVH).
- Echocardiogram, preferably colour Doppler echo.
- Cardiac catheterisation in some cases.

Complications

- Left ventricular failure.
- Infective endocarditis (10% cases).
- Sudden death due to ventricular fibrillation.
- Complete heart block (in calcification of aortic valve).
- Systemic embolism.

Signs of Severe AS

- Pulse is feeble or absent.
- Absent or soft A2 (or single S2).
- Harsh, loud, prolonged murmur with late peaking.
- Reverse splitting of second heart sound.
- Presence of fourth heart sound.
- Presence of heart failure or LVF (late sign).

Treatment

- If aymptomatic—follow-up with periodic echocardiogram. Avoid strenuous activity or exercise.
- If symptomatic or syncopal attack—valve replacement.
- If asymptomatic with severe AS—valve replacement.
- If the patient is unfit for surgery—percutaneous valvuloplasty.
- In children, elderly or pregnancy—valvotomy.

Indications of Surgery

- All symptomatic patients (such as syncope).
- If mean systolic pressure gradient is >50 mmHg (left ventricular systolic pressure > aorta).
- If the valve area is <0.7 cm^2.
- Abnormal BP in response to exercise.

AORTIC REGURGITATION (AR)

Causes

- Chronic rheumatic heart disease.
- Infective endocarditis.
- Syphilitic aortitis.
- Bicuspid aortic valve.
- Dissecting aneurysm affecting ascending aorta.
- Hypertension (by aortic dilatation).
- Marfan's syndrome.
- Seronegative arthritis (ankylosing spondylitis, Reiter's syndrome).
- Rheumatoid arthritis.
- Cystic medial necrosis.
- Congenital.

Symptoms

- May be asymptomatic.
- Symptoms may be—palpitation, shortness of breath on exertion, occasional cough, anginal pain.

Signs

- Pulse—high volume, collapsing.
- Dancing carotid pulse in the neck (Corrigan's sign).
- BP—High systolic, low diastolic and wide pulse pressure.

Precordium

- Inspection:
  - Visible cardiac impulse.
- Palpation
  - Apex beat—shifted, thrusting in nature.
  - Diastolic thrill may be present in left parasternal area.
- Auscultation
  - 1st heart sound—normal in all the areas.
  - 2nd heart sound—A2 is absent and P2 is normal.
  - Early diastolic murmur in left lower parasternal area with patient bending forward and breathing hold after expiration.
  - ESM may be present in aortic area due to increased flow.

Formula of 3 to Diagnose AR

- 3 pulse—collapsing (water hammer), dancing carotid and capillary pulsation.
- 3 BP—rise of systolic, fall of diastolic and wide pulse pressure.
- 3 murmur—early diastolic murmur, Austin Flint murmur and ejection systolic murmur.

Investigations

- X-ray chest shows cardiomegaly.
- ECG (LVH).
- Echocardiogram, preferably colour Doppler.
- Cardiac catheterisation.
- Other investigations to find out cause.

Complications

- Acute LVF.
- Infective endocarditis.
- Arrhythmia.

Treatment

- In mild asymptomatic case—follow-up.
- In asymptomatic moderate to severe AR with normal LV function—long acting nifedipine.
- In symptomatic patient with—
  - Normal LV function—long acting nifedipine.
  - LV dysfunction—digitalis, ACE inhibitor, diuretic.
  - Heart failure—digitalis, ACE inhibitor, diuretic.
- In severe case—valve replacement.

Indications of Surgery

- Symptomatic patient.
- Asymptomatic patient with—
  - LV systolic dysfunction (EF <50%)
  - LV dilatation (LV end-systolic dimension >55 mm or LV end-diastolic dimension >75 mm).
  - Aortic root dilatation >50 mm.

HEART FAILURE

Definition

It is the failure of the heart to maintain adequate cardiac output to meet the demand of the tissue or can do so only at the expense of an elevated filling pressure.

Types

- Left-sided heart failure.
- Right-sided heart failure.
- Biventricular failure.

ACUTE LEFT VENTRICULAR FAILURE (LVF)

Definition

Acute left ventricular failure (LVF) is the failure of left ventricle to propel blood in the systemic circulation. As a result, there is accumulation of blood in pulmonary circulation resulting in pulmonary oedema (Table 2).

Causes of LVF (Pulmonary Oedema)

- Systemic hypertension.
- Acute myocardial infarction.
- Aortic valvular disease (stenosis and regurgitation).
- Mitral regurgitation.
- Cardiomyopathy.
- Coarctation of aorta.
- Rapid or excess infusion of fluid or blood or plasma.
- Hyperdynamic circulation.

Symptoms

- Breathlessness, may be orthopnoea.
- Cough with frothy sputum, occasional haemoptysis.
- Palpitation.
- Features of low cardiac output—restlessness, sweating, oliguria.

Signs

- Patient looks dyspnoeic with propped up position.
- Cyanosis.
- Pulse—tachycardia, may be pulsus alternans.
- BP—low but may be high if the patient is hypertensive.

Precordium

- Apex beat—may be shifted, thrusting or heaving in character.
- On auscultation—Gallop rhythm (tachycardia with 3rd or 4th heart sound. It resembles the sound produced by galloping horse).

- In lungs—bilateral basal crepitations.
- Signs of primary cause may be present.

Cardinal Features of LVF

- Bilateral basal crepitations.
- Gallop rhythm.
- Pulsus alternans.

Investigations

- Chest X-ray—shows pulmonary oedema (perihilar bats wing appearance, Kerleys B line, cardiomegaly).
- ECG—may show myocardial infarction, LVH.
- Echocardiogram.

Treatment of Acute LVF (Pulmonary Oedema)

- Bed rest.
- Propped up position.

Table 2
Differences between cardiac asthma and bronchial asthma

Features	Cardiac asthma	Bronchial asthma
History	• Hypertension, IHD, vulvular disease • Family history of hypertension	• History of previous attack of asthma, allergy or rhinitis • Family history of asthma or allergy
Age	• Usually elderly	• Young, but may be any age
Symptoms	• Dyspnoea • Cough with frothy sputum • Wheeze—rare • Sweating—common	• Dyspnoea • Cough with little mucoid sputum • Wheeze—common • Sweating—less
Signs	• Pulse—pulsus alternans • BP—high (if hypertensive) Heart— • Cardiomegaly (apex is shifted) • Gollop rhythm may be present • Primary cause (mitral or aortic valvular disease) may be present Lungs— • Bilateral basal crepitations. In severe case, extensive crepitations • No or little rhonchi	• Pulse—may be pulsus paradoxus • BP—Normal, low in severe case • Heart— • Absent • No • No • Lungs— • Plenty of rhonchi all over the lungs • No or little crepitations
CXR	• Pulmonary oedema—perihilar opacities (Bat's wing appearance) • Cardiomegaly	• Relatively clear, evidence of infection may be present
ECG	• Left ventricular hypertrophy, MI, arrhythmia	• Normal, only tachycardia may be present

- High-flow oxygen inhalation (60–100%).
- Diuretic—frusemide IV 80–120 mg. May be repeated.
- Morphine (if no contraindication, such as bronchial asthma, COPD, emphysema, chronic bronchitis)—10–20 mg IV slowly with antiemetic metochlopramide or cyclizine.
- ACE inhibitor—ramipril, captopril, enalapril.
- If no response, inotropic agents like dopamine, dobutamine may be added.
- Treatment of primary cause.
- Antiarrhythmic drug, if arrhythmia.

CONGESTIVE CARDIAC FAILURE

Definition

Congestive cardiac failure (CCF) actually means right-sided heart failure. There is inability of the right ventricle to propel blood resulting in backflow of blood to systemic veins causing engorged vein, enlarged liver and dependent oedema (Table 2).

Causes of CCF

- Secondary to left sided heart failure (common cause).
- Mitral stenosis with pulmonary hypertension.
- Chronic cor pulmonale due to any cause.
- Pulmonary hypertension.
- Pulmonary valve disease (stenosis or regurgitation).
- Tricuspid regurgitation.
- Shunt anomaly (ASD, VSD), when there is reversal of shunt (Eisenmenger's syndrome).
- Cardiomyopathy.
- Right ventricular myocardial infarction.

Symptoms

- Breathlessness on exertion, cough with mucoid sputum.
- Palpitation.
- Pain in right upper abdomen (due to hepatomegaly).
- Swelling in legs.
- Weakness, weight loss.
- Anorexia, nausea, vomiting.
- Oliguria, nocturia.

Signs

- Pulse—low volume.
- BP—may be low.
- JVP—engorged and pulsatile.
- Dependent pitting oedema—in legs or sacral oedema if lying.

Precordium

- Visible cardiac impulse.
- Apex beat—may be shifted.

- Thrill—absent or present, according to the cause.
- Heart sounds according to the vulvular lesion .
- Murmur, according to the vulvular lesion.

Abdomen

- Liver is enlarged and tender.

Cardinal Signs of Congestive Cardiac Failure

- Engorged and pulsatile neck veins.
- Enlarged and tender liver.
- Dependent pitting oedema.

Investigations

- X-ray chest—shows cardiomegaly.
- ECG.
- Echocardiogram.
- Others—CBC, ESR, urea, creatinine, electrolytes, lung function test (if COPD).

Treatment

- Complete rest.
- Restriction of fluid and salt.
- Diuretic—frusemide, bumetanide, aldosterone antagonist (e.g. spironolactone, eplerenone).
- Vasodilator (ACE inhibitor or ARB).
- Beta-blocker (bisoprolol 1.25 mg daily and gradually increase the dose over 12 weeks up to 10 mg daily).
- Digoxin (helpful in CCF with atrial fibrillation).
- Treatment of arrhythmia (e.g. amiodarone).
- Treatment of the underlying cause.
- Heart transplantation—if all above measures fail.

Complications of Digoxin

- Extracardiac—
  - Gastrointestinal—anorexia, nausea, vomiting, diarrhoea.
  - Altered colour vision (xanthopsia).
  - Others—weight loss, confusion, headache, gynaecomastia.
- Cardiac—
  - Bradycardia.
  - Multiple ventricular ectopics.
  - Ventricular bigeminy.
  - Atrial tachycardia with variable block.
  - Ventricular tachycardia.
  - Ventricular fibrillation.

Treatment of Digoxin Toxicity

- Digoxin should be stopped.
- Serum electrolytes, creatinine and digoxin level should be checked.

- Correction of electrolytes, if any.
- If bradycardia—IV atropine, sometimes pacing may be needed.
- Correction of arrhythmia.

Causes of Biventricular Failure

- Cardiomyopathy (dilated cardiomyopathy).
- Myocarditis.
- Ischaemic heart disease (such as extensive myocardial infarction).
- Right-sided heart failure secondary to left-sided heart failure (e.g. MR, AS or AR).
- Hyperdynamic circulation (in severe anaemia, thyrotoxicosis, arteriovenous shunt, beri- beri).
- Myxoedema (called myxoedema heart).
- Multiple vulvular diseases.

HYPERTENSION

Definition

Persistent rise of arterial BP above the arbitrarily normal range. If systolic blood pressure > 140 mm Hg, diastolic BP > 90 mm Hg, the patient is diagnosed as hypertensive.

Causes

1. Primary or essential hypertension (95%)—cause unknown.
2. Secondary (5%)—
   a. Renal (most common secondary cause)—
      - Chronic glomerulonephritis.
      - Chronic pyelonephritis.
      - Diabetic nephropathy.
      - Adult polycystic kidney disease.
      - Renal artery stenosis.

   b. Endocrine—
      - Cushing's syndrome.
      - Conn's syndrome (primary aldosteronism).
      - Phaeochromocytoma.
      - Congenital adrenal hyperplasia.
      - Hyperparathyroidism.
      - Primary hypothyroidism.
      - Hyperthyroidism.
      - Acromegaly.

   c. Drugs—
      - Alcohol.
      - Oral contraceptive pill.
      - Steroid.
      - Erythropoietin.
3. Others—
   - Preeclampsia and eclampsia (toxaemia of pregnancy).
   - Pregnancy induced hypertension.
   - Coarctation of aorta.
   - Cerebral tumour.

Clinical Features

Symptoms

- May be asymptomatic, detected during routine examination.
- Headache, dizziness, giddiness, insomnia, blurring of vision.
- Features of complication—heart failure, CVD, renal failure etc.

Complications of Hypertension

1. Cardiovascular—
   - Ischaemic heart disease.
   - Acute left ventricular failure.
   - Dissecting aneurysm.
2. Renal—
   - Renal failure.
3. Ocular—
   - Retinopathy.
4. Neurological—
   - CVD (intracerebral haemorrhage)
   - Subarachnoid haemorrhage.
   - Hypertensive encephalopathy.

NB: Following points are important—

- A single reading is not sufficient. At least three readings in different times should be taken to label as hypertensive.
- BP should be measured at least 5 minutes after the patient has taken rest comfortably in sitting or supine position.
- BP should be measured at least 30 minutes after smoking or coffee ingestion (Table 3).

Table 3
Grade of hypertension

Grade	Systolic	Diastolic
Grade 1 (mild)	140–159 mm of Hg and/or	90–99 mm of Hg
Grade 2 (moderate)	160–179 mm of Hg and/or	100–109 mm of Hg
Grade 3 (severe)	≥180 mm of Hg and/or	≥110 mm of Hg

White Coat Hypertension

When blood pressure is recorded in a hospital set-up or in the physician's clinic, there may be transient rise in BP in a normal individual. This is called white coat hypertension.

Hypertensive Encephalopathy

It is characterised by very high BP with neurological abnormalities, such as severe headache, loss of consciousness, convulsion, paraesthesia, transient disturbance of speech or vision, retinopathy, etc.

Malignant Hypertension

It is characterized by severe hypertension with diastolic BP >130 mmHg, associated with grade III or IV retinopathy (retinal haemorrhage or exudates and papilloedema) and renal failure or encephalopathy. If untreated, death occurs within months.

Treatment

Slow, controlled reduction of BP over a period of 24-48 hours is ideal. (Rapid reduction is avoided as it reduces tissue perfusion and can cause cerebral damage including occipital blindness, may even precipitate coronary or renal insufficiency).

The treatment include:
- Complete rest.
- Oral antihypertensive is sufficient to control BP.
- Sometimes IV or IM labetalol, IV glycerine trinitrate, IM hydralazine.

Refractory Hypertension

When there is no response to antihypertensive drugs, it is called refractory hypertension. The causes are:
- Nonadherence to drug therapy (most common cause).
- Inadequate therapy.
- Failure to recognize an underlying cause like renal artery stenosis or phaeochromocytoma.

Resistant Hypertension

Means failure to control BP with full doses of appropriate three drug regimen including a diuretic. The following things should be carefully excluded:
- Improper BP measurement.
- Volume overload which may be due to excess sodium intake, renal disease or inadequate diuretic therapy.
- Inadequate dose, inappropriate combination of drugs or noncompliance.
- Whether patient is taking drugs like NSAIDs, steroid, oral contraceptive pills, ciclosproin, erythropoietin.
- Other secondary causes of hypertension.
- Associated conditions like obesity, excess alcohol intake etc.

Investigations in Hypertension

History

1. Age: If young, likely to be secondary cause. If elderly, likely to be primary.
2. Family history: Family history of hypertension, hyperlipidaemia, diabetes mellitus, obesity, etc. may be present in primary hypertension. In some secondary hypertension, there may be positive family history, e.g. polycystic kidney disease.
3. Past medical history: Previous history of renal disease (haematuria, UTI, renal trauma, pain, pyelonephritis), toxaemia of pregnancy (in female).
4. Drug history: Prolong use of NSAIDs, steroids, oral contraceptive pill, etc.
5. Smoking and alcohol.
6. Symptoms to find out secondary cause:
   - Symptoms of renal disease like polyuria, frequency, haematuria, loin pain.
   - Paroxysmal attack of headache, palpitation, flushing and sweating (phaeochromocytoma).
   - Polyuria, polydipsia, extreme muscular weakness, tingling (Conn's syndrome).
   - Weight gain, hirsutism, striae, menstrual abnormality in female (Cushing's syndrome).
   - Claudication and cramp in lower limbs in young patient (coarctation of aorta).
   - Frequent attack of headache, vomiting, visual disturbance, neurological features (intracranial tumour).

Physical findings which indicates specific cause—
- Puffy face—renal failure.
- Central obesity with plethoric moon face, hirsutism, striae—Cushing's syndrome.

- Pulse—bradycardia suggests raised intracranial pressure, feeble pulse in lower limbs with radiofemoral delay found in coarctation of aorta.
- BP—high BP in upper limbs but low in lower limbs suggest coarctation of aorta.
- Anaemia—suggests chronic renal failure.
- Oedema—may be present in renal failure.
- Cardiovascular system—apex beat may be heaving and shifted (left ventricular hypertrophy), murmur may be present in coarctation of aorta.
- Abdomen—bilateral renal mass in polycystic kidney disease, renal bruit in renal artery stenosis.
- Fundoscopy.
- Other finding according to suspicion of cause like intracranial mass.
- Bed side urine examination for haematuria and proteinuria.

Laboratory Investigations

1. Routine—
   - Urine R/M/E—to see protein, RBC cast, pus cell.
   - Blood urea, creatinine.
   - Serum electrolytes.
   - Fasting blood sugar.
   - Serum lipid profile (total serum cholesterol, VLDL, LDL, HDL, triglyceride).
   - X-ray chest PA view.
   - ECG.
   - Echocardiogram.
2. Other investigations according to suspicion of cause—
   - If renal cause—ultrasonogram of kidney, IVU, CT scan of renal system, isotope renogram.
   - Cushing's syndrome—serum cortisol level, 24-hour urinary cortisol, ACTH, dexamethasone suppression test, etc.
   - Phaeochromocytoma—24 hours urinary VMA, serum catecholamines, USG, CT/MRI of suprarenal gland.
   - Conn's syndrome—plasma aldosterone and renin.
   - Coarctation of aorta—CT scan, aortogram.

Treatment of Hypertension

1. General measures (nondrug treatment):
   - Salt restriction (<6 g/day).
   - Smoking should be stopped.
   - Weight reduction in obese patient.
   - Dietary modification—low fat, consumption of more fruits and vegetables.
   - Regular exercise (at least 30 minutes daily).
   - Avoid anxiety and tension.
   - Control of diabetes mellitus.
   - Restriction of tea and coffee.
   - Restriction of alcohol intake (<21 units/week for men and <14 units/week for women).
   - Control of other modifiable risk factors.

2. Drug treatment:
   - Diuretic—thiazide (bendroflumethiazide).
   - ACE inhibitor- enalapril, lisinopril, ramipril.
   - ARB—losartan, valsartan, irbesartan.
   - Calcium channel blocker—amlodipine, nifedipine, diltiazem, verapamil.
   - Beta-blocker—atenolol, metoprolol, bisoprolol.
   - Combined alpha- and beta-blocker—labetalol, carvedilol.
   - Alpha-blocker—prazosin.
   - Others—Methyldopa (used in pregnancy).
3. Management of primary cause, if any.

How to Start Drug in Treatment of Hypertension?

- Single drug is started—diuretic or beta-blocker or calcium channel blocker or ACE inhibitor.
- If no response, combination therapy is given diuretic plus beta-blocker or diuretic plus ACE inhibitor or ACE inhibitor calcium channel blocker or beta-blocker plus calcium channel blocker.

Contraindications of Beta-blocker

- Respiratory—bronchial asthma, COPD, emphysema, chronic bronchitis.
- CVS—bradycardia, partial or complete heart block, CCF, peripheral vascular disease (Raynaud's phenomenon).
- Endocrine—phaemochromocytoma (beta-blocker alone is avoided), DM receiving insulin (masks the features of hypoglycaemia).

Treatment of Hypertension in Specific Conditions

Hypertension in bronchial asthma

- Diuretics, calcium channel blocker, ARB, ACE inhibitor (it may cause cough) may be used.
- Avoid β-blockers.

Hypertension in chronic kidney disease (Target BP is <130/80 mmHg)

- ACE inhibitors and ARB may delay progression of kidney disease (if creatinine is >2.5 mmol/L, these should be avoided).
- Calcium channel blockers may be used.
- Loop diuretic (Frusemide).

Hypertension in pregnancy

- Methyldopa or labetalol.
- Calcium channel blocker (nifedipine) may be used. Beta- blocker may be used (avoid in first trimester).
- ACE inhibitor is contraindicated.
- Diuretic is also avoided.
- More severe hypertension or eclampsia may be treated with intravenous hydralazine.

Hypertension in diabetes mellitus

- ACE inhibitor, ARB, calcium channel blocker may be used.

- Avoid thiazide (it aggravates diabetes).
- Avoid β-blocker in patient who is on insulin (it masks symptoms of hypoglycaemia).

Hypertension in peripheral vascular disease

- Calcium channel blocker.
- Alpha-blocker may be an alternative.
- Avoid beta-blocker.
- ACE inhibitor should be used carefully (as the patient may have renal artery stenosis also).

Hypertension in dyslipidaemia

- Alpha-blocker, ACE inhibitor, ARB, calcium channel blocker.
- Avoid beta-blocker and diuretic (which worsen lipid profile).

Hypertension in psoriasis

- Calcium channel blocker may be used.
- Avoid β-blocker, ACE inhibitor (which aggravates).

Hypertension in angina

- Beta-blocker, calcium channel blocker, nitrate.

RHEUMATIC FEVER

Definition

It is a multisystem disorder that occurs as a sequele to pharyngitis by group A beta-haemolytic streptococcus.

Mechanism

It is due to autoimmune reaction due to molecular mimicry between the antigen (M protein) of streptococcus beta- haemolyticus and cardiac myosin and sarcolemal membrane protein (laminin). As a result, antibody produced against streptococcal enzyme causes 'cross reaction' against endocardium, myocardium and pericardium as well as joints and skin. There is a formation of "Aschoff's nodule" in heart which is pathognomonic of rheumatic fever.

Rheumatic fever is usually common in children and young adults, 5–15 years of age. There is usually the history of sore throat 1–3 weeks prior to the fever.

Diagnostic Criteria of Rheumatic Fever

It is diagnosed by revised **Jones' criteria.** Following an attack of streptococcus pharyngitis, there is usually a latent period of 1–3 weeks.

1. Major criteria:
   - Carditis.
   - Shifting or migrating polyarthritis involving the big joints (knee, elbow, ankle, wrist).
   - Rheumatic chorea.
   - Erythema marginatum.
   - Subcutaneous nodule.
2. Minor criteria:
   - Fever.
   - Arthralgia.
   - Previous history of rheumatic fever.
   - High ESR or CRP.
   - Leucocytosis.
   - First or second degree AV block in ECG.

In addition, supportive evidence of previous streptococcal infection, like recent streptococcal infection, history of scarlet fever, raised ASO titre (>200) or other streptococcal antibody titre (anti-DNAse or antihyaluronidase) or positive throat swab culture.

Diagnosis is made by two or more major criteria, or one major and two or more minor criteria plus supportive evidence of streptococcal infection.

Signs of carditis: RF can cause carditis involving all the layers of the heart (endocardium, myocardium and pericardium), called pancarditis.

Signs of Endocarditis

- Soft heart sounds.
- Pansystolic murmur (due to MR).
- Mid-diastolic murmur (Carey Coomb's murmur).
- Early diastolic murmur (due to AR which is due to valvulitis with nodules on the valve).

Signs of Myocarditis

- Tachycardia.
- Soft heart sounds, S3 gallop.
- Cardiomegaly.
- Features of heart failure.

Signs of Pericarditis

- Pericardial rub (patient usually complains of chest pain).
- Pericardial effusion may be present.

Erythema Marginatum

It is a transient, geographical type rash with pink or red-raised edges, round margin and clear centre. It is found mostly on the trunk and proximal limbs (not in face).

Subcutaneous Nodule

These are small, mobile, firm, painless, pea-shaped nodules, felt over bony prominences, tendons or joints on the extensor surface.

Sydenham's Chorea (St. Vitus' Dance)

It is a neurological manifestation of acute RF, which usually occurs after 3 months of an acute attack, when almost all other signs have disappeared.

- Common in children and adolescents, more in female of 5–15 years of age.
- Usually associated with emotional instability, irritability, inattentiveness and confusion.
- May occur without any feature of acute RF.
- Carditis is common.
- Speech may be explosive and halting.
- ESR, ASO titre and CRP are usually normal.
- Rheumatic chorea is usually self-limiting, recovers within few months.
- Treatment—sedation (haloperidol) along with other treatment and prophylaxis of rheumatic fever.

Signs of Activity in Rheumatic Fever

- Persistent fever.
- Tachycardia.
- High ESR.
- Leucocytosis.
- Evidence of carditis.

Investigations of RF

- CBC, ESR (there is high ESR and leucocytosis).
- CRP—high.
- ASO titre—high (in adult >200, in children >300).
- Throat swab culture (to find streptococcus beta- haemolyticus).
- Chest X-ray—cardiomegaly, pulmonary oedema.
- ECG.
- Echocardiography.

Complications

- CCF.
- Arrythmia.
- Pericarditis and pericardial effusion.
- Rheumatic heart disease causing vulvular stenosis and regurgitation.

Treatment of Acute RF

1. Complete bed rest.
2. Oral phenoxymethylpenicillin 250 mg 6 hourly for 10 days or single injection of benzathine penicillin 1.2 million units, deep IM in the buttock. Erythromycin may be given, if allergic to penicillin.
3. Analgesic (to relieve pain). Aspirin 60 mg/kg per day in divided dose. Higher dose may be required.
4. Other treatment—
   - If carditis or severe arthritis—prednisolone 1–2 mg/kg daily.
   - If chorea—diazepam for mild case or haloperidol in severe case.
5. Treatment of complications like cardiac failure, valvular lesion, heart block, arrhythmia, etc., if needed.

Prophylactic Treatment of RF

Recurrence is common in patient who had carditis during initial episode. In children, 20% recurrence occurs within 5 years. Recurrence is uncommon after 5 years and in patient over 25 years of age.

To prevent recurrence—oral phenoxymethylpenicillin 250 mg 12 hourly or injection benzathine penicillin 1.2 million units deep IM in the buttock every 4 weeks should be given. In penicillin sensitive cases, erythromycin (250 mg 12 hourly) may be used.

Prophylactic drug should be continued up to 21 years of age or 5 years after the last attack (recurrence after 5 years is rare), whichever comes last. After this, antibiotic prophylaxis should be given for dental or surgical procedure. However, in high-risk streptococcal infection or if the attack occurs in the 5 years or patient lives in high area of prevalence, treatment may need to be extended. If there is documented recurrence or documented rheumatic valvular heart disease, life-long prophylaxis should be considered.

NB: Following points are important—

- Skin infection with streptococci is not associated with RF.
- Streptococcal sore throat may not be present in some cases.
- More than 50% patients of RF with carditis will develop chronic valvular disease after 10–20 years. All the cardiac valves may be involved, but most commonly the mitral valve is affected (90%). Also aortic valve may be involved. Involvement of the tricuspid and pulmonary valves is rare (5%).
- In chronic rheumatic heart disease, there may not be any history of rhematic fever in 50%–60% cases.
- Arthritis is rheumatic fever that recovers completely without any residual change (rheumatic fever licks the joints, kills the heart).

CONGENITAL HEART DISEASES

Types

Cyanotic

- Tetralogy of Fallot.
- Transposition of great vessels.
- Truncus arteriosus.
- Pulmonary atresia.
- Tricuspid atresia.
- Ebstein's anomaly.

Acyanotic

- Left to right shunt—ASD, VSD, PDA.
- Obstructive lesion—coarctation of aorta, aortic stenosis, pulmonary stenosis.
- Abnormal position of heart—dextrocardia.

Ventricular Septal Defect (VSD)

Causes

- Commonly congenital (most common congenital heart disease).
- Acquired—rupture of interventricular septum after acute myocardial infarction, rarely trauma.

Site of VSD

Common in perimembranous part of intraventricular septum (in 90% cases).

Types

Vary with the size of VSD—3 types according to the size.
- Small (maladie de Roger)—It is asymptomatic, closes spontaneously. The systolic murmur is loud and prolonged.
- Moderate—Patient presents with fatigue and dyspnoea.
- Large—The murmur is soft.

Clinical Features

Symptoms
- May be asymptomatic.
- Breathlessness, palpitation, fatigue, weakness.

Signs

In Precordium

Inspection: Visible cardiac impulse in left parasternal area.
Palpation: Systolic thrill—in left parasternal area (4th or 5th intercostal space).
Auscultation: Pansystolic murmur in left parasternal area in 4th or 5th intercostal space.

NB: When there is reversal of shunt (called Eisenmenger's syndrome), features of pulmonary hypertension will be present (see later).

Complications

- Infective endocarditis (more common in small VSD).
- Pulmonary hypertension with reversal of shunt (Eisenmenger's syndrome).
- Heart failure.

Investigations

- ECG.
- X-ray chest shows cardiomegaly.
- Echocardiography, preferably colour Doppler.
- Cardiac catheterisation.
- CMR (cardiac magnetic resonance angiography) may be helpful.

Treatment

1. Small VSD—Surgery is not needed, only follow-up. Prophylactic penicillin for SBE may be given.
2. Moderate to large VSD—Surgical correction.
3. When Eisenmenger's syndrome develops—Surgery is contraindicated, as it aggravates right-sided heart failure. Then, following treatments are given:
   - Diuretic.
   - Digoxin in some cases.
   - Venesection, especially if there is polycythaemia.
   - Heart lung transplantation may be done.

ATRIAL SEPTAL DEFECT (ASD)

Common in females M:F = 1:2.

Types: 2 Types

1. Ostium primum (15% cases)—results from atrioventricular defect in septum.
2. Ostium secundum (75% cases)—defect mainly at the fossa ovalis in the atrial mid septum.

Clinical Features

Symptoms

- May be asymptomatic.
- Breathlessness on exertion.
- Palpitation, weakness.

Signs

In precordium
Auscultation

- First heart sound is normal.
- Wide and fixed splitting of 2nd heart sound.
- An ejection systolic murmur in left 2nd and 3rd intercostal space.
- There is also a high-pitched MDM in tricuspid area.

NB: When there is reversal of shunt, features of Eisenmenger's syndrome will be found.

Investigations

- X ray chest—shows cardiomegaly.
- ECG.
- 2D echocardiography and colour Doppler.
- Cardiac catheterisation in some cases.
- MRI (or CMR) may be helpful.

ECG finding in ASD

- In primum type—RBBB with left-axis deviation.
- In secundum type—RBBB with right-axis deviation.

Complications of ASD

- Pulmonary hypertension with reversal of shunt (Eisenmenger's syndrome).
- Arrhythmia—atrial fibrillation (most common).
- Embolism (pulmonary and systemic) and brain abscess.

Treatment

- Small ASD—Surgery is not needed, only follow-up.
- Moderate to large—Surgical closure.
- Angiographic closure is possible with transcatheter clamshell device.
- If Eisenmenger's syndrome develops—surgical closer is contraindicated (see in Eisenmenger's syndrome).

PATENT DUCTUS ARTERIOSUS (PDA)

Causes

Common in females M:F = 1:3. Probable etiological factors are:
- Maternal rubella in the first trimester.
- Birth at high-altitude.
- Prematurity.

Mechanism

During foetal life, ductus arteriosus connects pulmonary artery at its bifurcation to the descending aorta just below the origin of left subclavian artery and permits blood flow from pulmonary artery to aorta. After birth, within hours or days, it closes spontaneously and remains as ligamentum arteriosum.

In PDA, it allows blood to flow from aorta to pulmonary artery. Up to 50% of left ventricular output may enter into pulmonary artery, because pressure in aorta is higher.

Clinical Features

Symptoms

- May be asymptomatic.
- Breathlessness on exertion.
- Palpitation, weakness and loss of appetite.

Signs

- Pulse—may be high volume.
- BP—wide pulse pressure.
- JVP—normal

In Precordium

Palpation
- Apex beat—thrusting or heaving in nature.
- Systolic thrill—present in pulmonary area.

Auscultation
- Continuous murmur in left 2nd and 3rd intercostal space, called machinery murmur like 'train in a tunnel.'

Complications

- Pulmonary hypertension with reversal of shunt (Eisenmenger's syndrome).
- CCF.
- Infective endocarditis.
- Arrhythmia (atrial fibrillation).
- Duct may rupture or calcify.

Investigations

- ECG.
- X-ray chest shows cardiomegaly.
- 2D and colour Doppler echocardiography.
- MRI or CMR .
- Cardiac catheterisation.

Treatment

- Majority of PDA are small and can be closed at cardiac catheterisation by using implantable occlusive device.
- In large PDA—surgical closure
- Prophylaxis for infective endocarditis.
- In neonate (1–3 weeks old), indomethacin (0.2 mg/kg IV) or ibuprofen may be given to constrict and close PDA by inhibiting prostaglandin E synthesis. It is not helpful in older children.
- If Eisenmenger's syndrome develops, surgery is contraindicated (see Eisenmenger's syndrome).

EISENMENGER'S SYNDROME

Definition

Pulmonary hypertension with reversal of shunt is called Eisenmenger's syndrome.

Causes

VSD, ASD, PDA.
In these cases, persistently raised pulmonary flow (due to left to right shunt) causes increased pulmonary resistance followed by pulmonary hypertension. This increases the pressure in right ventricle leading to reversal of shunt (from right to left side).

Clinical Features

Symptoms

- Dyspnoea.
- Fatigue.
- Syncope.
- Angina.
- Haemoptysis.
- Features of CCF.

Signs

- Central cyanosis. But in PDA, differential cyanosis occurs (cyanosis in toes, not in the hands).
- Clubbing. But in PDA, differential clubbing occurs (clubbing in toes, not in the hands).
- Pulse—low volume.
- Prominent **'a'** wave in JVP.
- Other signs of pulmonary hypertension—palpable P2, left parasternal lift, epigastric pulsation.
- TR may occur.
- Original murmur of VSD, ASD or PDA—decrease in intensity, may disappear.

Treatment

- Diuretic.
- Digoxin may be given in some cases.
- Venesection may be required, especially if there is polycythaemia.
- Heart lung transplantation may be done.
- Surgery is contraindicated in Eisenmenger's syndrome, as it aggravates right-sided heart failure.

Causes of Death

- Right heart failure.
- Infective endocarditis.
- Pulmonary infarction.
- Cerebral thrombosis or abscess.
- Arrhythmia.

TETRALOGY OF FALLOT (TOF)

Definition

It is a cyanotic congenital heart disease consisting of the following:
1. Pulmonary stenosis (right ventricular outflow tract obstruction).
2. Overriding and dextroposition of aorta (aortic origin—two-thirds from left ventricle and one-third from right ventricle).
3. Right ventricular hypertrophy.
4. Ventricular septal defect (VSD).

Clinical Features

Symptoms

- Breathlessness.
- Bluish discolouration of lips and fingers during exertion.
- Weakness, cough, chest pain, palpitation.
- Young child usually presents with cyanotic spell (Fallot's spell) during exertion, feeding or crying. The child becomes apnoeic and unconscious. Squatting relieves cyanosis.
- Growth retardation.
- Syncope, seizure, cerebrovascular events or even sudden death.

Signs

- Short stature.
- Cyanosis (both central and peripheral).
- Generalized clubbing involve fingers and toes.
- Pulse—low volume.
- BP—low.
- JVP—prominent 'a' wave (due to RVH).

Precordium

Inspection
- Visible cardiac impulse in the apical and epigastric region.

Palpation
- Left parasternal lift and epigastric pulsation (due to RVH).
- Systolic thrill—present in the pulmonary area.

Auscultation
- 1st heart sound—normal in all the areas.
- 2nd heart sound—P2 is soft (or absent) in pulmonary area, A2 is normal.
- Ejection systolic murmur in pulmonary area, which radiates to the neck, more on inspiration.

Cardinal Features of TOF

- Child with growth retardation.
- Generalised clubbing and cyanosis.
- Pulmonary ejection systolic murmur.
- History of cyanotic spells during exercise (relieved by squatting).

Investigations

- CBC, ESR—polycythemia, ESR may be low.
- Chest X-ray—boot-shaped heart.
- Echocardiogram—2D and colour Doppler.
- ECG—RVH.
- Cardiac catheterisation.

Complications

- Infective endocarditis (common).
- Paradoxical emboli.
- Cerebral abscess (10% cases).
- Polycythaemia (due to hypoxaemia, and may lead to cerebrovascular accident and myocardial infarction).
- Coagulation abnormality.

Pentalogy of Fallot—When TOF is associated with ASD.

Triology of Fallot—ASD with PS with RVH.

Acyanotic Fallot—When the TOF is associated with infundibular pulmonary stenosis. Outflow obstruction is mild and there is no cyanosis.

Treatment

- Total surgical correction is the definitive treatment, ideally should be done prior to the age of 5.
- If pulmonary artery is hypoplastic or anatomy is unfavourable, then temporarily palliative surgery called Blalock-Taussig shunt is performed. Corrective surgery is done later on.
- Prophylactic antibiotic to prevent infective endocarditis.
- Treatment of cyanotic spell (see below)

Blalock Taussig Shunt

It is the anastomosis between left subclavian artery with left pulmonary artery. This improves pulmonary blood flow and pulmonary artery development and may facilitate definitive surgery later on.

Treatment during cyanotic spell

- Knee-chest position of child.
- High concentration of O_2.
- Morphine or diamorphine injection (it relaxes right ventricular outflow obstruction).
- Beta-blocker may be used.
- If medical therapy fails, emergency surgical shunt may be considered.

Prognosis of TOF

Prognosis is good after surgery, especially if operation is done in childhood. Restenosis, recurrence of septal defect and rhythm disorder may occur after surgery. So, regular follow-up is required in every case.

COARCTATION OF AORTA

Definition

Coarctation of aorta (COA) is the narrowing of the aorta.

Types: 2 Types

1. Postductal (adult type): Below the origin of left subclavian artery, where ductus arteriosus joins the aorta.
2. Preductal (infantile type, 2%): Above the origin of left subclavian artery.

Causes

- Congenital (most common).
- Rarely, may be acquired in trauma, Takayasu's disease.

Clinical Features

Symptoms

- More common in male.
- May be asymptomatic.
- Headache, nose bleeding, claudication of lower limbs and cold legs (due to poor blood flow in lower limbs).

Signs

- BP—High in the upper limb and low in the lower limb.
- Pulse—Normal in upper limb, feeble in lower limb and radiofemoral delay.

Precordium

Inspection
- Visible cardiac impulse.
- Visible dilated tortuous artery around the scapula, anterior axilla and over the left sternal border (due to collateral vessels).

Palpation
- Heaving Apex beat.
- There may be thrill over the collateral vessels.

Auscultation
- Both first and second heart sounds—normal.
- Murmur—systolic murmur audible close to the sternum and better heard in 4th intercostal space posteriorly (site of coarctation).

Investigations

1. X-ray of chest P/A view—
   - Heart is enlarged.
   - Rib notching.
   - Figure of '**3**' (constriction at coarctation, prestenotic and poststenotic dilatation).

2. ECG (LVH).
3. Echocardiogram.
4. CT scan and CMR.

Reverse Coarctation

When pulse is absent in upper limb, but present in lower limb, it is called reverse coarctation. It occurs in Takayasu's disease.

Complications of COA

- Hypertension and its complication (LVF, CVA).
- Infective endocarditis.
- Rupture at the coarctation site.
- Dissecting aneurysm.
- Aneurysm of aorta.
- Subarachnoid haemorrhage (rupture of Berry aneurysm of circle of Willis).

Causes of Death

- Acute LVF.
- Dissecting aneurysm of aorta.
- Subarachnoid haemorrhage.
- Cerebral haemorrhage.

Treatment of COA

It should be treated surgically as early as possible, preferably before the age of 5.

- Surgical resection and end to end anastomosis is usually done.
- If coarctation is extensive—prosthetic vascular graft may be done.
- If surgery is done in early childhood, hypertension usually resolves completely but if done in adolescence or adulthood, hypertension may persist in 70% cases, because of irreversible changes in arterioles or renal damage.
- Balloon angioplasty may be helpful. It is particularly effective after restenosis.

Prognosis after Surgery

- Surgical correction in childhood—25-year survival is 83%. But if delayed until adulthood, 25-year survival rate drops to 75%. Without surgery, only 25% live up to 50 years of age, while cardiac failure occurs in two-thirds of surviving patients over 40.
- In few cases, there is restenosis as the child grows. This can be treated by balloon angioplasty.
- If operation is delayed, patient may have persistent hypertension because of irreversible changes in the arterioles.
- May develop paradoxical hypertension, due to baroreceptor-induced increased sympathetic activity (detected by increased serum and urinary catecholamines).
- Coexistent bicuspid aortic valve is present in 50% cases, may lead to progressive aortic stenosis or regurgitation.

ISCHAEMIC HEART DISEASE

Ischaemic heart disease (IHD) results from reduced coronary blood flow to the myocardium, when there is an imbalance between the supply of oxygen and myocardial demand. IHD includes angina pectoris and myocardial infarction.

Causes of IHD

Coronary blood flow to the myocardium may be reduced by obstruction due to the following:
- Atherosclerosis—most common.
- Thrombosis.
- Spasm.
- Embolus.
- Coronary ostial stenosis.
- Coronary arteritis (e.g. in SLE).

Common Presentations of IHD

- Angina pectoris.
- Acute myocardial infarction.
- Arrythmia.
- Heart failure.
- Sudden death.

Risk Factors for Coronary Artery Disease

Following factors are responsible for atherosclerosis:

Nonmodifiable

- Age—Common in elderly.
- Sex—Common in male. After menopause in female, incidence is same.
- Family history—More common, if there is a family history of IHD.
- Genetic factors—A number of genetic factors have been linked with coronary artery disease.

Modifiable

- Smoking—IHD is more in smokers.
- Alcohol—Moderate alcohol consumption is associated with a reduced risk but high-intake increases the risk.
- Diet—High fats are associated with IHD. Diet low in fresh fruits, vegetables and polyunsaturated fatty acids are associated with increased risk.
- Obesity—Overweight have an increased risk.
- Exercise—More in sedentary workers.
- Hypertension.
- Diabetes mellitus.
- Hyperlipidaemia—High-serum cholesterol, triglyceride and low high-density lipoproteins (HDL), is associated with coronary atheroma.
- Psychosocial factors—stress, lack of social support, depression, anxiety.

Angina Pectoris

Definition

It is defined as paroxysomal precordial pain of short-duration due to transient myocardial ischaemia.

Symptoms

Main symptom is pain which has the following characters—
- Site—central, retrosternal chest.
- Character—stabbing or squeezing or constricting.
- Radiation—lower jaw, neck, inner-side of the left arm up to the finger.
- Precipitated by exertion, eating or emotion (3 E).
- Relieved by rest and nitroglycerine.
- Duration—5–10 minutes (<1/2 hour).

Signs

Usually no definitive physical sign.

Types of Angina Pectoris

- Stable angina or classical angina see as above).
- Unstable angina—It is characterized by angina of new onset or rapidly worsening angina, angina at rest or minimal activity. It is more severe, lasting for longer duration, occurs more frequently, not improved by rest or nitroglycerine. It is due to rupture, fissuring or ulceration of an atherosclerotic plaque or thrombus. ECG shows transient ST, T changes (depression) but enzymes are normal. May cause MI in 10–20% cases.
- Prinzmetal's angina—It occurs at rest without any provocating factor, usually in the early morning. More common in female. It occurs due to coronary artery spasm. ECG shows ST-elevation rather than depression during pain.
- Decubitus angina—It occurs when patient lies down due to impaired left ventricular function.

Investigations

1. ECG is often normal. During attack—ST-depression, T-inversion.
2. Chest X-ray.
3. Echocardiography.
4. ETT.
5. Coronary arteriography.
6. Other stress testing—
   - Myocardial perfusion scan.
   - Stress echocardiography
   - Transthoracic echocardiography.
7. For risk factor—Fasting lipid profile and blood sugar.

Tretament

During acute attack—
- Sublingual glyceryl trinitrate (GTN) administered from a metered-dose aerosol or as tablet allowed to dissolve under the tongue and retained in the mouth will usually relieve an attack of angina in 2–3 minutes.

- If no response, it can be repeated. But if still no response, myocardial infarction should be excluded.

Prevention of further attack—

1. Antiplatelet therapy—low-dose (75–150 mg) aspirin, clopidogrel (75 mg daily).
2. Antianginal drugs—
   - To prevent angina pain—oral nitrates, such as isosorbide dinitrate (10–20 mg 8 hourly), isosorbide mononitrate (20–60 mg once or twice a day) can be given by mouth.
   - Other drugs—Beta-blocker (atenolol, metoprolol, bisoprolol). Calcium antagonists (nifedipine, nicardipine, verapamil and diltiazem), potassium channel activators like nicorandil may be used.
   - If recurrent or persistent pain, coronary angiogram should be done. If coronary artery blockage, then stenting or percutaneous transluminal coronary angioplasty (PTCA) or coronary artery bypass surgery (CABG) may be required.
3. Risk factors should be controlled:
   - Smoking must be stopped.
   - Reduction of weight, if obese.
   - Regular exercise, at least for 30 minutes daily.
   - Avoid alcohol intake.
   - Control of hypertension and diabetes mellitus.
   - Lipid lowering drugs—atorvastatin, rosuvastatin.
   - Avoidance of anxiety, tension, and depression.
   - Lifestyle modification.

Treatment of Unstable Angina

- Hospitalisation.
- Complete bed rest, oxygen.
- Sedation, if needed.
- Aspirin or clopidogrel.
- Nitroglycerine.
- Beta-blocker.
- Calcium channel blocker.
- Heparin—LMW heparin (enoxaparin S/C) for 5–7 days.
- If pain persists, nitroglycerine infusion.
- If all measures fail, urgent coronary angiography and revuscularisation, if necessary.

Myocardial Infarction

Definition

Myocardial infarction (MI) It is defined as myocardial necrosis which occurs as a result of critical imbalance between coronary blood flow and myocardial demand due to occlusion of coronary artery by thrombus.

Types of MI

- Q-wave (Transmural) or ST-elevated MI.
- Non-Q-wave or non-ST-elevated (NSTEMI) or subendocardial MI.

Clinical Features

Symptoms

- Central chest pain which is severe, stabbing or squeezing or constricting, radiates to the lower jaw, neck, inner-side of the left arm up to the finger, not relieved by rest and nitroglycerine, persist more than 30 minutes.
- Sweating.
- Fear of impending death.
- Nausea and vomiting (more in inferior MI).
- Breathlessness.
- Collapse or cardiogenic shock.

Signs

- The patient is restless with pallor, sweating, tachycardia (bradycardia in inferior MI).
- Hypotension, oliguria, cold peripheries.
- Signs of complications, e.g. cardiogenic shock, acute left ventricular failure, arrhythmia, mitral regurgitation, pericarditis.

Investigations

1. ECG shows—
   - ST-elevation (with upward convexity).
   - Pathological Q-wave.
   - T-inversion.
2. Enzymatic changes in acute MI—
   - Troponin I—rise in 2–4 hours, may persist up to 7 days.
   - CPK—rise in 4–6 hours, peak in 12 hours, returns to normal within 48–72 hours. CK-MB is cardiac specific.
   - SGOT—increases after 12 hours, peak in 24 hours, returns to normal in 3–4 days.
   - LDH—rises after 12 hours, peak in 3–4 days, normal after 7–10 days.
3. Others—Chest X-ray, echocardiography may be done.

Sites of MI

- Inferior myocardial infarction.
- Anterior myocardial infarction.
- Anteroseptal myocardial infarction.
- Lateral myocardial infarction.
- Posterior (true) myocardial infarction.
- Subendocardial myocardial infarction.

Complications of MI

May be early and late:

1. Early complications—
   - Arrhythmia—Ventricular ectopics (more common), ventricular fibrillation, ventricular tachycardia, sinus bradycardia (common in inferior MI), sinus tachycardia, atrial fibrillation, heart block.

- Cardiogenic shock.
- Cardiac failure (LVF, biventricular failure).
- Acute pericarditis (common in 2nd or 3rd day).
- Thromboembolism (systemic and pulmonary).
- Rupture of papillary muscle or chordae tendineae resulting in MR.
- Rupture of interventricular septum causing VSD.
- Rupture of the ventricular wall.

2. Late complications—
   - Ventricular aneurysm (10%).
   - Postmyocardial infarction syndrome (Dressler's syndrome).
   - Frozen shoulder.
   - Postinfarct angina (may occur in up to 50% of patients).

Treatment of Acute Myocardial Infarction

- Admission in CCU.
- Complete bed rest.
- High-flow O_2 inhalation (60%)—2–4 L/min by nasal cannula.
- To relieve pain—Inject morphine (5–10 mg) or diamorphine (2.5–5 mg) plus antiemetic (cyclizine or metoclopramide) IV. May be repeated, if necessary.
- Chewable aspirin—300 mg and clopidogrel 300 mg.
- Primary PCI, if available—treatment of choice. Should be performed as early as possible.
- Or thrombolytic therapy—streptokinase, if no contraindication.
- Other therapy—β-blocker (if no contraindication)—IV bolus atenolol 5–10 mg or metoprolol 5–15 mg slowly over 5 minutes. Oral atenolol 25–50 mg BD, or bisoprolol 5 mg daily or metoprolol 25–50 mg BD or TDS may be given.
- Sublingual nitroglycerin—0.3–1 mg.
- Anticoagulants—Heparin 5000 IU IV bolus, then 0.25 U/Kg/hour. Or low molecular weight heparin (S/C enoxaparin 1 mg/kg body weight 12 hourly.
- ACE inhibitor.

Criteria of thrombolytic therapy

- Typical history of chest pain.
- ECG change—ST-elevation > 1 mm in limb leads or 2 mm in chest leads (in 2 or more contiguous leads) or new left bundle branch block.
- High cardiac enzyme.

Streptokinase

It is a protein synthesized by Streptococcus, produced by recombinant DNA technology, used as thrombolytic. It is more effective, if started particularly within 6 hours (greatest benefit within first 2 hours), may be given in 6–12 hours, unlikely to be beneficial after 12 hours. Reperfusion occurs in 50–70% of cases. Dose -1.5 million units in 100 cc normal saline given IV for 1 hour. Toxicity—allergic reaction, hypotension, bleeding (major hazard).

Other thrombolytic drugs are—alteplase, reteplase, tenecteplase. Thrombolytic therapy is not effective in non-ST elevated MI (NSTEMI).

Contraindications of thrombolytic therapy

1. Absolute contraindications—
   - Haemorrhagic stroke or stroke of unknown origin at any time.
   - Ischemic stroke in preceding 6 months.
   - Central nervous system damage or neoplasm.
   - Recent major trauma, surgery, head injury (within preceding 3 weeks).
   - Gastrointestinal bleeding in the last month.
   - Coagulation or bleeding abnormalities.
   - Dissecting aortic aneurysm.
   - Diabetic retinopathy (proliferative).
2. Relative contraindications—
   - Transient ischemic attack in the preceding 6 months.
   - Oral anticoagulant therapy.
   - Heavy vaginal bleeding, pregnancy or puerperal bleeding or within 1-week of postpartum.
   - Severe hypertension (malignant hypertension, systolic > 180 and diastolic > 120).
   - High probability of active peptic ulcer.
   - Advanced liver disease.
   - Infective endocarditis.

Follow-up after an acute myocardial infarction:

1. Patient should be reviewed after 6 to 8 weeks.
2. Risk factors should be reviewed and modified accordingly—
   - Lifestyle modification (avoid stress, heavy work).
   - Smoking should be stopped.
   - Regular exercise.
   - Diet—avoid fatty, oily food.
   - Weight control, if obese.
   - Good control of hypertension and diabetes mellitus.
   - Antiplatelet (aspirin or clopidogrel) should be continued indefinitely.
   - Beta-blocker.
   - ACE inhibitor should be continued indefinitely in patient with persistent LV dysfunction (EF <40%)
   - Lipid lowering agents.
   - Rehabilitation.

Secondary Prevention (after the attack)

- Antiplatelet therapy (aspirin and/or clopidogrel).
- β-blocker.
- ACE inhibitor.
- Statin.
- Control of diabetes and hypertension.

Post Myocardial Infarction Syndrome (Dressler's Syndrome)

It is a late complication of myocardial infarction that occurs usually after few weeks or even months (2–10 weeks) after acute MI. It is characterized by (5P's):

- Pain (chest pain).
- Pyrexia.

- Pleurisy.
- Pericarditis (or pericardial effusion).
- Pneumonitis (or pulmonary infiltrate).

Treatment

- High-dose aspirin (600–900 mg) every 4–6 hours or other NSAID.
- In severe or in recurrent case—corticosteroid may be given.
- Anticoagulant should be discontinued (unless strong evidence for high-risk of thromboembolism).

Ventricular Aneurysm

If in ECG, ST remains elevated after a few months of acute myocardial infarction, the diagnosis is ventricular aneurysm.

X-ray chest—enlarged heart, with a bulged or rounded protrusion from the left ventricular wall, calcification may occur at the wall of aneurysm. Confirmed by echocardiogram.

Complications of ventricular aneurysm

- Heart failure.
- Arrhythmia (ectopic, atrial fibrillation, occasionally serious ventricular arrhythmia, etc.).
- Systemic embolism from mural thrombus.

Treatment of ventricular aneurysm

1. Symptomatic treatment:
   - If heart failure—diuretic, ACE inhibitor, digoxin.
   - If arrhythmia—antiarrhythmic drugs.
   - Aspirin in low dose.
   - Treatment for embolism (anticoagulant, aspirin).
2. If difficult to control, surgery is indicated.

ACUTE PERICARDITIS

Definition

It is the acute inflammation of pericardium.

Causes

- Viral (coxsackie B, echovirus)—common cause.
- Acute rheumatic fever.
- After acute myocardial infarction (in 2nd or 3rd day).
- Bacterial (*Staph. aureus, H. influenzae*).
- Tuberculous pericarditis.
- Fungal (histoplasmosis, coccidioidomycosis).
- Acute renal failure.
- Malignancy (from carcinoma of bronchus, breast, lymphoma, leukemia).
- Trauma.
- Radiation
- Drugs (doxorubicin, cyclophosphamide).
- Collagen disease (SLE, scleroderma).

Clinical Features

Symptoms

- Main symptom is chest pain which is retrosternal, sharp or stabbing in nature, may radiate to the shoulder and neck.
- Aggravated by movement, lying down and deep breathing, exercise and swallowing.
- Pain may be relieved by sitting or bending forward.
- Other symptoms—according to cause (e.g. low grade evening rise of temperature, night sweat weight loss in TB).

Signs

Pericardial rub—

- It is a high-pitched, harsh, scratching, grating, leathery sound, to and fro in quality.
- Better heard over the left lower parasternal area with the patient leaning forward.
- Augmented by pressing the stethoscope.
- Usually heard in systole, but may be in diastole.
- Present after holding the breath (to differentiate from pleural rub).

Investigations

- ECG—ST-elevated with upward concavity (chair-shaped or saddle-shaped).
- CXR PA view.
- Echocardiography.
- CT and cardiac MRI may be done in some cases.
- Others—according to suspicion of cause.

Treatment

- To relieve pain—NSAIDs (indomethacin or ibuprofen).
- In severe or recurrent pain—corticosteroid.
- If no response to steroid—azathioprine or colchicine may be added.
- If recurrence with no response to medical treatment—pericardiotomy may be done.
- Treatment of primary cause—antibiotic, if bacterial infection. Anti-Koch's, if tuberculosis is suspected.

PERICARDIAL EFFUSION

Definition

Accumulation of fluid in the space between parietal and visceral pericardium.

Causes

- After acute pericarditis (bacterial, viral).
- Tuberculosis (most common).
- Collagen diseases (SLE, rheumatoid arthritis)
- Myxoedema.
- Lymphoma.
- Neoplasm (secondary from carcinoma of breast, bronchial carcinoma).
- Renal failure and dialysis.
- After radiotherapy.

Clinical Features

Symptoms

- Heaviness in chest or breathlessness.
- Palpitation.
- Symptoms of primary cause.

Signs

1. Pulse—low volume, tachycardia, there may be pulsus paradoxus (indicating cardiac tamponade).
2. JVP—raised, Kussmaul's sign positive (rise of JVP during inspiration. Normally, JVP falls during inspiration).
3. Blood pressure—low systolic, normal diastolic and narrow pulse pressure.
4. Precordium—
   - Area of cardiac dullness is increased (on percussion).
   - Apex beat is difficult to palpate. If palpable, it is within the area of cardiac dullness.
   - Heart sounds are muffled or distant.
   - Bronchial sound at the left inferior angle of scapula (Ewart's sign).
5. Liver is enlarged and tender.

Investigations

1. Chest X-ray—heart is enlarged, globular, pear-or pitcher- shaped with clear margin. Lung fields are oligaemic.
2. CBC (ESR high in tuberculosis, SLE, RA).
3. ECG (low-voltage tracing, tachycardia).
4. Echocardiogram (shows echo-free zone).
5. Paracentesis—see the colour, analysis of the pericardial fluid (Gram staining, AFB staining, C/S, viral study, cytology, biochemistry).
6. Magnetic resonance imaging (MRI) is very helpful.
7. Other investigations according to the suspicion of causes—
   - TB (MT, sputum for AFB).

- Collagen disease (RA test, ANA, Anti-ds-DNA).
- Hypothyroidism (FT3, FT4, TSH).

Confirmation of Diagnosis

By echocardiogram (shows the echo-free zone). Paracentesis is definitive.

Treatment

According to cause—

- If tuberculosis, antituberculosis drug plus prednisolone is given.
- If bacterial cause is suspected—broad spectrum antibiotic.
- Other treatment of primary cause (e.g. hypothyroidism, SLE, RA, lymphoma).
- Paracentesis, if cardiac temponade develops.

Cardiac Tamponade

It is a state of compression of heart in rapidly developing pericardial effusion. It interferes with the diastolic filling of heart and the patient develops features of shock.

Causes

- Trauma or cardiac surgery (causing haemopericardium).
- Malignancy (repeated effusion may occur).
- Myocardial rupture.
- Dissecting aortic aneurysm.
- Any cause of pericardial effusion can cause.

Symptoms

- Heaviness and compression in chest.
- Dyspnoea.
- Features of shock.

Signs

See above in pericardial effusion.

Treatment

- Immediate pericardiocentesis.
- Treatment of primary cause.

Pericardiocentesis

It is the aspiration of pericardial fluid. Done under ultrasonographic or echocardiographic guidance. Aspiration needle is introduced through left costoxiphoid junction, directed upwards, backwards and towards the left shoulder.

Complications

- Injury to the coronary artery and ventricles.
- Arrhythmia.
- Bleeding.

CHRONIC CONSTRICTIVE PERICARDITIS

Definition

It is a disease characterised by progressive thickening, fibrosis and calcification of pericardium. Commonly, involves right side of the heart.

Causes

- Infection—TB and coxsackie B infection.
- Haemopericardium (which may be due to trauma, myocardial rupture after infarction and dissecting aneurysm).
- Collagen disease (rheumatoid arthritis).
- Cardiac operation.
- Mediastinal irradiation.
- Fungal infection (histoplasmosis).
- Rarely, after acute purulent pericarditis.
- Idiopathic.

Clinical Features

Most features are due to systemic venous congestion.

Symptoms

- Cough, breathlessness on exertion, may be orthopnoea, paroxysmal nocturnal dyspnoea.
- Weakness, dizziness, giddiness, anorexia, nausea, and vomiting.
- Abdominal swelling, later ankle swelling.

Signs

- Tachycardia, low volume pulse. Pulsus paradoxus may be present.
- JVP—raised, fall of Y descent (Friedrich sign). Kussmaul sign positive (raised JVP on inspiration).
- Pericardial knock (a third heart sound due to rapid ventricular filling).
- Enlarged tender liver.
- Ascites.
- Peripheral oedema later on.

NB: Calcification commonly involves right side of the heart and can be seen by fluoroscopy. Calcification does not always means constriction. RF does not causes chronic constrictive pericarditis.

Complications

- Atrial fibrillation (in 30% cases).
- Ascites.
- Myocardial fibrosis.

Investigations

- Chest X-ray (PA and lateral view)—Relatively small heart, pericardial calcification in 50% cases.

- ECG—low-voltage tracing, tachycardia, and T inversion.
- Echocardiogram.
- CT scan or CMR.
- Cardiac catheterisation shows that diastolic pressure is equal in all chambers (left and right ventricles), end- diastolic pressure (EDP) is equal in left and right atrium.
- Other investigations according to suspicion of cause (e.g. MT, RA, ANA, etc.).
- Endomyocardial biopsy—may be necessary to differentiate from restrictive cardiomyopathy in difficult cases.

Treatment

- Surgery—Complete resection of pericardium (helpful in 50% cases).
- Treatment of primary cause should be done.
- After surgery, persistent constriction and myocardial fibrosis may be present. AF may occur after full recovery (Table 4).

Table 4
Difference between CCF and chronic constrictive pericarditis

Features	CCF	Chronic constrictive pericarditis
1. Breathlessness	Common, more on exertion	Not common in rest, marked only on exertion
2. Pulsus paradoxus	No	May be present
3. JVP	Raised, but no Kussmaul sign	Raised, Kussmaul sign positive, may be Y descent
4. Cardiomegaly	Present	Absent
5. Oedema	Early feature than ascites	Ascites early, oedema late feature
6. On auscultation	Murmur may be present	Pericardial knock is present

MYOCARDITIS

Definition

It is the inflammation of the myocardium of heart.

Causes

1. Infection:
   - Viral—Coxsackie A and B, influenza A and B.
   - Bacterial—Streptococcus, Pneumococcus, *Borrelia burgdorferi* (Lyme disease).
   - Protozoal—Trypanosoma cruzi (Chaga's disease).
   - Fungal—candida, actinomyces.
2. Rheumatic fever.
3. Diphtheric myocarditis.
4. Drugs and toxins—doxorubicin, lithium, cocaine, penicillin, sulphonamide.
5. Radiation.
6. Autoimmune—SLE, Rheumatoid arthritis.
7. Unknown cause.

Symptoms

- May be asymptomatic.
- Plapitation, breathlessness, chest pain.
- Features of cardiac failure.
- Features of primary disease, if any.

Signs

- Pulse—low volume, tachycardia.
- Apex beat may be displaced downwards and outwards due to cardiomegaly.
- First and second heart sounds may be soft.
- S3/S4 may be present.
- Mitral regurgitation may be present.
- Features of heart failure.
- Arrhythmia may be present.

Investigations

- Chest X-ray.
- ECG—nonspecific ST and T wave changes.
- Echocardiography—low ejection fraction and global hypokinesia.
- MRI.
- Endomyocardial biopsy may be needed for confirmation.

Treatment

- Complete bed rest.
- Low salt diet.
- Diuretics therapy.
- ACE inhibitors may be helpful.
- Treatment of arrhythmia.
- Treatment of primary cause, if any.

ENDOCARDITIS

Definition

It is the infection of the endocardium, mainly the lining of chamber or heart valve or congenital anomaly.

It usually occurs at the site of pre-existing heart disease or septal defect. Infection with virulent organism may cause acute endocarditis in normal heart (e.g. *Staphylococcus aureus*).

Acute Endocarditis

Causes

Usually by highly virulent and invasive organism, e.g. *S. aureus, Streptococcus, Pneumococcus*. It can affect damaged as well as normal heart. Vegetations are usually very large and valve destruction is more than in subacute endocarditis.

Clinical Features

Symptoms

- Fever, usually very high with chill and rigor.
- Headache, bodyache, malaise, weakness.
- Chest pain, breathlessness.

Signs

- Patient looks toxic with very high-temperature.
- Prominent and changing heart murmur.
- Stigmata of subacute or chronic endocarditis are usually absent.

Subacute Bacterial Endocarditis (SBE)

Usually caused by organisms of low-virulence, affecting rheumatic or congenitally abnormal valves.

Predisposing Factors or Causes of SBE

- Rheumatic valve lesion (e.g. AR, MR).
- Congenital heart disease (VSD, PDA, bicuspid aortic valve, coarctation of aorta, TOF).
- Prosthetic valve.
- Dental extraction.
- Instrumentation (IV canula, CV line, cardiac catheterization).
- Cardiac surgery.
- IV drug abuse (right sided endocarditis is more common, especially tricuspid valve).

Organisms Causing Infective Endocarditis

1. Subacute bacterial endocarditis—
   - *Strep. viridans*—most common (35–50%).
   - *Enterococcus faecalis, Enterococcus faecium.*
   - *S. bovis* (associated with large bowel carcinoma), *S. milleri* and other streptococci.
   - *Staphylococcus aureus* or epidermidis.
   - HACEK organisms (*Haemophilus, Actinobacillus, Cardiobacterium hominis, Eikenella, Kingella*).

2. Acute bacterial endocarditis—
   - *S. aureus* (most common).
   - Others—*Pseudomonas, Candida, Streptococcus pneumonae, Neisseria gonorrhoea.*
3. Postoperative endocarditis—
   - *Staphylococcus albus.*
   - *Candida.*
   - *Aspergillus.*
   - All other organisms causing subacute and acute endocarditis.

Clinical Features

Symptoms

- Fever, usually low-grade continuous which is persistent and does not respond to usual antibiotics.
- Chest pain and palpitation.
- Difficulty in breathing .
- Anorexia, weight loss, malaise, weakness, night sweat, arthralgia.
- Symptoms of embolism according to involvement like brain (CVD), kidney (renal infarction), lung (pulmonary infarction).

Signs

General Examination—

1. Appearance—Ill looking, emaciated and toxic, anaemia.
2. In hands—
   - Clubbing involving all the fingers and toes.
   - Osler's node (small painful violaceous raised nodule, present on the tip of the fingers).
   - Janeway lesion (large painless erythematous macules on the palm and sole).
   - Infarction at the tip of fingers or toes, petechiae on the dorsum or other parts.
   - Splinter haemorrage (subungual).
   - Infarction due to embolism.
3. Pulse—tachycardia.
4. BP may be low.
5. Precordium—
   - Signs of previous heart disease (AR, MR, ASD, VSD, PDA, etc.).
   - Murmur—appearance of new murmur or changing character of previous murmur.
6. Abdomen—splenomegaly may be present.
7. Fundoscopy—Roth's spot (white-centered retinal haemorrhage).

Investigations

- CBC, ESR—anaemia, neutrophilic leucocytosis, high ESR.
- CRP—high.
- Blood culture (both aerobic and anaerobic)—3 samples from different sites at 1-hour apart.
- Echocardiography—to see vegetation, valvular lesion or congenital anomaly. Transoesophageal echocardiography is more sensitive.
- Urine R/M/E (haematuria, proteinuria may be present).
- Chest X-ray shows cardiomegaly.
- ECG.
- Urea and creatinine.

Vegetation: It is a small solid mass composed of platelet, fibrin and organism, occurring at the site of endothelial damage in the valve or endocardium. It may result in embolism.

Complications of SBE

- Heart failure (LVF is a common cause of death).
- Valve destruction, regurgitation, obstruction.
- Aortic root abscess.
- Systemic embolism.
- Right-sided endocarditis involves the pulmonary valve and may cause septic pulmonary emboli, occasionally infarction and lung abscess.

Causes of Culture Negative Endocarditis

- Prior antibiotic treatment (common cause).
- Fungal, yeast, anaerobic infection or Q fever.
- Right-sided endocarditis.
- Noninfective endocarditis: **Libmann Sac's** (nonbacterial verrucous endocarditis in SLE), **marantic endocarditis** (nonbacterial thrombotic or verrucous endocarditis found in malignancy, such as bronchial carcinoma).

Treatment

Ideally antibiotic should be given according to culture and sensitivity. However, treatment should be started as soon as the blood sample is sent for culture and sensitivity.

- For viridans streptococci—Benzyl penicillin 1.2 g IV 4 hourly and gentamycin 1 mg/kg IV 8 hourly for 4 weeks or ceftriaxone 2 gm once daily IV for 4 weeks or vancomycin 15 mg/kg IV 12 hourly for 4 weeks.
- In acute case—flucloxacillin 2gm IV 6 hourly is added to cover staphylococci.
- In penicillin allergy or meticillin resistant Staph. aureus (MRSA) infection—triple therapy with vancomycin with gentamycin. Or another regimen—vancomycin 1 gm 12 hourly IV with ceftriaxone 2 g every 24 hours.
- In penicillin resistant case—Flucloxacillin plus gentamicin IV.
- In prosthetic valve endocarditis—IV penicillin 6 weeks and IV gentamicin 2 weeks should be given.
- For HACEK organisms—ceftriaxone 2 gm IV once daily for 4 weeks. If prosthetic valve is involved, then treatment should be given for 6 weeks.
- Q fever endocarditis—prolong treatment with doxycycline and rifampicin or ciprofloxacin.

Prevention during Dental Procedure

Routine antibiotic prophylaxis prior to dental procedure is no longer recommended which is not proved to be effective. However, in few high-risk cases, antibiotic prophylaxis may be considered. These are—

- Prosthetic cardiac valve.
- Previous infective endocarditis.
- Congenital heart disease.

Drugs used for prophylaxis are—

- Amoxicillin 2 gm 1 hour before procedure.
- If penicillin allergy—clindamycin 600 mg or cephalexin 2 gm or azithromycin or clarithromycin 500 mg 1 hour before procedure.
- If the patient is unable to take by mouth, parenteral therapy may be given with ampicillin 2 gm IV or IM 30 minutes before the procedure. In penicillin allergy, clindamycin 600 mg IV 1 hour before procedure or cefazolin 1 g IM or IV 30 minutes before procedure.

Indications of Cardiac Surgery

- Progressive heart failure from valve damage.
- Valvular obstruction.
- Repeated embolisation.
- Fungal endocarditis.
- Persistent bacteraemia inspite of adequate antibiotic therapy.
- Myocardial abscess.
- Endocarditis of prosthetic valve.
- Large vegetation in left-sided valve.

CARDIOMYOPATHY

Definition

Cardiomyopathies are a group of disease involving the heart muscle and not due to congenital, valvular, hypertension, coronary arterial or pericardial abnormalities.

Types

Cardiomyopathy is of 3 Types—
1. Hypertrophic cardiomyopathy.
2. Dilated cardiomyopathy (ischaemic).
3. Restrictive cardiomyopathy.

Hypertrophic Cardiomyopathy

Definition

Hypertrophic cardiomyopathy (HCM) is a disease of the heart muscle characterised by hypertrophy of cardiac muscle with misalignment of the cardiac fibers.

Hypertrophy may be generalized or localized to the interventricular septum (asymmetrical septal hypertrophy) or other regions (apical hypertrophic cardiomyopathy).

Types

- Asymmetrical septal hypertrophy (70%).
- Basal septal hyperatrophy (15–20%).
- Concentric (8–10%).
- Apical or lateral wall (<2%).

Clinical Features

Symptoms
- May be asymptomatic.
- Angina on exertion.
- Palpitation.
- Breathlessness on exertion.
- Presyncope or syncope on exertion.
- Sudden death.

Signs
- Pulse—Carotid pulse is jerky.
- BP—low systolic, normal diastolic, narrow pulse pressure.

Precordium

Palpation
- Apex beat—heaving (may be double apical impulse).
- A systolic thrill may be palpable at apex.

Auscultation
- Ejection systolic murmur at the left lower sternal border.
- Pansystolic murmur at the apex due to mitral regurgitation.

Investigations

- Chest X-ray (may be normal).
- ECG (may be LVH, infarction, deep T—bizarre pattern).
- Echocardiogram (diagnostic)—shows asymmetrical septal hypertrophy (ASH), systolic anterior motion (SAM) of anterior leaflet of mitral valve.
- Cardiac MR.
- Genetic analysis.

Treatment

1. In nonobstructive case—
   - Beta-blocker, rate limiting calcium channel blocker (verapamil, diltiazem) and disopyramide for symptomatic relief and prevention of syncope.
   - Amiodarone may be helpful in arrhythmia.
2. In significant left ventricular outflow obstruction—
   - Dual chamber pacing may be needed.
   - Outflow tract obstruction can be improved by partial surgical resection (myectomy).
   - Iatrogenic infarction of basal septum by injecting alcohol with cardiac catheter.
3. Other treatment—
   - ICD (Implantable Cardioverter Defibrillator) if there is clinical risk factors for sudden death (see below).
   - Cardiac transplantation may be needed in CHF not responding to treatment.
   - Infective endocarditis prophylaxis may be needed.

Advice to be Given in HCM

- Vigorous exercise and dehydration should be avoided.
- Genetic counselling, as in 50% cases it may be inherited as autosomal dominant.
- First degree family members should be screened by echocardiogram.

Risk Factors for Sudden Cardiac Death in HCM

- History of previous cardiac arrest or sustained VT.
- Recurrent VT.
- Adverse genotype or family history of sudden cardiac death (<50 years old).
- Failure of blood pressure to rise during exercise (no change or hypotension).
- Nonsustained VT on 24 hours Holter monitoring.
- Marked increase in left ventricular wall thickness (>30 mm on echocardiography).
- Delayed gadolinium enhancement on cardiac MRI.

Drugs to be Avoided in HCM

- Digoxin.
- Vasodilators.
- Diuretics.
- Nitrates.
- Dihydropyridine calcium channel blockers.
- Alcohol (may cause vasodilatation).

Effect of HCM in Pregnancy

Pregnancy is not contraindicated in HCM. Patient usually tolerates pregnancy well if not severely symptomatic. There is no risk of sudden cardiac death in pregnancy.

Following precautions should be taken—

- Prenatal counselling regarding risk of disease in offspring.
- The patient should have regular follow-up in well-equipped centre with expertise in high-risk pregnancies and cardiac disease.
- β-blockers or calcium blockers should be continued.

Dilated Cardiomyopathy

Definition

Dilated cardiomyopathy (DCM) is characterised by dilatation and impaired contraction of the left and sometimes the right ventricle leading to progressive left-sided later right-sided heart failure. Functional mitral or tricuspid regurgitation may occur.

Causes

- Alcohol.
- 25% cases are inherited as autosomal dominant trait.
- Autoimmune reaction to viral myocarditis.
- Ischaemic heart disease.
- Nutritional—thiamine (Vitamin B1) deficiency.
- Muscular dystrophies—Duchenne or Becker's.
- Others—thyrotoxicosis, pregnancy, infiltrative disease (haemochromatosis, sarcoidosis).
- Idiopathic in many cases.

Symptoms

- Breathlessness on exertion.
- Features of heart failure—palpitation, swelling of legs, fatigue.
- Sporadic chest pain.
- Sudden death.

Signs

- Signs of cardiac failure (left or right or biventricular)
- Arrhythmia.

Investigations

- ECG usually shows nonspecific changes.
- Chest X-ray (shows cardiomegaly).
- Echocardiography.

Treatment

Mainly of heart failure.

1. Rest, salt and fluid restriction, avoidance of exercise.

2. Medical therapy—
   - β-blockers.
   - ACE inhibitors or Angiotensin receptor blocker.
   - Diuretics.
   - Nitrates.
   - Antiarrhythmic drugs if arrhythmia—amiodarone.
3. In some patients—implantation of ICD.
4. Treatment of primary cause, if any.
5. Cardiac transplantation may be indicated.

Restrictive Cardiomyopathy

Restrictive cardiomyopathy (RCM) this rare condition, ventricular filling is impaired because the ventricles are 'stiff.' This leads to high atrial pressures with atrial hypertrophy, dilatation and later atrial fibrillation.

Diagnosis

- Doppler echocardiography.
- CT or MRI.
- Endomyocardial biopsy.

Treatment

Symptomatic but the prognosis is usually poor and transplantation may be indicated.

Postpartum Cardiomyopathy

Definition

If any patient develops cardiac failure in the last trimester of pregnancy or within 6 months after delivery in the absence of previous heart disease, it is called postpartum/peripartum cardiomyopathy.

It is a type of dilated cardiomyopathy and the cause is unknown. Immune and viral causes are postulated. Other factors are advanced age, multiple pregnancy, multiparity and hypertension in pregnancy. Commonly occurs immediately after or in the month before delivery (peripartum).

Symptoms

It occurs usually in multipara, age above 30 years.
- Respiratory distress, orthopnea.
- Features of heart failure—weakness, pain in abdomen, swelling in legs.
- Cough with frothy sputum due to pulmonary edema.

Signs

- Signs of heart failure.
- Atrial fibrillation or other arrhythmia may occur.

Diagnostic Criteria (four criteria)

1. Presentation in the last month of pregnancy or within 6 months of delivery.
2. Absence of an obvious cause for heart failure.

3. Previously normal cardiac status.
4. Echocardiographic evidence of systolic left ventricular dysfunction.

Treatment

- Symptomatic for heart failure (diuretics, ACE inhibitor, digoxin).
- Beta-blocker may be helpful in some cases.
- Inotropic agent may be given.

Prognosis

More than half cases have a complete or near complete recovery over several months. Immunosuppressive therapy has doubtful value. Mortality rate is 10 to 20%.

The patient should avoid subsequent pregnancy, due to risk of relapse. However, if the heart size is normal in the first episode following heart failure, subsequent pregnancy is tolerated in some cases. If the heart size remains enlarged, further pregnancy causes refractory chronic heart failure.

ARRHYTHMIA

Definition

It is defined as the disorder of rate, rhythm and conduction of cardiac impulse.

Types

1. Impulse arising from SA node (Sinus arrhythmia)—
   - Sinus arrhythmia.
   - Sinus tachycardia.
   - Sinus bradycardia.
   - Sick sinus syndrome.
2. Impulse arising from atria (atrial tachyarryhythmia)—
   - Atrial fibrillation.
   - Atrial flutter.
   - Atrial tachycardia.
   - Atrial ectopics.
3. Impulse aring from AV junction or nodal—
   - Nodal or junctional rhythm.
   - Nodal tachycardia.
   - Nodal ectopics.
4. Impulse arising from ventricles (ventricular tachyarrhythmia)—
   - Ventricular tachycardia.
   - Ventricular fibrillation.
   - Ventricular ectopics.
5. Heart block—
   - SA block.
   - AV block.
   - Bundle brunch block (LBBB, RBBB).

Sinus Arrhythmia

Definition

It is an arrhythmia in which heart rate increases in inspiration and decreases in expiration.

It is a benign condition, common in children and young adults. Sometimes, in healthy old person, absent in autonomic neuropathy.

Mechanism

It is the normal manifestation of autonomic activity which varies with respiration. During inspiration, parasympathetic activity diminishes, so heart rate increases. It reverses during expiration.

Investigation

ECG findings

- PP or RR interval: Short in inspiration and long in expiration.
- Rhythm: Irregular (PP or RR interval is irregular).

Sinus Tachycardia

Definition

When heart rate is greater than 100/min in sinus rhythm.

Causes

1. Physiological—anxiety, emotion, exercise, pain, pregnancy.
2. Pathological—
   - Anaemia.
   - Fever.
   - Thyrotoxicosis.
   - Shock (except vasovagal attack in which bradycardia is present).
   - Heart failure.
   - Sick sinus syndrome.
   - Bleeding and hypovolaemia.
   - Chronic constrictive pericarditis.
   - Acute anterior myocardial infarction (bradycardia is common in inferior myocardial infarction).
   - Drugs (salbutamol, atropine, adrenaline, isoprenaline, ephedrine, propantheline, thyroxine).

Symptoms

- Palpitation.
- Features of primary disease, if any.

ECG shows

- Heart rate— >100 beats/minute.
- P, QRS and T—normal.
- Rhythm—regular.

Treatment

- If symptomatic—beta-blocker (propranolol, atenolol) or rate limiting calcium channel blocker(verapamil).
- Treatment of primary cause, if any.

Sinus Bradycardia

Definition

When heart rate is less than 60/min in sinus rhythm.

Causes

1. Physiological (due to increased vagal tone)—
   - Athlete.
   - Sleep.
   - Occasionally, healthy elderly.
2. Pathological—
   - Hypothyroidism.

- Hypothermia.
- Raised intracranial pressure.
- Drugs (digoxin, β-blockers, verapamil).
- Acute inferior myocardial infarction.
- Obstructive jaundice.
- Sick sinus syndrome.
- Electrolyte imbalance (hypokalemia).

Causes of Bradycardia

- Sinus bradycardia due to any cause.
- Sick sinus syndrome.
- Second degree heart block (Mobitz type II).
- Complete heart block.
- Nodal rhythm.
- Idioventricular rhythm.
- Drugs (β-blocker, digoxin).

ECG Findings

- Heart rate—<60/minute.
- P, QRS and T- normal.
- Rhythm—regular.

Treatment

Treatment of primary cause.

SICK SINUS SYNDROME

Definition

It is the dysfunction of SA node characterised by attacks of sinus bradycardia, sinus arrest or junctional rhythm which may lead to dizziness or syncope, followed by episodes of paroxysmal tachycardia, so called tachy-brady syndrome.

It includes sinus arrest, SA block, persistent sinus bradycardia with tachycardia, paroxysomal junctional or atrial tachycardia.

Causes

Due to fibrosis, degenerative changes or ischaemia of sinoatrial node. Probable causes are as follows:

- Elderly (due to degeneration).
- Ischaemic heart disease.
- Drug (digoxin).
- Cardiomyopathy.
- Rheumatic heart disease.
- Idiopathic in many cases.

Symptoms

- May be asymptomatic.
- Dizziness, syncope, and palpitation.

Signs

- Pulse—bradycardia or tachycardia or drop beat.
- Features of primary disease.

Investigations

- ECG.
- Holter monitoring (single ECG may sometimes be normal).

Treatment

- If asymptomatic—no specific therapy. Follow-up.
- If symptomatic—permanent dual chamber pacemaker.
- Antiarrhythmic drug—may be required.

SUPRAVENTRICULAR TACHYCARDIA (SVT)

Definition

It is a type of tachycardia that occurs due to re-entry or rapidly firing ectopic focus in atria or AV node.

Causes

1. Physiological—anxiety, tension, tea, coffee, alcohol.
2. Pathological—
   - Thyrotoxicosis.
   - Ischaemic heart disease.
   - WPW syndrome.
   - Digitalis toxicity.

Symptoms

- Palpitation, dizziness, syncope, breathlessness, chest pain.
- Polyuria after the attack.

Complications

In SVT, because of rapid heart rate, there is short diastolic filling time. This results in reduction of stroke volume and precipitate heart failure.

ECG Findings

- P—absent.
- QRS—narrow.
- Rhythm—regular.
- Heart rate—high (150-250/minute).

Treatment

1. Rest and reassurance.
2. Carotid sinus massage or Valsalva manoeuver. It acts by increasing the vagal tone.
3. If no response—
   - IV adenosine—3 mg over 2 seconds. If no response in 1-2 minutes, then 6 mg IV. If still no response in 1-2 minutes, then 12 mg (maximum dose).
   - Or IV verapamil 10 mg slowly over 5-10 minutes (verapamil should be avoided if QRS > 0.12 second or history of WPW syndrome or if the patient is on β-blocker).
4. Other drugs—β-blocker, disopyramide or digoxin may be used.
5. If the patient is hemodynamically unstable (hypotension, pulmonary oedema)—DC shock should be given.
6. If the attack is frequent or disabling—prophylactic oral therapy with β-blocker, verapamil, disopyramide or digoxin may be given.
7. In WPW syndrome—transvenous radiofrequency catheter ablation is the treatment of choice.
8. In some cases—antitachycardial pacing is done (overdrive atrial pacing).

Adenosine

1. Mode of action—It causes transient AV block, lasting for few seconds.
2. Side effects (all are transient)—chest pain, dyspnea, bronchospasm, choking sensation, transient flushing, hypotension.
3. Contraindications—
   - History of bronchial asthma.
   - Second or third degree heart block.
   - Sick sinus syndrome.

WPW SYNDROME

Definition

It is a syndrome in which there is an accessory pathway that bypasses the AV node and connects the atrium and ventricle (by bundles of Kent). May be associated with other congenital anomaly, commonly Ebstein anomaly.

Types

It is of 2 types:

1. Type A—accessory pathway on the left side (in ECG, tall R in V1 and V2).
2. Type B—accessory pathway on the right side (in ECG, deep Q in V1 and V2).

Clinical Features

- May be asymptomatic.
- May present with palpitation, paroxysmal attack of atrial or supraventricular tachycardia (most common) due to re-entry circuit, atrial fibrillation.
- Syncope.
- Sudden death (due to atrial fibrillation).
- Rarely—features of ventricular tachycardia, ventricular fibrillation.

Investigations

1. ECG shows—
   - PR interval short (<0.12 second).
   - QRS—wide.
   - Delta wave—in the upstroke of QRS (slurred QRS).
   - Q wave—may be present in lead II, III and aVF (confused with inferior myocardial infarction).
2. Electrophysiological study.

Treatment

1. If asymptomatic—no treatment is required.
2. If symptomatic—
   - Transvenous radiofrequency catheter ablation of accessory pathway is the specific treatment.
   - If this is not available—prophylactic antiarrhythmic drug should be given (β-blocker, amiodarone, flecainide, propafenone). These drugs prolong refractory period of accessory pathway.
   - Previously, surgical resection of accessory pathway used to be done.
3. Treatment atrial fibrillation with WPW syndrome—It is a medical emergency. Sudden death may occur. Treatment is as follows:
   - If troublesome symptoms—DC shock should be given. If not available, IV flecainide.
   - Radiofrequency ablation of abnormal pathway.
   - Drugs that slow down the conduction of accessory pathway may be used—amiodarone, flecainide, disopyramide, sotalol, etc.

Drugs to be Avoided in WPW Syndrome

Digoxin and IV verapamil. These drugs shorten the refractory period of accessory pathway.

Digoxin blocks the AV node and increases the conduction through the accessory pathway. So, it increases the heart rate. Verapamil may cause same effect. It may precipitate ventricular fibrillation.

NODAL RHYTHM OR JUNCTIONAL RHYTHM

Definition

When the impulse originate from AV node, it is called nodal or junctional rhythm. If the rate is high, it is called junctional tachycardia. Usually, it occurs due to depressed activity of SA node.

Nodal rhythm may be transient or permanent.

1. Transient—may occur in normal people.
2. Also transient or permanent nodal rhythm may occur in—
   - Digitalis toxicity.
   - Ischaemic heart disease (commonly, inferior myocardial infarction).
   - Rheumatic myocarditis.
   - Myocarditis due to any cause.

Types

- High-nodal rhythm—small inverted P wave before QRS (simulate low atrial ectopic).
- Mid-nodal rhythm—P is not seen (buried in QRS).
- Low-nodal rhythm—P is present after QRS.

ECG Findings

- Heart rate—40-60/minute.
- P—small, inverted (P may not be seen, buried in QRS or after QRS).
- PR interval—short.

Treatment

Treatment of primary cause.

ATRIAL FIBRILLATION

Definition

Atrial fibrillation (AF) is an arrhythmia where atria beat rapidly, chaotically and ineffectively, while the ventricles respond at irregular intervals, producing the characteristic irregularly irregular pulse.

Types

AF is of 3 Types—

1. Paroxysmal—Discrete self-limiting episodes. May be persistent, if underlying disease progresses.
2. Persistent—Prolonged episode that can be terminated by electrical or chemical cardioversion.
3. Permanent—Sinus rhythm cannot be restored.

According to heart rate, AF is of 2 types—

1. Fast atrial fibrillation—Heart rate > 100 beats/min.
2. Slow atrial fibrillation—Heart rate < 100 beats/min.

Causes

- Chronic rheumatic heart disease with valvular lesions, commonly mitral stenosis.
- Coronary artery disease (commonly, acute myocardial infarction).
- Thyrotoxicosis.
- Hypertension.
- Lone atrial fibrillation (idiopathic in 10% cases).
- Others—ASD, chronic constrictive pericarditis, acute pericarditis, cardiomyopathy, myocarditis, sick sinus syndrome, coronary bypass surgery, pneumonia, thoracic surgery, electrolyte imbalance (hypokalaemia, hyponatraemia), alcohol, pulmonary embolism.

NB: First five causes are always the top most causes.

Complications

- Systemic and pulmonary embolism (systemic from left atrium and pulmonary from right atrium).
- Heart failure.

Lone Atrial Fibrillation

It means atrial fibrillation without any cause. Prognosis—low risk of CVD (0.5% per year). Usually, life span is normal.

Clinical Features of AF

Symptoms

- Palpitation, breathlessness, weakness.

Signs

- Pulse—irregularly irregular (irregular in rhythm and volume).
- Examination of heart (heart rate to see pulsus deficit, mitral valvular or other cardiac disease).

- Thyroid status (warm sweaty hands, tremor, tachycardia, exophthalmos, thyroid gland size).
- Check BP in hypertensive case.

Investigations

1. ECG—shows absent P wave (replaced by fibrillary 'f' wave) with Irregularly irregular (R-R interval is irregular).
2. Chest X-ray.
3. Echocardiography.
4. Thyroid function test, if thyrotoxicosis is suspected.

Treatment

Aim of treatment:
- Control of heart rate.
- Restoration of sinus rhythm and prevention of recurrence.
- Treatment of primary cause.

Treatment (according to the type)—

Paroxysmal AF
- If asymptomatic—no treatment, only follow-up.
- In troublesome symptoms—β-blocker.
- Amiodarone is effective in prevention.
- Low dose aspirin to prevent thromboembolism.
- If bradycardia is present (in sinoatrial disease)—Permanent overdrive atrial pacing.
- In intractable cases—Radiofrequency ablation may be required, who does not have structural heart disease.

Persistent AF
- To control heart rate—β-blocker, digoxin or calcium channel blocker (verapamil, diltiazem).
- To control rhythm—DC cardioversion may be done safely.
- β-blocker or amiodarone may be used to prevent recurrence.

Permanent AF
- Control of heart rate—digoxin, β-blocker, calcium channel blocker (verapamil or diltiazem).
- In intractable case—Transvenous radiofrequency ablation may be done, followed by permanent pacemaker.

ATRIAL FLUTTER

Definition

It is characterised by rapid atrial rate associated with 2:1, 3:1, 4:1 or more AV block.

Causes

Same like atrial fibrillation.

Symptoms

- Palpitation.
- Breathlessness.
- Fatigue, weakness, light headedness, dizziness, even syncope.

ECG Findings

- P—saw-toothed appearance (normal P is replaced by flutter or F wave).
- RR—regular (may be irregular, when there is variable block).

NB: Occasionally, atrial fibrillation and flutter may be present together, it is called flutter-fibrillation.

Treatment

- To control heart rate—digoxin, β-blocker or verapamil. Amiodarone, propafenone or flecainide may be used and these can be used to prevent recurrence.
- If no response and patient shows troublesome symptoms—DC cardioversion or atrial overdrive pacing may be done.
- In persistent or troublesome symptoms—radiofrequency catheter ablation.

ECTOPICS

Definition

Ectopic beat or extrasystole is a premature beat which arises from other than SA node and comes earlier than the normal beat.

It arises from abnormal focus—atria, AV node or ventricle.

Types of Ectopic

- Atrial.
- Nodal.
- Ventricular.

Atrial Ectopics

Causes

- Due to excess tea, coffee, smoking.
- Any organic heart disease (myocarditis, cardiomyopathy).
- Electrolyte imbalance.
- COPD.

ECG Findings

- P—small or inverted.
- PR interval—short.
- PP interval—irregular.

Ventricular Ectopics

Types

Ventricular ectopics may be—unifocal, multifocal, bigeminy, trigeminy, quadrigeminy.

Causes

- Normally found in young adults, due to anxiety, excess caffeine, and alcohol.
- Myocarditis.
- Cardiomyopathy.
- Valvular heart disease.
- Mitral valve prolapse.
- Hypertensive heart disease.
- Electrolyte imbalance (specially hypokalaemia).
- Digoxin toxicity.
- Hypoxemia.

ECG Findings

- P—absent.
- QRS—wide >0.12 second (3 small squares).
- T—opposite to major deflection.

Treatment

- In the absence of any heart disease and asymptomatic case—no treatment is necessary. β-blocker may be used.
- With organic heart disease—treatment of primary cause.
- Antiarrhythmic drug does not improve, and may even worsen the prognosis.

VENTRICULAR TACHYCARDIA

Definition

Ventricular tachycardia (VT) is defined as three or more consecutive ectopic beats, heart rate usually 140–220 beats/minute with regular rhythm.

Causes

- Acute myocardial infarction.
- Myocarditis.
- Cardiomyopathy.
- Chronic ischemic heart disease (specially with poor left ventricular function).
- Ventricular aneurysm.
- Mitral valve prolapse.
- Electrolyte imbalance (mainly hypokalemia and hypomagnesemia).
- Idiopathic.

Symptoms

Palpitation, dyspnoea, dizziness, giddiness.

ECG Findings

- P wave—absent.
- QRS—broad >0.14 second, abnormal or bizarre pattern.
- Rate >100 beats/minute (usually, 140–220 beats/min).

Types of VT

- Sustained ventricular tachycardia.
- Nonsustained ventricular tachycardia.

Treatment

- If patient is haemodynamically unstable (such as hypotension, systolic BP< 90 mm Hg or heart failure)—cardioversion (DC shock).
- If the patient is haemodynamically stable—IV amiodarone bolus followed by IV infusion. If fails, cardioversion should be done.
- To prevent recurrence- β-blocker, oral amiodarone may be used.
- Correction of hypokalaemia, hypomagnesemia, hypoxemia and acidosis should be done.
- If all fails—automatic implantable cardioverter defibrillator device (ICD) or radiofrequency ablation of focus should be done.

VENTRICULAR FIBRILLATION

Definition

Ventricular fibrillation (VF) is a type of ventricular arrhythmia characterised by rapid, irregular, ineffective and uncoordinated ventricular activation with no mechanical effect.

There is chaotic electrical disturbance of ventricles, with impulse occuring irregularly at rate of 300–500/min. Cardiac output falls to zero.

It is the most common cause of sudden death. It may occur as a primary arrhythmia or as a complication in acute myocardial infarction.

Causes

- Acute myocardial infarction.
- Electrolyte imbalance (hypokalemia, hypomagnesemia).
- Electrocution.
- Others—drowning, drug overdose (digitalis, adrenaline, isoprenaline).

ECG Findings

QRS—Chaotic, wide, bizarre, irregular.

Signs

- Patient—unconscious.
- Pulse—absent.
- BP—not recordable.
- Respiration—ceases or absent.
- Pupil—dilated, less or no reaction to light.
- Heart sounds-absent.

Treatment

- Immediate defibrillation—200 Joules. If no response, another shock with 200 Joules. If still no response, another shock with 360 Joules is given.
- If three shocks unsuccessful—adrenaline IV, followed by cardiopulmonary resuscitation.
- If defibrillator is not available—cardiopulmonary resuscitation should be given.
- The patient who survives from VF in the absence of identifiable cause is at high risk of sudden death. It is treated with ICD.

HEART BLOCK

Definition

It is defined as defect in either initiation or conduction of cardiac impulse.

Sites of Heart Block

- SA node.
- AV node.
- Bundle of His.
- Branches of bundle of His (left and right).

Types of Heart Block

1. SA block.
2. Atrioventricular block—It is of 3 types:
   - 1st degree AV block.
   - 2nd degree AV block. It is of 2 types:
     - Mobitz type 1 (Wenckebach's phenomenon).
     - Mobitz type 2.
   - Complete heart block or 3rd degree heart block.
3. Bundle branch block:
   - Right bundle branch block (RBBB).
   - Left bundle branch block (LBBB).

Hemiblock

It means when there is block involving one of the fascicles of left bundle branch. It is diagnosed by seeing the axis deviation in ECG.

- When there is left-axis deviation—it is called left anterior hemiblock.
- When there is right-axis deviation—it is called left posterior hemiblock.

NB: There may be more blocks either two or three. In that case, it is called bifascicular or trifascicular block.

SA Block (Sinoatrial Block)

Definition

Failure to inititate an impulse from SA node.

Causes of SA Block

- Degenerative changes in elderly.
- Ischaemic heart disease (involving SA node).
- Drugs (digoxin).
- Increased vagal tone (may present like sick sinus syndrome).

Symptoms

- May be asymptomatic.
- Dizziness, giddiness.

Signs

Drop beat and no heart sound at the time of drop beat.

Investigations

- ECG—complete absence of one complex (P-QRS-T).
- Holter monitoring—may show the block.

Treatment

- No treatment, if asymptomatic.
- Withdrawal of offensive drug, if any.
- If any syncopal attack or sick sinus syndrome—permanent pacemaker should be given.

First Degree AV Block

Definition

It is the prolongation of PR >0.22 sec. Every atrial depolarisation is followed by conduction to the ventricles, but with delay.

Causes

- Normally found in athletes (due to increased vagal tone).
- Drugs (digitalis toxicity).
- Acute myocardial infarction (common in inferior MI).
- Acute rheumatic carditis.
- In elderly (atherosclerosis).
- Hyperkalaemia.

Symptoms

Usually asymptomatic.

ECG findings

- PR interval—prolonged >0.22 second (normal 0.12–0.20 second).
- QRS—normal.
- Rhythm—normal.

Treatment

No specific treatment is required.

Second Degree AV Block

Types

It is of 3 types:

- Mobitz type I (Wenckebach's phenomenon).

- Mobitz type II.
- 2 : 1 or 3 : 1 heart block.

Mobitz Type I (Wenkebach's Phenomenon)

Definition

Progressive prolongation of PR interval followed by a drop beat.

ECG findings

Progressive lengthening of PR interval followed by absent QRS complex.

Site of block

Higher area of AV node (proximal to bundle of His).

Causes

- Physiological—in athlete, during rest, sleep (due to increased vagal tone).
- Drugs—digoxin toxicity.
- Acute myocardial infarction (commonly inferior MI).

Symptoms

- Usually, asymptomatic.
- Features of primary disease.

Sign

- Pulse is irregular (drop beat occurs).

Treatment

- No treatment is required.
- Primary cause should be treated.

Mobitz Type II AV block:

Site of lesion

Disease of His-Purkinje system.

ECG Criteria

- Some P waves are not followed by QRS complexes.
- PR interval is constant (also PP interval constant).
- QRS—wide.

(In 2 :1 AV block, alternate P wave is conducted. It may be 3:1, 4:1). This type of AV block is rare and more severe. It is generally a sign of severe conduction system disease.

Cause

Acute anterior myocardial infarction.

Treatment

1. If due to inferior myocardial infarction:
   - If asymptomatic—close monitoring and follow-up.
   - If symptomatic—Injection atropine 0.6 mg IV. If fails, temporary pacemaker. Majority will resolve in 7-10 days.
2. If due to anterior myocardial infarction—temporary pacing followed by permanent pacemaker is required (because complete heart block may develop).

COMPLETE HEART BLOCK

Definition

No impulse from atria transmitted to the ventricles. So, ventricles generate their own rhythm.

Causes of Complete Heart Block

1. Acute CHB—Acute MI (commonly inferior).
2. Chronic CHB—
   - Progressive fibrosis of distal His-Purkinje system (Lev's disease) in elderly.
   - Progressive fibrosis of proximal His-Purkinje system (Lenegre's disease) in younger.

Other Causes

- Cardiomyopathy.
- Myocarditis.
- Drugs (digoxin, β-blocker, amiodarone).
- Cardiac surgery (aortic valve replacement, VSD repair).
- Radiofrequency AV node ablation.
- Infiltrative disease (sarcoidosis, amyloidosis, haemochromatosis).
- Infection (infective endocarditis, Chaga's disease, Lyme's disease).
- Collagen disease (SLE, Rheumatoid arthritis).
- Congenital complete heart block. It is common in child of mother with SLE (due to transplacental transfer of anti-Ro antibody/SSA).

Symptoms

- Weakness, dizziness, giddiness, syncopal attack (Stokes-Adams attack).
- Breathlessness on exertion.

Signs

- Pulse—bradycardia, 20–40 beats/minute (<40 beats/min), high volume, does not increase by exercise or injection atropine.
- BP—high systolic, normal diastolic and high-pulse pressure.
- Neck vein—cannon waves (large 'a' wave) may be present.
- Heart sounds—variable intensity of first heart sound.
- Murmur—systolic flow murmur.

Mechanism of Cannon Wave

When the atria contracts against closed tricuspid valve, backward pressure produces cannon wave.

ECG Criteria

- Atrial rate more, ventricular rate <40.
- PP interval—constant.
- No relationship between P wave and QRS complex (PR looks variable, a clue).

Treatment

- If the patient is symptomatic—permanent pacemaker.
- In congenital complete heart block, pulse rate is high, no pacemaker is necessary.

Stokes–Adams Attack

It is the brief attack of syncope or blackout in a patient with complete heart block due to ventricular asystole.

Symptoms

- Syncope or blackout with or without preceding dizziness.
- During attack—the patient is unconscious, looks pale and may have convulsion.
- If asystole persists—there may be cyanosis, pulse is absent, pupil is fixed and dilated, incontinence of urine,
- Plantar is extensor.
- Usually, consciousness recovers rapidly followed by flushing.

Treatment

- Permanent pacemaker.

RIGHT BUNDLE BRANCH BLOCK (RBBB)

ECG Criteria

- RSR—in V1 and V2 (M pattern).
- QRS—wide, >0.12 second (3 small squares).

Causes

- Normal variant (common).
- Coronary artery disease- acute myocardial infarction.
- Atrial septal defect (ASD).
- Right ventricular hypertrophy.
- Chronic cor pulmonale.
- Pulmonary embolism.
- Cardiomyopathy.
- Conduction system fibrosis.

Fascicular Block (Hemiblock)

Left bundle divides into anterior and posterior fascicles.

- Anterior fascicle spreads in anterior and superior part of left ventricle.
- Posterior fascicle spreads in posterior and inferior part of left ventricle.
- Fascicular block is diagnosed by looking at the axis deviation.

Fascicular block are of two types:

- RBBB with left anterior hemiblock (block in anterior fascicle).
- RBBB with left posterior hemiblock (block in posterior fascicle).

ECG in RBBB with Left Anterior Hemiblock

- RBBB with left axis deviation.

ECG in RBBB with Left Posterior Hemiblock

- RBBB with right axis deviation.

Left Bundle Branch Block (LBBB)

ECG Criteria

- RSR′- in V5 and V6, also in LI and aVL (M pattern).
- QRS wide, >0.12 second (3 small squares).

Causes

- Severe coronary artery disease.
- Acute myocardial infarction.
- Cardiomyopathy.
- Aortic valve disease (stenosis or regurgitation).
- Left ventricular hypertrophy.
- Hypertension.
- Myocarditis.

Symptoms

- Features of primary disease.

Signs

On auscultation, there is reverse splitting of second heart sound.

Treatment

- Treatment of primary cause.
- In acute myocardial infarction—if there is new LBBB, temporary pacemaker is indicated.

TAKAYASU'S DISEASE

Definition

It is a chronic inflammatory, granulomatous panarteritis of unknown cause involving the elastic arteries.

It commonly involves aorta and its major branches, carotid, ulnar, brachial, radial and axillary. Occasionally, may involve pulmonary artery, rarely abdominal aorta, renal artery resulting in obstruction. Common in female at the age of 25-30 years. Mainly found in asians.

Clinical Features

- General- fever, malaise, weight loss, arthralgia, myalgia, dizziness, giddiness, headache, syncope, seizure, claudication in the upper limb.
- There may be aortic regurgitation, renal artery stenosis or anginal pain. Hypertension is found in 32-93%. There may be pericarditis, myocardial infarction, congestive cardiac failure, etc.

Ophthalmologic findings—Ophthalmologic examination may show retinal ischaemia, retinal hemorrhages, cotton-wool exudates, venous dilatation and beading, microaneurysms of peripheral retina, optic atrophy, vitreous hemorrhage, and classic, wreath like peripapillary arteriovenous anastomoses.

Signs

- Pulse—All peripheral pulses are absent or feeble in the upper limb. In the lower limbs, pulse is present.
- BP—Not recordable in upper limbs.
- Bruit—may be present over both carotids.
- Locomotor system—small joints of hands, wrists and elbows are mildly tender.

Investigations

- CBC (high ESR and normocytic normochromic anaemia).
- Chest X-ray shows cardiomegaly and widening of aorta.
- Aortography of aortic arch and its branches, renal angiogram shows narrowing, coarctation and aneurismal dilatation.
- Serum immunoglobulin is high.

Treatment

- High-dose prednisolone—40-60 mg daily or 1-2 mg/kg.
- If refractory to steroid or difficult to taper steroid, methotrexate up to 25 mg weekly.
- Reconstructive vascular surgery in selected case.

Prognosis

With appropriate treatment, the 5 year survival is 83%.

PACEMAKER

Pacemaker is an artificial device used to electrically stimulate the heart.

It is composed of two parts:

- Battery-powered generator.
- Wire electrode—which is attached to the heart chamber to be stimulated (atrium or ventricle or both).

Pacemaker may be single chamber or dual chamber. Two types of pacemaker—temporary and permanent.

Indications of Temporary Pacemaker

- Acute inferior myocardial infarction with second or third degree AV block or severe bradycardia with haemodynamic change.
- Acute extensive anterior MI with second or third degree AV block or new bifascicular block (LBBB or RBBB with left anterior hemiblock, RBBB with left posterior hemiblock).
- Patient awaiting for permanent pacing.
- Some tachycardia, such as AV re-entry tachycardia and ventricular tachycardia can be terminated by overdrive pacing.
- After open-heart surgery.
- Some cases of cardiac arrest.
- Severe digitalis toxicity.

Indications of Permanent Pacemaker

- Most common—complete heart block with syncope or Stokes-Adams syndrome and sick sinus syndrome.

Others

- Symptomatic or asymptomatic Mobitz type 2 second degree AV block.
- Symptomatic Mobitz type 1 second degree AV block.
- Bifascicular or trifascicular block with syncope.
- Carotid sinus syndrome with bradycardia.
- Repeated vasovagal syndrome with bradycardia.
- In some cases of permanent atrial fibrillation (when other treatment fails, radiofrequency ablation followed by permanent pacemaker).

ECG Findings (Atrial Pacing)

- There is a spike followed by P wave.
- QRS—normal.

ECG Findings (Ventricular Pacing)

- There is a spike followed by QRS.
- QRS -wide (looks like LBBB).

Complications of Pacemaker

1. Early—
   - Pneumothorax.
   - Infection.
   - Lead displacement.
   - Cardiac tamponade.
   - Pocket haematoma.
2. Late—
   - Infection.
   - Erosion of generator or lead.
   - Chronic pain at implant site.
   - Lead fracture.
   - Malfunction.
   - Perforation of ventricular wall.
   - Ventricular arrhythmia (PVC).
   - Electromagnetic interference.
   - Pacemaker failure.
   - Pacemaker mediated tachycardia (by dual-chamber pacing).
   - Pacemaker syndrome (by single-chamber pacing).

PULMONARY HYPERTENSION

Definition

It is defined as mean pulmonary arterial pressure > 25 mm Hg at rest and > 30 mm Hg during exercise.

Causes

1. Idiopathic pulmonary hypertension—no underlying cause. May have genetic predisposition.
2. Secondary pulmonary hypertension—it is more common than idiopathic pulmonary hypertension.
3. Respiratory—COPD, emphysema, chronic bronchitis, DPLD, pulmonary thromboembolism.
4. Cardiac—Left-sided heart failure, mitral stenosis, reversal of shunt (ASD, VSD, PDA).
5. Connective tissue disorders—scleroderma, SLE.
6. Sleep apnoea syndrome and other sleep disorders.
7. Drugs—such as cocaine.

Symptoms

- May be asymptomatic.
- Shortness of breath (orthopnea or paroxysmal nocturnal dyspnea).
- Chest pain, palpitations, cough.
- Haemoptysis (rarely).
- Fatigue.
- Ankle swelling.
- Dizziness, syncope.

Signs

- Palpable P2.
- Prominent 'a' wave in JVP.
- Left parasternal heave (indicates RVH).
- Epigastric pulsation (indicates RVH).
- Loud P2 on auscultation.
- Early diastolic murmur (Graham-Steel murmur due to pulmonary regurgitation).

Complications

- Right-sided heart failure and cor pulmonale.
- Arrhythmia.

Investigations

- CBC, ESR.
- CXR PA View (shows enlargement of pulmonary arteries).
- ECG—RVH, RAH.
- Doppler echocardiography.
- Pulmonary function test.
- Ventilation-perfusion (V/Q) scan.

- CT scan of chest.
- Other investigations according to suspicion of cause.
- Open-lung biopsy.
- Genetic tests.

Treatment

1. General—reduction of weight, avoid heavy exercise, smoking must be stopped.
2. Oxygen.
3. Diuretics.
4. Digoxin
5. Vasodilator drugs—ACE inhibitors: Sildenafil and Tadalafil.
6. Endothelin receptor antagonists—Bosentan, Ambrisentan.
7. Calcium channel blockers—Amlodipine, Nifedipine.
8. Anticoagulants—Warfarin.
9. Surgery—
   - Atrial septostomy.
   - Heart-lung transplantation in selected cases.
   - Pulmonary thromboendarterectomy.
   - Cardiac arrest.

CARDIAC ARREST

Definition

It is defined as sudden loss of cardiac function, when the heart abruptly stops beating.

Causes

1. Ventricular fibrillation (commonest cause).
2. Ventricular tachycardia (pulseless).
3. Asystole.
4. Electromechanical dissociation.
5. Others—
   - Myocardial rupture.
   - Cardiac tamponade.
   - Respiratory arrest (loss of breathing function).
   - Massive pulmonary embolism.
   - Tension pneumothorax.
   - Electrocution.
   - Drowning.

Clinical Features

- Sudden collapse, loss of consciousness.
- No pulse.
- No BP.
- No breathing.

Permanent brain damage and death can occur unless the flow of blood to the brain is restored within five minutes.

Treatment

- A - Airway restoration.
- B - Breathing should be ensured (mouth to mouth breathing).
- C - Circulation (CPR should be started—15 compression:2 breaths).
- Precordial thump.
- Defibrillation—in ventricular fibrillation.
- Other supportive therapy—injection adrenaline, transvenous pacemaker.

MARFAN'S SYNDROME

Definition

It is a connective tissue disorder inherited as autosomal dominant trait due to mutation in the fibrillin-1 gene, a component of extracellular matrix. The fibrillin gene is located in the long arm of chromosome 15 (15q21.1).

Clinical Features

Marfan's syndrome is characterized by triad of eye, skeletal and cardiac abnormalities.

Eye

- Blue sclera.
- Subluxation or dislocation of lens (ectopialentis).
- Iridodonesis (tremor of iris).
- Heterochromia iris (various colour of iris).
- Myopia.
- Retinal detachment.
- Glaucoma.

Skeletal

- Tall, lean and thin.
- Arachnodactyly.
- Hyperextensibility of joints.
- High-arch palate.
- Kyphosis, scoliosis or both, pesplanus.
- Pectusexcavatum or carinatum or asymmetry of chest.
- Arm span > height.
- Lower segment > upper segment.

CVS

- AR (due to aortic root dilatation, secondary to cystic medial necrosis involving aorta).
- MR (with mitral valve prolapse).

Complications

- Dissecting aneurysm.
- Infective endocarditis.
- Heart failure.

Associations in Marfan's Syndrome

- Cystic disease in lung (may cause recurrent spontaneous pneumothorax), bullae, apical fibrosis, aspergilloma, bronchiectasis.
- Inguinal or femoral hernia and decreased subcutaneous fat.
- Nodule or papule in skin of neck (Miescher'selastoma).
- Coarctation of aorta.

Table 5
Differences between homocystinuria and Marfan's syndrome

Features	Homocystinuria	Marfan's syndrome
Inheritance	AR	AD
Lens	Dislocated downward	Dislocated upward
Skeletal abnormality	Osteoporosis—common	Osteoporosis—less common, but flat foot, scoliosis, pectusexcavatum are common
Aortic regurgitation	Rare	Common
Mental retardation	Common	No
Vascular complication	Prone to develop thrombosis	No
Life expectancy	May be normal	Short due to cardiovascular risk
Test (urine)	Cyanide nitroprusside-positive	Cyanide nitroprusside-negative
Spectroscopic examination (urine)	Homocystine detected	No
Pyridoxine	May respond	No

Investigations

- X-ray chest (may be normal, aortic aneurysm and unfolding of aorta. Pneumothorax, scoliosis may be present).
- ECG (to see any arrhythmia).
- Echocardiogram (mitral valve prolapse, aortic regurgitation, mitral regurgitation, aortic root dilatation).
- CT or CMR (to see aortic dilatation).

Treatment

- β-blocker (propranolol) reduces aortic dilatation and prevents the risk of aortic rupture or dissecting aneurysm.
- ACE inhibitor—in Marfan syndrome there is upregulation of TNF-β which is specifically inhibited by ACE inhibitor. Also prevents aortic root dilatation.
- Avoid strenuous exercise to prevent aortic dissection.
- Surgery—elective replacement of ascending aorta and aortic valve in patient with progressive dilatation of aorta (>5 cm).
- Prophylaxis for infective endocarditis.
- Echocardiography annually.
- Genetic counselling and orthopaedic measures (Table 5).

Pregnancy in Marfan's Syndrome

- Pregnancy is well tolerated, if there is no serious cardiac problem. Avoided, if aortic root dilatation is >4 cm with AR.
- Maternal death may occur due to aortic dissection during pregnancy. Early premature abortion may also occur.
- Echocardiogram should be done every 6–8 weeks throughout pregnancy and 6 month postpartum.
- BP should be regularly monitored.
- Vaginal delivery is possible, caesarean section is not done routinely. If aortic root is >4.5 cm delivery should be done at 39 weeks by induction or Caesarean section. β-blocker should be continued throughout pregnancy.

CHAPTER

3 Respiratory Diseases

CHAPTER CONTENTS

LUNG FUNCTION TEST (SPIROMETRY)

Spirometry is a method of assessing lung function by measuring the volume of air after maximal expiration following maximal inspiration. FEV1 and FVC are measured, by maximum inspiration followed by forced expiration (as long as possible), into the spirometer. FEV1 is expressed as percentage of FVC.

It is done to diagnose and differentiate obstructive airway disorders (e.g. chronic obstructive pulmonary disease (COPD), asthma) from restrictive diseases (e.g. ILD). Spirometry can also be used to determine the severity of asthma and COPD.

By spirometry following are measured—

1. **FEV1 (forced expiratory volume in 1st second):** It is the volume of air in the first second of forced expiration after full inspiration.

2. **FVC (forced vital capacity):** It is the total volume of air expired forcibly in one breath after full inspiration.

3. **FEV1/FVC:** It is the ratio of FEV1 to FVC expressed as percentage.

4. **PEFR (peak expiratory flow rate):** It is the highest flow which can be achieved during forceful expiration. Long-term monitoring of asthma can be done by seeing diurnal variability of PEFR at patient's home by maintaining peak flow. The patient is asked to take a full inspiration as far as possible, then blow out forcefully into the peak flow meter. PEFR is best used to monitor progress of the disease and its treatment.

Regular measurement of PEFR on waking, in afternoon and before bed demonstrates the wide diurnal variations in airflow limitations that characterize bronchial asthma. PEF physiologically falls at late night or early morning. Fall of PEF >20% in early morning is known as 'morning dipping.' It is characteristic of uncontrolled asthma.

Spirometry indicates presence of airway abnormality, if recordings shows—

- FEV1— <80% of predicted value.
- FVC— <80% of predicted value.
- FEV1/FVC ratio— <75%.

Obstructive disorder shows (Table 1)—

- FEV1—reduced (<80% of predicted value).
- FVC—reduced.
- FEV1/FVC ratio—reduced (<75%).

Table 1

Differences between restrictive and obstructive airway disease

Points	Restrictive	Obstructive
1. Both FEV1 and FVC	Proportionately reduced	FEV1 is markedly reduced and FVC also reduced
2. Ratio between FEV1 and FVC	Normal	Reduced
3. RV	Reduced or normal	Increased
4. TLC	Reduced	Increased
5. Ratio between RV and TLC	Normal or slightly increased	Markedly increased

Restrictive disorder shows (Table 1)

- FEV1 and FVC—proportionately reduced.
- FEV/FVC ratio—normal (>75%).

1. **Baseline spirometry:** It means spirometric assessment when patient is asymptomatic or in his best condition. It is done without reversibility test to classify asthma into intermittent and persistent (mild, moderate or severe) varieties.

2. **Reversibility test:** Bronchodilator reversibility test can be used to differentiate between asthma and COPD. After bronchodilatation, both >12% and >200 mL increase in FEV1, over pre-bronchodilator levels indicates positive reversibility test, suggesting diagnosis of bronchial asthma. Negative result indicates COPD (or severe persistent asthma).

3. **Bronchoprovocation test:** Fall of FEV1 > 20% after inhalation of methacholine or hypertonic saline is used for diagnosis of hyperresponsiveness of airways in susceptible patients with normal spirometry. Susceptible patients are—(i) patient with cough-variant asthma, (ii) mild intermittent asthma, (iii) chronic bronchitis with hyperresponsive airways.

4. **Exercise challenge test:** Fall of FEV1 or PEFR > 15% from baseline value after vigorous exercise (i.e. running or climbing stairs for 6 minutes) indicates 'exercise-induced asthma'.

BRONCHIAL ASTHMA

Definition

It is a chronic airway inflammatory disorder characterized by hyperresponsiveness of the airways to various stimuli presenting with breathlessness, cough, chest tightness and wheeze. It is reversible.

Causes

1. Genetic factors—asthma and atopy are common in family members. Atopic individuals have higher incidence of developing asthma.
2. Allergens—
   - Indoor—house dust, mite, pet allergens, dander, cockroach allergen, fungal spores.
   - Outdoor—grass and flower pollens.
   - Food allergens—egg, crab, fish.
3. Irritants—
   - Tobacco smoke.
   - Wood smoke.
   - Strong odours, perfume, sprays, cosmetics, paints.
   - Vehicle smoke.
4. Upper respiratory tract infection—
   - Viral (RSV) or bacterial infection (H.influenzae).
   - Common cold.
5. Occupational asthma.
6. Others—
   - Exercise.
   - Psychological factors—anxiety, stress may exacerbate asthma.
   - Drugs—NSAID's, β-blockers.
   - Changes in weather, temperature.
7. Conditions associated with asthma—
   - Atopic dermatitis.
   - Allergic rhinitis.
   - Allergic conjunctivitis.

Symptoms

- Recurrent attacks of dyspnoea, cough with mucoid sputum and wheeze. Attack may be spontaneous or precipitated by exercise, cold weather, exposure to air-born allergens or pollens, viral respiratory infection.
- There is diurnal variation, symptoms may be more in the early morning. Occasionally, symptoms may be during sleep at night called 'nocturnal asthma.'
- In some patients, cough is the only symptom, no wheeze or breathlessness, called 'cough-variant asthma.'

Signs

- Breath sound—vesicular with prolonged expiration.
- Multiple rhonchi both in inspiration and expiration, present all over the lungs.

Investigations

1. X-ray chest—normal in early cases. Emphysematous changes in late cases.
2. Lung function tests—
   - Spirometry—to see FEV_1 and FVC (shows obstructive airway disease).
   - FEV_1 >15% increased after administration of bronchodilator (reversibility test).
   - PEFR—patient should record after rising in the morning and before retiring in the evening. Diurnal variation >20% (lowest value in the morning, called morning dipping).
   - FEV_1 >15% decrease after 6 minutes of exercise.
3. Others—
   - CBC—may be high eosinophil.
   - Sputum for eosinophil—high.
   - Serum IgE—high in atopic patient.
   - Skin prick test to identify allergic factors.
   - Methacholine provocation test—helpful when the main symptom is cough. This test indicates presence of airway hyperresponsiveness.

Diagnostic criteria of bronchial asthma: Typical clinical history plus either/or—
- FEV_1 >15% increased after administration of bronchodilator.
- PEFR >20% on >3 days in a week for 2 weeks (lowest value in morning).
- FEV_1 >15% decrease after 6 minutes of exercise.

Asthma may be Extrinsic or Intrinsic (Table 2)

- Intrinsic asthma (nonatopic or late onset asthma)—when no causative agent can be identified. It is not allergic, usually begins after the age of 30 years, tends to be more continuous and more severe.
- Extrinsic asthma (atopic or early onset asthma)—when a definite external cause is present. There is history of allergy to dust mite, animal danders, pollens, fungi, etc. It occurs commonly in childhood and usually shows seasonal variations.

Types of Bronchial Asthma: 4 groups

1. Intermittent or episodic asthma—occasional attack of asthma, between the episodes the patient remains symptom free.

Table 2
Differences between extrinsic and intrinsic bronchial asthma

Points	Extrinsic	Intrinsic
1. Age	Early or childhood	Middle age or late onset
2. History of allergy	Usually present	Absent
3. Precipitating allergen	Present	Absent
4. Atopy	Atopic individual	Nonatopic
5. Family history of asthma, rhinitis, eczema	Usually present	Usually absent
6. Skin prick test	Usually positive	Usually negative
7. Serum IgE	High	Normal

2. Persistent or chronic asthma—frequent asthmatic attacks, which are persistent or chronic (at least more than two occasions in a month).
3. Acute exacerbation—increased symptoms, loss of lung function, not controlled by use of standard medication.
4. Special variants. Five types—
   - Cough variant asthma.
   - Exercise induced asthma.
   - Occupational asthma.
   - Drug-induced asthma.
   - Seasonal asthma.

Cough Variant Asthma

It is a type of asthma in which there is chronic dry cough with or without sputum eosinophilia, but no abnormalities in airway function. Cough is the only symptom, mostly at night. Examination during day may not reveal any abnormality. Cough may be increased with exercise, exposure to dust, strong fragrances or cold air.

Treatment
- Allergic rhinitis should be treated, if present.
- Gastroesophageal reflux disease should be treated with proton-pump inhibitor (e.g. omeprazole) and prokinetic agent (e.g. domperidone).
- Environmental factors like cold, dust, fume should be avoided.
- Nedocromil sodium is effective.

Exercise-induced Asthma

Asthma produced by exercise is called exercise induced asthma.

Treatment
- Short-acting β2 agonist (salbutamol), sodium chromoglycate or nedocromil sodium immediately before exercise should be used.
- Inhaled corticosteroid twice daily for 8–12 weeks reduces severity.

Occupational Asthma

It may be defined as asthma induced at work by exposure to occupation related agents, which are mainly inhaled at the workplace. Main feature is symptoms that worsen on work days and improves on holidays. Commonly found in chemical workers, farmers, grain handlers, cigarette manufacturers, fabric, dye, press and printing workers, laboratory workers, poultry breeders, wood and bakery workers.

Treatment
- Avoidance of further exposure using mask at work.
- If no response, step care asthma management plan.

Drug-induced Asthma

Symptoms of asthma that occurs after use of certain drugs, such as aspirin, beta-blocker, some NSAIDs, etc. These drugs can cause bronchospasm.

ACUTE SEVERE ASTHMA

Definition

It is defined as severe acute persistent attack of asthma without any remission, not controlled by conventional bronchodilator. Previously it was called 'status asthmaticus'.

Signs of Severe Acute Bronchial Asthma

- Inability to complete a sentence in one breath.
- Respiratory rate ≥25/min.
- Pulse rate ≥110/min (pulsus paradoxus may be present)
- PEFR <50% of predicted normal (<200 L/min).

Signs of Life Threatening or Very Severe Asthma

- Exhaustion, confusion or coma.
- Silent chest, cyanosis, feeble respiratory effort.
- Bradycardia, hypotension or arrhythmia.
- PEFR <33% of predicted (<100 L/min).
- Blood gas analysis—
  - PaO_2 <8 kPa (60 mmHg) even with O_2
  - High $PaCO_2$ (>6 kPa)
  - Low or falling blood pH.

Treatment of Acute Severe Bronchial Asthma

- High flow O_2—40–60%.
- Inhaled salbutamol 2–10 puff (100 μg/metered inhalation) via large volume spacer or nebulizer. May be repeated after 10–20 minutes.
- In life threatening cases—nebulized salbutamol 5mg or terbutaline 10 mg. May be repeated every 20–30 minutes or if necessary.
- Nebulized ipratropium bromide 0.5 mg (500 μg) may be added every 4–6 hours.
- Prednisolone 30–60 mg orally or Inj. hydrocortisone 200mg IV 6 hourly. When improves, oral prednisolone 60 mg daily should be given for two weeks, then taper.
- If no response—magnesium sulphate IV 1.2–2 g over 20 minutes may be given.
- In some cases—injection aminophylline 5 mg/kg loading dose over 20 minutes, then continuous infusion at 1 mg/kg/h.
- If no response—the patient should be shifted to ICU for assisted ventilation.

Indications for Assisted Ventilation

1. Coma, exhaustion, confusion.
2. Respiratory arrest.
3. Blood gas analysis—
   - PaO_2 <8 kPa (60 mmHg) even with O_2
   - High $PaCO_2$ (>6 kPa)
   - Low or falling blood pH.

Management of Bronchial Asthma (Table 3)

1. General measures—
   - Avoidance of allergens (house dust, mite, pets, pollens).
   - Smoking must be stopped.
   - Drugs that aggravate asthma should be avoided.
   - In occupational asthma—use of mask, changes of occupation may be needed.
2. Drug therapy—bronchodilator therapy and preventive drug therapy.

Drug Used in Bronchial Asthma

- β2 adrenoceptor agonist.
- Methyl xanthines.
- Anticholenergic bronchodilator.
- Corticosteroid.
- Chromones.
- Leucotrine receptor antagonist (LTRA).
- Anti-IgE therapy (monoclonal antibody).
- Miscellaneous.

β_2 Adrenoceptor Agonist

2 groups—short acting (salbutamol, terbutaline) and long acting β2 agonist (salmeterol, formoterol).

These are bronchodilators, given as inhalation. Also in nebulized solution or dry powder form. Main side effects— tremor, palpitation. Levosalbutamol causes less tremor.

Anticholenergic (Antimuscarinic) Drug

Ipratropium bromide or oxitropium bromide, used as inhaler or in a nebulizer, may be combined with salbutamol. These drugs should be carefully used in patients with angle closure glaucoma, prostatic hyperplasia or urinary bladder outflow obstruction.

Methyl Xanthines

- Theophylline—given orally.
- Aminophylline—given orally or intravenously or as suppository.
- Doxophylline 400 mg given orally once or twice daily.

Corticosteroid

Given orally (prednisolone), hydrocortisone intravenously in acute attack. Mostly used as inhaled corticosteroid—beclomethasone dipropionate, budesonide, fruticasone propionate, momentasone furoate. Combined corticosterid and long-acting β2 agonist (budenoside plus formoterol or fluticasone and salmeterol are commonly used). Ciclesonide is given once daily.

Chromones

Sodium cromoglycate and nedocromil sodium, effective in mild asthma. They inhibit degradation of mast cells and preventive mediator release. Ketotifen is less effective.

Leucotrine Receptor Antagonist (LTRA)

Montelukast, zafirlukast—given orally. These are effective alone or with inhaled corticosteroid.

Table 3
Stepwise management of asthma

Step	*PEFR*	*Treatment*
Step 1. Occasional symptoms (< 1 in a week for 3 months and fewer than 2 nocturnal symptoms/month)	100% predicted	» Inhaled short-acting β2 agonist as required » If used more than once daily, move to step 2
Step 2. Daily symptoms. Also indicated in— - Exacerbation of asthma in the last 2 years - Uses inhaled β2 agonist 3 times a week or more - Symptoms 3 times a week or more - Awakened by asthma one night per week	≤80% predicted	Add any of the following— » Low-dose inhaled corticosteroid (ICS) —started at 400 µg beclomethasone (BDP) or equivalent (budesonide, fluticasone, ciclesonide) daily and may be increased to 800 µg daily » Leukotriene receptor antagonist (LTRA), theophylline or sodium cromoglicate (these are less effective) » If not controlled, move to step 3
Step 3. Severe symptoms or poorly controlled despite regular use of ICS	50–80% predicted	Add one of the following (add on therapy)— » Low-dose ICS + long-acting β2 agonist like salmeterol, formoterol » Low-dose ICS + LTRA » Low-dose ICS + sustained release theophylline » Medium or high-dose ICS » If not controlled, move to step 4
Step 4. Severe symptoms or poorly controlled with high-dose inhaled corticosteroids	50–80% predicted	High dose inhaled corticosteroid, up to 2000 µg daily Plus regular long-acting β2 agonist Plus either LTRA or modified release theophylline or β2 agonist
Step 5. Severe symptoms deteriorating	≤50% predicted	Regular oral corticosteroid—add prednisolone 40 mg daily to step 4 and or Anti-IgE treatment
Step 6. Severe symptoms deteriorating inspite of prednisolone	≤30% predicted	Hospital admission

Anti-IgE Therapy

Omalizumab, a monoclonal antibody against IgE is effective in allergic asthma.

Miscellaneous

Methotrexate, ciclosporin, IV immunoglobulin, etanercept, infliximab.

MANAGEMENT OF ASTHMA WITH OTHER DISEASES

Asthma with Diabetes Mellitus

Drugs are used as in other cases of bronchial asthma. However, the following points should be remembered—

- Corticosteroid can be used if necessary, but regular sugar monitoring should be done.
- In severe acute asthma, insulin therapy may be necessary.
- Metformin should be avoided in uncontrolled asthma and is contraindicated in acute severe asthma.
- Dose of oral hypoglycaemic drugs like sulfonylurea and pioglitazone should be adjusted if used with aminophylline, as it may cause hypoglycaemia.

Asthma in Pregnancy

1. During pregnancy:
   - All inhalers are safe and effective.
   - β2 agonist (both short and long acting), inhaled steroid, theophylline, oral prednisolone, chromone (sodium chromoglycate) are safe.
   - If the patient was getting leukotriene receptor blockers (e.g. montelukast, zafirlukast), it can be continued.
2. During labour—Treatment as usual should be continued. If the patient is on maintenance prednisolone >7.5 mg/day for >2 weeks prior to delivery, it should be changed to parenteral hydrocortisone, 100 mg 6–8 hourly during labour.
3. Breastfeeding should be continued.

Asthma with Hypertension

Management is same. Following points are important—

- β-blocker should be avoided—such as propranolol.
- Drug of choice—calcium channel blocker or ARB (losartan, valsartan).
- ACE inhibitor is avoided as it may induce cough.

BRONCHIECTASIS

Definition

It is the abnormal, permanent dilatation of one or more bronchi with destruction of bronchial wall proximal to the terminal bronchiole.

Causes

1. Congenital or hereditary—
   - Cystic fibrosis.
   - Kartagener's syndrome (triad of bronchiectasis, dextrocardia and sinusitis or frontal sinus agenesis).
   - Primary ciliary dyskinesia (including immotile ciliary syndrome).
   - Hypogammaglobulinaemia (of IgA and IgG. It causes recurrent infection and bronchiectasis).
   - Yellow nail syndrome.
   - Young's syndrome (obstructive azoospermia and chronic sinopulmonary infection, thought to be due to mercury intoxication).
   - Sequestrate segment of lung.
2. Acquired—
   - In children, pneumonia complicating measles, whooping cough, primary TB and foreign body.
   - In adults, bronchial neoplasm, pulmonary TB, recurrent aspiration or suppurative pneumonia.
   - Allergic bronchopulmonary aspergillosis (causes proximal bronchiectasis).

NB: In children, postmeasles or whooping cough are commonly associated with bronchiectasis. In adult, post-tubercular bronchiectasis is the common one.

Types of Bronchiectasis: 3 types

- Saccular or cystic (more severe form).
- Cylindrical.
- Fusiform.

Symptoms

- Recurrent cough with profuse expectoration of sputum, usually more marked in the morning after waking from sleep.
- Haemoptysis.

Signs

- Generalized clubbing in fingers and toes.
- In chest—multiple coarse crepitations in affected side, altered by cough.

Dry bronchiectasis (bronchiectasis sicca): It is a type of bronchiectasis in which dry cough is associated with intermittent episodes of haemoptysis.

Commonest site of bronchiectasis: Left lower lobe and lingula.

Investigations

1. Chest X-ray PA view—shows ring with or without fluid level, may be multiple (cystic bronchiectasis).
2. High-resolution CT scan (definitive).

Treatment

- Postural drainage, keeping the affected part remaining up and percussion over it. It is done for 5–10 min, once or twice daily.
- Antibiotic, if infection.
- Chest physiotherapy.
- Bronchodilator drugs. Also, nebulized salbutamol may be used.
- Inhaled or oral steroid can decrease the rate of progression.
- Surgery (lobectomy). Done in unilateral and localized to a single lobe or segment.

Indications of Surgery

- Unilateral and localized to a single lobe or segment.
- Severe and recurrent haemoptysis.

Complications

- Secondary infection.
- Lung abscess.
- Pleural effusion, empyema or pneumothorax.
- Pulmonary hypertension and cor pulmonale.
- Respiratory failure.
- Amyloidosis .
- Brain abscess (metastatic cerebral abscess).
- Aspergiloma in the bronchiectatic cavity.

BRONCHIAL CARCINOMA

Causes or Risk Factors

- Cigarette smoking is the major risk factor. Even passive smoking causes 1.5 times increase in the risk of bronchial carcinoma.
- Other factors are exposure to asbestos, silica, beryllium, cadmium, chromium, arsenic, iron oxide, radon, radiation, petroleum products and oils, coal tar, products of coal combustion.
- Adenocarcinoma may develop in nonsmokers and in old scar.

Symptoms: Usually in elderly patients with history of smoking.

1. Due to lung lesion—
   - Cough—dry or sputum production. Changing pattern of regular cough in a smoker is highly suspicious.
   - Haemoptysis.
   - Breathlessness.
   - Chest pain.
2. Due to local spread in mediastinum—
   - Hoarseness of voice and bovine cough (due to recurrent laryngeal nerve palsy).
   - Dysphagia (due to oesophageal involvement).
   - Puffiness with plethoric face—due to SVC obstruction.
   - Horner's syndrome—due to involvement of cervical sympathetic chain.
   - If pericardium is invaded, there may be pericardial effusion.
   - Stridor—when lower trachea, carina and main bronchi are compressed by tumor.
3. Features of distant metastasis (in liver, brain, bone).
4. Nonmetastatic extrapulmonary manifestations.
5. General features of malignancy—anorexia, weight loss, malaise, fatigue.

Nonmetastatic extrapulmonary manifestations (paraneoplastic syndrome): Occur in 15–20% cases of bronchial carcinoma due to secretory products by the tumour. These may precede, coincide or follow after the cancer. Treatment of carcinoma improves the features.

1. Endocrine (10%, usually in small cell carcinoma):
   - SIADH (syndrome of inappropriate ADH, usually in small-cell carcinoma).
   - ACTH secretion causing Cushing's syndrome (usually in small-cell carcinoma).
   - Carcinoid syndrome (usually in small-cell carcinoma).
   - Hypercalcaemia due to release of parathormone-like substance (usually in squamous cell carcinoma).
   - Gynaecomastia due to excess oestrogen (in large cell).
   - Rarely, hypoglycaemia and thyrotoxicosis.
2. Neurological (in any type):
   - Peripheral neuropathy (usually sensorimotor).
   - Cerebellar degeneration.
   - Cortical degeneration (dementia).
   - Myelopathy—motor neuron disease like feature.
   - Retinal blindness (small-cell carcinoma).
3. Musculoskeletal:
   - Polymyositis or dermatomyositis (in all types).

- Myasthenic myopathic syndrome (Eaton-Lambert syndrome).
- Clubbing and hypertrophic osteoarthropathy (non-small-cell type).

4. Haematological (in all types):
   - Migrating thrombophlebitis.
   - DIC.
   - Thrombotic thrombocytopenic purpura.
   - Normocytic normochromic anaemia, and occasionally haemolytic.
   - Eosinophilia.
5. Heart (in adenocarcinoma):
   - Marantic endocarditis (nonbacterial, thrombotic or verrucous endocarditis).
6. Skin (in all types):
   - Acanthosis nigricans.
   - Dermatomyositis.
   - Herpes zoster.
7. Renal:
   - Nephrotic syndrome due to membranous glomerulonephritis (rare).
8. Metabolic (universal at some stage):
   - Loss of weight.
   - Lassitude.
   - Anorexia.

Types of Bronchial Carcinoma: 4 types

1. Small cell carcinoma—20%.
2. Non-small cell carcinoma—
   - Squamous cell carcinoma—35%.
   - Adenocarcinoma—30%.
   - Large cell carcinoma—15%.

Investigations

- X-ray chest P/A view (homogeneous irregular opacity).
- CT scan of chest.
- Sputum for malignant cells.
- CT-guided FNAC.
- FNAC (or biopsy) of lymph nodes (if present).
- Fibre-optic bronchoscopy and biopsy.
- PET-CT scan.
- To see metastasis—USG of whole abdomen, X-ray skull, isotope bone scan.

Treatment: Staging should be done before therapy.

1. Non-small cell carcinoma—
   - Surgery should be done, if the tumour is localized to a lobe or segment.
   - If surgery is not possible—radiotherapy or chemotherapy or combined therapy should be given.
   - In squamous cell type- radiotherapy (specially indicated in SVC obstruction, repeated haemoptysis and chest pain caused by chest wall invasion or skeletal metastasis).
   - Chemotherapy is less helpful in non-small cell type.

2. Small cell carcinoma—
   - Even small, metastasis occurs early. Surgery is less helpful. Chemotherapy is usually given. Radiotherapy may be added.
   - Usual chemotherapy—IV CDV (cyclophosphamide, doxorubicin and vincristine) or CE (cisplatin plus etoposide). Chemotherapy is given every 3 weeks for 3–6 cycles.
3. Other treatments—usually palliative.
   - Laser therapy with fibreoptic bronchoscopy.
   - Endobronchial therapy—tracheobronchial stent, cryotherapy, laser, brachytherapy (a radioactive source is placed closed to the tumor).
   - RFT (radiofrequency thermal ablation).
   - Pleural drainage or pleurodesis (in pleural effusion).
   - Drug—steroid to improve appetite, morphine or diamorphine for pain (along with laxatives if constipated). Oral candidiasis should be treated.
   - Short courses of palliative radiotherapy are helpful for bone pain, severe cough or haemoptysis.

Contraindications of Surgery

- Distant metastasis.
- Involvement >2 cm of main carina.
- Invasion of central mediastinal structures including heart, great vessels, trachea and oesophagus.
- Malignant pleural effusion.
- Contralateral mediastinal lymph node involvement.
- FEV1 <0.8 L.
- Poor general condition, severe or unstable cardiac or other medical problem.

PNEUMONIA (CONSOLIDATION)

Definition

It is defined as "Inflammation of the lung parenchyma characterized by the accumulation of secretion and inflammatory cells in alveoli".

Types

1. Anatomically 2 types—
   - Lobar—commonly involves one or more lobe.
   - Lobular (bronchopneumonia)—it is characterized by nonpatchy alveolar opacity with bronchial and bronchiolar inflammation. Commonly, involves both lower lobes.
2. Clinically 4 types—
   - Community acquired pneumonia (CAP).
   - Nosocomial (hospital acquired).
   - Pneumonia in immunocompromised.
   - Suppurative and aspiration pneumonia.

Causes of Community Acquired Pneumonia (CAP)

- Common organisms—*Streptococcus pneumoniae* (50%), *Mycoplasma pneumoniae, Chlamydia pneumoniae* and *Legionella pneumophila.*
- Others - *Staphylococcus aureus, H. influenzae, Chlamydia psittaci, Coxiella burnetii* (*Q fever*), *Klebsiella, Actinomyces israelii* and viral (influenza, parainfluenza, measles, respiratory syncytial virus in infancy and varicella).

Pathological Stages of Pneumonia—Four Stages

- Stage of congestion—persists for 1-2 days.
- Stage of red hepatisation (red, solid like liver)—persists for 2-4 days.
- Stage of grey hepatisation—persists for 4-8 days.
- Stage of resolution—8-9 days or more.

Symptoms

- Fever, may be high with chill and rigor.
- Cough, initially dry. Later on, expectoration (during resolution). Rusty sputum (due to S*treptococcus pneumoniae*).
- May be dyspnoea, haemoptysis.
- Chest pain, pleuritic (may radiate to shoulder or abdomen)
- Other features—anorexia, nausea and vomiting.

Signs (On Affected Site)

- Inspection—Restricted movement.
- Palpation—Vocal fremitus is increased.
- Purcussion—Dullness (woody).
- Auscultation—Breath sound is bronchial. Vocal resonance is increased and there is whispering pectoriloquy. Pleural rub (due to pleurisy), crepitations (during resolution).

Complications of Pneumonia

- Pulmonary—lung abscess, pleurisy, pleural effusion, empyema thoracis, pneumothorax by *Staphylococcus aureus*, acute respiratory distress syndrome (ARDS).
- Cardiovascular—pericarditis, myocarditis, endocarditis, arrhythmia, peripheral circulatory failure.
- Neurological—meningism, meningoencephalitis.
- Musculoskeletal—septic arthritis.
- GIT—meteorism (gaseous distension of stomach, intestine or abdomen).

Causes of Slow or Delayed Resolution of Pneumonia

Delayed resolution means when the physical signs persist for more than 2 weeks and radiological features persist for more than 4 weeks after antibiotic therapy. Causes are—

- Incorrect microbiological diagnosis.
- Fungal, tubercular or atypical pneumonia.
- Improper antibiotic or insufficient dose.
- Bronchial obstruction (bronchial carcinoma, adenoma, foreign body).
- Empyema or atelectasis.
- Immunocompromised patient (HIV, DM, lymphoma, leukaemia, multiple myeloma).

Causes of recurrent pneumonia (3 or more separate attacks):

- Bronchial obstruction (bronchial carcinoma, adenoma, foreign body), bronchiectasis.
- Aspiration (achalasia cardia, pharyngeal pouch).
- Immunocompromised patient (HIV, DM, lymphoma, leukaemia, multiple myeloma).

Investigations

1. CBC, ESR
   - In bacterial pneumonia—polymorpho nuclear leucocytosis.
   - In atypical pneumonia—normal or slightly increased leucocytes.
   - In viral pneumonia—leucopenia.
2. X-ray chest—homogeneous opacity with air bronchogram.
3. Sputum—Gram staining, C/S (aerobic and anaerobic).
4. Blood C/S (positive in pneumococcal pneumonia).
5. Arterial blood gas analysis.
6. Others (according to aetiology)—
   - Pneumococcal antigen in serum.
   - Mycoplasma antibody (agglutination, CFT), Coomb's test, C/S in special media.
   - Antibody against virus, chlamydia, legionella.
   - Urinary legionella pneumophila antigen.
   - CRP (high).

Treatment of Pneumonia

Sputum should be sent for C/S before starting antibiotic.

- General treatment—rest, O2 therapy, adequate hydration and chest physiotherapy.
- Antibiotic (empirically with suspicion of cause)as follows—

Community Acquired Pneumonia (CAP)

1. Mild CAP—
   - Amoxicillin 500 mg 8 hourly orally or erythromycin 500 mg 6 hourly or clarithromycin 500 mg twice daily or azithromycin 500 mg daily.
   - If *Staph. aureus* is suspected—clarithromycin 500 mg twice daily orally or IV, **plus** flucloxacillin 1-2 g 6 hourly IV.
   - If Klebsiella is suspected—ciprofloxacin 200 mg IV 12 hourly, **plus** gentamycin 60-80 mg IV 8 hourly or gentamycin **plus** ceftazidime 1 g IV 8 hourly. Duration of treatment—7-10 days (up to 14 days).
   - If Mycoplasma, Legionella or atypical organism is suspected—clarithromycin 500 mg twice daily orally or erythromycin 500 mg 6 hourly orally. Tetracycline or doxycycline may be used. Duration of treatment—2-3 weeks.
2. Severe CAP—
   - Clarithromycin 500 mg twice daily IV or erythromycin 500 mg 6 hourly IV.
   - **Plus** one of the following—
     i. Co-amoxiclav 1-2 g 8 hourly IV.
     ii. Cefuroxime 1.5 g 8 hourly IV
     iii. Ceftriaxone 1-2 g IV daily.
     iv. Amoxicillin 1 g 6 hourly IV.
     v. If *staph. aureus* is suspected—flucloxacillin 2 g 6 hourly IV or sodium fusidate is added.

Nosocomial Pneumonia

New episode of pneumonia occurring at least 2 days after admission in the hospital is called nosocomial pneumonia.

Causes

If occurs within 4-5 days of admission (early onset), organisms are similar to CAP. If occurs later (late onset), common organisms are—

- Gram-negative enterobacteriaceae—*E.coli*, Klebsiella, *Pseudomonas aeruginosa* are common.
- *Staph. aureus* including methicillin resistant *Staph. aureus* (MRSA).
- Anaerobic organisms.

Predisposing Factors

- Elderly patient.
- Bed bound, unconscious (e.g. CVA).
- Postoperative case (thoracic or abdominal surgery).
- Malignancy.
- Diabetes mellitus.
- Use of steroid, cytotoxic drugs, antibiotics.
- Prolonged anaesthesia, intubation, tracheostomy, IV canula.
- Achalasia of cardia, dysphagia due to any cause, vomiting.
- Bulbar or vocal cord palsy.
- Nasogastric intubation.
- Abdominal sepsis, infected emboli.

Treatment of Nosocomial Pneumonia

Empirical antibiotic therapy should be started which should cover gram-negative organisms —

- A third generation cephalosporin (e.g. cefotaxime) with an aminoglycoside (gentamicin).
- Meropenem or A monocyclic beta lactam (e.g. aztreonam) and flucloxacillin.
- MRSA is treated with IV vancomycin. When possible, oral therapy may be considered with doxycycline, rifampicin or linezolid.
- If pseudomonas infection is suspected—IV ciprofloxacin or ceftazidime.

BRONCHOPNEUMONIA

Definition

It is defined as wide spread diffuse patchy alveolar opacity associated with bronchial and bronchiolar inflammation, often affecting both lower lobes. In children, it occurs as a complication of measles or whooping cough and in elderly, complication following bronchitis or influenza.

Atypical Pneumonia

When pneumonia is caused by mycoplasma, legionella, coxiella or chlamydia. In this case, constitutional symptoms are more then respiratory symptoms. Features are—

- Gradual onset.
- Dry cough.
- Low-grade fever.
- Constitutional symptoms—headache, myalgia, fatigue, nausea, vomiting.
- Less physical finding in the chest.

Investigations

- WBC (normal).
- Chest X-ray (commonly involves lower lobe , may be bilateral patchy consolidation).
- Cold agglutinin (positive in 50% cases).
- Rising antibody titre (CFT) for *Mycoplasma pneumoniae.*
- Others (CFT and haemagglutination test).

Extrapulmonary Complications of *Mycoplasma pneumoniae*

- Maculopapular skin rash, erythema multiforme , Stevens Johnson syndrome.
- Myocarditis and pericarditis.
- Haemolytic anaemia (Coombs test may be positive), thrombocytopenia.
- Meningoencephalitis, GBS and other neurological abnormalities.
- Myalgia and arthralgia.
- Gastrointestinal symptoms like vomiting, diarrhoea.

Treatment

- Clarithromycin 500 mg twice daily orally or I/V or erythromycin 500 mg 6 hourly orally or I/V for 7–10 days.
- Or, doxycycline 100 mg twice daily.
- Rifampicin 600 mg 12 hourly.

Legionella pneumophila

- Outbreak of infection is associated with contaminated water supply or cooling system, or from stagnant water in cistern or shower head.
- Sporadic case, source is unknown, common in middle aged and elderly, more in smokers.
- Outbreaks may occur in immunocompromised patient, e.g. those on corticosteroid therapy, diabetes and CKD.

Features are—Initially viral-like illness with high fever, chill and rigor, malaise, myalgia and headache, dry cough, later productive and purulent. There may be nausea, vomiting, diarrhoea and pain abdomen. Mental confusion and other neurological signs, even coma may be present. Occasionally, renal failure and haematuria may be seen.

Investigations

- WBC—lymphopenia without marked leucocytosis.
- Chest X-ray—shows lobar or multilobar shadow. Small pleural effusion may be present. Cavitation is rare.
- Hyponatraemia.
- Hypoalbuminaemia.
- High serum aminotransferases, CPK.
- Direct immunofluorescent for Legionella in pleural fluid, sputum or bronchial washings. Culture on special media can be done, but takes 3 weeks.
- Legionella serology—4 fold rise is highly suggestive.
- Urine for antigen (highly specific).
- Urine R/E shows haematuria.

Treatment

- Clarithromycin 500 mg twice daily orally or I/V or Erythromycin 500 mg 6 hourly orally or I/V for 7-10 days.
- Rifampicin 600 mg 12 hourly.

CHRONIC BRONCHITIS

Definition

It is defined as "presence of cough, productive of sputum, not attributable to other causes, on most of the days, for 3 consecutive months, at least for 2 successive years".

Causes

Multiple factors are responsible—
- Smoking.
- Exposure to dust, fume, foggy environment (may be occupational).
- Dampness, sudden change in temperature—all exaggerate chronic bronchitis.
- Infection (*H. influenzae, Streptococcus pneumonae, Moraxella catarrhalis*—exaggerate chronic bronchitis).

Symptoms

- Cough with sputum, which is mucoid or mucopurulent.
- Tightness of the chest and breathlessness on exertion.
- In advanced stage, features of pulmonary hypertension and cor pulmonale are present.

Signs (in Chest)

The patient looks blue bloater (cyanosed and oedematous).

On Auscultation—
- Breath sound—Vesicular with prolonged expiration, plenty of rhonchi in both lung fields, present in both inspiration and expiration.

Investigations

1. CBC.
2. Chest X-ray PA view.
3. ECG (usually normal. In cor pulmonale, there may be features of RVH).
4. Lung function tests—FEV1 (reduced), FVC (reduced). Ratio of FEV1: FVC is also reduced (indicates obstructive airway disease).
5. PEFR (reduced).
6. Blood gas analysis—PO_2 (reduced), PCO_2 (normal or increased), pH (acidosis).
7. CT scan of chest in some cases.

Treatment

1. Smoking must be stopped, avoid air pollution (dust, fume).
2. Control of infection with appropriate antibiotic.
3. Bronchodilator—
   - Inhaled β agonist—salbutamol (200 μg 4–6 hourly), terbutaline.
   - Inhaled antimuscarinic—ipratropium (40 μg 4 hourly), tiotropium (18 μg daily), oxitropium (200 μg BD).
   - Long-acting β agonist—salmeterol, formoterol.
   - Oral theophylline (in some cases).

4. Inhaled corticosteroid—beclomethasone (400 μg BD) or budenoside or fluticasone. In severe case—oral prednisolone 30 mg for 2 weeks, followed by maintenance dose.
5. Mucolytic agents like bromhexine or N-acetylcysteine (200 mg 8 hourly orally for 8 weeks) may be given.
6. Other measures—
   - Chest physiotherapy.
   - Exercise and weight reduction, if obese.
   - Long-term domiciliary oxygen.
   - Pulmonary rehabilitation.
   - Annual influenza vaccine, 5 yearly pneumococcal vaccine and H. influenzae vaccine may be given.

Treatment of Acute Exacerbations

- Nebulized bronchodilator like terbutaline, ipratropium bromide.
- I/V antibiotic to control infection.
- Oxygen inhalation (24%, 1–3 L/min).
- I/V hydrocortisone and oral steroid (steroid is only used in acute exacerbations and unlike in asthma, it does not influence the course of chronic bronchitis).

Complications of Chronic Bronchitis

- Emphysema.
- Pulmonary hypertension.
- Cor pulmonale.
- Respiratory failure.

ACUTE BRONCHITIS

Symptoms

- Cough, which may be dry or productive (mucoid or mucopurulent).
- Fever may be present if secondary infection.

Signs

- Breath sound is vesicular with prolonged expiration.
- Multiple rhonchi in both lung fields.

Treatment

- Smoking must be stopped.
- Hot drinks, such as tea, coffee to help expectoration.
- Steam or tincture benzoin co-inhalation to relieve cough.
- Antihistamine may be used.
- Antibiotic if secondary infection.

ACUTE RESPIRATORY DISTRESS SYNDROME

Definition

Acute respiratory distress syndrome (ARDS) is defined as severe diffuse acute inflammatory process in the lungs associated with hypoxaemia, in which there is damage of both capillary endothelium and alveolar epithelium resulting in noncardiogenic pulmonary oedema.

There is increased capillary permeability, accumulation of protein-rich cellular fluid within alveoli, alveolar collapse and reduced lung compliance which results in hypoxaemia due to ventilation-perfusion mismatch and increased pulmonary shunt.

Causes

1. Inhalation (direct)—
   - Aspiration of gastric contents.
   - Toxic gas or burn injury.
   - Pneumonia.
   - Blunt chest trauma.
   - Near-drowning.
2. Blood-borne (indirect)—
   - Septicaemia.
   - Multiple trauma.
   - Acute pancreatitis.
   - Cardiopulmonary bypass.
   - Drugs—heroin, barbiturates, thiazides.
   - Severe burns.
   - Major transfusion reaction.
   - Anaphylaxis.
   - Fat embolism.
   - Carcinomatosis.
   - Obstetric crises (amniotic fluid embolus, eclampsia).

Symptoms

- Dyspnea, cough, tachypnea, anxiety.

Investigations

- Arterial blood gas analysis—hypoxemia and hypocapnea.
- Chest X-ray—shows diffuse bilateral fluffy shadows.

Treatment

- Patient should be treated in ICU.
- High-flow oxygen via mask or endotracheal tube.
- Treatment of underlying cause.
- Broad-spectrum antibiotics in sepsis.
- Mechanical ventilation is usually necessary.
- Steroid—methylprednisolone 500mg–1gm in 5% DA 200cc IV for 3–5 days.

EMPHYSEMA

Definition

It is the permanent distension of alveoli with destruction of their walls distal to the terminal bronchioles.

Causes

- Smoking.
- Cold, dust (centrilobular).
- α_1-antitrypsin deficiency.
- Macleod's syndrome (unilateral emphysema).

Symptoms: Common in Elderly Smokers

- Breathlessness on exertion and minimum cough with lip pursing.

Signs

On inspection

- The patient is dyspnoeic with lip pursing.
- Barrel-shaped chest.
- Indrawing of lower intercostal space during inspiration.
- Horizontal ribs with wide intercostal spaces.
- Wide subcostal angle.
- Suprasternal and supraclavicular excavation during inspiration.
- Prominent sternomastoid and scalene muscles.
- Tracheal tug.

On plapation

- Reduced cricosternal distance (length of trachea above suprasternal notch).
- Apex beat cannot be palpated.
- Vocal fremitus is reduced on both sides.

On percussion

- Increased resonance in both lung fields.
- Upper border of liver dullness—lower down.
- Cardiac dullness—obliterated.

On auscultation

- Breath sound—reduced vesicular with prolonged expiration.
- No added sound (rhonchi may be present if associated with chronic bronchitis).

Investigations

1. X-ray chest P/A view shows—
   - Increased translucency of both lung fields with loss of peripheral vascular markings.
   - Low flat diaphragm.

- Tubular heart.
- Widening of intercostal space and ribs appear horizontal.

2. Lung function tests—
   - FEV1 and FVC are reduced.
   - Ratio of FEV1: FVC is reduced (obstructive type).
   - PEFR—reduced.
   - Lung volume with increased TLC and RV.
3. Arterial blood gas analysis—low PCO_2 (due to hyperventilation), low PO_2, impaired gas transfer of CO.
4. Other investigations—
   - TC, DC, Hb%, ESR (polycythaemia may be present).
   - HRCT of chest (highly suggestive).
   - To confirm—biopsy of lung tissue (not a routine test).
   - In young patient—serum α_1 antitrypsin may be done.
   - ECG shows—tall P, RVH, RAD in patient with cor-pulmonale.
   - Echocardiography.

Treatment

1. Smoking must be stopped.
2. For breathlessness—
   - Inhaled salbutamol (200 mg 4-6 hourly) or ipratropium (40 mg 4 hourly) or tiotropium (18 mg daily) or oxitropium (200 mg BD).
   - If no response—inhaled corticosteroid beclomethason (400 μgm BD).
   - In severe case—oral prednisolone 30 mg for 2 weeks, followed by maintenance dose.
3. Antibiotic, if secondary infection.
4. In chronic cough—mucolytic therapy (acetylcysteine 200 mg 8 hourly orally for 8 weeks).
5. Domiciliary O_2 may be given.
6. Vaccination, such as annual influenza vaccine, 5 yearly pneumococcal vaccine and *H. influenzae* vaccine may be given.
7. Other treatment—
   - Alpha1-antitrypsin in case of deficiency.
   - Lung transplantation in young patient.
   - Surgical intervention (if large bullae).

PLEURAL EFFUSION

Definition

Accumulation of excessive amount of fluid in pleural cavity is called pleural effusion.

Causes: Four Common Causes

- Tuberculosis.
- Parapneumonic.
- Bronchial carcinoma.
- Pulmonary infarction.

Other Causes

- Lymphoma.
- SLE.
- Liver abscess brusting in pleural cavity.
- Rheumatoid Arthritis.
- Congestive Cardiac Failure.
- Nephrotic Syndrome.
- Meig's syndrome (triad of ovarian fibroma, ascites & right- sided pleural effusion).

Causes of Bilateral Effusion

- All causes of transudative effusion (CCF, nephrotic syndrome, cirrhosis of liver, hypoproteinaemia).
- Collagen diseases (rheumatoid arthiritis, SLE).
- Lymphoma.
- Bilateral extensive pulmonary TB.

Causes of Recurrent Pleural Effusion

- Bronchial carcinoma (commonest cause).
- Lymphoma.
- Collagen diseases (rheumatoid arthritis and SLE).
- All causes of transudate.

Types of Pleural Effusion: According to Colour

- Serous (Hydrothorax)
- Straw.
- Purulent (empyema or pyothorax).
- Milky or chylous (chylothorax).

Pleural effusion may be exudative or transudative.

Causes of Exudative Effusion (Pleural Fluid Protein >3 g%)

- Tuberculosis.
- Parapneumonic.
- Bronchial carcinoma.

- Pulmonary infarction.
- Lymphoma.
- Collagen diseases (rheumatoid arthritis and SLE).

Causes of Transudative Effusion (Pleural Fluid Protein <3 g%)

- CCF.
- Nephrotic syndrome.
- Cirrhosis of liver.
- Hypoproteinaemia.

Clinical Features

Symptoms

- May by asymptomatic,
- Cough, chest pain, breathlessness, heaviness in the chest.

Signs (In Chest)

On inspection—Restricted movement in affected side.

On palpation—

- Trachea and apex beat—shifted to the opposite side.
- Vocal fremitus—reduced or absent in affected side.
- Chest expansion is reduced.

On percussion—stony dull in affected side.

On auscultation

- Breath sound—diminished or absent.
- Vocal resonance—diminished or absent.

Investigations

1. Chest X-ray PA view (if small effusion, lateral decubitus view).
2. Hb%, TC, DC, ESR (high ESR in TB, leucocytosis in pneumonia).
3. Mantoux test.
4. Aspiration of fluid for analysis—
   - Physical appearance (straw-coloured, serous, haemorrhagic, chylous).
   - Gram staining, cytology (routine), exfoliative cytology (malignant cells).
   - Biochemistry (protein and sugar), also simultaneous blood sugar, protein and LDH may be done.
   - ADA (high in tuberculosis).
   - Culture and sensitiviy.
   - AFB and mycobacterial C/S.
5. Others (of pleural fluid), according to suspicion of causes—
   - Cholesterol, LDH and rheumatoid factor (in RA).
   - Amylase(high in acute pancreatitis, oesophageal rupture, malignancy).
   - Triglyceride (in chylothorax).
6. Pleural biopsy (positive in 80% cases in TB, 40-60% cases in bronchial carcinoma).
7. If palpable lymph node—FNAC or biopsy (for lymphoma, metastasis).

8. Other investigations according to suspicion of causes—
   - ANF, anti-double stranded DNA (SLE).
   - LFT (CLD).
   - Urine for protein and serum total protein (nephrotic syndrome).
9 CT scan in some cases.

Treatment

- If tuberculosis—full course anti-tubercular therapy. Prednisolone 20-30 mg daily may be given for 4-6 weeks.
- If parapneumonic—aspiration of fluid. Antibiotic should be given. If empyema—thoracotomy may be done. Thoracotomy with decortication may be necessary.
- If malignancy—treatment given accordingly. Because of recurrent effusion, pleurodesis is necessary.

EMPYEMA

Definition

Presence of pus in the pleural space.

Causes

- Bacterial pneumonia.
- Lung abscess (bursting in pleural cavity).
- Bronchiectasis.
- Tuberculosis.
- Secondary infection after aspiration of pleural fluid.
- Rupture of subphrenic abscess or liver abscess.
- Infected haemothorax.

Symptoms

- High fever, sometimes hectic, may be associated with chill, rigor and sweating.
- Malaise, weight loss.
- Pleuritic chest pain, breathlessness, cough.
- Copious purulent sputum if empyema ruptures into a bronchus (broncho-pleural fistula).

Signs

- General feature—patient is toxic, emaciated, tachypnoic, tachycardia, clubbing.
- In chest—features of pleural effusion.

Investigations

- CXR P/A view.
- Hb%, TC, DC, ESR (high ESR in TB, leucocytosis in pneumonia).
- Mantoux test.
- Aspiration of fluid and analysis (as described in pleural fluid).

Treatment

1. **Nontuberculous**
   - Drainage of pus with wide bore intercostal tube using water seal drainage.
   - Antibiotic for 2–6 weeks. I/V Co-amoxyclav or cefuroxime plus metronidazole. May be given according to C/S.
   - Surgical intervention if pus is thick or loculated. Surgical decortication of the lung may be needed, if visceral pleura is grossly thickened.

2. **Tuberculous empyema**
   - Antitubercular drug.
   - Wide-bore needle aspiration or intercostal tube drainage.
   - Sometimes surgical ablation of pleura.

LUNG ABSCESS

Definition

It is the localised area of suppuration within the lung parenchyma that leads to parenchymal destruction, manifested radiologically as a cavity with air–fluid level.

Causes

- Aspiration of nasopharyngeal or oropharyngeal contents, such as in vomiting, anaesthesia, tooth extraction, tonsillectomy, unconscious patient, alcoholism and achalasia of cardia. Organisms are aerobic and anaerobic.
- Specific infections (*Strepto. pneumoniae* type 3, *Staph. aureus, Klebsiella pneumoniae* and fungal). In HIV, *Pneumocystis jiroveci, Cryptococcus neoformans* and *Rhodococcus equi.*
- Obstruction by bronchial carcinoma, adenoma and foreign body.
- Infection in pulmonary infarction (by *Strepto. pneumoniae, Staph. aureus, H. influenzae* and *anaerobic*).
- Spread from liver abscess and subphrenic abscess (due to transdiaphragmatic spread).
- Haematogenous from other infection as septic emboli (pelvic abscess, salpingitis, right-sided endocarditis, I/V drug abuse).

Symptoms

- Cough with profuse foul-smelling sputum, may be foetid (due to anaerobic infection).
- Haemoptysis.
- Chest pain (pleuritic).
- Fever, usually high with chill and rigor, with profuse sweating.
- Malaise, weakness and loss of weight.

Signs

Depends on site. If deep seated within the lung parenchyma, there may not be any physical findings. If it is near the surface, findings are—

- Features of consolidation, usually.
- Rarely, features of cavitation.
- Sometimes, combined features of consolidation and cavitation, if large abscess.

Investigations

- CBC (leucocytosis).
- X-ray chest (cavity with air–fluid level).
- Sputum examination—Gram staining, C/S (both aerobic and anaerobic), AFB, fungus, malignant cells.
- Bronchoscopy (to exclude mass and foreign body).
- CT or MRI (in some cases).
- Blood sugar.

Treatment

Sputum is sent for C/S and broad-spectrum antibiotic should be started.

- Amoxicillin or co-amoxiclav or erythromycin **plus** metronidazole. Or, cefuroxime 1 g IV 6 hourly **plus** metronidazole 500 mg IV 8 hourly for 5 days, followed by cefaclor **plus** metronidazole (in 70% cases anaerobic organisms are present, but mixed organisms are also common).
- If improves, continue as above. If no response, antibiotic is given according to C/S. Treatment should be continued for 4–6 weeks.
- Postural drainage and chest physiotherapy.
- If no response to medical therapy (occurs in 1–10% cases), percutaneous aspiration (USG or CT guided).
- Sometimes, surgery (lobectomy) may be done.
- Treatment of the cause, if present.

Indications of Surgery

- No clinical response.
- Increasing size of the abscess.
- Massive haemorrhage or haemoptysis.

MEDIASTINAL MASS

Mediastinum is divided into four groups:

- Superior mediastinum—above the line drawn below the lower border of 4th thoracic vertebra and upper end of body of sternum.
- Anterior mediastinum—part in front of the heart.
- Middle mediastinum—part between anterior and posterior compartment.
- Posterior mediastinum—part behind the heart.

Differential diagnosis of mediastinal mass according to following sites:

Mass in Superior Mediastinum

- Retrosternal goitre.
- Thymic tumour.
- Dermoid cyst, teratoma.
- Lymphoma.
- Aortic aneurysm.

Mass in Anterior Mediastinum

- Retrosternal goitre.
- Thymic tumour or cyst, aneurysm of ascending aorta.
- Dermoid cyst, teratoma.
- Pericardial cyst or pad of fat, Morgagni hernia.

Mass in Middle Mediastinum

- Bronchial carcinoma, hilar gland enlargement (lymphoma, sarcoidosis), bronchial cyst, hiatus hernia.

Mass in Posterior Mediastinum

- Neurogenic tumour (neurofibroma), paravertebralmass.
- Dilated oesophagus (achalasia cardia), aortic aneurysm.
- Hiatus hernia, Bochdalek hernia.

Bochdalek hernia: Foramen Bochdalek persists as a developmental defect in the diaphragm posteriorly. Around 90% remain on the left side.

Morgagni hernia: Foramen Morgagni persist as a developmental defect in the diaphragm anteriorly. Around 90% remain on the right side.

Features of Mediastinal Mass

Signs and symptoms of mediastinal mass occur due to involvement and pressure effect on different structures present in mediastinum. Examples:

- Trachea and main bronchus—stridor, breathlessness, collapse of lung.
- Oesophagus—dysphagia.
- Phrenic nerve—diaphragmatic palsy.
- Left recurrent laryngeal nerve—palsy leads to left vocalcord paralysis, causing hoarseness of voice and bovine cough.

- Sympathetic trunk—Horner's syndrome.
- Superior vena cava—SVC obstruction (puffy, plethoric face, engorged, nonpulsatile neck veins).
- Pericardium—pericarditis and pericardial effusion.

Dermoid cyst: It is a benign teratoma arising from totipotent stem cells, comprising derivatives from all the three germ layers. Mainly, it contains tissue of ectodermal origin. Calcification may be seen. About 30% of the cases are malignant. CT or MRI and CT-guided FNAC may be helpful for diagnosis.

SUPERIOR VENA CAVAL OBSTRUCTION

Causes of SVC Obstruction

1. Bronchial carcinoma (commonest, in 75%).
2. Lymphoma (in early age, also in the elderly).
3. Other causes—
   - Retrosternal thyroid.
   - Thymoma.
   - Mediastinal fibrosis (its causes are—idiopathic, radiation, methysergide used in migraine, histoplasmosis).

- Metastasis to the mediastinum.
- Giant aortic aneurysm.
- Carcinoma of oesophagus.
- Rarely thrombosis, invasion by malignancy and chronic constrictive pericarditis.

Symptoms

- Breathlessness, cough, hoarseness of voice, stridor and dysphagia.
- Flushing, red, puffy and oedematous face.
- Headache (early morning), which becomes severe with coughing. May be syncope, dizziness or blackout, stupor, seizure (due to increased intracranial pressure).

Signs

1. Face—oedematous or puffy, red, plethoric and cyanosed.
2. Eyes:
   - Periorbital oedema.
   - Red eyes, congested conjunctiva (blood shot eyes).
   - Chemosis (conjunctival oedema).
3. Neck—swollen, neck veins are engorged and nonpulsatile.
4. Visible tortuous veins in chest wall and abdomen, flow is downward.
5. Upper limb may be oedematous with prominent engorged veins.

Investigations

- Chest X-ray.
- Sputum for malignant cells.
- CT or MRI of chest.
- If palpable lymph node—FNAC or biopsy.

Treatment: According to cause

- If cause is bronchial carcinoma—radiotherapy in non-small cell carcinoma and chemotherapy for small cell carcinoma.
- Lymphoma—treatment should be given accordingly (usually chemotherapy).
- To relieve oedema—intravenous frusemide, head should be raised. Dexamethasone may be used.

PNEUMOTHORAX

Definition

Presence of air in the pleural cavity.

Causes

1. **Spontaneous:**
   a. Primary—Without underlying lung disease. It is due to—
      - Rupture of apical subpleural bleb due to congenital defect in connective tissue of alveolar walls. Common in young, 15–30 years of age.
      - Rupture of subpleural emphysematous bullae or pulmonary end of pleural adhesion.

   b. Secondary—due to preexisting lung disease. Causes are—
      - Commonly COPD and tuberculosis.
      - Others—lung abscess, acute severe asthma, bronchial carcinoma, pulmonary infarction.
2. **Traumatic:**
   - Iatrogenic—during aspiration of pleural fluid, thoracic surgery, lung biopsy or pleural biopsy.
   - Chest wall injury.

Symptoms

- Sudden unilateral pleuritic chest pain.
- Breathlessness.

Signs (in chest): In affected side

Inspection

Restricted movement of chest

Pulpation

- Trachea and apex beat—shifted to the opposite side.
- Vocal fremitus reduced in affected side.
- Chest expansion—reduced in affected side.

Purcussion

Hyperresonance.

Auscultation

- Breath sound diminished or absent.
- Vocal resonance diminished or absent.

Investigations

- Chest X-ray P/A view (shows translucent shadow with collapse lung margin, trachea & heart shifted to the opposite side).
- Sometimes, CT scan of chest.
- Other investigations according to the suspicion of cause.

Treatment

1. In small pneumothorax—
   - Spontaneous resolution occurs. Follow up at 2 weeks interval (repeat chest X-ray).
   - Avoid strenuous exercise.
2. In moderate to large with breathlessness—Percutaneous needle aspiration of air (2–5 litre).
3. In secondary pneumothorax—Water seal drainage should be given.
4. Open pneumothorax—Surgery.
5. Tension pneumothorax (see below).

Advise to the Patient

- Must stop smoking.
- Avoid air travel for 6 weeks after normal chest X-ray.
- Diving should be permanently avoided

TENSION PNEUMOTHORAX

Definition

It is a valvular type of pneumothorax, in which there is a communication between lung and pleural cavity with one way valve, which allows air to enter during inspiration and prevents to leave during expiration. It causes shifting of mediastinum to the opposite side, compresses opposite lung and heart.

Causes

- Traumatic.
- Mechanical ventilation at high pressure.
- Rarely, spontaneous pneumothorax.

Features of Tension Pneumothorax

- Severe and progressively increasing dyspnoea.
- Features of shock (hypotension, central cyanosis and tachycardia).
- Severe chest pain.
- Tachycardia, pulsus paradoxus.

Treatment

- Immediate insertion of wide-bore needle in second intercostal space in mid-clavicular line.
- Intrathoracic tube is inserted in fourth or fifth or sixth intercostal space in midaxillary line.
- Patient should be kept propped up .
- If bubbling ceases, repeat chest X-ray. If the lung re-expands, tube may be removed after 24 hours.
- If no response or continued bubbling for 5–7 days, surgical treatment may be necessary.
- Advise to the patient—never raise the bottle above the chest wall, it must be kept below the level of chest.

SARCOIDOSIS

Definition

It is a multisystem granulomatous disease of unknown aetiology characterized by noncaseating granuloma in different organs.

Cause

Unknown. There is an imbalance between subset of T lymphocyte and disturbance of cell-mediated immunity.

Symptoms

Common in young , in 3rd or 4th decade, more in females.

- May be asymptomatic.
- Constitutional symptoms—fever, arthralgia, polyarthritis.
- Pulmonary symptom—cough, breathlessness on exertion.
- Other features—according to the involvement of organ.

Sign

1. In skin—erythema nodosum, lupus pernio, maculopapular rash, plaque, subcutaneous nodules, hypo- or hyperpigmentation
2. Generalized lymphadenopathy, bilateral parotid enlargement.
3. Hepatosplenomegaly.
4. Others—according to the involvement of organ (see below).
   - Ocular—episcleritis, scleritis, uveitis, keratoconjunctivitis sicca, lacrimal gland enlargement.
   - Metabolic manifestations—hypercalcaemia (in 10% cases).
   - Central nervous system—rare (2%), called neurosarcoid. There may be cranial nerve palsy, meningism, seizure, psychosis, diabetes insipidus.
   - Bone and joint involvement—arthralgia, bone cysts (in the digits).
   - Cardiac involvement—arrhythmias, conduction defects, cardiomyopathy, congestive cardiac failure.

NB: Presence of fever, arthritis or arthralgia, erythema nodosum with BHL in chest X-ray is highly suggestive of sarcoidosis.

Investigations

- CBC, ESR (lymphopenia, high ESR).
- MT (usually negative).
- Serum calcium and γ-globulin (usually high).
- X-ray chest (shows BHL, reticulonodular shadow, pulmonary fibrosis, honeycomb shadow, miliary mottling).
- X-ray of hands or feet (cyst may be found in the phalanges).
- X-ray kidney (may show nephrocalcinosis).
- HRCT of chest.
- Lung function tests (restrictive lung disease, reduction of gas transfer).

- Liver function tests (usually abnormal).
- Bronchoscopy (shows cobble-stone appearance of mucosa).
- Bronchoalveolar lavage (shows increased CD4:CD8 T-cell ratio. Increase neutrophil in pulmonary fibrosis).
- Lung biopsy—transbronchial or percutaneous or open biopsy (shows noncaseating granuloma).
- FNAC or biopsy from other involved site—Lymph node, skin nodule, liver, lacrimal gland.
- Others:
  - ACE in blood (increased level indicates active sarcoidosis).
  - 67Gallium scanning of lung (abnormal diffuse uptake).

Radiological Stages in Sarcoidosis

Stage I: Bilataral hilar lymphadenopathy (BHL)

Stage II: BHL and parenchymal lung involvement.

Stage III: Lung parenchymal involvement without BHL.

Stage IV: Pulmonary fibrosis.

Treatment

1. Acute with erythema nodosum—Bed rest with NSAID. Spontaneous resolution occurs usually.
2. If no improvement in 6 months—prednisolone should be given, 20–40 mg for 6 weeks, then alternate day 15 mg for 6–12 months.
3. Other treatment:
   - Avoid strong sunlight
   - Topical steroid for uveitis.
   - Inhaled corticosteroid.
   - Chloroquine, hydroxychloroquine, low-dose thalidomide may be useful in cutaneous sarcoid.
   - In severe disease with no response to steroid—Methotrexate 10–20 mg weekly or azathioprine 50–100 mg daily or TNF-a blocker (infliximab, etanercept).
   - Single lung transplantation may be done in selected case.

Indications of Steroid

- Severe symptoms, such as persistent erythema nodosum, fever, arthritis or arthralgia.
- Parenchymal lung disease.
- Vital organ involvement (eye, central nervous system, heart, kidney).
- Hypercalcaemia.

Two Syndrome in Sarcoidosis

1. **Lofgren syndrome**—When there is erythema nodosum, polyarthralgia and BHL, it is called Lofgren syndrome.
2. **Heerfordt-Waldenström syndrome** (also called uveoparotid fever)—It is characterized by fever, bilateral parotid enlargement, anterior uveitis and lower motor neuron facial palsy.

CHRONIC OBSTRUCTIVE PULMONARY DISEASE

Definition

Chronic obstructive pulmonary disease (COPD) is a disease characterised by airflow limitation, which is chronic, slowly progressive and not fully reversible.

It is diagnosed by history and spirometry. Postbronchodilator shows FEV1 <80% predicted and FEV1: FVC <70% predicted.

Risk factors or causes of COPD: Multiple factors may be responsible, such as—

1. Exposure to—
   - Smoking (commonest)—active or passive.
   - Indoor and outdoor air pollution.
   - Occupation—exposure to dust, fumes, smokes, chemicals (e.g. coal miners and those who work with cadmium).
   - Urban dweller.
   - Low socioeconomic status.
   - Low birth weight.
   - Poor lung growth which may be due to childhood infections or maternal smoking.
   - Infections—recurrent lung infection, persistent adenovirus in lung tissue.
2. Host factors—
   - Genetic factors—α_1 antitrypsin deficiency.
   - Airway hyperreactivity.

Symptoms

Usually, the patient is above 40 years, male and smoker.

- Chronic cough and sputum production, which is progressively increasing.
- Progressively increasing breathlessness.

Signs (in Chest)

On inspection—

- The patient is dyspnoeic, respiratory rate is high.
- The chest is barrel shaped.
- Indrawing of lower intercostal space on inspiration.
- Suprasternal and supraclavicular space excavation.
- Prominent accessory muscles of respiration.

On Palpation—

- Tracheal tug is present (descent of trachea during inspiration).
- Crico-sternal distance is reduced (normally three fingers or more).
- Chest expansion is reduced and chest movement is vertical.
- Vocal fremitus is reduced on both sides.

On Percussion—

- Increased resonance in both lung fields.
- Obliteration of liver and cardiac dullness.

On auscultation—
- Breath sound is diminished vesicular with prolonged expiration.
- Rhonchi may be present.
- Vocal resonance—normal.

Investigations
1. CBC—may be polycythaemia.
2. Chest X-ray PA view.
3. Lung function tests—
   - FEV1 and FVC are reduced. Ratio of FEV1:FVC is also reduced (indicates obstructive airway disease).
   - Postbronchodilator FEV1 <80% of the predicted value and FEV1/FVC is <70%.
4. Arterial blood gas analysis—Often normal at rest, PO_2 (reduced), PCO_2 (normal or increased), pH (acidosis).
5. HRCT.

Treatment
1. Smoking must be stopped.
2. Avoidance of dust, fume, smoke.
3. Drug therapy—
   - Short-acting inhaled bronchodilator like β2 agonist (salbutamol, terbutaline) or anticholinergic (ipratropium) when needed.
   - Long acting bronchodilator like β2 agonist (e.g. salmeterol, formoterol).
   - Inhaled steroid (fluticasone).
   - Long-term oxygen, if chronic respiratory failure.
4. Other therapy—
   - Oxygen, if needed.
   - Mucolytic (N-acetylcysteine).
   - Antibiotics (if infection).
   - Diuretic (if oedema).
   - Pulmonary rehabilitation.
   - Pneumococcal and influenza vaccination.
   - Reduction of obesity.
5. Surgical intervention—
   - Bullectomy.
   - Lung volume reduction surgery (LVRS).
   - Lung transplantation.

Management of acute exacerbation of COPD (type II respiratory failure):
- Oxygen—continuous low-concentration oxygen via venturi mask to raise PaO_2 >8 kPa (60 mm Hg). Initially 24% or 28% oxygen is given and increased gradually provided $PaCO_2$ does not rise unacceptably. If $PaCO_2$ rises and pH falls below 7.25, artificial ventilation or a respiratory stimulant should be given.
- Bronchodilator—nebulized short-acting β2 agonist (e.g. salbutamol) with an anticholinergic agent (e.g. ipratropium).

- Oral prednisolone 30 mg daily for 10 days.
- Antibiotic—given if infection is suspected.
- Diuretic—if peripheral oedema.
- Chest physiotherapy. Secretions should be removed by suction.
- Respiratory support—If above treatment fail, noninvasive ventilatory technique like BiPAP or CPAP is occasionally needed.

DIFFUSE PARENCHYMAL LUNG DISEASE

Definition

Diffuse parenchymal lung disease (DPLD) are a heterogenous group of diseases characterized by diffuse lung injury and inflammation that can progress to lung fibrosis. Previously, it was called interstitial lung disease (ILD).

Causes

1. Granulomatous DPLD (e.g sarcoidosis).
2. Granulomatous DPLD with vasculitis (e.g. Wegener's granulomatosis, Churg-Strauss syndrome, microscopic vasculitis).
3. Idiopathic interstitial pneumonia (IIP)—
   a. Idiopathic pulmonary fibrosis (IPF), previously called cryptogenic fibrosing alveolitis.
   b. Idiopathic interstitial pneumonia other than IPF—
      - Desquamated interstitial pneumonia.
      - Acute interstitial pneumonia.
      - Nonspecific interstitial pneumonia.
      - Respiratory bronchiolitis.
      - Cryptogenic organizing pneumonia (COP, also called BOOP—bronchiolitis obliterans organizing pneumonia).
      - Lymphocytic interstitial pneumonia.
4. Rheumatic diseases—rheumatoid arthritis, SLE.
5. Drugs (busulfan, bleomycin, methotrexate, nitrofurantoin, amiodarone).
6. Other forms of DPLD, e.g. histiocytosis X (Langerhans' cell histiocytosis), Goodpasture's syndrome, idiopathic pulmonary haemosiderosis, diffuse alveolar haemorrhage, lymphangioleiomyomatosis, pulmonary alveolar proteinosis.

Symptoms

Patient is usually above 50 years.

- Cough, usually dry.
- Progressive breathlessness, usually exertional.

Signs

- The patient is dyspnoeic, hyperventilating with cyanosis and finger clubbing.
- Respiratory rate is high.
- Chest expansion on both sides is reduced symmetrically.
- Breath sound is vesicular with prolonged expiration.
- Bilateral basal end-inspiratory fine crepitations unaltered by coughing.

Investigations

1. CBC with ESR.
2. X-ray chest—ground glass appearance, bilateral reticulonodular shadow. In advanced stage, there may be a honeycomb appearance.
3. HRCT—helpful in early diagnosis, even when chest X-ray is normal.

4. Lung function tests—
   - Restrictive pattern (FVC and FEV1 are proportionately low and ratio is normal or high).
   - Reduced carbon monoxide (CO) transfer.
5. Arterial blood gas—hypoxaemia with normal or low $PaCO_2$ (due to hyperventilation).
6. Bronchoscopy.
7. Others (according to suspicion of cause).
8. For confirmation, lung biopsy is the definitive.

Treatment

- Smoking must be stopped.
- Avoid air pollution (dust, fume).
- Control of infection with appropriate antibiotic.
- Bronchodilator—salbutamol, Terbutaline, ipratropium, tiotropium, oxitropium. Long-acting β agonist—salmeterol, formoterol.
- Oral theophylline (in some cases).
- Prednisolone 0.5 mg/kg with azathioprine 2–3 mg/kg. Prednisolone is given for 2 months then tapered to maintenance dose of 10–12.5 mg daily.
- Antifibrotic therapy—Pirfenidone, N-acetyl cysteine.
- Single lung transplantation in young patient at advanced stage. Survival is 1 year in 60% cases.

HYPERSENSITIVITY PNEUMONITIS/EXTRINSIC ALLERGIC ALVEOLITIS

Definition

Hypersensitivity pneumonitis results from inhalation of wide variety of organic antigens which give rise to widespread diffuse inflammatory reaction in the alveoli and bronchioles. Commonest causes are farmer's lung and bird fancier's lung. Repeated episodes of pneumonitis progress to pulmonary fibrosis.

Symptoms

History of work in the firm.

- Breathlessness which is progressively increasing.
- Cough, usually dry.
- Weight loss, fever, night sweat.

Investigations

- CXR—shows fluffy nodular shadows in upper zone, honeycomb lung
- HRCT of chest.
- Lung function test—shows restrictive pattern with decrease CO transfer,
- CBC—No eosinophilia, may be leukocytosis.
- Antibodies in the serum
- Bronchoalveolar lavage—shows high T lymphocyte and granulocyte.

Diagnostic Features of Hypersensitivity Pneumonitis

1. Evidence of exposure to a recognized antigen.
2. Clinical and radiographic features (cough, wheeze, fever, micronodular shadows in upper, mid or lower zones, restrictive lung defect).
3. Bronchoalveolar lavage with lymphocytosis (with low CD4 to CD8 ratio).
4. Positive inhalation challenge test.
5. Compatible histopathological changes. The diagnosis is possible without histological confirmation, if criteria 1-3 are present.

Treatment

- Avoidance of allergen.
- Prednisolone 30-40 mg daily for 1-2 weeks and then tapered over the next 2-4 weeks.

RESPIRATORY FAILURE

Definition

It is defined as when pulmonary gas exchange fails to maintain normal arterial oxygen and carbon dioxide levels.

Types: Two Types

- Type I—there is hypoxaemia (PaO_2 <60 mmHg) with normal or low $PaCO_2$. There is exchange failure caused by ventilation-perfusion mismatch.
- Type II—there is hypoxaemia and hypercapnia ($PaCO_2$ >50 mmHg).There is alveolar hypoventilation with or without ventilation-perfusion mismatch.

Causes of Type I Respiratory Failure

- Acute bronchial asthma.
- Pulmonary oedema.
- Pneumonia.
- Pneumothorax.
- Pulmonary embolism.
- ARDS.
- Emphysema.

Treatment of Type I Respiratory Failure

- Oxygen inhalation in high concentration (40–60% via ventury mask).
- Treatment of underlying cause.
- Mechanical ventilation may be needed.

Causes of Type II Respiratory Failure

- COPD.
- Severe bronchial asthma.
- Obstructive sleep apnoea syndrome.
- Foreign body causing upper airway obstruction.
- Extrapulmonary causes—drugs causing CNS depression (narcotics, sedatives), respiratory muscle paralysis (GBS, myasthania gravis, poliomyelitis), kyphoscoliosis.

Clinical Features

1. Features of primary cause.
2. Features of CO2 retention—
   - Symptoms—headache, drowsiness, confusion, even coma.
   - Signs—warm periphery, bounding pulse, flapping tremor, twitching of the muscles, papilloedema.

Investigations

- Chest X-ray.
- ECG.

- Arterial blood gas analysis.
- Pulse oxymetry.
- Other investigations according to cause.

Treatment

- Oxygen in low concentration (24–28%).
- Treatment of underlying cause.
- Maintenance of airway, suction, chest physiotherapy.
- Mechanical ventilation may be required if the condition deteriorates.

NB: Respiratory centre becomes insensitive to persistent hypercapnoea in COPD patient, only hypoxia stimulates the respiratory centre. So, low flow oxygen is given (high flow oxygen is avoided, total hypoxia should not be corrected).

TUBERCULOSIS

Causative Organism: Three Types of Mycobacteria

1. *Mycobacterium tuberculosis* (causes TB in human)
2. *Mycobacterium bovis* (endemic in cattle, rarely infects human).
3. Atypical mycobacteria.

Types of Tuberculosis

- Primary.
- Postprimary or secondary.
- Miliary.

Sites of tuberculosis: Lung, lymph node, spine (Pott's disease), kidney, intestine (ileocaecal), fallopian tube, meninges, pericardium.

Primary Tuberculosis

Definition

First infection of the lung is called primary pulmonary tuberculosis. It is due to inhalation of the bacillus. Primary lesion in the lung is called 'Ghon focus', commonly occurs subpleural at the lower part of upper lobe or upper part of lower lobe. From the primary site, the bacili are carried to the hilar lymph nodes. The primary lesion with the hilar lymphadenopathy is called 'Ghon complex'.

Symptoms

- Mostly asymptomatic.
- May be low-grade fever, malaise, weakness, loss of weight.

Signs

Usually no physical sign. Erythema nodosum may be present.

Fate of Primary Pulmonary Tuberculosis

- Majority heals completely (80–90%). May calcify.
- Some cases remain dormant, reactivate later in immunosuppressed condition, e.g. lymphoma, leukaemia, chemotherapy, HIV infection.
- Some may be active, progress from the beginning.
- In few cases, bacilli may enter into the blood stream, cause miliary tuberculosis and also spread to the other organs.

Postprimary Tuberculosis

Definition

After primary infection, if there is again tuberculosis, it is called postprimary tuberculosis. It may occur due to—

- Reactivation of dormant primary lesion.
- Directly from the primary lesion.
- Reinfection after the primary lesion is healed.

Postprimary tuberculosis usually involves the lung, commonly apical segment. Cavitation may occur.

Pulmonary Tuberculosis

Symptoms

- Patient may be asymptomatic.
- Cough, dry or expectorant, haemoptysis.
- May present with PUO, pleural effusion, pneumothorax.
- General features—low-grade fever (evening rise), loss of weight, night sweating, weakness, loss of appetite.

Signs

- Emaciated.
- Clubbing.
- In lung, may be crepitation.

Investigations

- CBC, ESR (usually high).
- Chest X-ray.
- Tuberculin test (MT).
- Sputum for AFB staining, mycobacterial C/S.
- PCR.
- Xene xpert.
- In a child, sputum collected from gastric lavage or laryngeal swab (to see AFB).

Treatment

- First 2 months (intensive phase)—combination of rifampicin, isoniazide (INH), ethambutol and pyrazinamide.
- Next 4 months (continuation phase)—rifampicin and INH.
- Pyridoxine 10–20 mg to prevent peripheral neuropathy.

First and second line antitubercular drugs
- First line antitubercular drugs—rifampicin, INH, ethambutol, pyrazinamide (streptomycin and thiacetazone are less used).
- Second line antitubercular drugs—ethionamide, prothionamide, kanamycin, amikacin, ciprofloxacin, ofloxacin, clarithromycin, azithromycin, amoxiclav, PAS (para-amino-salicylate), cycloserine. These drugs are used only when first-line drugs fail or in multidrug resistant tuberculosis (MDR-TB).

Common side effects of antitubercular drugs
- Rifampicin—Hepatitis, skin rash.
- INH—Peripheral neuropathy.
- Ethambutol—Optic neuritis.
- Pyrazinamide—Hepatitis, gout.

MT (Tuberculin Test) with Its Interpretation

- MT is done by using 10 tuberculin unit (0.1 mL of 1:1000 strength PPD).
- Injection is given intradermally in forearm, reading is taken after 72 hours.
- It is positive, when induration (not erythema) is 10 mm or above.
- Only positive MT does not indicate tuberculosis.

MT positive may occur in the following cases:

- BCG vaccination.
- Previous sufferer of tuberculosis or exposure to TB bacillus.
- Present infection (should be correlated with clinical features).

MT negative may occur in (even patient may have TB):

- Immunocompromised patient (lymphoma, leukaemia, malignancy), HIV infection (if CD4 <200/mL).
- Immunosuppressive drugs (cytotoxic drug, steroid).
- Malnutrition.
- Elderly and also in newborn.
- Exanthematous disease (measles, chicken pox).
- Some cases of severe TB (negative in 25%).
- Sarcoidosis.

Treatment of Tuberculosis in Pregnancy

- INH, rifampicin, ethambutol and pyrazinamide are administered as the usual doses. These drugs do not cause harm to the foetus. Breast feeding should be continued
- Injection streptomycin should never be given in any stage of pregnancy, because it causes damage of the 8th cranial nerve of the foetus.

MDR-TB

When tubercular bacilli are resistant to both INH and rifampicin.

Diagnosis of MDR-TB

To diagnose MDR-TB, high degree of suspicion is the key point.

1. Clinically, the following features are suggestive:
   - Persistent symptoms till 2 months or more (fever, cough, haemoptysis).
   - History of contact with MDR-TB patient.
   - Worsening of symptoms with therapy.
2. Laboratory criteria for diagnosis:
   - With treatment, sputum for AFB is positive after 5 months.
   - Culture is positive after 3 months.
   - Culture and sensitivity show resistance.

Treatment of MDR-TB

Treatment of MDR-TB is expensive, difficult and lengthy, because of lack of available drugs, costs and side effects. The following combination therapy may be given:

- Ethambutol.
- Ethionamide.

- Ofloxacin or ciprofloxacin.
- Pyrazinamide.
- Streptomycin.

1. Initial phase—at least 6 months or till the culture is negative.
2. Continuation phase (sterilizing)—at least 18 months after culture becomes negative. Total duration may be 24 months, which may go up to 36 months.

Miliary Tuberculosis

Definition

It is the acute dissemination of pulmonary TB, characterized radiologically by multiple small nodules in the lungs. It is due to rupture of tuberculous focus through blood stream. It occurs in primary TB, not in postprimary TB.

Symptoms

- Fever, malaise, weight loss, night sweat.
- Cough, usually dry.
- Headache, drowsiness, confusion.
- Only PUO.

Signs

- May not be any sign.
- Hepatosplenomegaly (25% cases).
- Lung examination—may be normal, there may be few crepitations.
- Fundoscopy—choroid tubercle may be present.

Complications

- Tuberculous meningitis.
- Addisonian crisis.

Diagnosis tuberculous meningitis

It is diagnosed by:

- History of tuberculosis.
- On examination—neck rigidity, Kernig's sign.
- Fundoscopy shows choroid tubercle (in 5–10% cases).
- Lumbar puncture and CSF study (shows high pressure, high lymphocyte; biochemistry shows high protein and low sugar).

Investigations of Miliary Tuberculosis

- Chest X-ray—shows multiple military shadow in both lung fields.
- CBC, ESR (usually high).
- Sputum for AFB staining, mycobacterial C/S, PCR.
- MT.
- Other test—fibreoptic bronchoscopy, bronchial washing for AFB.
- Sometimes bone marrow study.

Miliary Mottling

It means multiple, small shadows, usually 1-2 mm, involving all the zones of both lung fields.

Nontuberculous Mycobacteria

These are usually environmental mycobacteria, also called atypical mycobacteria or mycobacteria other than tuberculosis (MOTT), rarely cause human disease. May cause disease in immunocompromised persons (HIV, previous disease with lung damage). Organisms in these groups are—

- *Mycobacterium scrofulaceum.*
- *Mycobacterium avium* complex (MAC)—both avium and intracellulare.
- *Mycobacterium fortuitum.*
- *Mycobacterium xenopi.*
- *Mycobacterium kansasii.*
- *Mycobacterium chelonei.*
- *Mycobacterium malmoense.*
- *Mycobacterium haemophilum.*
- *Mycobacterium marinum.*
- *Mycobacterium bovis.*

Treatment

- If localized lymph node involvement, excision is better.
- Most organisms are resistant to standard antitubercular drugs.
- Drugs used are combination of clarithromycin 500 mg twice daily or azithromycin 500 mg plus ethambutol 15 mg/kg plus rifabutin 300 mg/daily.

PULMONARY THROMBOEMBOLISM

Definition

It is the occlusion of main pulmonary artery or its branches by embolus arising from thrombus in right side of heart or systemic veins.

Causes

- Deep venous thrombosis from legs, also in pelvis.
- Thrombus in the right side of the heart (in atrial fibrillation).

Risk Factors for Thromboembolism

- Surgery—Abdominal or pelvic surgery, hip or knee surgery, postoperative cases.
- Obstetrical—Pregnancy, puerperium
- Cardiac—Atrial fibrillation
- Malignancy—Carcinoma of pancreas, ovary, stomach.
- Hypercoagulable diseases—Antiphospholipid syndrome, polycythaemia rubra vera, nephrotic syndrome.
- Miscellaneous—Prolonged immobility, trauma, oral contraceptive pill, fracture, varicose veins.

Types

- Acute massive pulmonary embolism—In which the embolus occlude the main pulmonary artery.
- Small pulmonary embolism—embolus occludes the small branches of pulmonary artery causing pulmonary infarction.

Acute Massive PE

Occlusion of major proximal artery causes—
- Reduced cardiac output.
- Acute right heart Failure.

Symptoms

- Severe central chest pain, crushing in nature.
- Severe dyspnoea.
- Faintness or syncope.
- Features of shock or sudden death.

Signs

- Tachycardia, tachypnoea.
- Cyanosis.
- Raised JVP.
- Loud P2, wide splitting of second heart sound.
- Right ventricular gallop.
- Features of shock.

Small or Medium Sized PE

Occlusion of segmental pulmonary or small pulmonary artery causing infarction of lung tissue.

Symptoms

- Pleuritic chest pain.
- Restricted breathing.
- Low-grade fever
- Haemoptysis.

Signs

- Tachycardia,
- Pleural rub.
- Raised hemidiaphragm.
- Crepitations (localized).
- Effusion (often bloodstained).

Investigations

1. Chest X-ray P/A view—
   - In massive PE—oligaemic lung field, enlarged pulmonary artery. May be normal X-ray.
   - Small or medium PE—wedge-shaped opacity due to pulmonary infarction, linear atelactasis, focal infiltration, raised hemidiaphragm.
2. ECG.
3. Blood gas analysis—low PaO2 and low PaCO2.
4. If pulmonary infarction—neutrophil leukocytosis, high ESR, high LDH.
5. Echocardiogram—vigorously contracting left ventricle and clot in right heart or main pulmonary artery.
6. Ventilation and perfusion scan (V/Q scan)—reduction of perfusion in major lung area.
7. Spiral CT angiography—it is sensitive and specific for medium-size embolism.
8. MRI (if CT is contraindicated).
9. Plasma D-dimer—if low or undetectable, it excludes pulmonary embolism.
10. CT pulmonary angiography(CTPA)—may be done in some cases. It is definitive.

ECG in PE

- Sinus tachycardia (common).
- P pulmonale (tall P wave in LII, LIII and aVF).
- RBBB (incomplete or complete).
- ST depression and T wave inversion in V1 and V2.
- Right axis deviation.
- SI, QIII, TIII pattern (S in LI, Q and T inversion in LIII). This is classic combination of ECG findings in pulmonary embolism.

Treatment

- High-flow oxygen (60–100%).
- Relief of pain by (morphine or pethidine).
- Anticoagulant—inj. heparin 10,000 units IV bolus, followed by continuous infusion 1000–2000 units/hour. Or low molecular heparin given subcutaneously.
- Oral anticoagulant (warfarin)—started after 48 hours of heparin therapy. Heparin is usually stopped after 5 days.
- Warfarin is continued for 6 weeks to 6 months. In recurrent pulmonary embolism, it may be required to continue for life long.
- Fibrinolytic therapy—streptokinase (2,50,000 units by IV infusion over 30 minute followed by streptokinase 1,00,000 units IV hourly for up to 12–72 hours). Or alteplase (60 mg IV over 15 minutes) is used following a major embolism. Heparin should be given subsequently.
- In massive pulmonary embolism with severe hemodynamic compromise—surgical embolectomy is necessary.
- In case of recurrent pulmonary embolism—insertion of a filter in inferior vena cava above the level of renal veins may be done.

PNEUMOCONIOSIS (OCCUPATIONAL LUNG DISEASE)

Definition

It is defined as fibrosis of the lung due to the inhalation of mineral dust.

Common Diseases are

- Coal worker's pneumoconiosis—due to coal dust.
- Silicosis—due to silica.
- Asbestosis—due to asbestos.
- Siderosis—due to iron oxide.
- Byssinosis—due to cotton dust.
- Stannosis—due to tin oxide.
- Berylliosis—due to beryllium.

NB: Symptoms are common in all pneumoconiosis, such as breathlessness, cough, with or without sputum, later pulmonary hypertension, cor pulmonale.

Coal-Worker's Pneumoconiosis

Causes

Coal-worker's pneumoconiosis (CWP) is due to prolonged inhalation of coal dust. 2 types—

1. Simple CWP—small radiographic nodules in an otherwise asymptomatic individual. Does not impair lung function and not progress once exposure ceases.
2. Progressive massive fibrosis (PMF)—formation of several fibrotic masses mainly in the upper lobes, which may cavitate.

Clinical Features

- Cough, sputum which may be black.
- Breathlessness.
- PMF leads to respiratory failure and right ventricular failure.
- Development of large fibrotic nodules in coal miners with rheumatoid arthritis (Caplan's syndrome).

Silicosis

Definition

Inhalation of crystalline silica usually in quartz by workers in cutting, grinding and polishing stone.

Usually manifests after 10–20 years of continuous silica exposure.

Clinical Features

- May be asymptomatic.
- Cough, breathlessness.

Investigation

- Chest X-ray—shows multiple well-circumscribed 3–5 mm nodular opacities, in mid and upper zones. Enlargement of hilar glands with an 'egg-shell' calcification.

Asbestosis

Definition

It is defined as fibrosis of the lung caused by asbestos dust, which may or may not be associated with fibrosis of parietal or visceral pleura.

Asbestosis related lung disease occurs in ship workers. Also, mining and milling of mineral.

Asbestosis related lung diseases are:

1. In the pleura—
   - Benign pleural plaques or calcification.
   - Pleural effusion.
   - Mesothelioma (blue asbestos is the common cause).
2. In the lungs—
   - ILD (progressive pulmonary fibrosis).
   - Carcinoma.
   - Honeycomb lung.
3. Others—carcinoma of larynx, mesothelioma of peritoneum.

Types of Asbestosis: 3 Types

1. Chrysotile (white asbestos)—90%.
2. Crocidolite (blue asbestos).
3. Amosite (brown asbestos).

PLEURAL MESOTHELIOMA

Definition

It is the primary malignant tumour of pleura due to blue asbestos.

Causes

Prolonged exposure to asbestos, commonly blue (crocidolite). Latent period between the first exposure to asbestos and development of mesothelioma is usually 20–40 years. Not related to smoking.

Clinical Features

- Chest pain (pleuritic).
- Features of pleural effusion (bloodstained).
- Breathlessness.

Investigations

- Chest X-ray
- CT scan or MRI.
- FNAC and biopsy (this may be complicated by tumour seeding along the biopsy or chest drain tract).

Treatment

- No satisfactory treatment. Does not respond to chemotherapy.
- Radiotherapy may be given.

SLEEP APNOEA

Definition

It is defined as intermittent cessation of airflow in nose and mouth during sleep. Apnoea means cessation of airflow through the nose for at least 10 seconds.

Types—Two Types

- Obstructive sleep apnea.
- Central sleep apnea.

Obstructive Sleep Apnoea (OSA)

Causes

During sleep apnoea occurs due to obstruction of upper airway. Common in obese, middle aged male.

Risk Factors

- Obesity.
- Craniofacial abnormalities.
- Upper airway soft tissue abnormalities.
- Nasal obstruction.
- Current smokers, alcoholism.
- Associated with certain medical illnesses, such as heart failure, stroke, hypothyroidism, acromegaly.

Diagnosis

Overnight polysomnography.

Clinical Features

- Nocturnal symptoms—loud snoring, cessation of breathing, insomnia with frequent awakening with choking, vivid dreams, restlessness, witnessed apnea by bed partner.
- Daytime symptoms—sleepiness, morning headache, lack of concentration, fatigue, cognitive deficit, changes in mood.

Treatment

- If obese—weight loss should be done.
- Correction of any cause—Nasal polyp, DNS, enlarged tonsil, hypothyroidism, acromegaly.
- Avoidance of alcohol, sedatives.
- Specific therapy—Continuous positive airway pressure (CPAP), oral appliances,
- In some cases, surgery, e.g. uvulo-palato-pharyngo-plasty.

Central Sleep Apnoea

Definition

It is a disorder in which apnoea occurs during sleep without obstruction of airway. Common in elderly, male, or comorbid conditions.

Causes

- Central nervous system diseases—stroke or CVD, central nervous system suppressing drugs or substances.
- Neuromuscular diseases.
- Acromegaly.
- Renal failure.
- Severe abnormalities in pulmonary mechanics (e.g. kyphoscoliosis).
- High altitude.
- Cardiovascular diseases.

Clinical Features

- Disrupted sleep, excessive daytime sleepiness, poor sleep quality, insomnia, inattention, poor concentration, fatigue, decreased libido, impotence.
- Feature of primary disease.

Treatment

- O2 during sleep.
- CPAP.
- Treatment of primary cause.

CHAPTER

4 Gastrointestinal System

CHAPTER CONTENTS

CAUSES OF MOUTH ULCER

- Aphthous ulcer.
- Trauma.
- Local infection—viral (herpes simplex), candidiasis, Vincent's angina, syphilis (chancre in primary and snail tract ulcer in secondary syphilis).
- GIT disease—Crohn's disease, ulcerative colitis, coeliac disease.
- Rheumatological disease—SLE, Behcet's syndrome, Reiter's syndrome.
- Drugs—hypersensitivity (Stevens-Johnson syndrome), cytotoxic drugs.
- Dermatological—pemphigus vulgaris, pemphigoid, lichen planus.
- Neoplastic—carcinoma, leukaemia, Kaposi's sarcoma.

APHTHOUS ULCER

Definition

It is characterized by superficial, painful, round or ovoid ulcer in any part of the mouth, usually recurrent.

Cause

Unknown. Common in young female, prior to menstruation and nonsmokers, family members may be affected. Deficiency of iron, B12 or folic acid are sometimes found.

- Single or multiple round or oval oral ulcers with inflammatory hallo often painful and usually recurrent.
- May be associated with inflammatory bowel disease, emotional stress.

Treatment

- Avoid trauma, tobacco, spicy and hot food.
- Maintenance of oral hygiene.
- Chlorhexidine 0.2% mouth wash.
- Topical triamcinolone 0.1%—applied 2–3 times daily.
- Tetracycline mouth wash.
- In severe and recurrent case—oral prednisolone may be given for a short period.
- Sometimes dapsone, colchicine, thalidomide, azathioprine may be used.
- Pain may be relieved by using local anaesthetic mouth wash, anaesthetic lozenge.

CANDIDIASIS (ORAL THRUSH)

Definition

It is characterized by multiple white patches over the surface of the tongue with some denuded area on the margin, caused by *Candida albicans*.

Underlying Diseases Associated with Oral Candidiasis

- Poor oral hygiene.
- Diabetes mellitus.

- Immunosuppressive disease, e.g. lymphoma, leukaemia, malignancy, HIV.
- Prolonged use of antibiotic, steroid and immunosuppressive drug.
- Steroid inhaler use.

Typical finding in mouth in HIV—Hairy leukoplakia (commonly on the lateral margin of tongue).

Clinical Features

Creamy white curd-like patches in the mouth and tongue.

Treatment

- Topical antifungal—nystatin, econazole, miconazole.
- Systemic antifungal—fluconazole or clotrimazole.
- Maintenance of oral hygiene.
- Antiseptic mouth wash.
- Treatment of underlying disease.

Causes of Halitosis (Bad Breath)

- Poor oral hygiene.
- Fetor hepaticus (like dead mouse. It is due to methylmercaptan, found in hepatic precoma).
- Acetone breath (sweetish, found in diabetic ketoacidosis).
- Fishy amoniacal (present in renal failure).
- Others—smoking, alcoholism, lung abscess (foetid), bronchiectasis, offensive faecal smell in gastrocolic fistula.

Causes of Gum Hypertrophy

- Pregnancy.
- Drug—phenytoin, nifedipine, ciclosporin, oral contraceptive pill with high oestrogen.
- Acute leukaemia (mainly myelomonocytic leukaemia).
- Gingivitis.
- Scurvy.

TONGUE

By looking or examining the tongue, many diseases may be diagnosed, as follows:

1. Dry or moist:
   - Dry—dehydration, mouth breathing, xerostomia (in Sjogren's syndrome), anticholinergic drug.
   - Moist—sialorrhoea in postencephalitic parkinsonism, local mouth infection, gastro-esophageal reflux disease (GERD), heavy metal poisoning.
2. Colour:
   - Pale—anaemia.
   - Yellow—jaundice (mainly undersurface of tongue).
   - Bluish—central cyanosis, methaemoglobinaemia, sulphaemoglobinaemia (involves the sides of tongue), blue-coloured food material.
   - Bluish red—polycythaemia.
   - Black tongue (lingua nigra)—ingestion of bismuth, liquorice, charcoal, Addison's disease (pigmented).
   - Brownish—CKD.
   - Magenta coloured—riboflavin (vit. B2) deficiency.
   - Raw beefy tongue (red, swollen and painful)—vit. B12 deficiency, niacin deficiency (pellagra).
   - White patches over tongue—candidiasis, leukoplakia, chronic superficial glossitis.
   - Black hairy tongue—smoking, fungal infection, tetracycline, penicillin.
   - White or greyish coating or "furred tongue"—smoking, chronic debilitating disease.
   - White and red strawberry tongue—scarlet fever.
   - Blotting paper like pallor with black pigmentation in the margin—hookworm infestation.
3. Mass or ulcers:
   - Ulcers—aphthous, malignant, tuberculous, snail track ulcer in secondary syphilis, Crohn's disease.
   - Bite mark—convulsion.
   - Squamous cell carcinoma.
   - Hairy leukoplakia—found in AIDS.
   - Papilloma (viral wart).
   - Median rhomboid glossitis (lozenge-shaped area with loss of papillae and fissuring in the midline of the tongue, anterior to the foramen caecum). It is a congenital anomaly.
4. Size and shape:
   - Macroglossia—found in Down's syndrome, acromegaly, cretinism, myxoedema, primary amyloidosis, mucopolysaccharidosis (e.g. Hurler syndrome), lymphangioma, tumour infiltration.
   - Microglossia (atrophy or hemiatrophy)—found in bulbar and pseudobulbar palsy, LMN lesion of XII cranial nerve.
   - Tongue tie (ankyloglossia).
   - Acute swelling—infection, angioneurotic oedema.
5. Neurological disease:
   - Flaccid wasted tongue with fasciculation—bulbar palsy.
   - Spastic tongue without fasciculation—pseudobulbar palsy.
   - 'Jack in the box' sign—rheumatic chorea.

- Tremor—anxiety neurosis, thyrotoxicosis, chronic alcoholism, parkinsonism.
- Fasciculation—bulbar palsy, LMN palsy of XII cranial nerve.

6. Others:
   - Geographical tongue (there is irregular red and white patches on the tongue. These lesions look like a geographic map. Slowly changing red rings and lines that occur on the surface of the tongue). It has no clinical significance but can be a sign of riboflavin deficiency.
   - Scrotal tongue (deep horizontal fissure)—no clinical significance.
   - Glossitis or bald tongue (total loss or atrophy of papillae, smooth tongue)—vitamin B12 deficiency, iron deficiency anaemia, Coeliac disease, pellagra, tropical sprue.
   - Mushroom-like tongue (sore tongue with white slough)—corrosive poisoning.
   - Central coating with red tip and margins—enteric fever.
   - Tongue tie—unable to protrude.

DISEASES OF OESOPHAGUS

Dysphagia

It means difficulty in swallowing.

Causes

1. Oropharyngeal disease:
   - Acute tonsillitis.
   - Peritonsilar abscess.
   - Pharyngeal web.
   - Carcinoma of pharynx.
   - Plummer-Vinson syndrome.
   - Pharyngeal diverticulum.
   - Disease of mouth and pharynx (stomatitis, aphthous ulcer).
2. Oesophageal causes:
   - Cause in the lumen—foreign body.
   - Cause in the wall—achalasia cardia, carcinoma of oesophagus, stricture, oesophagitis due to candidiasis, peptic oesophagitis, diffuse oesophageal spasm, scleroderma, Chaga's disease.
   - Pressure from outside—retrosternal goiter, mediastinal mass, enlarged left atrium due to mitral stenosis (Ortner's syndrome), giant aortic aneurysm.
3. Neurogenic causes—bulbar or pseudobulbar palsy, myasthenia gravis.

Odynophagia

It means pain during swallowing.

Causes

- Oesophagitis due to herpes simplex infection, candidiasis.
- Drugs—doxycycline, aspirin, nonsteroidal anti-inflammatory drug (NSAID), ferrous sulfate, bisphosphonate, slow-release potassium
- Oesophageal ulceration due to corrosive poisoning, radiation.
- Oesophageal perforation.
- Reflux oesophagitis.

Globus Hystericus

It means feeling of a lump in the throat without any organic cause. It is found in conversion disorder (HCR).

Haematemesis

It means vomiting of blood.

Causes

- Chroinc duodenal ulcer.
- Chronic gastric ulcer.
- Gastric erosion—due to NSAID, steroid.

- Rupture of oesophageal varices.
- Carcinoma of stomach.
- Mallory-Weiss syndrome.
- Bleeding disorder—haemophilia, ITP.
- Others—dengue haemorrhagic fever, hereditary haemorrhagic telangiectasia, prolong use of antiplatelet (aspirin, clopidogrel), anticoagulant (warfarin).

Factors that Affect Adversely in Upper GIT Bleeding

1. Age >60.
2. Presence of shock (pulse >100, Systolic BP <100).
3. Comorbidity—IHD, CCF, renal or liver failure.
4. Presence of oesophageal varices or malignancy.
5. Evidence of rebleeding—haematemesis or melaena.
6. Endoscopy—if active bleeding, visible or spurting vessel.

Haematochezia

It means passage of fresh blood per rectum. It indicates bleeding from lower GIT (usually large gut, also small intestine).

Causes

- Haemorrhoid, anal fissure.
- Bacillary dysentery.
- Diverticular disease.
- Angiodysplasia of colon.
- Inflammatory bowel disease (commonly ulcerative colitis).
- Carcinoma of rectum.
- Ischaemic colitis.

Melaena

It means passage of black tarry stool per rectum. It indicates bleeding from upper GIT.

Causes

As in haematemesis.

GASTROESOPHAGEAL REFLUX DISEASE

Definition

Gastroesophageal reflux disease (GERD) means regurgitation of gastroduodenal contents into the oesophagus. In some patients of GERD, there is reduced lower oesophageal sphincter tone, allowing reflux when intra-abdominal pressure rises.

Causes

- Obesity.
- Pregnancy.
- Smoking and alcohol.
- Food—chocolate, coffee, fatty food, large meal.
- Drug—anticholinergics, nitrates, calcium channel blocker.
- Dilatation by pneumatic bougie in achalasia cardia.
- Systemic sclerosis.
- Hiatus hernia.

Symptoms

- Retrosternal burning (heart burn), pain, regurgitation.
- Symptoms aggravated by bending, straining or lying down.
- Nocturnal regurgitation with cough and dyspnoea.
- Atypical chest pain which confuses with anginal pain.

Investigations

- Barium swallow X-ray of oesophagus in trendelenburg position—shows hiatus hernia.
- Endoscopy.

Treatment

1. General
   - Weight reduction if obese and avoidance of tight belts or corsets.
   - Diet aggravating symptoms should be avoided.
   - Smoking, alcohol intake should be avoided.
   - Patient is advised not to lie down immediately after food, also should avoid drinking of water while eating (should be taken sometimes after food).
   - Straining during defaecation, lifting heavy object should be avoided.
   - Head end of the bed should be raised, specially who have nocturnal symptoms.
2. Drug treatment:
   - Antacid gives symptomatic relief.
   - Proton pump inhibitors (PPI)—omeprazole, lansoprazole, etc.
   - H2 receptor blocker—ranitidine, famotidine, etc.
   - Domperidone may be given.
   - If medical treatment fails—laparoscopic anti reflux surgery may be considered. Large hiatus hernia may require surgery.

BARRETT'S OESOPHGUS

Definition

It is the metaplasia of normal squamous epithelium to columnar epithelium of lower oesophagus. More in males above 50 years.

Causes

- Usually, secondary to reflux oesophagitis. Hiatus hernia is common.
- Smoking (but not alcohol).

Investigations

Endoscopy and biopsy. If dysplastic change is found, endoscopy and biopsy should be done every 6 months.

Complication

Malignant change, usually adenocarcinoma.

Treatment

Regular follow-up. If there is dysplastic change, surgical intervention may be necessary.

HIATUS HERNIA

Definition

It is the herniation of part of the stomach into the chest through the oesophageal hiatus of diaphragm.

Types: 3 types

1. **Sliding or oesophagogastric**—In this type, gastro-oesophageal junction and part of stomach are situated above the diaphragm. This type of hernia may be present in 30% people above 50 years age and may remain asymptomatic. The sphincter is usually incompetent and symptoms of reflux oesophagitis may occur.
2. **Rolling or paraoesophageal**—less common, a part of fundus of stomach is herniated or rolled up into the chest along the side of oesophagus. Gastroesophageal junction remains in its normal position below the diaphragm and the sphincter remains competent. This type of hernia may be severe. Occasionally, it may produce severe pain due to gastric volvulus or strangulation, requiring surgery.
3. **Rarely, a mixed type**—combination of both sliding and rolling types may be found.

Clinical Features

- May be asymptomatic.
- Heart burn, regurgitation of food.
- Retrosternal chest pain.
- Dysphagia, if oesophageal stricture develops.

Investigations

- Barium swallow X-ray of oesophagus in trendelenburg position.
- Endoscopy.

Treatment

- As in GERD.
- Surgery—if symptoms persist despite adequate medical therapy (fundoplication).

ACHALASIA CARDIA

Definition

Achalasia of oesophagus or cardia is a motility disorder, characterized by failure of relaxation of the lower oesophageal sphincter due to absence or reduction of ganglion cells of Auerbach's plexus. As a result, food is collected in the oesophagus resulting in progressive dilalation.

Cause

Unknown. There is failure of nonadrenergic noncholinergic (NANC) innervation related to abnormal nitric oxide synthesis within the lower oesophageal sphincter. Degeneration of ganglion cells within the sphincter and body of oesophagus occurs.

Symptoms

- Dysphagia, both for solid and liquid.
- Regurgitation of food.
- Retrosternal chest pain (due to oesophageal spasm), may be severe.
- Repeated respiratory infection, aspiration pneumonia.
- Cough and dyspnoea due to pressure of dilated oesophagus on trachea and bronchi.
- Loss of weight.

Investigations

- Barium swallow X-ray of oesophagus—shows smooth tapering of the lower end with dilatation above, with loss of peristalsis.
- Endoscopy and biopsy.
- Oesophageal manometry—gold standard investigation.

Complications

- Respiratory—recurrent aspiration pneumonia, bronchiectasis, collapse of lung.
- Carcinoma of oesophagus (squamous type in 5–10%).
- Malnutrition (due to dysphagia).

Treatment

1. Endoscopic dilatation by pneumatic bougie.
2. If repeated dilatation fails—surgery, open or laparoscopic.
   - Heller's cardiomyotomy (circular muscle layer is cut). This may be complicated by perforation and reflux oesophagitis. So, sometimes myotomy plus partial fundoplication (modified Heller's) may be done to prevent reflux esophagitis. Proton pump inhibitor (e.g. omeprazole) should be used for long time.
   - Per oral endoscopic myomectomy may be done.
3. Medical treatment—long-acting nitrate, calcium channel blocker (nifedipine) may be used. Injection botulinum toxin in lower esophageal sphincter may be given.

CARCINOMA OF OESOPHAGUS

Types: Mainly 2 types

1. Squamous cell carcinoma (involves upper and middle parts).
2. Adenocarcinoma (involves lower third, from Barrett's oesophagus or cardia of stomach).

Sites

- Upper part—15%.
- Middle part—45%.
- Lower part—40%.

Causes

Unknown. Predisposing factors are:

- Smoking.
- Chewing of betel nuts or tobacco.
- Alcoholism.
- Achalasia of oesophagus.
- Plummer-Vinson syndrome.
- Barrett's oesophagus.
- Postcricoid web.
- Postcaustic stricture.
- Tylosis (familial hyperkeratosis of palm and sole, dysphagia).
- Coeliac disease.

Symptoms

- Dysphagia initially for solid, later for both solid and liquid diets. It is progressive and painless.
- Retrosternal discomfort or chest pain at the site of obstruction (patient can localise the site).
- Anorexia, regurgitation, weight loss.
- Features of metastases (lymph node, lung, liver, brain, bone) and tracheaesophageal fistula (cough, dyspnea, pneumonia).

Signs

- Patient is emaciated or cachexic.
- Anaemia.
- Signs of metastasis—lymphadenopathy, hepatomegaly, etc.

Investigations

1. Barium swallow of oesophagus—shows irregular filling defect, shouldering, narrowing like rat-tail appearance.
2. Endoscopy and biopsy.
3. Others—to see metastasis.
   - CXR
   - Ultrasonography of whole abdomen.

- CT scan or MRI of chest and abdomen.
- Endoscopic USG.

4. Complete blood count (CBC), erythrocyte sedimentation rate (ESR).

Treatment

1. Upper and middle parts—high-voltage radiotherapy.
2. Lower part—surgery (oesophagogastrectomy).
3. Chemotherapy (using 5-fluorouracil and cisplatin may be tried).
4. Palliative therapy—
   - Endoscopic laser therapy.
   - Repeated dilatation of stricture,
   - Endoscopic insertion of plastic or metallic stent into the oesophagus.
   - Endoscopic gastrostomy and tube feeding.
5. Palliative radiotherapy.

DISEASE OF THE STOMACH AND DUODENUM

Acute Gastritis

Definition

It means inflammation associated with mucosal injury of stomach. It is often erosive and haemorrhagic.

Causes

Mostly due to pain killers like aspirin, indomethacin, diclofenac or other NSAID's. Also due to corticosteroid, alcohol.

Symptoms

- Anorexia, nausea, vomiting, epigastric fullness or pain.
- Haematemesis, melaena.

Signs

Epigastric tenderness.

Investigations

Endoscopy—differentiates acute simple gastritis from erosive gastritis, peptic ulcer, mucosal laceration (Mallory-Weiss syndrome).

Treatment

- Antacid, proton pump inhibitor (omeprazole, lansoprazole, esomoprazole), H2 receptor blockers (ranitidine, famotidine) are given.
- Prokinetic drug (domperidone).
- Sucralfate 1g TDS in NSAID-induced erosions.
- Diet—soft or liquid.

Chronic Gastritis

Causes

- Mostly associated with *Helicobacter pylori* infection.

Symptoms

- Asymptomatic.
- Anorexia, nausea, vomiting, epigastric fullness or pain.
- Haematemesis, melaena.

Signs

Epigastric tenderness.

Investigations

- Endoscopy and biopsy.

- Biopsy shows varying degrees of atrophy and infiltration of lamina propria with lymphocytes and plasma cells.

Treatment

- Antiulcer regimen, i.e. antacid, anticholinergic, H_2 receptor blockers and mild tranquilizer.
- Avoidance of alcohol, tobacco, spices and hot foods.
- Helicobacter therapy may be given.

PEPTIC ULCER DISEASE

Definition

Peptic ulcer disease (PUD) is the break of superficial epithelial cells either in the stomach or duodenum.

Sites

- First part of duodenum.
- Lesser curvature of stomach.
- Lower end of oesophagus.
- In gastrojejunostomy stoma.
- Rarely, in Meckel's diverticulum.

Causes

1. *H. pylori* infection.
2. Drugs—aspirin or other NSAIDs, steroid, bisphosphonate.
3. Smoking, alcohol.
4. Others—
   - Acid hypersecretory disorder (e.g. Zollinger-Elison syndrome).
   - Hyperparathyroidism.
   - Crohn's disease.
   - Genetic.
   - Blood group 'O'.
   - Other associated disease—COPD, cirrhosis of liver, chronic renal failure.

Helicobacter pylori

Helicobacter pylori is a spiral-shaped Gram-negative multi-flagellete bacilli. It is slow growing and produces urease. It colonizes in the mucosal layer of gastric antrum, also found in duodenum only in areas of gastric metaplasia. Its prevalence is high in developing countries (80–90%) and low in developed countries (20–50%).

Mode of Transmission

It spreads from person to person by faeco-oral or oro-oral, either by kissing or ingestion of contaminated vomit. Infection is acquired in childhood, persist for life unless treated. Majority of the infected case remain healthy and asymptomatic, only few develop clinical disease, specially in smokers.

H. pylori associated PUD

It is associated with 90% duodenal ulcers and 70% gastric ulcers. After infection, *H. pylori* causes the following:

1. Duodenal ulcer (DU)—*H. pylori* increases acid secretion due to excess gastrin secretion and also increased parietal cell mass.
2. Gastric ulcer (GU)—also it is associated with gastritis, gastric atrophy, parietal cell loss and reduced acid production (hypochlorhydria).

Diagnosis H. pylori infection

1. Noninvasive tests—
   - Serology—anti *H. pylori* antibody (IgG), 90% sensitive, 83% specific.
   - ^{13}C urea breath test.
2. Invasive tests (antral biopsy by endoscopy)—
   - Rapid urease tests, e.g. CLO, Pyloritek.
   - Histology (modified Giemsa stain of gastric biopsy specimen)—H. pylori can be detected from the gastric mucosa.
   - Microbiological culture (biopsy material in a special media).

Indications of H. pylori Eradication Therapy

- All patients with proven gastric or duodenal ulcer.
- *H. pylori* positive dyspepsia.
- MALToma.
- Atrophic gastritis.
- After gastric cancer resection.
- First degree relatives of patients with gastric cancer.
- *H. pylori* infection should be sought for and treatment in unexplained iron deficiency anaemia, ITP.

NB: In asymptomatic case with *H. pylori* infection, there is controversy. Treatment may be considered with the hope that symptoms will be reduced and also to prevent gastric cancer.

Treatment H. pylori Infection

1. First line therapy—following combination is given for **7 days**—
   - Omeprazole 20 mg 12 hourly plus
   - Clarithromycin 500 mg 12 hourly plus
   - Amoxycillin 1 g 12 hourly or Metronidazole 400 mg 12 hourly.
2. Second line therapy—given if failure of first line therapy. Following combination is given for **14 days**—
   - PPI 20–40 mg 12 hourly.
   - Bismuth citrate 120 mg 6 hourly.
   - Metronidazole 400 mg 8 hourly.
   - Tetracyline 500 mg 6 hourly.

Duodenal Ulcer

Symptoms

- Pain in the epigastrium, burning in nature, more in empty stomach (hunger pain), also late hours of night. Pain is relieved by taking food, antacid or after vomiting.
- Heart burn, dyspepsia and sometimes vomiting.
- Periodicity—pain comes and goes every 2–3 months.

Sign

Tenderness at duodenal point which is 2.5 cm from the midpoint of transpyloric plane to the right of the midline.

Investigations

- Barium meal X-ray of stomach and duodenum—shows ulcer crater or deformity of bulb.
- Endoscopy—definitive investigation.

Complications of Chronic Duodenal Ulcer

- Bleeding (haematemesis and melaena).
- Perforation.
- Gastric outlet obstruction (pyloric stenosis).

Management: Aims of Treatment

- To relieve symptoms.
- To induce healing.
- To prevent recurrence.
- To prevent future complication.

Treatment

1. *H. pylori* eradication (see above).
2. General measures—
   - Avoid smoking, aspirin and NSAIDs (moderate alcohol is not harmful).
   - No special dietary advice.
3. Other drugs—antacid, H_2 antagonist, PPI, sucralfate, prostaglandin analogue may be given for short-term therapy.
4. Maintenance treatment may be needed in some cases.
5. Surgical treatment—Less needed nowadays. Indications are:
   - Emergency—Perforation or haemorrhage.
   - Elective—Complications, such as pyloric stenosis, recurrent ulcer following gastric surgery.

Gastrojejunostomy with vagotomy is usually done. Sometimes partial gastrectomy may be done.

Management of Peptic Ulcer Bleeding

1. I/V access and resuscitation—I/V fluid, normal saline. Intravenous PPI therapy (omeprazole 80 mg followed by infusion 8 mg/hour for 72 hours) followed by oral therapy according to improvement.
2. Initial clinical assessment—
   - Check circulatory status—see pulse and BP, urine output, other features of shock like cold clammy extremities. Central venous pressure should be monitored in patient with severe bleeding.
   - Other systems—cardiorespiratory, cerebrovascular or renal diseases, evidence of liver disease should be assessed.
3. Blood tests—
   - Blood grouping and cross matching.
   - Full blood count.
   - Urea and electrolytes.
   - Liver function tests.
   - Prothrombin time.
4. Blood transfusion—if Hb is < 10 g/dl or the patient is in shock.
5. Oxygen—if shock (pallor, cold nose, systolic BP <100 mmHg, pulse >100/min).

6. Endoscopy of upper GIT after resuscitation. When applicable, patient may be treated with heater probe, injection of dilute adrenaline or by metallic clips to stop bleeding.
7. Surgical management—urgent surgery is indicated when—
   - Endoscopic management fails to stop active bleeding.
   - Rebleeding occurs on one occasion in an elderly or frail patient, or twice in younger fit patient.

NB:

- If patient is suffering from chronic peptic ulcer, eradication therapy for *H. pylori* should be started as early as possible.
- Proton pump inhibitors should be continued for 4 weeks to ensure healing.

Complications of peptic ulcer surgery (gastric resection or vagotomy)

1. Recurrent ulcer (check for *H. pylori* and also rule out Zollinger-Ellison syndrome).
2. Dumping syndrome—This occurs following gastrectomy or gastrojejunostomy.
   - Early dumping syndrome—occurs 15-30 minutes after a meal, specially sweet food. Rapid gastric emptying of food into the jejunum causes rapid fluid shift from plasma into the lumen, resulting in reduction of blood volume. Patient presents with nausea, abdominal distension, flushing, palpitation, faintness, sweating, tachycardia and hypotension. It is usually mild, patient adapts himself. Reassurance is sufficient.
   - Late dumping syndrome—occurs 2-3 hours after meal which is due to hypoglycaemia. Patient complains of sweating, light headedness, palpitations and occasional syncope. In such case, the patient should avoid taking large meal with high carbohydrate content. Instead, patient should take small amounts of food at frequent intervals. Anticholinergic agents or subcutaneous octreotide may be given.
3. Bile reflux gastritis.
4. Diarrhoea, mostly after vagotomy.
5. Nutritional—
   - Iron deficiency anaemia due to poor absorption.
   - Vitamin B12 deficiency anaemia due to lack of intrinsic factor.
   - Folic acid deficiency due to poor intake and absorption of food.
   - Osteomalacia and osteoporosis due to vitamin D and calcium deficiency respectively.
   - Weight loss due to less intake of food or malabsorption.
6. Carcinoma stomach after partial gastrectomy.

Gastric Ulcer

Symptoms

- Epigastric distress, pain which is relieved by vomiting, antacid.
- Dyspepsia or early satiety. Even after small amount of eating, patient feels fullness of abdomen. There may be pain after eating (Table 1).

Signs

Epigastric tenderness.

Investigations

- Barium meal X-ray of stomach.
- Endoscopy.

Treatment

As above.

Table 1

Difference between duodenal ulcer and gastric ulcer:

Points	Duodenal ulcer	Gastric ulcer
Pain	Epigastrium, mainly duodenal point.	Epigastrium.
Relation with food	More in empty stomach. Relieved after taking food (hunger pain).	More after taking food. Patient may be afraid to take food.
Periodicity	Present.	Absent or less marked.
Vomiting	Absent	May be present.
Bleeding	Less haematemesis	More
Appetite	Good	Poor
Malignant change	No	May occur.

Nonulcer Dyspepsia

Definition

It is defined as chronic dyspepsia characterized by pain or upper abdominal discomfort without any organic cause.

Cause

Unknown, probably due to spectrum of mucosal motility and psychiatric disorder. Patient is usually young <40 years, women are twice more affected.

Symptoms

- Upper abdominal pain or discomfort.
- Early satiety, fullness, bloating and nausea after meal.
- Symptoms are more in the morning. There is no weight loss.
- Symptoms like IBS may be present. Sometimes, these two conditions may exist together.
- Patient looks anxious. Symptoms may be disproportionate to clinical wellbeing. Abdomen may be inappropriately tender.

Diagnosis is often from history. No investigation is needed in young patient. For older patients or with alarming symptoms, endoscopy should be done to exclude other disease. In young female, pregnancy should be excluded.

Other investigations—ultrasonography of whole abdomen (to exclude hepatobiliary or pancreatic disease), liver function test, CBC, OBT, colonoscopy, CT abdomen when appropriate.

Treatment

- In most cases—explanation, reassurance, life style change.
- Restriction of fat, coffee, alcohol.
- Smoking must be stopped.

- Drugs—antacid, prokinetic drug (metoclopramide, domperidone) if nausea, vomiting or bloating is prominent, H_2 blocker or PPI may be given if night pain or heartburn is prominent. Amitriptyline may be helpful.
- Sometimes *H. pylori* eradication regimen may be given but the role is controversial.
- Psychotherapy should be given.

Functional Disorders of GIT

It may be in the oesophagus, small gut or large gut—

1. Functional oesophageal disorder—
   - Heart burn.
   - Chest pain.
   - Dysphagia.
   - Globus.
2. Functional gastroduodenal disorder—
   - Nonulcer dyspepsia.
   - Nausea and vomiting disorder.
   - Rumination syndrome (persistent effortless regurgitation of recently swallowed food into the mouth with subsequent remastication and reswallowing).
   - Belching disorder.
3. Functional bowel disorder—
   - Irritable bowel syndrome.
   - Functional bloating.
   - Functional constipation.
   - Functional diarrhoea.
   - Unspecified functional bowel disorder.
4. Functional abdominal pain syndrome.
5. Functional gallbladder and sphincter of Oddi disorder.

Zollinger–Ellison Syndrome (Gastrinoma)

Definition

It is a syndrome characterized by severe peptic ulceration due to excess secretion of gastrin from a nonbeta cell tumour of pancreas arising from G-cells that stimulates gastric acid hypersecretion. It is also called gastrinoma.

Pathology

The tumour secrets excessive gastrin, which stimulates excessive acid secretion. Acid output may be very high, which inactivates pancreatic lipase and precipitates bile acids, resulting in diarrhoea. 90% tumour involves the head of the pancreas, half are multiple. It may occur as a part of MEN type 1 (adenoma of parathyroid and pituitary glands). Half to two-thirds of tumours are malignant.

Symptoms

- Epigastric pain due to multiple and severe ulcers in stomach, duodenum, jejunum and oesophagus.

- Nausea, vomiting.
- Chronic diarrhoea.
- Weight loss.
- Ulcer does not respond to standard therapy or recurrence of ulcer after standard surgery.
- Bleeding and perforation are common.

Complications

- GI haemorrhage.
- GI perforation.
- Gastric outlet obstruction or stricture.
- Metastasis (commonly in liver).

Investigations:

- Barium meal X-ray—shows coarse gastric mucosa.
- Upper GI endoscopy—shows multiple ulcers.
- High basal gastric acid secretion, no or little increase after pentagastrin.
- Serum gastrin is high.
- CT scan and selective arteriography of pancreas.
- Somatostatin receptor scintigraphy combined with endoscopic ultrasound—to exclude metastatic disease.

Treatment

- High-dose PPI—Omeprazole 60–80 mg daily.
- Octreotide—subcutaneously reduces gastrin secretion.
- Surgical resection, if tumour is single. Occasionally, total gastrectomy.
- If wide metastasis or incurable gastrinoma—debulking surgery and chemotherapy are indicated.

Pyloric Stenosis (Gastric Outlet Obstruction)

Causes

- Chronic duodenal ulcer (commonest cause).
- Carcinoma of the pylorus.
- Others (rare)—congenital hypertrophic pyloric stenosis.

Symptoms

- History of duodenal ulcer.
- Loss of pain and periodicity.
- Anorexia, nausea.
- Vomiting—which is recurrent, projectile, large in volume, contains previous day's food, but there is no blood or bile. History of self-induced vomiting, which relieves abdominal discomfort.
- Food habit—patient eats breakfast, little lunch and little or nothing at dinner.
- Constipation.
- Weight loss.

Signs

- Patient looks emaciated with signs of dehydration.
- Abdomen is distended with visible peristalsis.
- Succussion splash—present 4 hours or more after the last meal or drink.

Investigations

- CBC with ESR.
- Serum electrolytes—low sodium, low potassium and high bicarbonate (metabolic alkalosis).
- Blood urea, serum creatinine.
- Endoscopy of upper GIT with biopsy (if needed).
- Barium meal X-ray of the stomach and duodenum.

Treatment

- Resuscitation of the patient—correction of dehydration and electrolyte imbalance (normal saline 3–4 L and potassium).
- Nasogastric aspiration may be given.
- Surgery—partial gastrectomy or gastrojejunostomy with vagotomy followed by PPI to prevent stomal ulcer.

CARCINOMA OF STOMACH

Sites

- Antrum—50%.
- Body of the stomach (greater curvature)—20-30%.
- Cardiac end of stomach—20%.

Benign tumour of stomach—Leiomyoma.

Types of Carcinoma of Stomach

1. Macroscopic—4 types: polypoid, ulcerative, fungating or cauliflower, diffuse infiltrative (also called linitus plastica).
2. Microscopic—Adenocarcinoma (95%). Others—squamous cell carcinoma, Hodgkin's lymphoma, leiomyosarcoma.

Causes

Unknown. Predisposing factors are—

1. Diet:
   - Preservatives in diet—nitrites and nitrates which are converted to N-nitroso compounds which are carcinogenic.
   - Diet rich in salted, smoked or prickled food.
   - Diet lacking fresh fruits, vegetables, vitamin C and A may be a contributing factor. Diet with high vegetables, fruits and low salt protects carcinoma stomach.
2. Smoking.
3. Alcohol.
4. Gastric surgery (partial gastrectomy).
5. *H. pylori* Infection—causes chronic atrophic gastritis and intestinal metaplasia which is precancerous, mostly associated with achlorhydria.
6. Others—pernicious anaemia, familial adenomatous polyposis, Ménétrier's disease, blood group A and first degree relatives.
7. Rarely—familial.

Clinical Features

1. Any patient above 40 years of age presenting with **'3A'** (anaemia, anorexia, asthenia).
2. Vomiting (if tumour at the pyloric end).
3. Epigastric pain or discomfort—not relieved by antacid, food or vomiting.
4. Dysphagia (if tumour at the cardiac end).
5. Haematemesis and melaena.
6. Mass in the epigastrium.
7. Features of anaemia (unexplained).
8. Features of metastasis—
   - Hepatomegaly.
   - Ascites due to peritoneal metastasis.
   - Virchow's gland—enlarged left supraclavicular lymph node (Troisier's sign).
   - Hard nodule around umbilicus (Sister Mary Joseph's nodule).

  - Ovarian involvement (Krukenberg's tumour).
  - Prerectal pouch—a shelf-like mass (Blumer's shelf).
9. Paraneoplastic syndrome (acanthosis nigricans, dermatomyositis, thrombophlebitis migrans).

Investigations

- Hb%, TC, DC and ESR.
- Barium meal double contrast—shows filling defect, irregular ulcer, in infiltrating type—stomach looks like tube.
- Endoscopy and biopsy.
- Ultrasonography of whole abdomen (to see any metastasis). Computed tomography scan may be needed.
- Stool for occult blood test.
- To monitor recurrence—carcinoembryonic antigen (CEA).

Treatment

1. Surgery is the only curative treatment. 5 year survival is 90% if surgery is done in early gastric cancer, but only 10% if done in advanced cases.
2. Perioperative chemotherapy—**ECF** (epirubicin, cisplatin and fluorouracil) has improved 5 year survival in operable gastric and lower oesophageal adenocarcinoma.
3. Chemotherapy—not much helpful. **FAM** (combination of 5-fluorouracil, adriamycin, mitomycin C) may be given.
4. Palliative—
   - Radiotherapy—very little role.
   - Endoscopic laser ablation of tumour tissue if surgery is not possible (palliative therapy).
   - Endoscopic dilatation or insertion of expandable metallic stent may be used for relief of dysphagia or vomiting.

Early Gastric Cancer

When carcinoma is confined to mucosa or submucosa regardless of lymph node involvement, it is called early gastric cancer. It is associated with 5 years survival in 90%. Many may survive 5 years even without treatment. It may be cured by endoscopic mucosal resection or endoscopic submucosal dissection.

Gastric Lymphoma

It is the second commonest neoplasm of stomach. Among the GIT lymphoma, 60% occur in the stomach. 95% is low-grade non-Hodgkin's B-cell type. Gastric lymphoma may be—

- Primary—arise from mucosa-associated lymphoid tissue (MALT).
- Secondary to lymph node involvement in other parts of the body.

Primary gastric lymphoma may be due to *H. pylori* infection. 85% are low grade, 40% are high grade when associated with *H. pylori* infection. Chronic antigenic stimulation result in monoclonal lymphoproliferation that may cause low-grade MALT lymphoma.

Symptoms

Similar to that of gastric cancer. Patient with primary gastric lymphoma has stomach pain, ulcers or other localized symptoms but systemic complaints, such as fatigue or fever are rare.

Investigations

Endoscopy and biopsy.

Treatment

- Primary type—anti helicobacter therapy may regress the tumour. If no response, radiotherapy or chemotherapy should be given.
- Secondary type—usual therapy for lymphoma.

DISEASE OF THE PANCREAS

Acute Pancreatitis

Definition

It is the acute inflammation of the pancreas in which activated pancreatic enzymes leak into the substance of pancreas causing autodigestion of the gland.

Causes

1. Common (90%)—Gallstones, alcohol, idiopathic, post endoscopic retrograde cholangiopancreatography (ERCP).
2. Rare—
   - Postsurgical (abdominal, cardiopulmonary bypass).
   - Trauma.
   - Drugs—azathioprine, thiazide diuretics, sodium valproate.
   - Metabolic—hypercalcaemia, hypertriglyceridaemia.
   - Sphincter of Oddi dysfunction.
   - Infection—mumps, Coxsackie B virus.
   - Hereditary.

Symptoms

- Abdominal pain mainly in upper abdomen which is severe, agonizing, radiating to the back and reduced by bending forward (called Mohammedan's prayer position).
- Nausea, vomiting, fainting attack, sweating.
- In severe case, the patient becomes hypoxic and develops hypovolaemic shock.

Signs

- Patient looks exhausted and distressed.
- Features of shock (cold clammy skin, tachycardia, low BP).
- Tenderness in the upper abdomen.
- Bluish-red or green-brown discolouration of the flanks (Grey Turner's sign) or bluish discolouration around the periumbilical region (Cullen's sign) are features of severe pancreatitis with haemorrhage.
- Mass due to pseudocyst may be found.

Investigations

- Serum amylase and lipase—high.
- Ultrasonography or CT scan of abdomen.
- Blood sugar—high.
- Serum calcium—low.
- Serum electrolytes.
- Complete blood count, CXR, plain X-ray abdomen.
- Blood gas analysis.

Complications

- Pancreatic—pseudocyst, abscess, necrosis.
- Systemic—shock, multiorgan dysfunction, systemic inflammatory response syndrome (SIRS).
- Respiratory—ARDS, pleural effusion.
- Kidney—acute renal failure
- GIT- bleeding from gastric or duodenal erosion, paralytic ileus.
- Hepatobiliary—jaundice, common bile duct obstruction.
- Metabolic—hypoglycaemia or hyperglycaemia, hypocalcaemia, hypoalbuminaemia.
- Haematologic—DIC.

Treatment

- Nil per os (NPO), nasogastric suction.
- O_2 inhalation.
- IV fluid and correction of electrolytes.
- Control of blood sugar.
- Relief of pain by tramadol or other opiates (meperidine or fentanyl). Injection pethidine 100 mg IM or morphine 15 mg IM with atropine may be necessary in severe case.
- Broad-spectrum antibiotic—imipenem, cefuroxime with metronidazole.
- LMW heparin for DVT prophylaxis.
- Treatment of primary cause, if any.
- Treatment of complications.
- Early enteral nutrition in the first 72 hours through a nasojejunal tube placed endoscopically or radiologically .
- In patients with gallstone pancreatitis, ERCP may be done to remove stone in common bile duct and sphincterotomy for those who have a high suspicion of cholestasis.
- Cholecystectomy should be performed after recovery in all patients with gallstone pancreatitis.

CHRONIC PANCREATITIS

Definition

It is a chronic inflammatory disease of the pancreas characterized by fibrosis, permanent and progressive morphologic or functional damage of the pancreas.

Causes

- Alcohol.
- Tropical or idiopathic.
- Severe chronic calcific pancreatitis (possibly due to malnutrition or cassava consumption).
- Hereditary.
- Autoimmune.
- Cystic fibrosis.
- Recurrent and severe acute pancreatitis.
- Obstructive—stenosis of ampulla of Vater, pancreas divisum.

Symptoms

- Epigastric pain—recurrent or chronic persistent.
- Recurrent attack of pancreatitis.
- Diarrhoea.
- Steatorrhoea.
- Weight loss.
- Diabetes mellitus.

Investigations

- Serum amylase and lipase may be high specially during acute attack.
- Ultrasonography, CT scan of abdomen (may show atrophy, calcification or ductal dilatation.
- Abdominal X-ray (may show calcification).
- Magnetic resonance cholangiopancreatography (MRCP).
- Endoscopic ultrasound.
- Blood sugar to see diabetes mellitus.

Treatment

- Alcohol must be stopped.
- Pain relief by tramadol. Sometimes in chronic pain, amitriptyline or pregabalin may be used. If still no response, coeliac axis nerve block may be tried.
- Endoscopic therapy—dilatation or stenting of pancreatic duct strictures, removal of calculi.
- Surgical—surgical interventions may be necessary, such as partial pancreatic resection, pancreaticojejunostomy.
- For steatorrhoea—oral pancreatic enzyme supplements, H_2 receptor antagonist or PPI may be given.

Complications

- Pseudocyst and pancreatic ascites.
- Pleural effusion.
- Obstructive jaundice.
- Portal or splenic vein thrombosis.
- Risk of pancreatic cancer.

CARCINOMA OF PANCREAS

Types

Usually adenocarcinoma (90%), which arises from the epithelium of pancreatic duct.

Sites

- 60% in head.
- 25% in body.
- 15% in tail.

Causes

Actual causes are unknown. Following factors are responsible:

- Age—above 70 years.
- Common in male.
- Chronic pancreatitis.
- Alcohol.
- Smoking.
- Environmental factors—such as petroleum product and naphthylamine.
- Genetic—in 5-10% cases. There may be hereditary pancreatitis, multiple endocrine neoplasia (MEN) and hereditary non-polyposis colon cancer (HNPCC).

Symptoms

- Painless obstructive jaundice, with palpable gallbladder—in carcinoma of head of pancreas.
- Carcinoma involving the body and tail—usually presents with pain in the epigastrium, which is deep seated, dull aching, radiates to the back, more on lying flat, feels better with bending forward.
- Weight loss, anorexia, nausea.
- Mass in upper abdomen (in 20% cases).
- Others—diabetes mellitus, acute pancreatitis.
- Rare features are—thrombophlebitis migrans, venous thrombosis, portal hypertension and marantic endocarditis.

Signs

- Patient is emaciated.
- Jaundice (if carcinoma of head).
- May be anaemic.
- Mass in the epigastrium.
- Hepatomegaly, enlarged lymph nodes, etc.

Courvoisier's law: In a jaundiced patient with palpable gall-bladder, the cause is unlikely to be gallstones, rather it is due to carcinoma head of pancreas and extrinsic pressure in bile duct (Reverse of the law—Obstructive jaundice without palpable gallbladder is unlikely to be due to carcinoma head of pancreas and extrinsic pressure in common bile duct.).

Investigations

- Ultrasonography of abdomen.
- Contrast enhanced CT scan.
- Endoscopic ultrasonography.
- Magnetic resonance imaging.
- Endoscopic retrograde cholangiopancreatography or MRCP.
- Ultrasonography guided FNAC.
- Other tests—liver function test, blood sugar, CA19-9.

Treatment

- In early stage—surgical resection (Whipple's operation—in this operation pancreas, duodenum, draining lymph node and part of mesentery are removed).
- Other treatment (usually palliative)—
  - Endoscopic insertion of stent to relieve intractable itching.
  - For pain—analgesic, injection of alcohol in coeliac plexus (USG guided or endoscopic USG guided).
  - Chemotherapy—5FU, adriamycin and cisplatin may be given. 5FU plus gemcitabine may help improve survival in advanced disease. FOLFIRINOX (5-fluorouracil, leucovorin, irinotecan, oxaliplatin) improves survival to 11 months.
  - Radiotherapy is not much helpful.

Prognosis

- Usually bad, mean survival is <6 months. Prognosis is better if tumour size <3 cm, no lymph node involvement.
- Usual 5 year survival is 2–5%.
- Following Whipples' operation, 5 year survival is 5–15%.
- If adjuvant chemotherapy is given with 5-fluorouracil, then 5-year survival becomes 21–29%.

ACUTE APPENDICITIS

Definition

It is the acute inflammation of appendix.

Cause

Obstruction of the lumen of appendics by faecolith, inflammation, worm. Infection by *E.coli* enterococci, proteus, anaerobes may be cause.

Symptoms

- Abdominal pain, colicky, initially felt in the umbilical region. After few hours, pain is shifted to the right iliac fossa.
- Vomiting—once or twice (due to reflex pylorospasm).
- Low-grade fever.

Signs

- Tenderness at Mcburney's point (it is the point in the medial two third and lateral one third of the line joining right anterior superior iliac spine and umbilicus).
- Rebound tenderness.
- Rovsing's sign—pressure over left iliac fossa produces pain over right iliac fossa.
- If not treated in time—appendicular lump may develop.

Investigations

Diagnosis is clinical.

- CBC—polymorphonuclear leucocytosis.
- USG of abdomen.
- Contrast-enhanced CT scan (CECT) may be done if diagnosis is doubtful.

Treatment

Appendicectomy should be done after resuscitation of the patient.

- NPO.
- IV fluids.
- Nasogastric suction.
- Antibiotic—IV broad-spectrum antibiotic with metronidazole.

Treatment of Appendicular Lump

Usually conservative. Surgery is done later on.

- Nothing by mouth.
- Nasogastric suction by Ryle's tube.
- IV fluid—5% DNS.
- Broad-spectrum antibiotic plus metronidazole—IV.
- After 3-4 days—when abdomen is soft, tenderness is less, stool has passed, then Ryle's tube remove, oral liquid is given followed by soft diet.
- Appendicectomy should be done after 6-8 weeks.

NB: No purgative, no exploratory laparotomy.

INTESTINAL OBSTRUCTION

Definition

It is the failure of onward propulsion of the contents of intestine.

Causes

1. Cause in the lumen:
   - Impacted faecal matter.
   - Ascariasis.
2. Cause in the wall:
   - Carcinoma of colon.
   - Stricture due to tuberculosis (TB), Crohn's disease.
   - Adhesions.
3. Cause outside the wall:
   - Hernia, band, adhesion.
   - Volvulus.
   - Intussusception.

Commonest cause According to Age

- Neonate—imperforate anus.
- Children—ascariasis, intussusception.
- Younger age—hernia.
- Elder patient—malignancy (carcinoma of colon, rectum).

Symptoms

- Abdominal pain, colicky—central abdominal in small gut obstruction, peripheral in large gut obstruction.
- Vomiting.
- Abdominal distension.
- Absolute constipation (no flatus, no faeces).

Signs

- Visible peristalsis.
- Distended abdomen.
- On auscultation—excess borborygmi.
- When paralytic ileus develops—no bowel sound.

Investigations

- Plain X-ray of abdomen in erect posture—shows multiple air-fluid level.
- CBC, ESR.
- Serum electrolytes.
- Ultrasonography of whole abdomen.
- CT scan.

Treatment

- NPO.
- Nasogastric suction by Ryle's tube.
- IV fluid—5% DNS.
- Correction electrolytes.
- Broad-spectrum antibiotic with metronidazole.
- Exploratory surgery, according to suspicion of cause.

INFLAMMATORY BOWEL DISEASE

It includes Crohn's disease and ulcerative colitis.

Crohn's Disease

Definition

It is a chronic inflammatory bowel disease of unknown cause characterized by localized areas of nonspecific granulomatous inflammation of bowel.

Common in female, M:F = 1:1.2, more in young (mean age is 26 years).

Sites

Any part of GI tract from mouth to anus, but commonly involves terminal ileum (hence, it was previously called regional ileitis). In order of frequency, sites of involvement are:

- Ileum and right side of colon.
- Colon alone.
- Terminal ileum alone.
- Ileum and jejunum.

Pathology

Lesion is transmural (all layers are involved). The disease can involve a small area of the gut, or multiple areas with relatively normal bowel in between them, called "skip lesion". There are deep ulcers which often appear as linear fissure, the mucosa between them is called "cobblestone". These may penetrate through the bowel wall forming abscess or fistula involving bowel, bladder, uterus, vagina and skin of perineum.

Causes

Unknown. Probable factors are:

- Genetic and familial.
- Diet—high sugar and fat, but low-residue diet.
- Smoking.
- Probable association with mycobacteria and measles virus (not proved).
- Abnormal immunological response.

NB: Following points are important—

- Appendicectomy protects ulcerative colitis, but increases the risk of Crohn's disease or may result in more aggressive disease.
- Oral contraceptive pill increases the risk of Crohn's disease.

Smoking in IBD

- Crohn's disease is high in smokers.
- Ulcerative colitis is more in nonsmoker or ex-smokers.

Symptoms

- Frequent diarrhoea.
- Colicky abdominal pain.

- Weight loss.
- Subacute or acute intestinal obstruction.
- General features—malaise, lethargy, low-grade fever, anorexia, nausea, vomiting.
- Patient may present like acute appendicitis. If laparotomy is done, terminal ileum looks oedematous and red.
- There may be recurrent aphthous ulceration of mouth, mass in right iliac fossa, anal fissures or perianal abscess.
- Crohn's colitis may present with bloody diarrhoea.
- Extraintestinal manifestations.

Extraintestinal Features of Crohn's diseases

- Eyes—conjunctivitis, episcleritis, uveitis or iritis.
- Mouth—aphthous ulcer, thickened lip.
- Skin—erythema nodosum, pyoderma gangrenosum, fistula in abdominal wall.
- Bones and joints—acute peripheral arthritis, ankylosing spondylitis or sacroilitis and clubbing.
- Perianal region—perianal fistula, skin tag and abscess.
- Liver or hepatobiliary—fatty liver, pericholangitis, sclerosing cholangitis (common in ulcerative colitis), autoimmune hepatitis, cirrhosis of liver, granuloma, liver abscess or portal pyaemia, gallstone and cholangiocarcinoma.
- Kidney—nephrolithiasis (oxalate stone), hydronephrosis and pyelonephritis.
- Others—amyloidosis and venous thrombosis.

Investigations

- CBC (anaemia—normocytic, may be megaloblastic due to vitamin B_{12} deficiency).
- ESR and CRP (both high).
- Total protein and A/G ratio (low albumin).
- Liver function tests (may be abnormal).
- Stool for R/E and C/S (to exclude infective cause like salmonella, shigella, campylobacter, *E. coli, Clostridium difficile*).
- USG of whole abdomen.
- Barium follow through or small bowel enema (shows narrowing of the affected segment, called '**string sign'** which is pathognomonic of Crohn's disease).
- Barium enema.
- Colonoscopy (in colonic Crohn's disease) with biopsy.
- Enteroscopy.
- Capsule endoscopy (in assessing small bowel disease).
- CT scan or MRI of abdomen.

Complications of Crohn's Disease

- Intestinal obstruction.
- Enteric fistula.
- Perianal disease (fissure, skin tag, fistula, perianal abscess, haemorrhoid).
- Carcinoma (rare, may occur if Crohn's disease involves the colon).
- Toxic dilatation of the colon (more common in ulcerative colitis).
- Malabsorption syndrome.

Treatment of Crohn's Disease

Induction of remission in active disease and maintenance of remission.

Induction of Remission

1. General measures—
   - Diet—high protein, low fat and milk free. If needed, enteral or parenteral feeding.
   - For anaemia—iron, B12, folic acid and zinc. Erythropoietin may be given.
   - Symptomatic treatment for diarrhoea (loperamide, codeine phosphate orcophenotrope). In long-standing diarrhoea, cholestyramine may be helpful.
2. Drugs:
   - Prednisolone—40-60 mg/day.
   - Combination of prednisolone and azathioprine or 6 mercaptopurine (6 MP) may be used.
   - For perianal disease—metronidazole (400 mg bd for 14 days) **plus** ciprofloxacin. 6 MP or azathioprine may be used in chronic case. Infliximab and adalimumab are effective in healing fistula and perianal disease.
   - In active and moderate to severe total Crohn's colitis or ileocolitis, treatment is like active ulcerative colitis—
     - Oral and per-rectal aminosalicylate plus per-rectal steroid should be given.
     - Oral prednisolone is indicated for more active disease or when aminosalicylate is ineffective.
     - In more severe colitis or in patient who fails to maximum oral therapy—patient should be hospitalized and treated as follows—
       - » I/V fluid and nutritional support.
       - » I/V methyl prednisolone or hydrocortisone 100 mg 6 hourly.
       - » Topical and oral aminosalicylates.
       - » If the patient does not respond to steroid therapy—I/V ciclosporin or infliximab may be given. Otherwise urgent surgery should be done.

Maintenance of Remission

- Smoking must be stopped.
- Aminosalicylate may be given, but has minimal efficacy.
- Thiopurines (azathioprine or 6-MP) is given in patient who relapses more than once a year.
- If it fails—weekly MTX should be given.
- In aggressive disease—combination of immuosuppressive and anti-TNF therapy should be given.

In resistant cases or failure of above therapy:
- Methotrexate.
- IV ciclosporin.
- Anti-TNF antibody, e.g. infliximab may be given. Relapse usually occurs after 12 weeks. So, MTX or azathioprine or 6-MP should be added to maintain remission.

Surgical Treatment

Surgery should be avoided if possible and minimum resection should be done, as the disease is multicentric and recurrence is common. Indications of surgery are as follows—
- Failure of medical therapy, intractable disease or fulminant disease.

- Complications like toxic megacolon, obstruction, perforation, massive haemorrhage, refractory fistula and abscess, etc.
- Extraintestinal complications like severe arthritis or pyoderma gangrenosum, not responding to medical treatment.
- Failure to grow in children despite medical treatment.
- Suspicion of malignancy or severe dysplasia.

Ulcerative Colitis

Definition

It is a type of inflammatory bowel disease characterized by ulceration of mucosa of colon.

Inflammatory process is limited to the mucosa, not the deeper layers of the bowel wall. There is crypt distortion, cryptitis, crypt abscess, loss of goblet cells, pseudopolyp formation.

Sites of Involvement

Large gut commonly rectum, invariably involved in 95% cases. Occasionally terminal ileum may be involved called backwash ileitis.

Types of Ulcerative Colitis

According to the site of involvement:
- Proctitis (when the disease is limited to rectum).
- Distal colitis (when sigmoid and descending colon are involved).
- Pancolitis or total colitis (when the whole colon is involved).

Symptoms

- Frequent bloody diarrhoea with passage of mucus.
- Tenesmus.
- In severe case—anorexia, weight loss, abdominal pain. Patient is toxic with fever, tachycardia.
- Extraintestinal features like Crohn's disease.

Investigations

Same as Crohn's disease.
- Barium enema—in early stage, mucosal irregularity, pseudopolyp, stricture may be seen. In chronic case, there is shortening and narrowing of the bowel with loss of haustrations.
- Sigmoidoscopy—uniform continuous involvement of the mucosa, loss of mucosal vascularity, diffuse erythema, multiple ulcers, blood, mucous or pus, pseudopolyp.

Pseudopolyp

These are formed by swollen residual mucosa in between the areas of ulceration.

Complications

1. Intestinal:
   - Perforation of colon.
   - Toxic megacolon.
   - Severe haemorrhage.
   - Malignant change.
2. Extraintestinal—similar to that for Crohn's disease.

Toxic Megacolon

It is characterized by huge dilatation of colon with severe colitis associated with fever, tachycardia, shock and cessation of diarrhoea. There is free passage of bacterial toxin through the diseased mucosa into the portal circulation. It usually occurs in the first attack of ulcerative colitis. The patient is toxic and abdomen is distended, commonly involve transverse colon.

In plain X-ray, if transverse colon is >6 cm, colonic perforation with peritonitis may occur. Barium enema is contraindicated. Computed tomography scan may be done.

Causes

- Ulcerative colitis (common cause).
- Rarely, Crohn's disease.
- Other causes are ischaemic colitis and pseudomembranous colitis.

Plain X-ray abdomen should be taken daily.

Treatment

- Nothing by mouth.
- IV fluid and correction of electrolytes.
- Blood transfusion, if Hb <10 g%.
- Hydrocortisone 100–200 mg 6 hourly IV or methylprednisolone.
- Antibiotic, if infection.
- Nutritional support.
- If no response within 5–7 days, or if the condition deteriorates, surgery should be done.

Suspicion of Malignancy in Ulcerative Colitis

Extensive ulcerative colitis of more than 10 years duration is at high risk of colorectal cancer (5% after 20 years, 12% after 25 years, 20% after 30 years). Dysplastic changes in colonic biopsy may be the early feature. Oral mesalazine therapy reduces the risk of dysplastic change. Azathioprine reduces the risk of colorectal cancer.

Treatment of Ulcerative Colitis

Objective of treatment is control of active disease and maintenance of remission.

Control of Active Disease

1. Active proctitis—
   - Oral aminosalicylate (mesalazine) plus mesalazine enema or suppository.
   - Rectal steroid (10% hydrocortisone foam or prednisolone 20 mg enema or foam) may be used.
   - If no response—then oral prednisolone 40 mg daily.
2. Active left sided or extensive proctocolitis—
   - In mild case—oral aminosalicylate (mesalazine) plus mesalazine enema or suppository and rectal steroid.
   - In moderate to severe case—oral prednisolone 40 mg daily.
3. In severe ulcerative colitis—patient should be hospitalized.
   - Intravenous methylprednisolone 60 mg or hydrocortisone 100 mg 6 hourly **plus** oral and topical aminosalicylate.

- Intravenous antibiotic, if necessary.
- General measures—intravenous fluid, blood transfusion and nutrition.
- If no response—IV ciclosporin or infliximab may be given.
- In patient with colonic dilatation >6 cm, or if the clinical condition deteriorates or who do not respond after 7–10 days with maximum conservative therapy, urgent surgery (colectomy) may be needed.
- After recovery—oral prednisolone should be given. Once remission, it should be tapered 5–10 mg weekly.

Following features indicate failure of medical therapy:
- Persistent fever.
- Tachycardia.
- Falling haemoglobin.
- Rising WBC.
- Falling potassium.
- Falling albumin.
- Persistently raised stool volume >500 g/day with loose bloody stool.

In such cases, surgery is indicated.

Maintenance of Remission

- After recovery—oral aminosalicylate either mesalazine or balsalazide is given to prevent relapse.
- In chronic cases with frequent relapse or which require steroid in high dose—azathioprine (1.5–2 mg/kg) may be given. Ciclosporin may also help.

Note: Prednisolone is used only in active disease, no role in preventing relapse. 5-aminosalicylates are mesalazine or olsalazine or balsalazide.

Inflammatory bowel disease in pregnancy:
- Pregnancy is affected adversely in case of active IBD.
- Disease should be in remission or optimized before pregnancy.
- 2/3 cases in remission will remain so in pregnancy.
- In active disease during pregnancy, role of 3 may be possible—1/3 improved, 1/3 get worse and 1/3 remain stable.
- Exacerbation may occur in puerperium, sometimes in first trimester of pregnancy.
- Drug treatment with corticosteroid, aminosalicylate or azathioprine is safe and can be continued during pregnancy.

CARCINOMA OF COLON (COLORECTAL CANCER)

Sites

- Commonest site is rectosigmoid.
- May occur in rectum, caecum, ascending, transverse and descending colon.

Types

1. Macroscopically—
   - Polypoid and fungating.
   - Annular and constricting.
2. Microscopically—adenocarcinoma.

Causes

Unknown. Predisposing factors are:

1. Dietary factors:
   - Excess consumption of red meat, saturated animal fat.
   - Less dietary fibres.
   - Less intake of vegetables and fruits (high vegetables and fruits may be preventive for carcinoma).
   - Excess and prolonged sugar consumption.
2. Nondietary factors:
   - Increasing age.
   - Genetic factors—benign adenomatous polyp or familial adenomatous polyposis.
   - Hereditary nonpolyposis colonic cancer.
   - Family history of colon cancer.
   - Long-standing extensive ulcerative colitis or Crohn's colitis, especially if associated with primary sclerosing cholangitis.
   - History of breast cancer.
   - Ureterosigmoidostomy.
   - Acromegaly.
   - Pelvic radiotherapy.
   - Alcohol (weak association)
   - Smoking (relative risk 1.5–3.0).
   - Obesity and sedentary lifestyle.
   - Cholecystectomy.
   - Type 2 diabetes (hyperinsulinaemia).

Factors which Decrease Risk of Colorectal Carcinoma

- Diet—increased fiber, fruits, vegetables, garlic, milk.
- Exercise.
- Drugs—aspirin or other NSAID, calcium, folic acid, omega3 fatty acid, combined oestrogen and progesterone hormone replacement therapy.

Symptoms

Depend on the site (may be asymptomatic):

1. If on the left side—
   - Bleeding per rectum.
   - Alteration of bowel habit.
   - Mass in left iliac fossa.
2. If on the right side—
   - Alteration of bowel habit.
   - Intestinal obstruction.
   - Mass in right iliac fossa.

Signs

Depend on site:

- Mass in left iliac fossa or right iliac fossa.
- Hepatomegaly, if metastasis.
- Others—anaemia, lymphadenopathy, etc.

Investigations

- USG of whole abdomen.
- Sigmoidoscopy or colonoscopy and biopsy (gold standard).
- CT colonography.
- CT scan of whole abdomen.
- Endo-anal ultrasound or pelvic MRI (used for staging of rectal cancer).
- PET scan is useful for detecting occult metastases.
- Barium enema (double contrast).
- Others—CBC, stool for occult blood, CEA (to see recurrence), X-ray chest.
- FNAC (CT guided or USG guided).
- Sometimes, laparotomy may be needed.

Treatment

1. Curative—surgical resection of the tumour with pericolic lymph nodes. Adjuvant postoperative chemotherapy (with 5 fluorouracil and folinic acid).
2. Palliative—palliative chemotherapy with 5FU may improve survival. If this fails, second line drug, such as irinotecan may be given. Endoscopic laser therapy or insertion of an expandable metal stent can be used to relieve obstruction.

Screening in carcinoma of colon :

- Any person >50 years of age, stool for OBT.
- Colonoscopy (gold standard).
- Flexible sigmoidoscopy is an alternative to colonoscopy.
- CT colonoscopy may be used in screening programme.

ILEOCAECAL TUBERCULOSIS

Causes

It is caused by reactivation of primary disease by Myco*bacterium tuberculosis*. May be secondary to pulmonary TB (by swallowing of sputum). Sometimes, primary TB due to *Mycobacterium bovis* (rare nowadays).

After involvement of mucosa and submucosa, intense inflammation with necrosis occurs in the bowel wall and lymphatic. Caseation is often found.

Type of Lesion and Type of Ulcer in Ileocaecal Tuberculosis

Types of lesion—ulcerative, hypertrophic or mixed.
Ulcer is transverse (in typhoid and Crohn's disease, the ulcer is longitudinal).

Symptoms

- History of pulmonary TB may be present.
- Abdominal pain is the commonest (usually in right iliac fossa, occasionally generalised), colicky in nature.
- Features of intestinal obstruction (acute or subacute).
- Tuberculous peritonitis or ascites.
- Diarrhoea or malabsorption syndrome.
- Mass in right iliac fossa.
- General features of TB—low-grade fever with evening rise, night sweat, malaise, weight loss.

Differential Diagnosis of Mass in Right Iliac Fossa

1. If the patient is young:
   - Appendicular lump (tender).
   - Ileocaecal TB.
   - Crohn's disease.
   - Lymphoma.
   - Amoeboma (less common nowadays, because of wide use of metronidazole).
   - Others—actinomycosis, yersinia, tubo-ovarian mass in females, pelvic kidney.
2. If the patient is elderly or middle aged—
   - Appendicular lump.
   - Ileocaecal TB.
   - Carcinoma of caecum (hard, irregular and nontender).
   - Lymphoma.
   - Others may be as above.

Investigations

- CBC with ESR.
- Ultrasonogram of whole abdomen.
- X-ray chest (shows TB in 50%).
- MT.
- Colonoscopy.
- Barium follow through with spot film in ileocaecal region.

- CT scan of abdomen.
- Laparoscopy to see tubercle in peritoneum and biopsy.

Complications of Ileocaecal Tuberculosis

- Intestinal obstruction.
- Fistula (entero-enteric or entero-cutaneous).
- Malabsorption.
- Perforation (rare).

Treatment

- Standard anti-TB chemotherapy (using four drugs).
- Treatment to be continued for at least 1 year.
- Occasionally, surgery (if intestinal obstruction or fistula).

TUBERCULOUS PERITONITIS

Definition

Infection of the peritoneum due to *M. tuberculosis*. It may be secondary to pulmonary TB.

Pathogenesis

Tuberculosis peritonitis may occur from direct spread of tubercular bacilli from ruptured abdominal lymph nodes or haematogenous seedling secondary to intestinal TB.

Symptoms

- Fever, weight loss, night sweat.
- Diffuse abdominal pain.
- Unexplained ascites.

Signs

- Abdomen is distended due to ascites.
- Doughy feeling.

Investigations

- CBC with ESR.
- Ultrasonogram of whole abdomen.
- X-ray chest (shows TB in 50%).
- MT.
- CT scan of abdomen.
- Ascitic fluid analysis (cytology, biochemistry, ADA, AFB, PCR),
- Laparoscopy—shows tubercle which is taken for biopsy.

Finding in Ascitic Fluid

Straw coloured, exudative (high protein and low glucose), high lymphocyte and high ADA. AFB and PCR may be positive.

Treatment

Anti-Koch's therapy, continued for one year. Steroid may be added.

IRRITABLE BOWEL SYNDROME

Definition

Irritable bowel syndrome (IBS) is characterized by recurrent abdominal pain associated with abnormal defaecations in the absence of any structural abnormality of the gut.

More common in female. Coexisting conditions, such as nonulcer dyspepsia, chronic fatigue syndrome, fibromyalgia, dysmenorrhoea may be present.

Cause

Unknown. Some factors may trigger—
- Affective disorder—anxiety, depression.
- Psychological factors (e.g. stress, trauma).
- Gastrointestinal infection.
- Antibiotic therapy.
- Sexual, physical, verbal abuse.
- Eating disorder.
- Dietary factors—lactose, fructose containing diet may be responsible.
- May be triggered by some organisms like Salmonella, Campylobacter, etc.

IBS may be—
- IBS with diarrhoea.
- IBS with constipation.
- Mixed—alternate constipation and diarrhoea.

Symptoms

- Usual symptoms are abdominal pain, bloating, alternate diarrhoea and constipation. Pain is relieved after defecation.
- Diarrhoea is usually painless, sometimes in the morning, usually not at night.
- Stools are usually pellet or ribbon like, mixed with mucous.
- Feeling of incomplete evacuation of bowel, dyspepsia, flatulence, heart burn or pain in the upper abdomen.
- Sometimes, frequency of micturition, urgency may be present.

Signs

- No abnormality, may be tenderness in the left iliac fossa
- Palpable sigmoid colon.

Investigations

No specific investigation. However, some tests are done to exclude any organic disease—
- Stool to see ova, cyst, parasite, occult blood.
- USG of whole abdomen.
- Sigmoidoscopy or colonoscopy.
- Barium enema.
- CT scan of abdomen.
- Thyroid function tests, if necessary.

Treatment

1. General measures—
   - Reassurance and explanation about the nature of illness.
   - Psychotherapy, behaviour therapy, hypnotherapy may be needed.
   - Avoid stress, depression.
   - Avoid fried foods, milk and milk products, alcohol, tea, coffee.
   - Regular meals and adequate sleep is essential.
2. If pain and distension or bloating—
   - Dietary modification, spasmolytic (mebeverine, alverine or pipperment oil or hyoscine).
   - Probiotic.
   - Rifaximin may be given.
   - Amitriptyline or imipramine may be added at night.
3. If diarrhoea is predominant—
   - Dietary modification (gluten free, milk or milk product free),
   - Loperamide or codeine or cholestyramine may be given.
   - Spasmolytic (mebeverine, alverine or pipperment oil or hyoscine).
4. If constipation is predominant—
   - High-fibre diet,
   - Isapgula husk, lactulose may be given.
   - 5-HT receptor agonist (prucalopride or linaclotide) may be given.
   - If symptoms persist, duloxetine or paroxetine may be tried.

VOMITING

Causes of Vomiting

- Physiological—pregnancy.
- GIT disorders—gastroenteritis, pyloric stenosis, PUD, carcinoma of stomach, acute cholecystitis, acute appendicitis, acute pancreatitis, intestinal obstruction.
- Hepatic—acute hepatitis.
- Renal—AKI, CKD.
- CNS—raised intracranial pressure, migraine, meningitis, encephalitis, vestibular neuronitis.
- Endocrine disorders—diabetic ketoacidosis, lactic acidosis, Addisonian crisis.
- Drugs—morphine, digoxin, cytotoxic drugs, NSAID, alcohol.
- Psychogenic vomiting.
- HCR, anorexia nervosa.

Investigations

According to suspicion of cause.

Treatment

According to cause.

- Symptomatic—antiemetic (e.g. prochlorperazine, ondansatron, metoclopramide, domperidone) may be given.
- Psychotherapy in psychogenic vomiting.
- Treatment of primary cause.

CONSTIPATION

Definition

It means passage of hard stool or bowel movement <3 times a week. Patient may complain of straining, sensation of incomplete evacuation of stool or anorectal blockage.

Causes

1. General:
   - Lack of fibre diet and fluid intake.
   - Pregnancy.
   - Immobility.
2. GIT Causes:
   - IBS.
   - Intestinal obstruction.
   - Diverticular disease.
   - Carcinoma of colon.
   - Hirschprung's disease.
   - Anorectal diseases (Crohn's disease, anal fissures, haemorrhoids).
3. Neurological causes:
   - Multiple sclerosis.
   - CVD.

   - Parkinsonism.
   - Spinal cord disease.
4. Endocrine and metabolic causes:
   - Hypothyroidism.
   - Diabetes mellitus.
   - Hyperparathyroidism and hypercalcaemia.
5. Drugs:
   - Opiates.
   - Anticholinergics.
   - Iron and calcium supplements.
   - Calcium antagonist (verapamil).
   - Aluminium containing antacids.
6. Psychological: Depression, anxiety, anorexia nervosa.

Symptoms

- Infrequent bowel movement, abdominal pain, fullness, nausea, vomiting.
- Features of underlying disease.

Investigations

Should be done according to suspicion of cause.

Treatment

- Diet—high fibre, such as bran, raw fruits, vegetables.
- Plenty of fluids.
- Ispaghula husk.
- Laxatives in some cases.
- Glycerin suppository or sometimes enema.
- Treatment of primary cause.

DIARRHOEA

Definition

It means frequent passage of loose stool more than 200g/day or passage of frequent stool 3 times per day.

Types

2 types:
- Acute diarrhoea—persists less than 2 weeks.
- Chronic diarrhoea—persists more than 4 weeks.

Acute Diarrhoea

Causes

1. Infection:
   - Bacterial—Enterotoxegenic *E. coli, Vibrio cholerae, Shigella, Salmonella, Campylobacter, Bacillus cereus, S. aureus, Clostridium difficile.*

- Viruses—Rota virus, Norwalk virus, Corona virus.
- Parasitic—*Entamoeba histolytica, Giardia lamblia, Cryptosporidium.*

2. Drugs:
   - Antibiotics—commonest cause.
   - Laxatives, prokinetic agents (domperidone), antacid, digitalis, colchicine, chemotherapeutic agents.

Symptoms

- Passage of loose stool, abdominal discomfort or pain, vomiting
- Fever if infective cause.
- Increased thirst.
- Decreased urination.
- Fatigue.
- Altered consciousness.

Signs

- Signs of dehydration (dry tongue, loss of skin turgor, tachycardia, low BP).
- Localized or diffuse abdominal tenderness.

Complications

- Hypovolaemia and shock.
- Renal failure.
- Electrolyte imbalance—hypokalaemia, hypernatremia, metabolic acidosis.

Investigations

- CBC.
- Stool for R/M/E & C/S
- Serum electrolytes.
- Blood urea and serum creatinine.
- In chronic case—investigation should be done according to suspicion of cause.

Treatment

- Fluid and electrolyte replacement—ORS, IV cholera saline.
- Antibiotic therapy (if bacterial infection is suspected).
- Treatment of cause.

Chronic Diarrhoea

Diarrhoea more than weeks or months, usually >4 weeks, which may be persistent or intermittent.

Causes

1. GIT causes:
   - IBS.
   - Inflammatory bowel disease.
   - Infectious—giardiasis, amoebiasis, intestinal tuberculosis.
   - Radiation colitis.
   - Colon cancer.

- Diverticulitis.
- Ischaemic colitis.
- Malabsorption syndrome.
- Postsurgical.
- Chronic pancreatitis.
- Coeliac disease, tropical sprue.
- Intestinal lymphoma.
- Gastrinoma.
- VIPoma.

2. Extraintestinal causes:
   - Zollinger-Ellison syndrome.
   - Hyperthyroidism.
   - Addison's disease (Addisonian crisis).
   - Medullary carcinoma of thyroid.
   - Diabetes mellitus (due to autonomic neuropathy).
   - Drugs—laxative, statin, metformin, anticancer drug, PPI.
   - Factitious diarrhoea (due to purgative abuse).

Investigations

As above.

Treatment

- Symptomatic and supportive.
- Treatment of cause.

Causes of Bloody Diarrhoea

- Bacillary dysentery.
- Ulcerative colitis.
- Carcinoma of large gut.
- Pseudomembranous colitis.
- Mesenteric vasculitis.
- Angiodysplasia of colon.
- Ischaemic colitis.
- Radiation enteritis.

MALABSORPTION SYNDROME

Definition

It is a group of disorders associated with disturbance of digestion and defective mucosal absorption of essentials constituents of food-like nutrients, electrolytes, minerals and vitamins. It is usually associated with chronic diarrhoea and features of malnutrition.

Causes

According to the organ involved:

1. Stomach
   - Gastrectomy (partial or total).
   - Carcinoma of stomach.
   - Menetrier's disease.
   - Bariatric surgery.
2. Intestine:
   - Coeliac disease.
   - Tropical sprue.
   - Whipple's disease.
   - Intestinal TB.
   - Carcinoid syndrome.
   - Intestinal resection—ileal resection or massive intestinal resection (short bowel syndrome).
   - Bacterial overgrowth.
   - Inflammatory bowel disease.
   - Parasites—*Giardia lamblia, Diphyllobothrium latum* (B12 malabsorption).
   - Radiation enteritis.
   - Fistulae, diverticular disease and strictures.
   - Infiltrative disease—amyloidosis, lymphoma, eosinophilic gastroenteritis.
3. Pancreatic causes:
   - Fibrocystic disease of the pancreas.
   - Chronic pancreatitis.
   - Carcinoma of pancreas.
   - Zollinger-Ellison Syndrome.
4. Liver disease:
   - Obstructive jaundice.
   - Primary biliary cirrhosis.
5. Systemic causes:
   - Hyperthyroidism.
   - Addison's disease.
   - Diabetes mellitus (due to autonomic neuropathy).
   - Systemic sclerosis.
6. Due to enzyme deficiencies:
   - Lactase deficiency causing lactose intolerance.
   - Intestinal disaccharidase deficiency.
   - Intestinal enteropeptidase deficiency.
   - Sucrose intolerance.

7. Drugs:
   - Cholestyramine.
   - Neomycin.
   - Orlistat.
   - Colchicine.
   - Cytotoxic drugs.
8. Miscellaneous:
   - HIV.
   - Intestinal lymphoma.
   - Abetalipoproteinemia.

Clinical Features

1. Diarrhoea or steatorrhoea (frothy, bulky, pale and offensive which floats on the toilet), abdominal discomfort, bloating, undigested food in stool, mucous and blood in stool are the commonest presentation.
2. Other features are due to defective absorption of specific nutrients.
   - Protein malabsorption—muscle wasting, oedema, weight loss, leuconychia.
   - Fat malabsorption—weight loss, bulky pale frothy stool.
   - Carbohydrate malabsorption—bloating, abdominal distension, borborygmi, flatus.
   - Growth retardation.
   - Iron, folic acid—anaemia, glossitis, koilonychia.
   - Vitamin B1 and B2—angular stomatitis, cheilosis, glossitis.
   - B12—anaemia, smooth shiny tongue, peripheral neuropathy, subacute combined degeneration of spinal cord.
   - Vitamin K—bleeding tendency (bruise, ecchymosis).
   - Vitamin A—night blindness, xerosis, xerophthalmia, toad skin.
   - Vitamin D and calcium—ricket or osteomalacia, bone and muscle pain, tetany.
   - Zinc—acrodermatitis enteropathica, poor wound healing, tingling.
   - Magnesium—weakness, tetany, paraesthesia.
   - Potassium—muscular weakness, abdominal distension, arrhythmia.
   - Sodium—weakness, hypotension, muscle cramp.

Investigations

1. Routine investigations:
   - CBC, ESR, PBF.
   - Blood sugar.
   - Stool—microscopy to see ova, cyst, larva. Also stool C/S.
   - Liver function tests.
   - Total protein and A:G ratio.
   - Serum iron, folic acid, B12, calcium, magnesium, electrolytes.
   - USG of whole abdomen.
   - Plain X-ray abdomen (to see pancreatic calcification).
   - CT scan of abdomen.
   - Barium meal and follow through.
   - Endoscopy.

2. Specific—according to suspicion of cause, e.g.
   - Coeliac disease (IgA anti-transglutaminase antibodies or IgA anti-endomysial antibodies for Coeliac disease).
   - IBD.
   - ERCP and/or MRCP.
   - Other tests—duodenal or jejunal biopsy, capsule endoscopy, colonoscopy.

Treatment

According to the cause.

- Replacement of nutrients, electrolytes and fluids.
- Pancreatic enzyme in pancreatic insufficiency.
- Dietary modification—gluten-free diet in coeliac disease, lactose avoidance in lactose intolerance
- Antibiotic therapy in bowel infection.
- Cholestyramine in bile acid malabsorption.
- Treatment of specific disease like Crohn's disease, ulcerative colitis.

COELIAC DISEASE

Definition

It is a gluten-sensitive enteropathy characterized by mucosal destruction mainly of jejunum due to hypersensitivity to gliadin fraction of gluten protein.

There is atrophy of villi, crypt hypertrophy, infiltration of plasma cells and lymphocytes in lamina propria.

Symptoms

- Diarrhoea or steatorrhoea.
- Anorexia, nausea, weight loss, abdominal pain, bloating, flatulence and distension.
- May be associated with itchy vascular rash due to dermatitis herpetiformis.
- Features of intestinal malabsorption—anaemia, muscle cramps, bone pain, osteomalacia, bleeding manifestation, ankle oedema.
- Failure to thrive (in children).

Investigations

- Stool RME.
- CBC—shows dimorphic anemia (both macrocytic and microcytic), due to deficiency of iron, folic acid and rarely B12.
- PBF—shows Howel-Jolly body, target cells.
- USG of whole abdomen (to exclude other disease).
- Antibody—anti-endomysial antibody, tissue transglutaminase antibody (anti-tTG) may be present in the serum. Antireticulin antibody which is very sensitive, but less specific. Anti-gliadin antibody is also less sensitive.
- Endoscopic jejunal biopsy—subtotal villous atrophy and crypts hyperplasia.
- Low-serum albumin, calcium, iron or folate level.

Complications

- Hyposplenism.
- Gastric or small bowel T cell lymphoma.
- Oesophageal squamous cell and small bowel carcinoma.
- Ulcerative jejunoileitis.
- Dermatitis herpetiformis may be associated with coeliac disease.

Treatment

- Avoid gluten-free diet (wheat, rye, barley, and oat).
- Iron, folic acid, calcium, magesium should be given.
- There is lactose intolerance, so milk and milk products should be avoided.

TROPICAL SPRUE

Definition

Tropical sprue is a chronic, progressive malabsorption in a patient residing in and from the tropical region, characterized by inflammation and flattening of villi of small intestine.

Cause is unknown. Probably due to bacterial, viral, amoebial or parasitic infection. Small bowel bacterial overgrowth with *E. coli*, Enterobacter and Klebsiella is frequently seen.

Clinical Features

Like coeliac disease. Relapse and remission may occur.

Investigations

- CBC- like coeliac disease.
- Endoscopy with small bowel biopsy—shows inflammation of the lining and flattening of villi of small intestine. Jejunal biopsy reveals presence of inflammatory cells (mostly lymphocytes).
- Low-serum albumin, calcium, iron or folate level.
- Low vitamin A, B12, E, D and K level.
- Stool examination—to exclude other disease.

Treatment

- Antibiotic—Tetracycline 250 mg four-times daily for 28 days, more may be required (up to 6 month).
- Folic acid 5 mg daily.
- In severely ill patient, correction of fluid and electrolytes.
- Other deficiencies should be corrected, e.g. iron, vitamin B12, etc.

DIVERTICULAR DISEASES

Diverticula are the sac-like out pouching of the colonic mucosa and submucosa through weaknesses of muscle layers in the colon wall. Presence of diverticula is called diverticulosis and inflammation of the diverticula is called diverticulitis.

Diverticulosis

Definition

Diverticulosis is characterized by presence of diverticula in the colon. These are associated with hypertrophy of circular muscle layer.

Site

Any part of colon, but commonly in the sigmoid colon.

Risk Factors

- Diet—Low-fibre diets. Refined diet and relative deficiency of fibres is thought to be responsible for diverticula.
- Positive family history.

Mechanism

High intracolonic pressure that occurs due to low-fiber diet causes herniation of mucosa through areas of weakness in colonic muscular wall where blood vessels penetrate the muscle.

Diverticula are common in elderly, occurs in 50% of the people over 50 years.

Symptoms

- Asymptomatic in 95% cases.
- In symptomatic case–pain or discomfort in the left iliac fossa, bloating, constipation or diarrhoea.
- During severe episode—there may be diarrhoea, bleeding per rectum, fever.

Signs

Tenderness in the left iliac fossa.

Complications

- Rectal bleeding.
- Perforation.
- Pericolic abscess.
- Fistula formation (into bladder, small bowel,vagina) .
- Diverticulitis.

Investigations

- Barium enema (avoided in acute attack).
- Sigmoidoscopy or colonoscopy.

- USG of abdomen to exclude other disease.
- CT scan of abdomen.

Treatment

In asymptomatic case—high-fibre diet and plenty of fluids are sufficient.
In acute attack—metronidazole 400 mg 8 hourly plus antibiotic (ciprofloxacin or ampicillin) for 7 days.

Diverticulitis

Definition

It means inflammation of diverticula are inflamed. Diverticulitis occurs when faecal matter obstructs the neck of the diverticulum causing stagnation, allowing bacteria to multiply and produce inflammation.

Symptoms

- Fever.
- Pain in left iliac fossa.
- Vomiting.
- Alternation in bowel habits (constipation or diarrhoea).

Signs

- Tenderness and rigidity in left iliac fossa.
- Colonic mass may be felt.

Complications

- Abscess formation.
- Obstruction.
- Bowel perforation.
- Fistula into the adjacent organ.
- Generalized peritonitis.

Investigations

- CBC—shows leukocytosis.
- CT scan (abdomen and pelvis)—reveals swollen, oedematous bowel wall or an abscess.
- Abdominal radiograph (to exclude other potential causes).
- Colonoscopy.

NB: Barium enema is contraindicated in acute diverticulitis due to the risk of perforation.

Treatment

- NPO.
- IV fluids.
- IV broad-spectrum antibiotic with metronidazole.

Surgery is recommended (resection of involved segment) once acute inflammation resolves.

CHAPTER

5 Haematology

CHAPTER CONTENTS

- Anaemia
  - Dimorphic anaemia
  - Sideroblastic anaemia
- Iron deficiency anaemia
- Megaloblastic anaemia
- Haemolytic anaemia
- Hereditary haemolytic anaemia
  - Beta thalassaemia major
  - Thalassaemia minor
  - Alpha thalassaemia
- Autoimmune haemolytic anaemia
- Sickle-cell anaemia
- Microangiopathic haemolytic anaemia
- Paroxysmal nocturnal haemoglobinuria
- Aplastic anaemia
- Polycythaemia
- Myeloproliferative disorder
  - Myelofibrosis
  - Polycythaemia rubra vera
- Myelodysplastic syndrome
  - Leukaemia
  - Acute leukaemia
  - Chronic myeloid leukaemia
  - Chronic lymphatic leukaemia
- Leukaemoid reaction
- Purpura
- Idiopathic thrombocytopenic purpura
- Henoch schonlein purpura
- Haemophilia
  - Christmas disease (Haemophilia B)
- Von willebrand's disease
- Lymphoma
  - Hodgkin's disease
  - Non-Hodgkin's lymphoma
- Multiple myeloma
- Disseminated intravascular coagulation
- Blood transfusion
- Stem cell transplantation (bone marrow transplantation)
- Haemolytic uraemic syndrome
- Thrombotic thrombocytopenic purpura

ANAEMIA

Definition

It is a clinical condition characterised by reduced haemoglobin concentration according to the age and sex of the individual.

Classification

Anaemia is classified in two ways:
- Etiological (based on cause).
- Morphological (based on morphology of RBC).

Etiological

1. Haemorrhagic anaemia (due to blood loss):
   - Acute—trauma, postpartum bleeding, haematemesis, melaena, epistaxis.
   - Chronic—hook worm, haemorrhoid, excessive menstrual loss, bleeding peptic ulcer.
2. Deficiency anaemias:
   - Iron deficiency anaemia.
   - Vitamin B12 and folic acid deficiency (megaloblastic anaemia).
3. Dyshaemopoietic anaemia (less production of RBC):
   - Aplastic anaemia (bone marrow failure which may be primary or secondary to some other diseases or drugs).
   - Anaemia of chronic disorder (ACD)—SLE, rheumatoid arthritis, sideroblastic anaemia, CKD, hypothyroidism, malignancy.
4. Haemolytic anaemia (due to break down of RBC):
   - Genetic—Red cell membrane defect (e.g. hereditary spherocytosis, eliptocytosis, stomatocytosis), haemoglobin abnormality (thalassaemia, sickle cell anaemia) or enzyme defects (glucose 6 phosphate dehydrogenase deficiency, pyruvate kinase deficiency).
   - Acquired—Autoimmune, toxic, mechanical and infectious causes.

Morphological (depending on MCV and MCHC)

1. Normocytic normochromic anaemia (normal mean corpuscular volume [MCV] and mean corpuscular haemoglobin concentration [MCHC]).
2. Microcytic hypochromic anaemia (low MCV < 76 fl, low MCHC < 30 g/dL).
3. Macrocytic anaemia (high MCV > 96 fL).
4. Dimorphic anaemia (combination of two cell lines—macrocytes and microcytes).

Causes of Normocytic Normochromic Anaemia

- Haemorrhagic.
- Haemolytic anaemia.
- Aplastic anaemia.
- Anaemia of chronic disorder.
- Malignancy.
- Endocrine disease.
- Sideroblastic anaemia.

Causes of Microcytic Hypochromic Anaemia

- Iron deficiency anaemia.
- Thalassaemia.
- Sideroblastic anaemia.
- Anaemia of chronic disorder (ACD).

Causes of Macrocytic Anaemia

- Macrocytosis with megaloblastic marrow:
  - Vitamin B12 deficiency.
  - Folic acid deficiency.
- Macrocytosis with normoblastic marrow:
  - Chronic liver disease.
  - Chronic alcoholism.
  - Hypothyroidism.
  - Haemorrhage.
  - Haemolysis.
  - Others—sideroblastic anaemia, pure red cell aplasia, azathioprine therapy.

Dimorphic Anaemia

When both microcytes and macrocytes are found in peripheral blood film, this is called dimorphic anaemia.

Causes

- Combined iron, B12 or folate deficiency.
- Sideroblastic anaemia.
- During treatment of anaemia.

Mechanisms of Anaemia of Chronic Disorder

Actual mechanism is unknown. It is due to abnormality of iron metabolism and erythropoiesis. There is less erythropoietin. Also red cell survival is short.

Investigations of Anaemia

Detailed history, physical examination and relevant laboratory investigations are done.

History

- Dietary history (to diagnose deficiency anaemia like iron, vitamin B12 and folic acid deficiency).
- Malabsorption (history of chronic diarrhoea).
- History of bleeding (haemorrhoid, epistaxis, haematemesis, melaena, menorrhagia in female).
- In female—multiple pregnancies, repeated abortion, menorrhagia.
- Drug history—NSAIDs, steroid, drugs causing bone marrow suppression (e.g. cytotoxic drugs), drugs causing haemolysis (e.g. sulfasalazine, methyldopa).
- History of surgery—gastrectomy or partial gastrectomy, ileal surgery (responsible for vitamin B12 absorption).

Table 1
Signs that may point to a specific cause of anaemia

Sign	Cause of anaemia
1. Triad of anaemia, jaundice and splenomegaly	Haemolytic anaemia
2. Angular stomatitis, cheilitis, glossitis, koilonychia	Iron deficiency anaemia
3. Glossitis	Iron deficiency anaemia, vitamin B12 deficiency, folate deficiency
4. Splenomegaly	Malaria, chronic haemolytic anaemia, acute infection, leukaemia, lymphoma, portal hypertension
5. Neurological changes (dementia, optic atrophy and features of subacute combined degeneration of spinal cord) and lemon yellow tint.	Vitamin B12 deficiency (megaloblastic anaemia)
6. Change (frontal and parietal bossing)	Hereditary haemolytic anaemia
7. Leg ulcer	Sickle cell anaemia, PNH
8. Bony tenderness	Acute leukaemia, multiple myeloma, lymphoma, myelofibrosis

- Family history (in hereditary haemolytic anaemia).
- History of chronic disease (e.g. SLE, RA, CKD, CLD).

Clinical examination

See in the Table 1.

Laboratory investigations

1. Hb%, TC, DC, ESR, platelet—
   - Pancytopenia—may be due to aplastic anaemia, hypersplenism, megaloblastic anaemia, aleukemic leukaemia.
   - Leucocytosis (abnormally high)—in leukaemia.
2. PBF examination—to see normocytic, microcytic, macrocytic or dimorphic (Table 2).
3. Reticulocyte count—High in haemolytic anaemia.
4. MCV and MCHC.
5. Bone marrow examination—to detect megaloblastic anaemia, aplastic anaemia, bone marrow infiltration (secondary deposit), ring sideroblasts (in sideroblastic anaemia).
6. Other investigations according to suspicion of cause.

Further investigations of microcytic hypochromic anaemia (low MCV and low MCHC)

- For iron deficiency anaemia—Serum iron, TIBC, serum ferritin.
- For hereditary haemolytic anaemia—Haemoglobin electrophoresis, skeletal survey.
- For sideroblastic anaemia—according to history, bone marrow examination (to see ring sideroblasts)
- For anaemia of chronic disease—test should be done according to the cause.

Further investigations for macrocytic anaemia (high MCV)

Bone marrow study should be done—

- If megaloblast is seen, serum B12 and folic acid assay should be done.
- If normoblast is seen, further investigation should be according to the cause (see above).

Table 2
Diseases may be diagnosed from PBF

Finding	Description	Common diagnoses
Anisocytosis	Variation in size of RBC	Iron deficiency anaemia, megaloblastic anaemia, sideroblastic anaemia
Poikilocytosis	Variation in shape of RBC	Iron deficiency anaemia, thalassaemia, sideroblastic anaemia
Microcytosis	MCV <76 fL	Iron deficiency anaemia, thalassaemia, sideroblastic anaemia, anaemia of chronic disorder
Macrocytosis	MCV >100 fL	Vitamin B12 and folic acid deficiency, chronic liver disease, alcohol, hypothyroidism, zidovudine
Hypochromia	Central pallor of RBC (lower haemoglobin content)	Iron deficiency anaemia, thalassaemia, sideroblastic anaemia, anaemia of chronic disorder
Basophilic stippling or punctate basophilia	Deep blue dots scattered in cytoplasm of RBC (seen with Romanowsky staining)	Chronic lead poisoning, dyshaemopoiesis
Target cells	Red cells with central dense area surrounded by a ring of pale area and an outer ring of dense area	Iron deficiency anaemia, thalassaemia, haemoglobic C disease, CLD, splenectomy
Howell-Jolly bodies	Small round remnants of nuclear material in RBC	Hyposplenism, postsplenectomy, dyshaemopoiesis
Heinz bodies (Ehrlich's bodies)	Formed from denatured aggregated haemoglobin in red cells (seen with supravital staining with brilliant cresyl blue)	Thalassaemia, haemolysis in glucose 6 phosphate dehydrogenase deficiency, asplenia and CLD, drug like sulfasalazine, dapsone
Acanthocytes (spur cells)	RBC with irregular spicules	Abetalipoproteinaemia
Burr cells	RBC with regularly placed spicules	CKD
Schistocytes	Fragmented RBC. These are found in microangiopathic haemolytic anaemia	Causes—DIC, HUS, TTP, disseminated carcinomatosis, malignant or pregnancy induced hypertension (eclampsia)
Spherocytes	Small, densely packed RBC with loss of central pallor	Hereditary spherocytosis, autoimmune haemolytic anaemia, postsplenectomy
Sickle cell	Sickle-shaped	Sickle cell anaemia
Blister cells	Swollen cell	Glucose 6 phosphate dehydrogenase deficiency
Nucleated RBC	Normoblasts	Bone marrow infiltration, severe haemolysis, myelofibrosis, acute haemorrhage
Polychromasia	Young red cells, reticulocytes (bluish tinge)	Haemolysis, acute haemorrhage, increased red cell turnover

Sideroblastic Anaemia

It is defined as a group of anaemia characterised by refractory anaemia, a variable number of hypochromic cells in the peripheral blood and excess iron and ring sideroblast.

Types

1. Hereditary.
2. Acquired, which may be primary and secondary.
   - Primary sideroblastic anaemia is one of the types of myelodysplastic syndrome, a refractory anaemia with ring sideroblast.
   - Secondary sideroblastic anaemia may be due to (i) drugs and chemicals (INH, cycloserine, alcohol, chloramphenicol, lead); (ii) haematological disease (myelofibrosis, polycythemia rubra vera, myeloma, Hodgkin's lymphoma, hemolytic anemia, leukemia); (iii) inflammatory disease (rheumatoid arthritis, SLE); (iv) others (carcinoma, myxedema, malabsorption).

Treatment

- Treatment of primary cause, e.g. withdrawal of drug, stop alcohol.
- Some cases may respond to pyridoxine, folic acid.
- Correction of anaemia by blood transfusion.

IRON DEFICIENCY ANAEMIA

Definition

Anaemia secondary to deficiency of iron.

Causes

- Bleeding due to any cause—GIT (haemorrhoid, colorectal carcinoma, carcinoma of stomach, diverticulitis, angiodysplasia of colon), menorrhagia in female.
- Hookworm (also schistosomiasis).
- Less intake of food.
- Malabsorption.
- More demand (pregnancy).

Symptoms

- Weakness, vertigo, dizziness, light headedness.
- Tingling and numbness.
- Anorexia, weight loss and palpitation.
- Breathlessness on exertion.
- Pica (eating of unusual material, e.g. dirt or paint)

Signs

- The patient is pale, anaemic.
- Koilonychia.
- Glossistis, angular stomatitis.

Investigations

1. Test to confirm iron deficiency anaemia:
   - CBC with PBF (microcytic hypochromic blood picture).
   - Serum iron, TIBC and ferritin (low iron, low ferritin, increased TIBC).
2. Test to find out causes:
   - Stool for ova or cyst of hookworm and occult blood test.
   - Upper GI endoscopy (to see oesophageal varices, peptic ulcer, carcinoma stomach).
   - Proctoscopy (haemorrhoid), sigmoidoscopy or colonoscopy (neoplasm, polyp, diverticulum, ulcer, angiodysplasia of colon).
   - USG of abdomen (any mass, fibroid uterus).
3. Bone marrow—shows erythroid hyperplasia, also to see stainable iron (by Prussian blue shows empty stain), not a routine, may be done in some cases.

Treatment

Severe anaemia should be corrected by blood transfusion.

Iron therapy—oral ferrous sulphate, ferrous gluconate or ferrous fumarate to be given for 3–6 months after haemoglobin is normal to replenish the iron store. If the patient is unable to take orally, it can be given parenteraly.

Treatment of cause (e.g. menorrhagia, haemorrhoid).

MEGALOBLASTIC ANAEMIA

Definition

Megaloblastic anaemia is a type of anaemia due to deficiency of vitamin B12, folic acid or both. It is characterised by macrocyte in peripheral blood and megaloblast in bone marrow.

Megaloblastic Anaemia due to Vitamin B12 Defciency

Causes of Vitamin B12 Deficiency

1. Diet—Strict vegetarians.
2. Stomach pathology—hypochlorhydria, total or partial gastrectomy, carcinoma of stomach.
3. Pernicious anaemia—in this condition, there is gastric mucosal atrophy causing intrinsic factor deficiency.
4. Small bowel pathology:
   - Ileal disease—Crohn's disease, ileal resection.
   - Pancreatic exocrine insufficiency—Vitamin B12 deficiency occurs in 30% patients,.
   - Motility disorders—can cause bacterial overgrowth and vitamin B12 deficiency.
   - Fish tapeworm (Diphyllobothrium latum).

Pernicious Anaemia: It is an autoimmune disease in which there is atrophy of gastric mucosa, with loss of parietal cells causing intrinsic factor deficiency. So, vitamin B12 is not absorbed due to the deficiency of intrinsic factor. There is anti-intrinsic factor antibodies and also antiparietal cell antibodies.

Symptoms of Megaloblastic Anaemia

- Weakness, malaise, weight loss, breathlessness, sore mouth.
- Paraesthesiae, poor memory, depression, hallucinations.
- Visual disturbance.

Signs

1. Tongue—smooth, shiny with atrophy of papilla.
2. Angular cheilosis.
3. Skin pigmentation, lemon yellow tint, vitiligo.
4. Neuropathy—
   - Peripheral nerves—neuropathy (Gloves and stocking pattern)
   - Spinal cord (causing subacute combined degeneration)—there is loss of vibration and position sense (posterior column lesion), upper motor neuron sings (due to corticospinal tract lesion).
   - Cerebral—dementia.
   - Optic atropy.

Investigations

- CBC—low Hb%, may be pancytopenia.
- PBF—shows macrocytes, hypersegmented neutrophils.
- Serum vitamin B12 (low).

- Parietal cell and intrinsic factor antibodies for pernicious anaemia.
- Bone marrow aspiration—shows increase cellularity, megaloblasts.
- Others—low reticulocyte count and high LDH.

Treatment

1. Blood transfusion—in severe anaemia.
2. Injection Hydroxycobalamine 1000 μg I.M daily 6 dose, for 2 or 3 days apart. Then 1000 μg every 3 months (life-long therapy should be given for pernicious anaemia).

Megaloblastic Anaemia due to Folic Acid Deficiency

Causes of folate deficiency are as follows:

1. Less intake of vegetables.
2. Malabsorption—due to any cause (e.g. coeliac disease, tropical sprue).
3. Increased demand—pregnancy, haemolysis.
4. Drugs—methotrexate, phenytoin.

Investigation of Folic Acid Deficiency

- Serum folate levels—low.
- Red cell folate level—low.

Treatment

1. Tablet folic acid 5 mg daily for 3 weeks. Then 5 mg weekly.
2. Prophylactic folic acid in pregnancy should be given, also in haemolytic anaemia.

NB: Folic acid alone should not be given, if there is Vitamin B12 deficiency, otherwise may aggravate neurological lesion. In such cases, both should be given.

HAEMOLYTIC ANAEMIA

Definition

Anaemia due to destruction or breakdown of RBC.

Classification

Haemolytic anaemia is classified as follows:

1. Inherited
   - Red cell membrane abnormality—hereditary sperocytosis, eliptocytosis.
   - Red cell enzyme deficiency—G6PD (Glucose 6 Phosphatase) deficiency, pyruvate kinase deficiency.
   - Haemoglbinopathy—thalassaemia, sickle cell disease and other haemoglobinopathies.
2. Acquired
   a. Autoimmune—
      - Warm antibodies (primary or idiopathic and secondary, such as SLE, rheumatoid arthritis: drugs including methyldopa, quinidine, CLL, lymphoma).
      - Cold antibodies (primary or idiopathic, secondary in mycoplasma pneumoniae, lymphoma).

   b. Nonimmune—
      - Mechanical (microangiopathic haemolytic anaemia, prosthetic valve).
      - Infection (falciparum malaria).
      - Chemical—dapsone, sulphasalazine, maloprim.
      - Acquired membrane abnormality—Paroxysmal nocturnal haemoglobinuria.

Evidence of Haemolysis

1. Clinical: Triad of anaemia, jaundice and splenomegaly (usually in hereditary haemolytic anaemia).
2. In the blood:
   - High serum bilirubin.
   - High urinary urobilinigen.
   - Low haptoglobin.
   - High LDH.
   - High reticulocytes.
   - Erythoid hyperplasia in bone marrow.

HEREDITARY HAEMOLYTIC ANAEMIA

Thalassaemia

It is an inherited disorder in which there is an impairment of haemoglobin production due to partial or complete failure to synthesize the specific type of globin chain. It is of two types:

1. **β-thalassaemia**—there is less production of β-chain, causing less production of HbA. Further, it is also classified as follows:
   - β-thalassaemia major—HbA is less, HbF is high.
   - β-thalassaemia minor—HbA2 is high.

2. **α-thalassaemia**—there is an inadequate production of α-chain, so less HbA, HbF and HbA2, as all of them contain α-chain.

Following points are important:
- Two α and two β chains of globin combine with haem to form hemoglobin. So, if synthesis of globin is reduced, there is less hemoglobin.
- Normal adult hemoglobin contains mainly HbA (98%), contains two α and two β chains.
- HbA2 contains two α and two δ chains.
- HbF contains two α and two γ chains.

BETA THALASSAEMIA MAJOR

Definition

It is characterised by reduced or absent synthesis of β-chain of globin. Family history may be present.

Symptoms

- Symptoms of anaemia—weakness, palpitation, dizziness.
- Yellow colouration of eyes and high-coloured urine.
- Feeling of a mass in the left upper abdomen.

NB: If the patient develops severe abdominal pain, likely cause is cholelithiasis. There may also be splenic infarction, acute pancreatitis.

Signs

- Triad of haemolytic anaemia—Anaemia, Jaundice and Splenomegaly.
- Frontal, parietal bossing and Mongoloid facies with prominent malar bones.
- Short stature and retardation of growth.

Investigations

1. CBC and PBF (microcytic hypochromic blood picture).
2. Reticulocyte count (by supravital stain)—high.
3. Haemoglobin electrophoresis.
4. Others:
   - X-ray of skull, hand and other skeletal survey.
   - Serum bilirubin—high.
   - Serum iron profile—ferritin (high), iron, TIBC.

Radiological Findings in Skull in β-thalassaemia Major

- Widening of diploic space.
- Thinning of outer table.
- Thickening and coarsening of trabeculae giving rise to hair-on-end appearance.

Treatment

1. Correction of anaemia—Blood transfusion to keep Hb% above 10 g/dL, every 4 months (because life span of RBC is 4 months).

2. Folic acid 5 mg daily, to be continued.
3. Iron containing drugs and diet are avoided (iron can only be given, if there is deficiency).
4. Repeated blood transfusion may cause haemosiderosis, which can be prevented by chelating agent.(See below)
5. Other treatment:
   - Injection erythropoietin.
   - Hydroxyurea 1-2 g daily may be helpful.
6. Specific therapy—Allogenic bone marrow transplantation. Also, gene therapy.
7. Splenectomy may be needed in some cases.
8. Genetic counselling should be offered.

Indications of Splenectomy

- Huge splenomegaly with pressure symptoms.
- Hypersplenism—as suggested by repeated transfusion in a short-interval.
- Full blood count shows pancytopenia.

Complications of Repeated Blood Transfusion

- Haemosiderosis (usually when more than 30–50 L of blood is transfused).
- Infections, such as hepatitis B, C, D and HIV.

Prevention of Haemosiderosis

Haemosiderosis can be prevented by using chelating agent desferrioxamine (1.5–2 gm with each unit of blood). It is usually given subcutaneously in the anterior abdominal wall with infusion pump for 12 hours. It may also be given with infusion drip (normal saline or aqua). Oral chelating agent, such as deferiprone, 75 mg/kg in 2–4 divided doses, is also available. Other oral chelating agent include deferasirox. Vitamin C 200 mg daily orally also helps in iron excretion.

THALASSAEMIA MINOR

Symptoms

- May be asymptomatic.
- May be features of anaemia.

Sign

Only anaemia.

Investigations

- Blood count—microcytic hypochromic blood picture.
- Haemoglobin electrophoresis shows high A2.

Differential Diagnoses

Thalassaemia minor confuses with iron deficiency anaemia. However, anaemia is more marked in iron deficiency and relatively less in thalassaemia minor. Also, in iron deficiency, there is low iron, low ferritin and high TIBC.

ALPHA THALASSAEMIA

Definition

This is characterised by reduced or absent alpha globin chain synthesis. Normally, adults have four alpha globin chain genes.

- When one alpha gene is absent—the patient is haematologically normal (silent carrier).
- When two alpha genes are absent—it is called alpha thalassaemia trait. The patient is clinically normal, life expectancy is normal.
- When three alpha genes are absent—the patient has Hb-H disease. There is chronic haemolytic anaemia with variable severity. Examination shows severe anaemia with splenomegaly.
- If all four alpha globin chains are absent—affected foetus is stillborn due to hydrops foetalis.

AUTOIMMUNE HAEMOLYTIC ANAEMIA

Definition

It is group of haemolytic anaemias that occurs due to red cell autoantibodies causing increased red cell destruction. Antibodies may be IgG or IgM. It is of two types depending on the temperature at which the antibody reacts with red cells.

- Warm antibodies bind at 37°C, common (80% of cases). Antibody is IgG.
- Cold antibodies bind at 4°C, but can bind up to 37°C in some cases. Antibody is IgM. Less common (20% cases).

Warm Autoimmune Haemolytic Anaemia

Occurs at all ages, common in middle age females.

Causes

1. Primary or idiopathic (50% cases).
2. Secondary:
   - Infection—mycoplasma pneumoniae, infectious mononucleosis, cytomegalovirus.
   - Collagen diseases—SLE, rheumatoid arthritis.
   - Drugs—methyldopa, quinidine.
   - Neoplastic—CLL, lymphoma.
   - Others—carcinoma, sarcoidosis.

Clinical Features

- Features of primary cause.
- May be asymptomatic.
- Features of haemolytic anaemia (anaemia, jaundice and splenomegaly).

Investigations

- CBC with PBF—macrocytes and spherocytes.
- Direct Coombs or antiglobulin test—positive.
- Serum IgG is high.

Treatment

- Treatment of underlying cause, offending drugs must be stopped.
- Prednisolone 1 mg/kg orally. When Hb and reticulocyte count are normal, prednisolone dose can be reduced slowly over 10 weeks.
- Blood transfusion for severe anaemia.
- If no response to prednisolone—splenectomy should be considered.
- If splenectomy is not possible—immunosuppressive therapy with azathioprine or cyclophosphamide may be given. Anti-CD20 monoclonal antibody, rituximab is helpful in some cases.

Cold Agglutinin Disease

It is the autoimmune haemolytic anaemia due to cold antibody. It is of two types: Cold haemagglutinin disease (CHAD) and paroxysmal cold hemoglobinuria (PCH).

Chronic cold agglutinin disease occurs in elderly and may be associated with an underlying low-grade B cell lymphoma. It causes low-grade intravascular haemolysis with cold, painful, blue fingers, toes, ears or nose (called acrocyanosis).

Causes

1. Idiopathic in most cases.
2. Secondary—Found in Lymphoma, CLL, SLE, Walderstrome macroglobunia. Also, may occur in mycoplasma pneumoniae, infectious mononucleosis.

Investigation

- CBC with PBF—shows cold agglutination at low- temperature.
- Direct Coombs test is positive with complements.
- Serum IgM is high.

Treatment

- Treatment of underlying causes.
- If idiopathic—patients must keep extremities warm, specially in winters.
- Some patients respond to corticosteroid therapy and blood transfusion may be needed in severe anaemia.
- Folic acid should be given.

SICKLE-CELL ANAEMIA

Definition

It is a hereditary disorder, inherited as an autosomal recessive trait, in which the red cells contains an abnormal haemoglobin called HbS. It is of two types:

- Homozygotes—produce abnormal beta chains that make haemoglobin S (called SS). This causes clinical syndrome of sickle cell disease.
- Heterozygotes—produce normal and abnormal beta chains that make normal HbA and HbS (called AS). This causes sickle-cell trait, clinically asymptomatic.

When haemoglobin S is deoxygenated, red cell membrane is distorted and produce sickle-shaped cells.

Clinical Features

- Usually, present in childhood before 2 years.
- Features of haemolytic anaemia, frequent infection, leg ulcers, gall stone, dactylitis (due to microinfraction of the medulla of the carpal and metatarsal bones).
- Splenomegaly is present, but repeated infarction of the spleen causes atropy (autosplenectomy) at the age of eight years. So spleen is no longer palpable.
- May present with following crises called sickle-cell crises:
  - *Vasoocclusive crisis:* Plugging of small vessels in the bone produces acute severe bone pain. Hands and feet in children (so-called dactylitis) or femur, humerus, ribs, pelvis and vertebrae in adults are most common sites. Mesenteric infarction causes acute abdominal pain. Papillary necrosis may occur in kidney. Cerebral infarction due to involvement of the brain.
  - *Sickle chest syndrome:* This may follow vasoocclusive crisis, common cause of death in adult sickle disease. Bone marrow infarction results in fat emboli to the lungs, which cause further infarction, leading to ventilatory failure.
  - *Sequestration crisis:* Vasoocclusion produces an acute painful enlargement of spleen. There is a splenic pooling of red cells and hypovolaemia, leading to circulatory collapse and death. Liver sequestration can also occur.
  - *Aplastic crisis:* Infection with human parvovirus B19 causes severe but self-limiting red cell aplasia. This causes very low haemoglobin, may cause heart failure.

Investigations

- CBC with PBF—shows sickle cells, target cells and features of hyposplenism.
- Reticulocyte count—high.
- Sickle solubility test—A mixture of Hb S in a reducing solution, such as sodium dithionite gives a turbid appearance because of precipitation of Hb S (normal Hb gives a clear solution).
- Definitive diagnosis—haemoglobin electrophoresis shows high Hb S, absence of HbA, 2–20% HbF.

Treatment

- Penicillin V to protect pneumococcal infection.
- Vaccination against pneumococcus, meningococcus, Haemophilus influenzae B, hepatitis B and seasonal influenza.

- Folic acid.
- Transfusion—if severe anaemia.
- Hydroxurea—may be helpful.
- Allogeneic stem cell transplants from HLA-matched siblings may be curative.
- Vasoocclusive crises are managed by aggressive rehydration, oxygen therapy, adequate analgesia and antibiotics.

MICROANGIOPATHIC HAEMOLYTIC ANAEMIA

Definition

It is a type of mechanical haemolytic anaemia in which anaemia is associated with fragmented RBC (schistocyte, helmet cell).

Causes

- Disseminated intravascular coagulation (DIC).
- Thrombotic thrombocytopenic purpura (TTP).
- Haemolytic uraemic syndrome (HUS).
- Disseminated malignancy.
- Vasculitis.
- Metallic cardiac valve prosthesis.
- Malignant hypertension.

Mechanism

Red cell fragmentation is due to contact between red cells and abnormal intima of partially thrombosed, narrowed or necrotic vessels.

Investigations

- CBC with PBF—shows anemia with fragmented RBC.
- Others—jaundice, high reticulocyte count.

Treatment

- Treatment of primary cause.

PAROXYSMAL NOCTURNAL HAEMOGLOBINURIA

Definition

Paroxysmal nocturnal haemoglobinuria (PNH) is an acquired clonal abnormality of red cells, which are destroyed by activated complement resulting in intravascular hemolysis. Also, platelet and granulocyte are involved, resulting in thrombocytopenia and leucopenia.

Clinical Features

Commonly, the urine voided at night and in the morning on waking from sleep, is dark-coloured. Haemolysis may be precipitated by infection, surgery or iron therapy.

Complications

- Venous thrombosis involving the mesenteric, portal (Budd-Chiari syndrome) or cerebral veins, also calf muscles. Cause of thrombosis is unknown, probably complement mediated activation of platelet deficient in CD55 and CD59, resulting in hypercoagulability.
- Aplastic anaemia may precede PNH in 25% cases and acute myeloid leukaemia may occur.
- Others—increased susceptibility to infection, iron deficiency, pigment gallstone, etc.

NB: Blood picture with pancytopenia, haemolysis and dark urine (due to presence of haemoglobin) is likely to be due to PNH.

Investigations

- CBC—anaemia, leucopenia, thrombocytopenia.
- Ham's acid serum test may be positive.
- Flow cytometric analysis of red cells with CD55 and CD59 has replaced Ham's test.
- Bone marrow may be hypoplastic or aplastic.

Treatment

- Supportive (blood transfusion, iron).
- Prednisolone (in some cases).
- In marrow failure—antithymocyte globulin, ciclosporin or bone marrow transplantation.
- A recombinant humanized monoclonal antibody (eculizumab) may be helpful.
- Long term anticoagulation may be used—aspirin, clopidogrel.
- Gene therapy.

Prognosis

Survival is 10-15 years.

APLASTIC ANAEMIA

Definition

Aplastic anemia is a disorder due to bone marrow failure leading to pancytopenia. The diagnosis is done by bone marrow aspiration and biopsy.

Causes

It may be primary and acquired or secondary.

1. Primary—cause unknown.
2. Acquired or secondary:
   - Drugs—cytotoxic drugs, antibiotics (chloramphenicol, sulfonamide), antithyroid drugs (carbimazole), carbamazepine, penicillamine.
   - Secondary deposits in bone marrow.
   - Radiotherapy.
   - Chemicals—benzene, lindane, DDT.
   - Infection—viral hepatitis, EBV infection, HIV, parboviral infection.
   - Others—lymphoma, multiple myeloma, paroxysmal nocturnal haemoglubinuria.

Symptoms (Primary)

- Features of anaemia—weakness, palpitation, dizziness, vertigo.
- Bleeding manifestations—gum bleeding, nasal bleeding, multiple bleeding spots, such as bruise, ecchymosis in different parts of the body.
- Infection—sore throat, other infections, septicaemia.

Signs

- Anaemia.
- Bleeding spots (e.g. purpura, ecchymosis, bruise).
- No lymphadenopathy, hepatomegaly, splenomegaly or bony tenderness (which may be present in secondary deposit or secondary causes of aplastic anaemia).

NB: In case of secondary aplastic anemia, features of primary are the predominant features.

Investigations

- CBC—shows pancytopenia (anaemia, leukopenia and thrombocytopenia).
- Bone marrow study (aspiration and trephine biopsy)—dry tap or markedly acellular or hypocellular marrow.

Treatment

1. Removal of causative agent, if any.
2. Supportive therapy—blood transfusion, control of infection.
3. Allogenic bone marrow transplantation (with HLA matched siblings)—if the patient is below 30 years with severe idiopathic aplastic anaemia.
4. In older patient or if HLA matched donor is not available—immunosuppressive therapy with ciclosporin and antithymocyte globulin (ATG) should be given. Tacrolimus may be used instead of ciclosporin.

5. Other treatment—if bone marrow transplantation is not possible:
   - Androgen (e.g. oxymetholone) is sometimes useful.
   - Prednisolone—In some cases.
   - If associated with thymoma in adult pure red cell aplasia—thymectomy may be done.

Causes of Pancytopenia

- Aplastic anaemia.
- Hypersplenism.
- Megaloblastic anaemia.
- Banti's disease.
- Aleukaemic leukaemia.
- Some myelodysplastic syndrome.
- Paroxysmal nocturnal haemoglobinuria.
- Others—SLE, myelofibrosis, hairy cell leukaemia, disseminated tuberculosis, leishmaniasis, brucellosis, HIV, multiple myeloma, lymphoma.

POLYCYTHAEMIA

Definition

It is defined as an increase in RBC, haemoglobin and haematocrit.

Types

Polycythaemia is of two types:
Relative (pseudopolycythaemia)—due to reduced plasma volume (e.g. dehydration, diuretic therapy).
True polycythaemia—red cell mass is increased. True polycythemia may be:
1. Primary—polycythaemia rubra vera (PRV).
2. Secondary—causes are:
   - Physiological (high altitude).
   - Cyanotic heart disease (TOF).
   - COPD, emphysema, chronic bronchitis.
   - Smoking.
   - Inappropriate and excess erythropoietin secretion (renal cyst, renal cell carcinoma, cerebellar haemangioblastoma, hepatoma, uterine fibroma).

MYELOPROLIFERATIVE DISORDER

Definition

It is a group of disorder characterised by clonal proliferation of bone marrow stem cells which gives rise to uncontrolled proliferation of erythroid, myeloid and megakaryocyte series.

It includes four diseases:
1. Polycyrhaemia rubra vera.
2. Essential thrombocythaemia.
3. Myelofibrosis.
4. Chronic myeloid leukaemia.

   All myeloproliferative disorders may lead to acute leukaemia.

MYELOFIBROSIS

Definition

It is a myeloproliferative disorder characterised by bone marrow fibrosis, extramedullary haemopoiesis and leuco-erythroblastic blood picture.

There is clonal proliferation of stem cells. Fibrosis in the marrow is due to hyperplasia of abnormal megakaryocyte, which releases fibroblast stimulating factors.

Clinical Features

Common in people above 50 years. History of polycythaemia rubra vera in 25% cases and 50% have JAK2 mutation seen in polycythaemia rubra vera (PRV). The clinical features are as follows:
- May be asymptomatic.
- Mass in the left hypochondrium or hepatosplenomegaly.
- General features—malaise, weakness, weight loss, night sweat, repeated infection and bleeding.
- There may be peptic ulcer, pruritus after hot bath and gout.

Investigations

1. CBC and PBF:
   - Leucocytosis, leucoerythroblastic blood picture (immature nucleated RBC and premature cells of WBC series—myelocytes and myeloblasts).
   - PBF shows tear drop RBCs (tear drop poikilocytes).
   - Platelets—very high, later decrease. Giant forms may be seen.
   - Anaemia—usually macrocytic, pancytopenia may occur.
2. Bone marrow—may be dry tap. Trephine biopsy should be done (which shows increased megakaryocyte, increased reticulin and fibrous tissue).
3. Others:
   - Leucocyte alkaline phosphatase (LAP) score—increased.
   - Uric acid is high and folic acid is low.
   - Genetic test may show JAK2 mutation.

Treatment

- Correction of anaemia by blood transfusion and folic acid.
- Hydroxyurea (it reduces WBC and splenomegaly).
- Radiotherapy for huge spleen.
- Splenectomy, if huge spleen with pressure symptoms and hypersplenism.
- Bone marrow transplantation (if the patient is young).
- A new drug ruxolitinib (inhibitor of JAK1 and JAK2) may be used in some patients.

Prognosis

Median survival is 4 years (ranges from 1 to 20 years).

Causes of Death

- Transformation to AML (10–20%).
- Infection.
- Bleeding (from GIT).
- Cardiovascular problem.

POLYCYTHAEMIA RUBRA VERA

Definition

Polycythaemia rubra vera (PRV) is a stem cell disorder in which there is excess proliferation of erythroid, myeloid and megakaryocyte progenitor cells.

PRV is characterised by increased hemoglobin, RBC, haematocrit, WBC and platelet. Also, increased LAP (leukocyte alkaline phosphatase), vitamin B12 and uric acid (may cause gout). Bone marrow is hypercellular with increased megakaryocyte.

Clinical Features

Polycythaemia rubra vera is common in males, after 40 years.

Symptoms

- Common features are hyperviscocity syndrome—headache, dizziness, black out, blurring of vision.
- Pruritus after hot bath or with warm body.
- Peptic ulcer is common, bleeding may occur.
- Thrombosis (CVD, peripheral vascular disease), hypertension, angina, intermittent claudication.

Signs

- Face—plethoric, deep dusky, cyanosed, redness of conjunctiva, engorged retinal vessels on fundoscopy.
- Splenomegaly (70%), hepatomegaly (50%).

Complications

- PRV may transform to myelofibrosis (15%), acute myeloid leukaemia and refractory state with anaemia.
- Thromboembolism (cerebral, coronary).
- Hypertension, gout, peptic ulcer.

Investigations

- CBC and platelet—high haemoglobin, RBC, WBC, platelet. Haematocrit is also high.
- Red cell mass measured with radioactive ^{51}Cr labelled red cells (increased).
- Erythropoietin is low or absent (high in secondary polycythaemia).
- Bone marrow shows erythroid hyperplasia and increased megakaryocyte.
- Others—high LAP score, high vitamin B12.

NB: Plethoric appearance, splenomegaly, increased RBC, WBC and platelets are highly suggestive of PRV.

Treatment

- Venesection (400–500 mL of blood, every 5–7 days) until haematocrit is <45% and platelet <400 × 10^9/L.
- Radioactive phosphorus for elderly (5 mCi of ^{32}P IV).
- Other drugs—hydroxyurea, interferon may be given.
- Aspirin reduces risk of thrombosis.
- Median survival—10 years, some 20 years.

MYELODYSPLASTIC SYNDROME

Definition

This is a group of acquired bone marrow disorders due to defect in stem cells, characterised by increasing marrow failure with quantitative and qualitative abnormality of all three cell lines. There is anaemia, neutropenia and thrombocytopenia, usually with hypercellular or normocellular marrow.

Secondary MDS may be found in any patient treated with radiotherapy, chemotherapy or combination (as in lymphoma).

Clinical Features

Common in elderly, transform to AML in 30% cases.

- May be asymptomatic.
- May present with anaemia, recurrent infection or bleeding manifestations.

Types of Diseases in MDS

1. Refractory anaemia (RA)—blast <5%, erythroid dysplasia only.
2. Refractory anaemia with sideroblast (blast <5%, ring sideroblast >15%).
3. Refractory cytopenias with multilineage dysplasia (blast <5%, 2-3 lineage dysplasia).
4. Refractory anaemia with excess blast (blast 5-20%, 2-3 lineage dysplasia).
5. Refractory anaemia with excess blast in transformation (blast 20-30%).
6. MDS with 5q-MDS with del (5q) cytogenetic abnormality blasts <5%, normal or increased blood platelet.
7. MDS unclassified—none of the above or inadequate material.

Investigations

- CBC—shows cytopenia (thrombocytopenia and leucopenia), hypogranular neutrophil, hyposegmented neutrophil (Pelger cells) or hypersegmented neutrophil. MCV—high (macrocytic) or normal.
- Bone marrow—hypercellular with dysplastic change despite pancytopenia. Megaloblastic changes, ring sideroblast in all types, dyserythropoiesis, granulocyte precursor and megakaryocyte show abnormal morphology.
- Chromosome analysis—abnormality in chromosome 5 or 7.

Treatment

1. If blast <5%—
   - Supportive therapy with platelet, red cell transfusion
   - Erythropoietin and G-CSF may be given.
2. If blast >5%—

- Supportive therapy.
- Chemotherapy—low dose hydroxyurea or etoposide.
- Lenalidomide (a thalidomide analogue) may be effective in early stage of MDS with chromosome 5q deletion
- Allogenic stem cell transplantation in young less than 55 years.
- A new hypomethylating agent Azacytidine may be given, its use especially is not eligible for transplantation.

LEUKAEMIA

Definition

Leukaemia is a malignant disorder of haemopoietic stem cell characterised by increased number of primitive WBC in marrow and peripheral blood.

Types

1. Acute—Characterised by presence of primitive blast cell in the marrow and blood. It is of two types:
   - Acute lymphoblastic (ALL)—more common in children, 80% is improved with chemotherapy. CNS involvement is common.
   - Acute myeloid (AML)—common in adult, CNS involvement is rare, cure rate is less.
2. Chronic—Characterised by presence of excess mature cells in the marrow and blood. It is of types:
   - Chronic lymphatic (CLL).
   - Chronic myeloid (CML).

Other types:

- Subleukaemic—when WBC count is normal but blast cells are seen in the blood.
- Aleukaemic—when WBC count is normal or subnormal but no blast cell in the blood. Diagnosis is done by bone marrow.

ACUTE LEUKAEMIA

Symptoms

- Features of anaemia—weakness, dizziness, giddiness.
- Fever, malaise.
- Bleeding—nasal, gum, persistent bleeding after operation.
- Infection—mouth, throat.
- Pain in the bones and joints (common in childhood).

Signs

- Anaemia.
- Bruise, ecchymosis, petechiae.
- Bony tenderness.
- Generalised lymphadenopathy, in ALL.
- Hepatosplenomegaly.

Investigations

- CBC and PBF—WBC is high, Hb and platelet are low. PBF shows blast cell (In ALL—mostly lymphoblast, in AML—myeloblast)
- Bone marrow—hypercellular with leukaemic blast cell.

Treatment

1. General measures—correction of anaemia, control of infection by antibiotics, control of bleeding, psychological support.
2. Specific—by chemotherapy.
   - Induction of remission.
   - Consolidation.
   - Maintenance.
3. Bone marrow transplantation—either allogenic or autologous may be done.

CHRONIC MYELOID LEUKAEMIA

Definition

Chronic myeloid leukaemia (CML) is a myeloproliferative stem cell disorder, characterised by proliferation of all haematopoeitic cells, predominantly granulocyte series.

Philadelphia chromosome is present in 95% cases. It is common in people of 40–60 years, peak age is 55 years.

Symptoms

- May be asymptomatic.
- Weakness, tiredness, lethargy, anorexia, weight loss.
- Patient may complain of mass or discomfort or heaviness or pain in left upper abdomen (due to splenomegaly).
- Fever, night sweat.
- Repeated infection.
- Bleeding.
- Priapism (painful erection of penis).

Signs

- Splenomegaly, may be huge.
- Hepatomegaly (in 50% cases).
- Bony tenderness.
- Lymphadenopathy, occurs in blastic crisis.

Investigations

1. CBC:
   - WBC—very high (50,000–500,000/cmm).
   - Differential count—high myelocyte, promyelocyte. Metamyelocyte. Myeloblast <10%, increase in neutrophil, also basophil and eosinophil.
   - Platelets are increased.
2. Bone marrow study—hypercellular marrow with increased myeloid precursors.
3. Cytogenetic analysis for Philadelphia chromosome, also RNA analysis to see the presence of BCR-ABL gene product.
4. Other tests:
   - Philadelphia chromosome (positive in 95% cases).
   - LAP score—low.
   - Serum uric acid—high.
   - Serum vitamin B12—high.
   - Serum LDH—high.

Clinical Phases or Types of CML

There are three phases:

- Chronic phase.
- Accelerated phase.
- Blastic crisis.

Blastic Crisis in CML

It means the disease is transformed to acute leukaemia. May be myeloid (70%) or lymphatic (30%). This condition is difficult to treat. Blastic crisis in CML can be suspected, if—

- Rapid deterioration of the patient.
- Increasing splenomegaly.
- Blood picture shows increase in number of blast cells and increasing basophil.

Causes of Death in CML

- Blastic crisis.
- Secondary infection.
- Myelofibrosis.

Treatment of CML

Depends on the phase of disease, chronic phase and accelerated or blastic crisis:

1. Treatment of chronic phase:
   - Imatinib—first line therapy. Dose is 400 mg daily. In some cases, 600–800 mg may be given, can be continued indefinitely.
   - If no response to imatinib—desatinib or nilotinib or allogenic bone marrow transplantation should be considered.
   - Hydroxyurea or alpha interferon are still useful.
   - Bone marrow transplantation from HLA matched sibling donor (usually below 40 years and in early chronic phase).
2. Treatment of accelerated phase and blastic crisis:
   - Treatment is difficult, imatinib is indicated if the patient has not received it.
   - Hydroxyurea can be effective.
   - Low dose cytarabine can be given.

CHRONIC LYMPHATIC LEUKAEMIA

Definition

Chronic lymphatic leukaemia (CLL) is a neoplastic disorder of lymphocyte, usually involving B lymphocytes (95%) and rarely T lymphocytes (5%). More in elderly male, of age 65–70 years.

Symptoms

- Asymptomatic in many cases, diagnosed incidentally during routine examination.
- General features—malaise, weakness, fatigue, weight loss and night sweating.
- Recurrent infections.

Signs

- Generalised lymphadenopathy.
- Hepatosplenomegaly.

Stages of CLL

There are three stages of CLL. These are as follows:

1. Stage A (60%)—survival >10 years:
   - No anaemia.
   - No thrombocytopenia.
   - Less than 3 areas of lymph nodes involvement.
2. Stage B (30%)—survival 7 years:
   - No anaemia.
   - No thrombocytopenia.
   - Three or more areas of lymph nodes involvement.
3. Stage C (10%)—survival 2 years:
   - Anaemia.
   - With or without thrombocytopenia.
   - Regardless of area of lymph nodes involvement.

Investigations

1. CBC—Hb% (low), WBC—very high (50 to 200 × $10^9/mm^3$). Differential count shows increased lymphocytes (95%) mostly small lymphocyte. Platelet is normal, low or slightly increased.
2. Bone marrow shows increased lymphocytes.
3. Others:
   - Reticulocyte (high in autoimmune haemolytic anaemia).
   - Coomb's test (positive in autoimmune haemolytic anaemia).
   - Uric acid—high.
   - Immunophenotyping of B cell antigen (CD19 and CD23) and T cell antigen (CD5).

Treatment

Early indolent case requires no treatment. Otherwise, treatment depends on stage:

- Stage A—No treatment, unless progression occurs. The patient survives for long time (reassurance and follow-up). Life expectancy is normal in older patient.

- Stage B—No treatment, if the patient is asymptomatic.
- Stage C—Usually treatment is necessary.

Modes of Treatment

1. Symptomatic:
   - For anaemia and thrombocytopenia—prednisolone, blood transfusion should be given.
   - Infection—antibiotic, immunoglobulin (gamma globulin 0.4 gm/kg/month).
   - Local radiotherapy for LN causing discomfort or local obstruction and symptomatic splenomegaly.
2. Specific:
   - Chlorambucil 5 mg daily, dose is adjusted according to blood count.
   - Fludarabine alone or with cyclophosphamide or mitoxantrone (with or without steroid) is very helpful. Combination therapy with rituximab (ineffective alone). Usually, rituximab plus fludarabine with or without cyclophosphamide is the treatment of choice.
   - Alemtuzumab may be used in patient that progress after fludarabine.
   - Allogenic stem cell transplantation may be curative, but only used in those patient whose disease cannot be controlled by standard therapies.

LEUKAEMOID REACTION

Definition

It means periphereal blood film resembles leukaemia but there is no leukaemia.

Types

There are two types of leukaemoid reaction—myeloid and lymphoid.

Myeloid

Blood picture resembles myeloid leukaemia.

Causes
- Leucoerythroblastic blood picture due to any cause.
- Infection—pneumonia, meningitis, disseminated tuberculosis.
- Acute haemolysis.
- Malignancy.

Lymphoid

Blood picture resembles lymphatic leukaemia.

Causes
- Viral infection—infectious mononucleosis, cytomegalovirus, measles, chicken pox.
- Hooping cough.
- Tuberculosis.
- Malignancy.

Leucoerythroblastic Blood Picture

It means presence of immature myeloid and nucleated RBC in peripheral blood due to involvement of the bone marrow by abnormal tissue. Its causes are as follows:
- Secondary carcinoma of bone.
- Myelofibrosis.
- Thalassaemia major, specially after splenectomy.
- Acitve haemolytic anaemia.
- Rarely—multiple myeloma, lymphoma.

PURPURA

Definition

It is the spontaneous bleeding or extravasation of blood from the capillary in the skin and mucous membrane that does not blanch on pressure and there is progressive colour change.

Causes of Purpura

- Thrombocytopenic.
- Vascular.
- Coagulation defect.

Thrombocytopenic Purpura

1. Primary or ITP.
2. Secondary:
   - Aplastic anaemia (due to any cause).
   - Leukaemia.
   - Secondary deposit in bone marrow.
   - SLE.
   - DIC.

Vascular Purpura

1. Congenital (hereditary haemorrhagic telangiectasia, Ehlers-Danlos syndrome).
2. Acquired:
   - Senility (in elderly).
   - Henoch-Schönlein purpura.
   - Drug-induced (NSAID, steroid, sulphonamide, penicillin).
   - Infections—SBE, meningococcal infection, septicaemia, dengue haemorrhagic fever.
   - Scurvy.
   - Metabolic disorder (CKD, Cushing's syndrome).
   - Collagen disease (RA, SLE).
   - Multiple myeloma.
   - Amyloidosis (periorbital).

Coagulation Defect

1. Haemophilia.
2. Christmas disease.
3. Anticoagulant therapy.

Investigations in Purpura

1. Hb%, TC, DC, ESR, platelet and PBF.
2. If pancytopenia or thrombocytopenia—bone marrow study (dry tap in aplastic anaemia, increased megakaryocyte in ITP).

3. Other investigations (according to suspicion of causes) -
   - Coagulation screen (BT, CT, PT, APTT and FDP) for haemophilia and Christmas disease and other coagulation factors, screening for DIC.
   - Blood culture (if septicaemia).
   - ANA, antidouble strand DNA (for SLE).
   - Anti phospholipid antibody.
   - Liver function tests (in CLD).
   - Renal function tests (in CKD).

IDIOPATHIC THROMBOCYTOPENIC PURPURA

Definition

Idiopathic thrombocytopenic purpura (ITP) is a type of thrombocytopenic purpura due to autoantibody against platelet (IgG type) which causes premature removal of platelet.

Types

1. Acute—common in children.
2. Chronic—common in adult women.

Symptoms

- In child—Common age is 2–6 years, usually acute presentation, previous history of viral infection followed by bleeding or purpura, easy bruising, etc.
- In adult—Common in adult female at the age of 20–40 years, usually insidious onset without preceding viral infection. There are purpura, easy bruising, epistaxis or menorrhagia. There may be relapse and remission.

Signs

Apart from bleeding points, no other physical findings.

NB: Following points are important:

- If platelet count is <20,000/cmm, spontaneous bleeding occurs.
- If platelet count is >50,000/cmm, there may not be any bleeding.

Investigations

- Full blood count—there is thrombocytopenia.
- Bone marrow—increased immature megakaryocytes.
- Bleeding time is prolonged, but clotting time is normal.
- Antiplatelet antibody is present in 60–70% cases.
- Anticardiolipin antibody is positive in 30% cases.

Treatment

In children—usually self-limiting, does not require treatment in most cases. If there is no improvement:

- Prednisolone (2 mg/kg) should be given, if platelet is <10,000/cmm and bruising, epistaxis or other bleeding.

- If still persistent bleeding, I/V immunoglobulin should be given.
- In some cases, platelet transfusion may be required when there is persistent bleeding (epistaxis, GIT bleeding, retinal haemorrhage, intracranial bleeding).

In adults—Persistent thrombocytopenia is common. Most patients with platelet count > 30,000/cmm are stable and do not require treatment. Even with low platelet, treatment is not necessary unless there is spontaneous bruise or bleeding.

1. First line therapy:
   - Prednisolone 1 mg/kg, given for 4–6 weeks, then taper. Relapse is common when the steroid dose is reduced or stopped. If relapse, steroid should be started again.
   - I/V immunoglobulin may be given, if there is severe haemostatic failure or slow response to steroid alone or surgery is required. Steroid may be added with immunoglobulin.
2. Second line therapy:
   If there is frequent relapse or require high dose of steroid, splenectomy should be done.
3. Third line therapy:
   - If failure after splenectomy—corticosteroid, IV immunoglobulin, danazol, dapsone, immunosuppressive drug (azathioprine, vincristine, vinblastine, ciclosporin), mycophenolate mofetil. Monoclonal antibody like rituximab, recombinant thrombopoietin may be given.
4. Platelet transfusion is not usually necessary. However, used only if persistent or potentially life threatening bleeding or where emergency splenectomy is done.

Causes of Thrombocytopenia

1. Less production:
   - Aplastic anaemia (primary or idiopathic).
   - Bone marrow infiltration—secondary deposit, multiple myeloma, leukaemia, lymphoma.
   - Marrow suppression by radiotherapy or cytotoxic drugs.
   - Megaloblastic anaemia.
   - Myelofibrosis.
   - HIV infection.
2. Excessive destruction or consumption:
   - Immune—ITP, drug-induced (heparin), SLE.
   - Nonimmune—DIC, thrombotic thrombocytopenic purpura, hypersplenism, massive blood transfusion (dilutional).

HENOCH-SCHONLEIN PURPURA (HSP)

Definition

It is a small vessel vasculitis characterised by purpura or skin rash, joint pain (in big joints), abdominal pain and glomerulonephritis. It occurs 1-3 weeks after upper respiratory infection (usually viral). Other factors responsible include food, drugs or vaccination.

Symptoms

More common in boys, 5-15 years of age, but may occur at any age.

1. Skin lesion—purpura is common in legs and buttock. Resolves in 2-4 weeks and fresh crops may appear.
2. Polyarthralgia—commonly involves knee and ankle, may be fleeting type.
3. Abdominal pain—colicky in nature, associated with nausea, vomiting, bloody diarrhoea.
4. Renal disease—may be haematuria and proteinuria. May be nephrotic syndrome and rarely renal failure.

Investigations

- CBC, platelet—normal (nonthrombocytopenic purpura).
- Urine (proteinuria and haematuria).
- Serum IgA is high in 50% cases.
- Skin biopsy from normal and involved skin (shows leukocytoclastic vasculitis).
- Kidney biopsy—shows focal and segmental proliferative glomerulonephritis. There is IgA deposition.

Treatment of HSP

- Usually self-limiting, spontaneous cure in most cases.
- Prednisolone is given, if GIT and joint symptoms. Abdominal pain may be improved in 24 hours following steroid therapy.
- In renal involvement—pulse IV steroid and cytotoxic drugs should be given.
- Recurrence may occur. If so, dapsone may help, specially in cutaneous recurrence.

HAEMOPHILIA

Definition

It is an X-linked inherited disorder due to deficiency of factor VIII or antihaemophilic factor, characterised by prolonged bleeding. Male is the sufferer, female is the carrier.

Types

Normal factor VIII level is 50–150 IU/dL. According to severity, it is of three types:
- Mild—factor VIII is 10–50% (>5 but <40 IU/dL). Bleeding occurs following injury or surgery.
- Moderate—factor VIII is 2–10% (1–5 IU/dL). There is severe bleeding following injury or surgery, also spontaneous bleeding sometimes.
- Severe—factor VIII is <2% (<1 IU/dL). There is frequent spontaneous bleeding, also bleeding into the joints and muscles.

Pedigree of Haemophilia

1. If father is affected:
   - All daughters are carriers.
   - All sons are normal.
2. If mother is carrier:
   - 50% daughters are carriers.
   - 50% sons are sufferers.

Conditions when a female can be a sufferer in haemophilia:
- If a carrier female is married to an affected male, the female baby may be a sufferer.
- Turner's syndrome (because there is XO, if the only X is affected).

Symptoms

Depends on whether factor VIII deficiency is mild, moderate or severe. Following are the symptoms:
- Prolonged and persistent bleeding after trauma or injury, tooth extraction.
- Spontaneous bleeding may occur in severe case.
- Bleeding into the large joints and muscles (psoas and calf muscle) is also common.

Complications

1. Due to repeated haemorrhage:
   - Arthropathy due to repeated bleeding in joints (e.g. knee, elbow).
   - Death may occur due to intracerebral haemorrhage.
2. Due to therapy:
   - Infections—hepatitis A, B, C, D. Also, HIV.
   - Factor VIII antibody (20–30%).

Treatment

1. Bleeding episodes are treated with intravenous infusion of factor VIII concentrate, usually two to three times daily.
2. If factor VIII is not available, cryoprecipitate, fresh frozen plasma or fresh blood can be given.

3. Synthetic vasopressin (desmopressin)—intravenous, subcutaneous or intranasal, increases factor VIII.
4. Genetic counselling.

Christmas Disease (Haemophilia B)

It is a coagulation disorder due to deficiency of factor IX. Features are like haemophilia.

Severe bleeding may occur if there is severe deficiency of factor IX. In such cases treatment with factor IX concentrate.

VON WILLEBRAND'S DISEASE

Definition

von Willebrand's disease is an inherited disorder of hemostasis, inherited as autosomal dominant, rarely recessive, equally affects both sexes. There is a defective platelet function and factor VIII: C deficiency, which is due to deficiency or abnormality of vWF. Coagulation defect is due to the deficiency of factor VIII activity in plasma.

Clinical Features

- Bleeding tendency is usually mild, such as easy bruising, epistaxis, which follow upper respiratory infection.
- Sometimes, severe bleeding may occur, prolonged bleeding up to 36 hours following minor laceration, tooth extraction may occur.

Investigations

- Platelet is normal and prothrombin time is also normal
- Bleeding time and APTT—prolonged.
- Failure of aggregation of platelet by ristocetin.
- Factor VIII: C activity may be reduced.
- von Willebrand's antigen is reduced or absent.
- Tourniquet test—positive.

Treatment

- Mild bleeding—synthetic vasopressin raises the vWF factor.
- Severe bleeding—factor VIII concentrate or cryoprecipitate. Fresh frozen plasma may be given.
- Oestrogen/progesterone may be used to control menorrhagia.

LYMPHOMA

Definition

It is defined as neoplastic disorder of lymphoid tissues.

Types

Lymphoma is of two types—Hodgkin's and non-Hodgkin's lymphoma.

Hodgkin's Disease

It is a type of lymphoma characterised by painless, progressive enlargement of LNs associated with Reed-Sternberg giant cell (hallmark of the disease).

It usually occurs in adolescence and young adults (20–35 years of age), also after 45 years of age (50–70 years, two peaks of incidence).

Symptoms

1. May be asymptomatic.
2. Lumps in the neck, axilla, inguinal region.
3. Systemic features:
   - Fever—may be low-grade, sometimes Pel-Ebstein type (recurrent bouts of pyrexia followed by apyrexial period).
   - Night sweat, cough, weight loss, anorexia, malaise, weakness and pruritus (10%), shortness of breath (due to mediastinal lymphadenopathy).
   - Pain at the site of disease after drinking alcohol.
   - Superior venacaval obstruction due to pressure by mediastinal lymph nodes.

Signs

- Generalised lymphadenopathy involving cervical, axillary and inguinal regions. Lymph nodes are soft, rubbery, discrete.
- Hepatosplenomegaly with abdominal para-aortic lymphadenopathy.

Investigations

1. CBC—anaemia, lymphopenia, high eosinophil, high ESR. Blood count may be normal.
2. Chest X-ray (shows bilateral hilar lymphadenopathy and widening of mediastinal shadow).
3. FNAC or biopsy of lymph node.
4. USG of whole abdomen.
5. CT scan of chest and abdomen including pelvis.
6. Others:
   - Bone marrow study (involved in advanced stage).
   - Renal function tests (serum creatinine).
   - Liver function tests (SGPT).
   - Serum uric acid.
   - Serum lactate dehydrogenase (LDH).

Staging of HD

For staging, following tests are done:

- Chest X-ray.

- Bone marrow.
- USG of whole abdomen.
- CT scan (whole abdomen and chest).

Stages of HD

Ann Arbor staging—4 stages.
- Stage I—Involvement of a single LN region (I) or extralymphatic site (IE).
- Stage II—Involvement of two or more LN regions (II) or an extralymphatic site and LN regions on the same side of diaphragm (IIE).
- Stage III—Involvement of LN regions on both sides of diaphragm with (IIIE) or without (III) localised extralymphatic involvement or involvement of spleen (IIIS) or both (IIISE).
- Stage IV—Diffuse involvement of one or more extralymphatic tissue with or without LN involvement (bone marrow, liver and lung).

Depending on systemic features, each stage is divided into:
- A symptoms—no systemic features.
- B symptoms, with systemic features—such as fever >38ºC, drenching sweats, unexplained loss of >10% of body weight in last 6 months.

Treatment

1. Chemotherapy and adjunctive radiotherapy—ABVD (Adriamycin or doxorubicin, Bleomycin, Vinblastine and Dacarbazine) regimen is widely used.
2. Patient with early stage HD (IA, IIA, no bulk) is treated with 2–4 cycles of ABVD followed by radiotherapy to the involved lymph nodes.
3. Patient with advanced disease is usually treated with chemotherapy alone. Usually 6–8 cycles of ABVD is given.
4. Patient who is resistant to chemotherapy may be considered for autologous bone marrow transplantation.
5. Other chemotherapeutic regimen that were previously used are as follows:
   - MOPP—Mechlorethamine, Oncovin (vincristine), Procarbazine and Prednisolone.
   - COPP—Cyclophosphamide, Oncovin (vincristine), Procarbazine and Prednisolone.

Non-Hodgkin's Lymphoma (NHL)

Non-hodgkin's lymphoma (NHL) is characterized by malignant proliferation of lymphoid cells, majority are B cells (70%) and few T cells (30%).

Types or Grading

1. Low-grade (indolent) shows following characteristics:
   - Low cell proliferation rate.
   - Asymptomatic for many years.
   - Slow indolent course.
   - Good response to minimal therapy.
   - Incurable, but the patient survives for long time.
   - No treatment is required, if the disease is not advanced and asymptomatic.
   - Median survival up to 10 years.

2. High-grade (aggressive)—shows following characteristics:
   - Cell divisions occur quickly.
   - Early symptoms are common.
   - Fatal, if untreated.
   - Responds to treatment and patient may achieve a long term remission if treated properly.

NB: Stages of NHL are similar to Hodgkin's lymphoma.

Symptoms

It can occur at any age, but common in 65–70 years.
- Generalised lymphadenopathy.
- B symptoms—fever, night sweats, weight loss may be present.
- Extranodal presentations are more common than Hodgkin's disease. May involve gastrointestinal tract (stomach), lung, thyroid, skin, testes and CNS.

Signs

- Discrete, painless, firm, lymph nodal enlargement.
- Hepatosplenomegaly.

Investigations: Similar to HL, plus the following:
- Routine bone marrow aspiration and trephine.
- Immunotyping of surface antigen—CD 20 should be done.

Treatment

1. *Low grade NHL:* No therapy if the patient is asymptomatic.
   Indications of treatment are:
   - Marked systemic symptoms.
   - Bone marrow failure.
   - Features of compression (superior vena caval obstruction, spinal cord, gut obstruction and ascites).

   Treatment options include:
   - Radiotherapy for stage I.
   - Chemotherapy is needed in most cases. Majority responds well to oral chlorambucil which is well-tolerated but not curative. More aggressive intravenous chemotherapy may be tried in younger age.
   - Monoclonal antibody—rituximab is effective in 60% cases. Rituximab in combination with cyclophosphamide, doxorubicin, oncovin (vincristine), prednisolone (R-CHOP) is recommended as first line therapy.
2. *High Grade NHL:* Always needs treatment. Options are:
   - CHOP (cyclophosphamide, hydroxydaunorubicin, vincristine and prednisolone). Rituximab may be combined with CHOP therapy (R-CHOP).
   - Radiotherapy may be given in stage I and compression syndrome.
   - Autologous bone marrow transplantation for relapse chemosensitive disease.

MULTIPLE MYELOMA

Definition

Multiple myeloma is a malignant disease characterised by malignant proliferation of plasma cells of bone marrow, associated with excessive production of paraprotein.

Plasma cells produce monoclonal paraprotein, which may be associated with the excretion of light chain in urine, called Bence-Jones protein, either kappa or lambda. In some cases, there is no paraprotein, only light chain in urine.

Types

- IgG—55%.
- IgA—21%.
- Light chains—22%.
- Others (D, E, nonsecretory)—2%.

Symptoms

Common in elderly, above 60 years, more in male, the ratio of male-female is M:F = 2:1. May be asymptomatic, diagnosis is suspected on routine blood test. Usual presentations are:

- Bone pain, commonly backache, generalised bodyache, bone pain, rheumatic like pain.
- Unexplained anaemia.
- Recurrent infection (respiratory, urinary tract).
- Spontaneous fracture, collapse of vertebrae (with shortening of stature).
- Bleeding manifestations.
- Renal failure.
- Features of hyperviscosity syndrome (dizziness, giddiness, headache, vertigo, blurring of vision, stupor, confusion, coma).

Diagnostic Criteria of Multiple Myeloma

Any two of the following three criteria:

- Lytic lesion in X-ray.
- Serum or urinary M protein.
- Increased atypical plasma cell in bone marrow.

Investigations

- CBC, ESR, PBF—high ESR, PBF—shows marked rouleaux formation.
- Bone marrow (to see atypical plasma cells).
- Plasma protein electrophoresis or immunoelectrophoresis (myeloma band).
- Urine for Bence-Jones protein.
- Serum total protein—high, Albumin—low.
- X-ray of Skull and other bones.
- Serum calcium (high), C-reactive protein (high), lactate dehydrogenase (high), uric acid (normal or high).
- Renal function (urea, creatinine and electrolytes).

- Serum alkaline phosphatase normal (May be high if there is fracture).
- Serum β2 microglobulin (high).

Treatment

In asymptomatic case with no evidence of organ damage (e.g. Kidney, bone marrow or bone), no treatment is necessary. Only follow-up. Treatment is given in symptomatic patient.

1. Supportive therapy—correction of anaemia, control of infection, control of renal failure. Allopurinol to prevent urate nephropathy. Plasmapheresis may be given for hyperviscosity; analgesic and bisphosphonate (e.g. Zolendronate) for bone pain.
2. Specific therapy—
   - Thalidomide or bortezomib are the first line treatment (Thalidomide can cause constipation, oversedation, peripheral neuropathy, venous thrombosis, also teratogenic).
   - Bortezomib followed by lenalidomide (a derivative thalidomide) may be given .
   - In older patients—thalidomide combined with melphalan plus prednisolone has improved survival > 4 years.
   - In young patients—first line chemotherapy up to maximum response then autologus hematopoietic stem cell transplantation improves survival.
   - Thalidomide, lenalidomide, and bortezomib shows good response with dexamethasone.
   - Radiotherapy in localised bone pain or spinal cord compression.
   - Patients whose disease progresses despite thalidomide or lenalidomide and bortezomib are candidates for carfilzomib.

NB: Therapy should be continued until a plateau phase is attained, characterised by the following points:

- The patient is clinically improved.
- Hb%, paraprotein, β2-microglobulin are stable for 3 months.

Bad Prognostic factors

- Low albumin.
- High β2-microglobulin.
- High LDH.

Paraprotein

Paraprotein is an abnormal immunoglobulin produced by atypical plasma cells. Causes of paraproteinaemia are as follows:

- Multiple myeloma.
- Waldenstrom's macroglobulinaemia.
- Benign monoclonal gammopathy of uncertain origin.
- Heavy chain disease.
- Chronic lymphatic leukaemia.
- Lymphoma (non-Hodgkin's).
- Amyloidosis.

DISSEMINATED INTRAVASCULAR COAGULATION

Definition

Disseminated intravascular coagulation (DIC) is a haemorrhagic disorder in which diffuse intravascular clotting causes a haemostatic defect resulting from utilisation of coagulation factor and platelet in the clotting process. For this reason, this is also called consumption coagulopathy.

There is secondary activation of fibrinolysis, leading to production of fibrin degradation products (FDP). The consequence of these changes is a mixture of initial thrombosis, followed by bleeding tendency due to consumption of coagulation factors and fibrinolytic activity.

Causes

1. Obstetrical -
   - Abruptio placenta.
   - Amniotic fluid embolism.
   - Abortion.
2. Surgery, especially heart and lung.
3. Haemolytic transfusion reaction.
4. Septicaemia (which is due to gram-negative and meningococcal).
5. Pulmonary embolism.
6. Others—falciparum malaria, malignant disease, liver disease, trauma, burn, snake bite, heat stroke, etc.

NB: Chronic DIC may occur in—acute leukaemia (usually promyelocytic), IUD, septicaemia, disseminated malignancy.

Investigations

1. CBC—thrombocytopenia.
2. Prothrombin time—prolonged.
3. APTT—prolonged.
4. Fibrinogen—low.
5. D-dimer—high.
6. FDP—high.

Treatment

- Treatment of underlying cause.
- Broad spectrum antibiotic, if septicaemia.
- Fresh frozen plasma
- Platelet transfusion.

BLOOD TRANSFUSION

Complications

- Allergic reaction—itching, urticaria, anaphylaxis.
- Febrile reaction/pyrogenic reaction—rise of temperature, chill and rigor.
- Circulatory overload—leading to pulmonary oedema or acute LVF.
- Infection—hepatitis B and C, HIV, CMV, EBV.
- Transmission of disease—malaria, kala-azar, toxoplasma, brucella.
- Haemolytic transfusion reaction, mostly due incompatibility.
- Repeated transmission may cause haemosidarosis.
- Thrombophlebitis.
- Air embolism.

Treatment during Reaction

- Transfusion should be stopped.
- Grouping and cross matching must be ckecked.
- Injection hydrocortisone 100 mg IV or dexamethasone IV.
- Antihistamine—chlorpheniramine IV.

Indication

- Severe anaemia
- Bleeding due to any cause.

Before Transfusion

- Always check grouping and cross matching
- Check the bag to see name of patient grouping, etc.
- Injection furosemide may be given, if chance of heart failure.

STEM CELL TRANSPLANTATION (BONE MARROW TRANSPLANTATION)

Stem cell transplantation (SCT) achieves reconstitution of haematopoiesis by transfusion of pluripotent haemopoietic stem cells.

It involves eliminating the patient's haemopoietic and immune system by chemotherapy and/or radiotherapy, then replacing with stem cells either from another individual (allogenic) or with previously harvested portion of patient's own haemopoietic stem cells (autologous).

In bone marrow translplantation, stem cells are collected from the bone marrow and transfused.

Types

- Allogeneic—stem cells are obtained from a donor, e.g. a matched sibling, identical twin or volunteer (matched unrelated donor).
- Autologous—patient's own stem cells from his bone marrow are collected and harvested, then it is transfused.

Indications

Autologous SCT

- Relapse aggressive NHL.
- Relapsed Hodgkin's lymphoma.
- Multiple myeloma (stage II/III).
- AML.
- Primary amyloidosis.

Allogeneic or Synergic SCT

- AML.
- ALL.
- CML.
- Myelodysplastic syndrome (MDS).
- Multiple myeloma.
- Severe aplastic anaemia (including Fanconi's anaemia).
- Thalassaemia major.
- Sickle-cell anaemia.
- Lymphoma.
- Severe acquired marrow disease—PNH, red cell aplasia.

Potential Donor

Allogenic/Synergic

- HLA matched sibling, identical twin.
- Unrelated HLA matched volunteer.
- Umbilical cord blood.

Autologous—Self

Process

- First step—bone marrow collection.
- Then—stem cell processing.
- Then—conditioning.
- Finally—stem cell infusion.

Complications

Early

If <100 days.

Due to chemoradiotherapy
- Nausea, vomiting.
- Reversible alopecia.
- Fatigue.
- Dry skin.
- Mucositis.

Due to transplantation
- Infection—bacterial (Gram negative and positive), viral (HZV, CMV), fungal (candida, *Aspergillus*, mucormycosis), pneumocystis pneumonia, toxoplasma, *Mycoplasma*, *Legionella*.
- Haemorrhage.
- Graft failure.
- Venoocclusive disease.
- Acute pattern of graft versus host disease (rash, erythroderma, bullae, desquamation).
- Cardiac failure (in autologous).
- Recurrence of original disease.

Late

If >100 days.
- Infection—specially varicella zoster, capsulated bacteria.
- Chronic graft versus host disease (arthritis, malabsorption, hepatitis, sicca syndrome, lichen planus, pulmonary disease, serous effusion).
- Infertility.
- Hypothyroidism.
- Secondary malignancy (allogenic).
- Cataract.
- Autoimmune disorder.
- Immunodeficiency.
- Graft failure.

HAEMOLYTIC URAEMIC SYNDROME

Definition

Haemolytic uraemic syndrome (HUS) is characterised by rapid onset of microangiopathichaemolyticanaemia, thrombocytopenia and acute renal failure (triad) due to thrombosis in small arteries and arteriole.

Causes

Caused by verotoxinproducing organism, such as EnterohaemorrhagicE. coli0157:H7. Recently, a new toxin producing E. coli 0104:H4 is found to be responsible in some countries. It occurs in up to 6% patients infected with this organism, by infected food (undercooked beef) or unpasteurized milk.

Pathogenesis

Infection triggers damage to the endothelial cells of microcirculation and derangement of haemostatic coagulation system. This is followed by cell swelling, platelet clumping, fibrinogen deposition, thrombosis and occlusion. Common in glomerular capillaries and renal arterioles.

HUS may be diarrhea associated (D+HUS) or nondiarrhoeal HUS (D-HUS or atypical HUS).

Clinical Features

Common in children, <3 years. It usually follows gastroenteritis.

- Fever.
- Vomiting and diarrhoea, often bloody called diarrhoea associated HUS (D+HUS).
- Intravascular hemolysis is followed by oliguria or anuria.
- Purpura, anaemia, bleeding, drowsiness and hypertension may occur.

Investigations

- CBC—anaemia, marked thrombocytopenia.
- PBF—shows features of microangiopathichaemilyticanaemia (schistocyte), spherocyte and thrombocytopenia.
- Creatinine—very high.
- Other features of intravascular haemolysis—high bilirubin, high LDH, reduced haptoglobin and increased reticulocyte count.
- Confused with DIC, but coagulation tests are normal in HUS.

Treatment

In diarrhoeal HUS, treatment is mainly supportive—

- Correction of water and electrolyte balance.
- Maintenance of nutrition.
- Control of hypertension.
- FFP.
- Dialysis.
- Heparin or antiplatelet drug may be helpful.

- Plasmapheresis—not helpful.
- No role of antibiotic.

In atypical HUS—
- Supportive, as above.
- Plasmapheresis or plasma transfusion.
- Monoclonal antibody anti-CD5 antibody—eculizumab may be effective.

Prognosis

Five percent die in acute episode, 5% develop CRF and 30% develop persistent proteinuria.

THROMBOTIC THROMBOCYTOPENIC PURPURA

Definition

Thrombotic thrombocytopenic purpura (TTP) is a disorder of unknown etiology characterised by fever, microangiopathic hemolytic anemia, thrombocytopenia, neurological signs and renal failure.

Pathophysiology of TTP

This is due to reduction of ADAMTS-13 which is normally responsible for regulating the size of vWF. Initially, endothelial damage, cell swelling, platelet adherence and thrombosis. There is severe microangiopathichaemolytic anaemia with thrombocytopenia.

Renal disease is due to hyaline occlusion of capillaries and arterioles and proliferative change in glomeruli. Microscopically, there is microvascular hyaline thrombi.

Clinical Features

Common in young female. The clinical features are as follows:
- Fever.
- Purpuric spot due to thrombocytopenia.
- Fluctuating neurological features.
- Microangiopathichaemolytic anaemia.
- Renal failure.

It confuses with haemolyticuraemic syndrome, but neurological features are absent in HUS. These two conditions are probably a part of the same disorder.

Diagnosis

Diagnostic pentad in TTP—
- Fever.
- Neurological features—headache, seizure and coma.
- Thrombocytopenia.
- Microangiopathic hemolytic anemia.
- Renal failure.

Investigations

- CBC—thrombocytopenia is invariable.
- PBF—shows presence of fragmented RBC (schistocyte)
- Reticulocytes—increased.
- Bleeding time—prolonged/
- Bilirubin and LDH—high, reduced haptoglobin.
- Coagulation screen (APTT, D-dimer, FDP and PT) are all normal. Usually no DIC.

Treatment

- Plasma exchange.
- Fresh-frozen plasma or cryoprecipitate infusion.

- Pulse IV methylprednisolone may be given.
- Rituximab is also very helpful.
- Platelet transfusion is contraindicated, as it may aggravate the disease.

Prognosis

Mortality 90% in untreated, 10–30% in treated cases.

CHAPTER

6 Hepatology

CHAPTER CONTENTS

- Jaundice
- Alcoholic liver disease
- Nonalcoholic fatty liver disease (NAFLD)
- Acute viral hepatitis
- Obstructive jaundice
- Liver abscess
  - Pyogenic liver abscess
  - Amoebic liver abscess
- Primary biliary cirrhosis (PBC)
- Ascites
- Cirrhosis of liver
- Portosystemic encephalopathy (PSE) or hepatic precoma
- Fulminating hepatic failure
- Oesophageal varices
- Portal hypertension
- Haemochromatosis
  - Primary or hereditary haemochromatosis
- Hepatoma
- Secondaries in the liver
- Primary sclerosing cholangitis
- Acute cholecystitis
- Chronic cholecystitis
- Carcinoma of gallbladder
- Liver transplantation

Investigations of hepatobiliary disease: Done for the following reasons:

1. Diagnosis of liver disease.
2. To find out the cause.
3. Severity and prognosis.

Liver Blood Biochemistry

Liver Function Tests (LFT's)

1. Serum bilirubin.
2. Enzymes—indicate hepatocellular damage.
   - SGOT/Aspertate aminotransferase (AST), high in acute hepatitis.
   - SGPT/Alanine aminotransferase (ALT) high in acute hepatitis.
   - Alkaline phosphatase—indicates cholestasis or obstruction of the biliary tree.
3. Gamma-glutamyl transferase (GGT)—It is sensitive marker for cholestatic damage. GGT is raised in chronic alcohol toxicity.
4. Prothrombin time (PT)—indicates acute or chronic hepatocellular damage.
5. Albumin—low level indicates chronic liver disease (cirrhosis of liver).

Imaging

Several imaging techniques can be used to determine the site and structural lesions in the liver and billiary tree.

- Ultrasound: Ultrasound most commonly use noninvasive test. It can be used to identify gallstones, biliary obstruction or thrombosis in the hepatic vasculature, splenomegally, abnormalities in the liver texture, focal lesion (tumours, abscess).
- CT scan.
- MRI.
- MRCP.
- ERCP.
- Fibroscan: It is a noninvasive test to differentiate severe fibrosis from mild scanning.

To Find Out Cause

- For Hepatitis A—anti-HAV IgM.
- For Hepatitis B—HBsAg, HBeAg, anti-HBc, HBV DNA, anti HBS.
- Hepatitis E—anti-HEV IgM and IgG.
- For Hepatitis C—anti-HCV.

Histological Examination

Liver biopsy—can confirm the severity of liver damage and provide aetiological information. It is performed percutaneously with a Trucut or Menghini needle or radiologically using a transjugular approach or during laparoscopy or laparotomy.

Immunological

Antimitochondrial antibody—for primary biliary cirrhosis.
ANA, antismooth muscle antibody (ASMA)—for autoimmune hepatitis.

JAUNDICE

Definition

It is a clinical condition characterised by yellow discolouration of skin and mucous membrane due to excess bilirubin in the blood.

Clinically, jaundice is seen when serum bilirubin is >3 mg/dL.

Types

Jaundice is of three types:

- Prehepatic (predominantly unconjugated hyperbilirubinemia).
- Hepatocellular (both conjugated and unconjugated hyperbilirubinemia).
- Posthepatic or obstructive (predominantly conjugated hyperbilirubinemia).

Causes

Prehepatic (Unconjugated Hyperbilirubinemia)

1. Excess production of bilirubin (due breakdown of RBC)—
   - Haemolytic anaemia due to any cause.
2. Reduced hepatic uptake of bilirubin or impaired conjugation—
   - Gilbert syndrome.
   - Drugs—sulfonamides, penicillin, rifampicin.
   - Crigler-Najjar syndrome Type 1 and 2.
   - Physiological jaundice of newborn.

Hepatocellular (Conjugated Hyperbilirubinemia)

1. Hepatitis—viral A, B, C, D, E and others—EBV, CMV, Yellow fever, dengue). Nonviral infections—leptospirosis, Q fever.
2. Drugs—
   - Antitubercular drugs—rifampicin, pyrazinamide, INH.
   - Phenothiazines—chlorpromazine, haloperidol.
   - Ciclosporine.
   - Alcohol
3. Metabolic—Wilson's disease, haemochromatosis.
4. Autoimmune.
5. Inherited disorders (Dubin-Johnson syndrome, Rotor syndrome).

Posthepatic or Obstructive

1. Extrahepatic:
   - Choledocholithiasis.
   - Carcinoma of head of pancreas.
   - Cholangiocarcinoma.
   - Periampullary carcinoma.
   - Extrahepatic biliary atresia.
   - Round worm in the common bile duct.
   - Biliary stricture—trauma, sclerosing cholangitis.

2. Intrahepatic:
   - Primary biliary cirrhosis (PBC).
   - Primary sclerosing cholangitis.
   - Viral hepatitis—causes transient intrahepatic cholestasis.

History to be taken in jaundice patient:

- Anorexia, nausea and vomiting (indicate viral hepatitis).
- History of contact with jaundiced patient or sexual exposure.
- Colour of the stool (yellowish, pale, dark), itching—indicate obstructive jaundice.
- History of injection, infusion or blood transfusion, I/V drug abuse, tattooing or surgery (HBV or HCV).
- History of alcohol or any drugs.
- Family history of jaundice, consanguinity of marriage among parents, associated pallor (indicate hereditary haemolytic anaemia).
- Associated history of high fever, urinary complain (indicate leptospirosis).
- Recurrent jaundice associated with any neurological abnormality (indicates Wilson's disease).
- Associated abdominal pain and fluctuating jaundice (indicates bile duct stricture or stone).
- History of travelling abroad (hepatitis B).

Features of Different Types of Jaundice

Features of Prehapatic Jaundice

- Usually in hereditary haemolytic anaemia. There is triad of anaemia, jaundice and splenomegaly. Other features—frontal and parietal bossing, mongoliod facies.
- Other causes of haemolytic anaemia—malaria, autoimmune haemolytic anaemia.

Features of Hepatocellular Jaundice

- Anorexia, nausea, vomiting, weakness.
- Stool is yellow in early stage, but may be dark or clay coloured in later stage due to intrahepatic cholestasis.
- Liver—enlarged and tender.

Features of Obstructive Jaundice

- Pale, dark or clay coloured stool.
- Itching of whole body.
- May be abdominal pain, mass in the epigastrium.
- Other features depent upon cause (xanthelasma or xanthoma in PBC).
- Bleeding tendency (due to deficiency of Vitamin K, resulting in deficiency in Vitamin K dependent clotting factors—factor II, VII, IX, X).
- Bone pain (due to osteomalacia).

Investigations of Jaundice

1. Liver function tests:
   - Serum bilirubin.
   - SGPT, SGOT.

 - Alkaline phosphatase.
 - Prothrombin time.
2. USG of hepatobiliary system.
3. Viral markers:
 - For A—anti-HAV IgM.
 - For E—anti-HEV IgM.
 - For B—HBsAg, HBeAg, anti-HBc.
 - For C—anti-HCV.
4. Other investigation should be done according to the suspicion of cause.

ALCOHOLIC LIVER DISEASE (ALD)

One unit of alcohol contains 8 gram ethanol. Effects of alcohol are worsen in women. Alcohol intake 21 units/week in male and 14 units/week in female is considered to be safe. Alcoholic liver disease occurs when the intake begins 30 g/day of ethanol. Consumption of > 80 g/day for more than 5 years is associated with significant risk of advance liver disease. Average alcohol consumption of a man with cirrhosis is 160g/day for over 8 years.

Definition

ALD means hepatic manifestations due to excess alcohol consumption. Disease depends on duration and amount of alcohol intake. Alcohol can produce the following liver disease:

- Fatty liver.
- Alcoholic hepatitis.
- Alcoholic cirrhosis.

Clinical Features

Depends on type of hepatic involvement:

- General—loss of appetite, fatigue, weight loss, nausea, vomiting, upper abdominal pain.
- Alcoholic fatty liver disease (AFLD)—may be asymptomatic. There is high aminotransferase on routine investigation. Prognosis is good after 3 months of alcohol abstinence.
- Acute alcoholic hepatitis—features like acute viral hepatitis.
- In chronic hepatitis or CLD or cirrhosis—stigmata of CLD (bilateral parotid enlargement, Dupuytran's contracture, spider angioma, etc).

Investigations

- CBC (shows macrocytosis).
- Liver function tests (AST is > ALT).
- Gamma GT—high.
- USG of HBS.
- CT of HBS.
- Liver biopsy.

Treatment

- Alcohol should be stopped.
- Nutritional supplementation—adequate vitamin B1, folic acid, protein.
- Corticosteroid is helpful acute alcoholic hepatitis.
- Pentoxifylline may be given in severe acute alcoholic hepatitis.
- If cirrhosis—manage accordingly. Liver transplantation should be considered but the patient must stop alcohol.

NON-ALCOHOLIC FATTY LIVER DISEASE

Definition

Non-alcoholic fatty liver disease (NAFLD) is defined as spectrum of liver disease in the absence of excessive alcohol consumption (<20 g/day for woman and <30 g/day in man.

It is often asymptomatic, but liver is enlarged due to lipid deposition within hepatocytes.

NAFLD is strongly associated with obesity, insulin resistance, dyslipidemia and type 2 DM. So, the patients with NAFLD are at high risk of developing cardiovascular disease.

NAFLD is of two types:

1. Nonalcoholic fatty liver (NAFL)—here hepatic steatosis is present without evidence of inflammation.
2. Nonalcoholic steatohepatitis (NASH)—here hepatic steatosis is associated with hepatic inflammation. May lead to progressive liver fibrosis, cirrhosis and liver cancer, also cardiovascular risk.

Investigations

- LFT.
- USG or CT scan of HBS.
- Liver biopsy—confirmatory.
- Other investigations to exclude other cause of liver disease.

Treatment

- Reduction of weight.
- Exercise program is effective in reducing weight and insulin resistance.
- Good control of diabetes melitus and hypertension. Metformin is given for insulin resistance associated with NAFLD.
- Orlistat for obesity.
- Atorvastatin for dyslipidaemia.
- Omega-3 fatty acids may also be used.

ACUTE VIRAL HEPATITIS

Definition

Hepatitis caused by the virus.

Causes

- Hepatotrophic viruses—A, B, C, D and E virus.
- Nonhepatotrophic viruses—Epstein-Barr virus, cytomegalo virus, yellow fever virus and dengue virus.

Symptoms

- Anorexia, nausea, vomiting.
- Yellow colouration of skin and sclera.
- High-coloured urine.
- Fever, malaise, weakness.
- Pain in the right upper abdomen,
- Pale stools may develop later (due to intrahepatic cholestasis).

Signs

- Jaundice—mild to moderate.
- Liver—enlarged, tender.

NB

- In hepatitis due to B virus—features of acute viral infection are same but certain extra features may be present, such as—serum sickness like illness characterised by skin rash (urticaria, maculo-papular rash), polyarthritis affecting small joints, fever, extrahepatic immune complex mediated arteritis or glomerulonephritis.
- Hepatitis E infection is only serious during pregnancy.

Investigations

1. CBC (may be leucopenia with relative lymphocytosis).
2. LFT:
   - Serum bilirubin—high.
   - SGPT—high.
   - SGOT—may be high (SGOT is raised in drug-induced hepatitis).
   - Alkaline phosphatase may be slightly high. In cholestatic hepatitis, alkaline phosphatase may be high.
   - Prothrombin time—prolonged in severe hepatitis.
3. Viral markers:
   - Virus A (anti-HAV, IgM indicates acute infection).
   - Virus B (HBsAg, HBeAg, anti-HBc).
   - Virus E (anti-HEV, IgM indicates acute infection)
   - Virus C—Anti HCV.
4. USG of HBS.
5. Others—blood sugar, urine R/E.

Complications

- Acute fulminating hepatic failure (by B and sometimes with E viral infection in pregnancy. It is rare by HAV).
- Relapsing hepatitis.
- Cholestatic hepatitis mostly by HAV, may persist for 7–20 weeks.
- Posthepatitis syndrome is seen in anxious patient.
- Chronic liver disease (due to B and C virus), which may lead to cirrhosis of liver and ultimately to hepatoma.
- Others—aplastic anaemia (usually reversible), rarely Coomb's positive haemolytic anaemia, polyarteritis nodosa, Henoch-Schönlein purpura, glomerulonephritis and collagen vascular disease.

Management

- Symptomatic and supportive.
- No specific dietary modifications are needed.
- Alcohol and hepatotoxic drugs should be avoided during acute illness.

OBSTRUCTIVE JAUNDICE

Causes

Obstruction usually occurs in common bile duct. Causes may be in the lumen, in the wall and outside the wall.

1. Causes in the lumen:
   - Stone in CBD (choledocholithiasis).
   - Worms (ascariasis).
2. Causes in the wall:
   - Sclerosing cholangitis.
   - Cholangiocarcinoma.
   - Periampulary carcinoma.
   - Stricture (may be due to surgery, trauma).
3. Causes outside the wall:
   - Carcinoma of head of the pancreas.
   - Lymphoma.
   - Enlargement of lymph node in porta hepatis.

Intrahepatic Causes of Cholestatic (obstructive) Jaundice

- Primary biliary cirrhosis.
- Primary sclerosing cholangitis.
- Viral hepatitis.
- Drugs and alcohol.
- Autoimmune hepatitis.
- Cystic fibrosis.
- Postoperative.
- Benign recurrent intrahepatic cholestasis.
- Pregnancy.

Features of Obstructive Jaundice

- Deep jaundice, dark yellow skin, deep yellow or mustard oil like urine.
- Pale or clay-coloured stool.
- Generalised itching with scratch mark.
- Weight loss, steatorrhoea.
- Deep seated abdominal pain due to stone in the common bile duct (choledocholithiasis), pancreatitis, choledochal cyst, sometimes due to carcinoma head of the pancreas.
- In prolonged case, osteomalacia due to vitamin D deficiency, bleeding disorder due to vitamin K deficiency, night blindness due to vitamin A deficiency.
- Palpable gallbladder, mass due to carcinoma of head of pancreas.

Investigations

1. Liver function tests:
   - Serum bilirubin.
   - SGPT—slightly high.
   - Alkaline phosphatase (very high).

- γ–glutamyl transferase (very high).
- PT (prolong).
- Serum total protein and A:G ratio.

2. USG of HBS and pancreas.
3. CT scan or MRI of upper abdomen.
4. ERCP, MRCP.

Treatment

- Rest, maintanence of nutrition.
- If patient can't take orally—I/V fluid.
- Injection vitamin K to prevent bleeding.
- For itching—cholestyramine.
- Treatment of primary cause.

LIVER ABSCESS

Types: There are two types of liver abscess (Table 1):
- Pyogenic liver abscess.
- Amoebic liver abscess.

Pyogenic Liver Abscess

Causes

1. Ascending cholangitis in biliary obstruction.
2. Haematogenous:
   - Portal pyaemia from intra-abdominal sepsis, suppurative appendicitis and perforation.
   - Septicaemia or bacteraemia (along the hepatic artery).
3. Direct extension from peripheral abscess.
4. Trauma—penetrating injury.
5. Infection of liver tumour or cyst.

Organisms

E. coli, S. milleri, S. faecalis or other *Streptococcus* species, *S. aureus,* anaerobic organisms or bacteroids.

Symptoms

- Fever, may be high with chill and rigor, malaise, anorexia and weight loss.
- Pain in right upper abdomen, may radiate to right shoulder.
- Pleuritic right lower chest pain (may be small pleural effusion, pleural rub).
- Jaundice is usually mild, may be severe in multiple abscesses causing biliary obstruction.
- Only pyrexia of unknown origin (PUO) may be present.

Investigations

1. CBC—neutrophilic leucocytosis.
2. USG of abdomen.
3. LFT (High alkaline phosphatase. SGPT is normal, may be slightly high).

Table 1
Differences between pyogenic and amoebic liver abscess

Points	Pyogenic	Amoebic
1. Organism	*E. coli* and others	*E. histolytica*
2. History	Cholangitis, septicaemia	Amoebiasis
3. Symptoms	High fever with chill and rigor	Fever mild to moderate, no chill and rigor
4. Neutrophil leucocytosis	Common	Less
5. Ultrasonography	Multiple lesion	Usually single
6. Aspiration	Frank pus	Chocolate and anchovy sauce
7. Prognosis	More fatal (mortality 16%)	Less fatal (<1%)

4. Serum albumin (low).
5. Chest X-ray (PA view) shows raised right dome of diaphragm, small right-sided pleural effusion.
6. Blood for C/S—positive in 30% cases.
7. CT scan or MRI of the upper abdomen may be done.

Treatment

- Antibiotic—Amoxicillin plus gentamicin plus metronidazole. Or Cefoperazone (1–2 g I/V 12 hourly) with metronidazole (500 mg every 6 hours for 2–3 weeks, sometimes up to 6 weeks.
- If larger liver abscess or not responding to antibiotic therapy—USG-guided aspiration should be done.

Amoebic Liver Abscess

Caused by *Entamoeba hystolytica* carried from the bowel to liver through portal circulation. Common in right lobe, usually single.

Symptoms

- History of diarrhoea (absent in 50% cases).
- Fever (low-grade), malaise, pain in the right upper abdomen.
- Anorexia, nausea, weight loss.

Signs

- Liver—enlarged and tender.
- Local oedema in the right lower chest with fullness in the intercostal space.
- Right lower chest is tender (punched tenderness).

Investigations

1. CBC—leukocytosis.
2. USG of abdomen.
3. Serum albumin (low).
4. Chest X-ray (PA view) shows raised right dome of diaphragm, small right-sided pleural effusion.
5. CT scan or MRI of the upper abdomen may be done.
6. Stool RME—to see cyst on *E. histolytica*.
7. Others:
   - Immunofluorescent antibody test (positive in 95%).
   - Indirect haemagglutination test (positive in 95%).
   - Complement fixation test.
   - ELISA.

Complication

- Abscess may rupture into pleural cavity, pericardial sac or peritoneal cavity.
- Hepatobronchial fistula.

Treatment

- Metronidazole 800 mg 8 hourly for 10 days or secnidazole 2 g daily for 5 days or tinidazole or ornidazole 2 g daily for 3 days. Or Nitaxozanide 500 mg 12 hourly for 3 days.
- After the treatment of amoebic liver abscess—diloxanide furoate 500 mg 8 hourly for 10 days for intestinal infection.
- If larger liver abscess or not responding to antibiotic therapy—USG-guided aspiration should be done.

Other Treatment

- Mixed infections may be found in many cases. Hence, antibiotic plus antiamoebic drugs may be needed.
- Abscess may rupture into pleural cavity, pericardial sac or peritoneal cavity. In such cases, immediate aspiration or surgical drainage is needed.

NB: Character of pus in amoebic liver abscess—chocolate or anchovy sauce colour.

PRIMARY BILIARY CIRRHOSIS

Definition

Primary biliary cirrhosis (PBC) is a chronic, progressive, cholestatic liver disease characterised by granulomatous destruction of interlobular bile ducts, inflammatory damage with fibrosis spreading from portal tract to liver parenchyma and eventual cirrhosis.

Causes

Actual cause is unknown. It is probably an autoimmune disease occurring in a genetically predisposed person.

Symptoms

Common in middle-aged 40–60 year females.

- May be asymptomatic. Incidental finding like isolated hepatomegaly on routine examination or during investigation (high alkaline phosphatase).
- Pruritus may be the early feature, may precede jaundice by many months or years.
- Jaundice usually with pruritus.
- Abdominal pain or discomfort.
- Malabsorption (steatorrhoea).
- Malaise, weakness, loss of weight, hyperpigmentation.
- Others—hepatic osteodystrophy (characterised by bony pain or fracture due to osteoporosis or osteomalacia from malabsorption).

Signs

- Ill looking, emaciated and hyperpigmented.
- Jaundice—moderate.
- Xanthelasma around both eyes (xanthomatous deposit may also be present in elbow, knee, buttock, hand crease and tendocalcaneus).
- Multiple scratch marks (due to pruritus).
- Spider angioma may be present.
- Generalised clubbing, leuconychia, palmer erythema.
- Liver—enlarged.
- Spleen may be palpable.

Investigations

- LFT—alkaline phosphatase is very high. SGPT—may be slightly elevated. γ-GT is also high. Serum total protein and albumin is reduced.
- USG—shows hepatomegaly with cirrhotic change, splenomegaly and ascites.
- Antimitochondrial antibody (AMA)—positive in 95% cases. Other antibodies, such as anti-smooth muscle antibody and antinuclear antibody may be present.
- Serum IgM may be very high.
- Liver biopsy.
- ERCP or MRCP (to rule out extrahepatic biliary obstruction).
- Others—serum cholesterol and triglyceride (high).

Treatment

- Urso-deoxycholic acid 10–15 mg/kg.
- For pruritus—cholestyramine 4–16 g/day orally, usually with orange juice. Main dose (8 g) is given before and after breakfast.
- Vitamins A, D, K and calcium supplement, alfacalcidol (1 mg/day orally).
- If osteoporosis—bisphosphonate (risedronate may be used).
- Liver transplantation should be considered in liver failure. (Indications are—advanced liver disease, intractable pruritus).
- Steroid improves biochemical and histological disease, but aggravates osteoporosis and other side effect, so should not be used.
- Azathioprine, penicillamine, cyclosporin have no beneficial role.
- In asymptomatic patient, follow-up should be done.

Secondary biliary cirrhosis: When cirrhosis develops due to prolonged obstruction of the large biliary ducts. Causes are stone, strictures and sclerosing cholangitis. Ultrasonography will give the diagnosis.

ASCITES

Definition

It is the pathological accumulation of free fluid in peritoneal cavity. Usually, 2 litre fluid is necessary to detect clinically (1 litre is necessary, in thin person).

Causes of Ascites

1. Liver diseases—cirrhosis of liver with portal hypertension, hepatoma with secondary in peritoneum, Budd-Chiari syndrome.
2. Abdominal causes—intra-abdominal malignancy with peritoneal metastasis, such as carcinoma of kidney, stomach, colon and ovary.
3. Peritoneal causes—peritonitis (tuberculous or pyogenic) and secondaries in the peritoneum.
4. Cardiovascular—chronic constrictive pericarditis (early ascites) and CCF (ascites occurs later).
5. Hypoproteinaemia due to nephrotic syndrome, malnutrition and malabsorption.
6. Others:
   - Collagen disease (SLE and polyarteritis nodosa).
   - Lymphoma and leukaemia.
   - Meig's syndrome (ovarian fibroma, ascites and right-sided pleural effusion).
   - Acute pancreatitis.
   - Myxoedema.
   - Chylous ascites.

Common Causes of Ascites

- Cirrhosis of liver with portal hypertension (in 80% cases).
- Intra-abdominal malignancy with peritoneal metastasis (usually ovarian and gastrointestinal tract malignancy).
- CCF.

Investigations

1. USG of abdomen.
2. If CLD—LFT should be done.
3. CBC (high ESR in TB and leucocytosis in pyogenic infection).
4. Chest X-ray (there may be TB, cardiomegaly or chronic constrictive pericarditis).
5. Ascitic fluid aspiration for the following tests:
   - Naked eye examination (straw coloured, blood-stained, serous or chylous).
   - Gram staining and C/S (in pyogenic infection).
   - Cytology (neutrophil >250 cells/mm^3 or WBC >500 cell/mm^3 in SBP, high lymphocyte in tuberculous peritonitis).
   - Biochemistry for protein and sugar shows high protein in exudative and low protein in transudative. Simultaneous serum albumin to see serum ascitic albumin gradient (see below).
   - In tuberculous peritonitis—fluid for AFB, ADA, mycobacterial C/S, PCR.
   - Exfoliative cytology (to see malignant cells).

6. Other tests (according to suspicion of causes):
   - For tuberculous peritonitis—MT.
   - Urine for proteinuria and serum total protein (nephrotic syndrome).
   - Ascitic fluid amylase in acute pancreatitis (>1000 is highly suggestive).
7. CT scan or MRI (if any growth or mass suspected).
8. Laparoscopy and biopsy in some cases.

Ascitic fluid colour indicates the following

- Serous—cirrhosis of liver.
- Straw—tuberculosis.
- Purulent or hazy—pyogenic.
- Blood-stained—malignancy.
- Chylous—lymphatic obstruction.

Treatment

1. Bedrest is suggested as it improves renal flow and increases diuresis.
2. Sodium and water restriction:
   - Sodium 100 mmol/day, in severe case 40 mmol/day.
   - Water 0.5–1 L/day.
   - Avoid salt containing and salt retaining diets and drugs (NSAIDs, steroid and antacid).
3. Weight, abdominal girth and urinary output should be monitored daily. Weight loss should be 0.5–1 kg/day (fluid loss should not be more than 1 litre daily).
4. If no response with above therapy—diuretic should be given. Spironolactone 100–400 mg/day. If no response, frusemide (20–40 mg daily) or bumetanide (1 mg daily) is added. If no response with spironolactone 400 mg plus frusemide 160 mg daily, it is considered as refractory ascites.
5. If no response or refractory ascites:
   - Ensure that patient is not taking any salt or salt containing diet or drugs.
   - If serum albumin is low, diuretics may not respond. Then IV salt-poor albumin followed by IV frusemide may be given.
6. Paracentesis (aspiration of ascitic fluid) -
   - Done in huge ascites with cardiorespiratory embarrassment or resistant ascites.
   - 3–5 L of fluid can be removed. After aspiration, IV albumin should be given. Dextran or haemaccel may be used.
7. Other modes of treatment (in resistant ascites) -
   - LeVeen shunt (peritoneovenous).
   - TIPSS (transjugular intrahepatic portosystemic stent shunt)
   - Portosystemic shunt surgery—rarely done now a days.
8. Liver transplantation may be considered, if all measures fail.

Serum Ascites Albumin Gradient (SAAG)

It is the difference of albumin between serum and ascitic fluid (calculated by serum albumin minus ascitic albumin, from samples taken at the same time). This gradient correlates directly with portal pressure. It is the single test to differentiate ascites due to portal hypertension from nonportal hypertension.

- If the gradient is >1.1 g/dL, it indicates CLD with portal hypertension.
- If <1, no portal hypertension (ascites is likely to be caused other than portal hypertension). It is 97% accurate.

NB: Ascites protein <25 g/L and SAAG >1.1 g/dL is usually suggestive of portal hypertension.

CIRRHOSIS OF LIVER

Definition

It is a chronic diffuse liver disease characterised by destruction of liver cells with fibrosis, distortion of normal liver architecture and nodular regeneration due to proliferation of surviving hepatocytes.

There are three types of cirrhosis:

- Micronodular—regenerative nodule is usually small, 1 mm size, involving every lobule, also called Laennec's cirrhosis. It is common in alcoholics.
- Macronodular—large nodules, common in postnecrotic cirrhosis, found in HBV.
- Rarely, mixed type (micronodular and macronodular).

Causes of Cirrhosis of Liver

- Chronic viral hepatitis (B or C).
- Chronic alcoholism.
- Nonalcoholic fatty liver disease (NAFLD).
- Immunological (autoimmune liver disease, primary sclerosing cholangitis).
- Biliary (PBC, secondary biliary cirrhosis).
- Genetic (haemochromatosis, Wilson's disease, α1-antitrypsin deficiency).
- Budd-Chiari syndrome.
- Drugs—methotrexate.
- Idiopathic or cryptogenic.

Symptoms

- May be asymptomatic.
- Weakness, fatigue, anorexia, nausea, vomiting, weight loss, upper abdominal discomfort.
- Others—abdominal distention due to ascites, isolated hepatomegaly.

Signs

Various signs of cirrhosis of liver are due to hepatocellular failure and portal hypertension.

Signs of Hepatocellular Failure or Stigmata of CLD

In hands:

- Palmar erythema (liver palm).
- Dupuytren's contracture.
- Leuconychia.
- Clubbing.
- Flapping tremor.
- Others—spider angioma, xanthoma, pigmentation, jaundice and cyanosis.

In face:

- Parotid enlargement (bilateral).
- Xanthelasma.
- Spider angioma (also in neck, arm, forearm, hand and any part above the nipple line).
- Pigmentation.

- Hepatic facies.
- Jaundice.
- Cyanosis.

In chest and abdomen:
- Gynaecomastia (also spider angioma).
- Less hair in chest or body, scanty axillary (also pubic hair).
- Engorged veins in chest and also abdomen (due to portal hypertension).
- In abdomen—splenomegaly, ascites, engorged veins and caput medusae.
- Testis—small and atrophied.

Others:
- Generalised pigmentation.
- Purpura, bruise and ecchymosis.

Signs of Portal Hypertension

- Splenomegaly.
- Ascites.
- Collateral circulation—oesophageal varices, haemorrhoid, venous hum (between xiphisternum and umbilicus).
- Portosystemic encephalopathy.
- Endoscopy shows oesophageal varices.

Signs of Decompensated Cirrhosis

- Ascites.
- Increasing jaundice.
- Hepatic encephalopathy.
- Portal hypertension with variceal bleeding.
- Worsening liver function (prolonged PT and low albumin).

Complications of Cirrhosis of Liver

- Portal hypertension with rupture of oesophageal varices (causing hematemesis and melaena).
- Portosystemic encephalopathy (hepatic precoma) and hepatic coma.
- Hepatorenal syndrome.
- Hepatopulmonary syndrome.
- Hepatoma.
- SBP.

Investigations in CLD

1. LFT (total protein and A/G ratio and prothrombin time are the two most important tests for CLD. Others—serum bilirubin, SGPT and alkaline phosphatase).
2. USG of whole abdomen (in cirrhosis, liver may be small, shrunken, coarse and high echogenic texture, splenomegaly, ascites and dilated portal vein).
3. Viral markers for HBV (HBsAg, HBeAg, anti-HBc) and for HCV (anti-HCV).
4. Proctoscopy (to see haemorrhoid).
5. Endoscopy (to see oesophageal varices).
6. CT scan of hepatobiliary system.

7. Liver biopsy under USG control (confirmatory).
8. If CLD is due to other cause, investigation should be done accordingly, such as:
   - For haemochromatosis—serum iron, TIBC and ferritin.
   - For PBC—antimitochondrial antibody and other autoantibodies.
   - For Wilson's disease—serum copper, caeruloplasmin and urinary copper.
   - For α_1 antitrypsin deficiency—serum α_1 antitrypsin.
9. If ascites—aspiration and test for cytology, biochemistry, SAAG.
10. Other routine investigations—
   - CBC, ESR.
   - Serum urea and creatinine, electrolytes, blood sugar.

Treatment

General Treatment

- Avoidance of alcohol, hepatotoxic drugs.
- Good nutrition.
- Vitamin supplementation.
- Treatment of cause, if any.
- Ascites (see in the previous page)
- Treatment of complication—SBP, encephalopathy, portal hypertention, etc.
- Liver transplantation.

Spontaneous Bacterial Peritonitis (SBP)

It means infection of ascitic fluid in a patient with cirrhosis of liver, in the absence of any apparently primary source of infection. Infective organism gain access to the peritoneum by haematogenous spread, most are *E. coli, klebsiella* or *enterococci.*

Symptoms

In a patient with cirrhosis and ascites following symptoms are seen:
- Fever.
- Sudden abdominal pain.
- Rebound tenderness.
- Absent bowel sounds and increasing ascites, not responding to diuretic.

Investigations

- Ascitic fluid shows—cloudy appearance with neutrophil counts > 250/mm^3.
- Ascitic fluid culture.

Treatment

- Broad-spectrum antibiotics—cefotaxime 2 g 8–12 hourly for at least 5 days or piperacillin and tazobactam.
- Ceftriaxone plus amoxyclav is an alternative.
- Recurrent of SBP is common. This can be reduced by norfloxacin 400 mg daily or ciprofloxacin 750 mg weekly.
- SBP is an indication to refer the patient to a liver transplant centre.

PORTOSYSTEMIC ENCEPHALOPATHY (PSE) OR HEPATIC PRECOMA

Definition

Portosystemic encephalopathy (PSE) is a state of neuropsychiatric syndrome due to biochemical disturbance of brain function caused by chronic liver disease. It may progress from confusion to coma.

Mechanism of PSE

It is due to the involvement of brain by nitrogenous substances of gut origin. Normally, these substances are metabolised by healthy liver. In diseased liver, these are not metabolised and enters into the brain through portosystemic shunt.

Nitrogenous substances are:
- Ammonia.
- Gamma-aminobutyric acid (GABA).
- Mercaptan, fatty acids and octopamine, which act as false neurotransmitters.

Factors Precipitating PSE

- High dietary protein.
- Gastrointestinal bleeding.
- Constipation.
- Drugs (sedative, antidepressants and diuretics).
- Infection including spontaneous bacterial peritonitis.
- Fluid and electrolytes imbalance (hypokalaemia).
- Trauma including surgery.
- Portosystemic shunt operation, TIPS.

Clinical Features of PSE (remember the formula DPIST-F)

- **D: Disturbance** of consciousness (confusion, disorientation, drowsiness, delirium, stupor, coma).
- **Disorder** of sleep (hypersomnia, inversion of sleep—more sleep in daytime).
- **P: Personality** change (childish behaviour, abnormal behaviour, apathy, irritability).
- **I: Intellectual** deterioration, from simple mathematical calculation to organic mental function. Earliest is constructional apraxia (see below).
- **S: Speech** disturbance (slow, slurred, monotonous and dysphasia).
- **T: Tremor** (flapping tremor).
- **F: Foetor** hepaticus (sweet musty odour in breath).

Constructional Apraxia

It means inability to perform a known act in the absence of any motor or sensory disturbance. It is tested in the following way (patient will be unable to do):
- Ask the patient to draw a star.
- Writing disturbance (unable to write or disturbance of writing).
- Ask the patient to make triangle with three matchsticks or ask to lighten the cigarette by matchstick.
- Reitan's trail making test (it is the ability to join or connect the numbers with a pen in a certain fixed time). It becomes prolonged in PSE.

Investigations

Diagnosis is clinical:
- Early diagnosis by EEG which shows diffuse slowing of the normal α-wave with eventual development of δ-wave.
- Arterial blood ammonia—high.

Treatment of PSE

- Precipitating factors should be avoided (drugs, constipation, electrolyte imbalance, bleeding).
- No sedative, no diuretic.
- No protein restriction is recommended.
- Nutrition—glucose (300–400 g/day) orally. If the patient cannot take by mouth, then IV should be given.
- Lactulose—15–30 mL 8 hourly. Lactitol is an alternative.
- Low bowel wash (if no response to lactulose, then enema).
- Gut sterilizer—Rifaximin 400 mg TDS orally. Metronidazole (200 mg 8 hourly).
- Correction of electrolytes.
- Control of infection by antibiotic.
- In chronic or refractory encephalopathy—liver transplantation.
- Zinc deficiency should be corrected, if present.
- If the patient is agitated—oxazepam (10–30 mg) may be given by mouth.

FULMINATING HEPATIC FAILURE

Definition

It is a clinical syndrome of encephalopathy due to severe hepatic failure, occurring within 8 weeks in the absence of previous liver disease. It is also called acute liver failure.

It may be hyperacute (<7 days), acute (within 8–28 days) or subacute (29 days to 12 weeks), between the onset of jaundice and encephalopathy.

Two most common causes are viral hepatitis (commonly B) and paracetamol toxicity. Other causes are acute fatty liver in pregnancy, Wilson's disease, following shock and rarely extensive malignancy of liver.

Clinical features are similar to PSE. Other features:

1. The patient is restless with aggressive outburst.
2. Jaundice.
3. Features of cerebral oedema due to raised intracranial tension are as follows:
   - Pupil—unequal or abnormally reacting, fixed pupil.
   - Hyperventilation.
   - Profuse sweating.
   - Local or general myoclonus, focal fit or decerebrate posture.
   - Rarely papilloedema, a late feature.

Investigations

- LFT—high bilirubin, high SGPT and SGOT, prolong PT.
- USG of HBS.
- Viral screening for HBsAg, HAV, HEV, HCV.

- Routine test—blood glucose, serum electrolytes, calcium, magnesium, phosphate, urea and creatinine, ABG.
- Others—according to suspicion of cause (e.g. paracetamol).

Treatment

- Similar to PSE.
- If signs of raised intracranial pressure are present—20% mannitol 1g/kg body weight IV, may be repeated.
- Correction of hypoglycaemia, hypokalaemia, hypomagnesaemia, hypocalcaemia.
- Coagulopathy or bleeding—intravenous vitamin K, fresh blood or fresh frozen plasma, platelet may be given.
- Broad spectrum antibiotic to control infection.
- PPI to prevent gastrointestinal bleeding.
- Liver transplantation may be considered.

OESOPHAGEAL VARICES

Complication

- Rupture, causing haematemesis and melaena.

Grades of Oesophageal Varices

1. Grade 1—Appear and disappear during endoscopy. Can be depressed by endoscope. Varices seen on oesophageal contraction and not during relaxation.
2. Grade 2—Fixed and discrete during endoscopy. Cannot be depressed by endoscope. Varices seen on both contraction and relaxation.
3. Grade 3—Varices are confluent, around the circumference of oesophagus.
4. Grade 4 -Bleeding spot or cherry red colour. Varix on varix condition.

Investigation

- Barium swallow of oesophagus—shows irregular worm like filling defect.
- Upper GI endoscopy.

NB: Normally, varices are seen as opaque and white. Appearance of red column or red spot predicts bleeding.

Treatment of Rupture Oesophageal Varices

1. Resuscitation (i.v. channel, blood transfusion, plasma transfusion).
2. If possible, endoscopy should be done to find out the source of bleeding (in 20% cases, bleeding may be from gastric erosion).
3. Sclerotherapy may be given.
4. Other measures to stop bleeding are as follows:

Local measures

- Sclerotherapy or banding (treatment of choice).
- Balloon tamponade by using Sengstaken-Blakemore tube (it contains two balloons, one of which exerts pressure at the fundus of stomach and the other in the lower end of oesophagus. It is introduced through the mouth and then inflated. It should be deflated for about 10 minutes every 3 hours to avoid oesophageal mucosal damage).
- Oesophageal transection by using stapling gun (may cause stenosis later on).

Reduction of portal pressure

- Vasopressin causes constriction of splanchnic arterioles and reduces portal blood flow. Dose is IV infusion 0.4 U/minute until bleeding stops, then 0.2 U/minute for further 24 hours. It causes constriction of other vessels, so may cause angina, arrhythmia, or even myocardial infarction (avoided in ischaemic heart disease patients).
- Glypressin or Terlipressin IV 2 mg/6 hours until bleeding stops, then 1 mg/6 h for 24 h.
- Octreotide IV 50 μg followed by infusion of 50 μg/h.
- Transjugular intrahepatic portosystemic stent shunting (TIPSS) is used when all other measures fail.

NB: Emergency portosystemic shunt surgery (splenorenal, portocaval) is of less or no use as the mortality rate is 50% or more.

Prevention of Rebleeding

Rebleeding can be prevented by following measures:

1. Sclerotherapy—sclerosing agent is injected at every 1-2 weeks interval, until varices are occluded. This may cause transient chest or abdominal pain, dysphagia, perforation and oesophageal stricture.
2. Banding—this is the treatment of choice. It is more effective with less side effects.
3. Drug therapy:
   - Propranolol—drug of choice. Pulse and BP should be checked. Aim is to reduce pulse rate by 25%. It reduces portal pressure by reduction of cardiac output (β1 effect) and splanchnic vasoconstriction (blockade of β2).
   - Other drugs (less effective)—isosorbide mononitrate, pentoxifylline and captopril.
4. TIPSS.
5. Surgery—portosystemic shunting (portocaval or selective splenorenal). Owing to high mortality, this surgery is not done as much.
6. Liver transplantation should be considered.

NB: Sclerosing agents used are 5% ethanolamine in oleate, sodium morrhuate, bucrylate and sodium tetradecyl sulphate.

Prevention of Initial Bleeding from Varices

- The use of drugs, viz. propranolol and isosorbide mononitrate may be helpful.
- Sclerotherapy, though not helpful.

Treatment of Congestive Gastropathy

Portal hypertension causes chronic gastric congestion seen on endoscopy as multiple areas of punctate erythema, which may cause bleeding.

- Propranolol, 80–160 mg/day.
- If ineffective, TIPSS can be carried out.

PORTAL HYPERTENSION

Portal vein is formed by the superior mesenteric vein and splenic vein. Normal portal pressure is 5–8 mmHg. Symptoms or complications develop when portal venous pressure is > 12 mm Hg.

Causes of Portal Hypertension

1. Prehepatic:
   - Portal vein thrombosis (in neonatal sepsis, congenital absence of portal vein, umbilical vein transfusion, oral contraceptive use, idiopathic).
2. Intrahepatic:
   - Cirrhosis of liver (90%), schistosomiasis, congenital hepatic fibrosis.
3. Posthepatic:
   Budd-Chiari syndrome, veno-occlusive disease, cystic liver disease, rarely in right heart failure and chronic constrictive pericarditis.

Clinical Signs of Portal Hypertension

- Splenomegaly (cardinal sign). Mild in adults, markedly enlarged in children.
- Ascites.
- Collateral vessels in anterior abdominal wall and caput medusae (engorged veins radiating from the umbilicus).
- Haemorrhoid.
- Endoscopy shows oesophageal varices.

Complications of Portal Hypertension

- Rupture of varices, causing haematemesis and melaena.
- Congestive gastropathy.
- Ascites.
- Hypersplenism.
- Hepatic encephalopathy.

HAEMOCHROMATOSIS

Definition

It is a clinical condition in which the amount of total body iron is increased, which is deposited in different organs of the body causing damage of that organ. It may be primary or secondary.

Causes of Haemochromatosis

1. Primary.
2. Secondary—
   - Haemolytic anaemia—β thalassaemia, sideroblastic anaemia, other chronic haemolytic anaemias.
   - Exogenous iron overload—repeated blood transfusion (transfusion siderosis), prolonged iron therapy.
   - Porphyria cutanea tarda.
   - Alcoholic cirrhosis (in advanced stage).

Mechanism

Normal body iron is 3-4 gram. In haemochromatosis, it may be 20-60 gram.Iron is deposited in liver and pancreatic islets, also in endocrine glands (pituitary, adrenal), heart and skin.

Primary or Hereditary Haemochromatosis

Definition

This is a hereditary disorder, inherited as autosomal recessive, characterised by excess absorption of iron and deposition in various organs, leading to fibrosis and functional organ failure.

It is more in male than female (protected by iron loss in menstruation and pregnancy). In postmenopausal women, it is almost equal in both sexes.

Clinical Features

Common in male above 40 years.

- Liver involvement—hepatomegaly, features of CLD (about 30% may develop HCC).
- Skin pigmentation (leaden grey skin pigmentation due to melanin deposition, bronze like pigmentation).
- Diabetes mellitus.
- Cardiac dysfunction (dilated cardiomyopathy, CCF, arrhythmia).
- Arthritis and chondrocalcinosis.
- Hypogonadism (testicular atropy may occur early).

NB: Any patient with CLD, if there is combination of cardiac diseases, arthritis, skin pigmentation and diabetes, haemachromatosis is the likely diagnosis.

Type of diabetes in haemochromatosis—called "bronze diabetes" due to the bronze colouration of the skin.

Investigations

1. Liver function tests (shows evidence of CLD).

2. Iron profile:
   - Serum iron (increased).
   - Total iron binding capacity (>70% is saturated).
   - Serum ferritin (increased, >600 μg/L).
3. CT scan or MRI of hepatobiliary system.
4. Hepatic iron index (HII).
5. Liver biopsy (shows iron deposition, hepatic fibrosis, cirrhosis) and to measure the iron stores is the definitive test.
6. Others—blood sugar, ECG, X-ray chest, echocardiogram, X-ray of the involved joint (shows chondrocalcinosis).

Treatment

- Venesection—weekly or twice in a week, 500 mL of blood until serum ferritin is normal. Aim is to reduce ferritin to <50 μg/L. Thereafter, venesection is continued to keep serum ferritin normal (usually 3–4 venesections per year is needed).
- Chelating agent—desferrioxamine may be given. It is used if patient cannot tolerate venesection, specially those with cardiac disease or severe anaemia.
- Symptomatic treatment of cirrhosis, diabetes mellitus (usually by insulin), CCF and cardiac arrhythmia.
- Alcohol must be avoided.
- Vitamin C must be avoided as it increases iron absorption.
- First degree family members should be screened.

Complication or Cause of Death in Haemochromatosis

- Death is usually due to cardiac failure (30%).
- Hepatocellular failure or portal hypertension (25%).
- HCC (30%).

HEPATOMA

Definition

It is the primary carcinoma of liver, also called hepatocellular carcinoma (HCC).

Causes of Hepatoma

- Chronic hepatitis B infections. 75–90% are associated with cirrhosis of liver.
- Chronic hepatitis C infections. Risk of HCC is higher in HCV than HBV. Usually, associated with cirrhosis.
- Other causes of cirrhosis of liver—in alcoholic cirrhosis, nonalcoholic steatohepatitis (NASH), haemochromatosis, Wilson's disease, α1-antitrypsin deficiency and primary biliary cirrhosis. Macronodular variant is more prone to develop hepatoma.
- Aflatoxin produced by a fungus *Aspergillus flavus* (from contaminated groundnut grain, stored in tropical condition).
- Chronic arsenicosis.
- Chlonorsis sinensis (a parasitic infection).
- Prolonged androgen therapy, anabolic steroid and oral contraceptive pill (oestrogen) may cause hepatoma (usually adenoma, rarely hepatoma).
- Smoking (rare).

Symptoms

- May be asymptomatic.
- Anorexia, nausea, vomiting, weight loss, heaviness in the right upper abdomen.
- Abdominal distension.
- Features of metastasis.

Signs

- Liver is enlarged, hard, surface is irregular and nodular, usually single nodule.
- Hepatic bruit.

Investigations

1. USG (shows filling defects in 90% of cases).
2. α-fetoprotein—high (in 60% cases).
3. Others:
   - Contrast-enhanced CT or MRI.
   - Carcinoembryonic antigen (high in secondaries).
4. Liver biopsy under USG control—confirmatory.
5. Viral markers (HBV and HCV).

Treatment

- Surgical resection, in noncirrhotic patient. Recurrence in 50% after 5 years.
- In cirrhotic patient—resection may be done in small tumour and good liver function.
- Liver transplantation. Hepatitis B and C may recur in transplanted liver.
- Percutaneous injection of ethanol. Recurrence is 50% after 3 years. Repeated injection may be given. It causes tumour necrosis.

- Transcatheter radiofrequency ablation using a single electrode inserted into the tumour under radiological guidance.
- Transcatheter hepatic arterial embolisation by Gelfoam and doxorubicin.
- Chemotherapy—sorafenib prolong survival up to 10 months.

SECONDARIES IN THE LIVER

Secondary carcinoma (Table 2) is more common in the liver, because relatively blood flow in liver is more, due to double blood supply (by portal vein and hepatic artery).

Primary Site

- In male common sites—carcinoma of stomach, lung and colon.
- In female common sites—carcinoma of breast, colon, stomach and uterus.

Investigations

- Ultrasonography of whole abdomen (shows multiple space occupying lesions).
- CT or MRI of abdomen may be done.
- Liver function tests—usually alkaline phosphatase is high.
- Other investigation to find out the primary source according to the history. For example, X-ray chest P/A view, endoscopy of upper GIT, colonoscopy, etc.
- FNAC or USG-guided liver biopsy may be done.

Treatment

- Treatment of the primary cause, if possible.
- If single metastasis, surgery may be possible (in colorectal carcinoma).
- If surgery is not possible, radiofrequency ablation of the metastasis may be tried.
- Majority requires palliative treatment.

Table 2
Differences between primary and secondary carcinoma

Primary carcinoma	Secondary carcinoma
1. History of hepatitis B or C infection or cirrhosis of liver	1. History of primary carcinoma (GIT, bronchus, breast, thyroid, kidney). No primary source in 50% cases
2. Nodule usually single, may be more	2. Usually multiple nodules
3. No umbilication over the nodule	3. There is umbilication (due to necrosis)
4. Bruit present (due to increased vascularity)	4. No bruit (because of necrotic lesion)
5. Rub may be present	5. Rub is more common
6. Investigations: • α-fetoprotein is increased • Alkaline phosphatase is slightly increased • Carcinoembryonic antigen is normal	6. Investigations: • α-fetoprotein is not high • Alkaline phosphatase is very high • Carcinoembryonic antigen is high

PRIMARY SCLEROSING CHOLANGITIS

Definition

It is a chronic cholestatic liver disease characterized by inflammatory destruction of intra- and extrahepatic bile ducts with fibrosis that leads to gradual obliteration of biliary tree, biliary cirrhosis, portal hypertension and hepatic failure.

Clinical Features

Common in male. 75% is associated with inflammatory bowel disease, commonly ulcerative colitis. Cholangiocarcinoma may occur in 10–30% cases.

- Features of inflammatory bowel disease.
- Anorexia, nausea, vomiting, fatigue, malaise, weight loss.
- Pain in right hypochondrium.
- Pruritus.
- Features of malabsorption, cholestastasis (stool is clay or muddy-coloured).

Signs

- Scratch marks in whole body.
- Jaundice.
- Hepatomegaly.
- In advanced case—stigmata of CLD.

Investigations

- Liver function tests—High alkaline phosphatase is common.
- USG of hepatobiliary system.
- MRCP is diagnostic. ERCP may be done in some cases (if therapeutic intervention is indicated).
- Liver biopsy.
- P-ANCA—positive in 60–80% cases in ulcerative colitis.
- ANA and antismooth muscle antibody may be positive.

Treatment

- Supportive—Cholestyramine for pruritus, ursodeoxycholic acid, fat soluble vitamins supplementation.
- Immunosuppressive drugs, such as prednisolone, azathioprine, cyclosporin, tacrolimus, MTX. Anti-TNF agent, such as etanercept or infliximab may be given.
- Biliary stenting may improve biochemistry and symptoms.
- Orthotopic liver transplantation is the definitive treatment.

ACUTE CHOLECYSTITIS

Definition

It is the acute inflammation of the gallbladder, usually associated with gall stone.

Symptoms

- Pain in the right hypochondrium, which is colicky in nature, radiates to the right shoulder tip or interscapular region.
- Nausea, vomiting.
- Fever.

Signs

- Tenderness in the right hypochondrium with muscle guard or rigidity.
- Murphy's sign positive—if thumb is pressed over the tip of the 9th costal cartilage and patient is asked to take deep breath, there is pain and arrest of breathing at the height of inspiration.

Investigations

- CBC—leucocytosis.
- USG of hepatobiliary system.
- LFT—bilirubin, SGPT, alkaline phosphatase, all may be slightly high.
- Plain X-ray shows gallstones in 10% cases.
- CT scan may be done.

Treatment

- Bed rest.
- Nothing by mouth. Nasogastric suction may be necessary.
- IV fluid—5% Dextrose in normal saline, Ringer's lactate solution.
- Analgesics to relieve pain.
- Antibiotic—IV cephalosporin (cefuroxime), pipercillin plus tazobactum.
- Metronidazole 500 mg IV 8 hourly.
- Once acute attack subsides, oral feeding is started.
- Surgery-cholecystectomy may be done in acute attack.

CHRONIC CHOLECYSTITIS

Definition

It is the chronic inflammation of the gallbladder usually associated with gall stone.

Causes

- Calculus—most common cause.
- Noncalculus.
- Due to infection by *Salmonellae typhi*.

Symptoms

- History of frequent attacks of biliary colic (like acute cholecystitis).
- Flatulent dyspepsia with fatty food intolerance.

Investigation

USG is the simple test.

Treatment

- During acute attack—treatment followed should be same as in acute cholecystitis.
- Cholecystectomy should be done.

CARCINOMA OF GALLBLADDER

It is common in the elderly, more in females, over 70 years.

Types

- Adenocarcinomas (90%).
- Rarely—anaplastic, squamous cell carcinoma.

Risk Factors

- Gall stones.
- Porcelain (calcified) gallbladder.
- Gallbladder polyp >1 cm.
- Chronic infection with Salmonellae is a risk factor.

Clinical Features

- May be asymptomatic, diagnosed incidentally during cholecystectomy.
- Jaundice.
- Recurrent attack of right upper abdominal pain.
- Weight loss, anorexia, nausea.
- Right upper abdominal mass, which is hard and irregular.

Investigations

- USG abdomen.
- Liver function test (high bilirubin, high alkaline phosphatase).
- CBC.
- X-ray abdomen (may show gallbladder calcification).
- CT abdomen.

Treatment

Surgical excision, if possible. Chemotherapy may be given.

LIVER TRANSPLANTATION

Types

- Orthotopic transplantation: Whole liver is taken from a recently deceased donor.
- Live donor transplant*:* The donor is a willing living person.
- Split type liver transplant*:* Transplantation of liver from a recently deceased person to two recipients.
- Auxiliary liver transplant: Recipient's own liver is not fully removed.

Indications

- Acute liver failure.
- Cirrhosis of liver.
- End-stage liver disease due to chronic Hepatitis B or chronic hepatitis C infection.
- Primary biliary cirrhosis.
- Primary sclerosing cholangitis.
- Haemochromatosis.
- Wilson's disease.
- Autoimmune hepatitis.
- Alpha-1 antitrypsin deficiency.
- Budd-Chiari Syndrome.
- Hepatocellular carcinoma.
- Secondaries in liver

Contraindications

- Sepsis.
- Extrahepatic malignancy.
- Active alcohol abuse.
- Cardiorespiratory dysfunction.

Complications

- Graft rejection.
- Infection.

CHAPTER

7

Endocrinology

CHAPTER CONTENTS

ENDOCRINE GLANDS

- Pituitary gland.
- Thyroid gland.
- Parathyroid gland.
- Islets cells of pancreas.
- Adrenal or suprarenal glands.
- Gonads—ovary in females and testes in males.
- Placenta—temporary endocrine gland formed during pregnancy.

THYROID GLAND

Diseases of the thyroid gland:

- Hyperthyroidism—excess function by thyroid hormones (also called thyrotoxicosis).
- Hypothyroidism—insufficient secretion of thyroid hormones, so less function. When associated with mucopolysaccaride deposition in the skin, it is called myxoedema. When hypothyroidism is present from birth, it is called 'critinism.' If it occurs in early age, it is called 'Juvenile Hypothyroidism.'
- Goitre—it means enlargement of thyroid gland.
- Tumour—May be benign (adenoma) and malignant, also lymphoma.
- Infection or inflammation—subacute thyroiditis, also called de Quervain's thyroiditis. Pyogenic or bacterial thyroiditis (rare). Riedel's thyroiditis (unknown cause).
- Autoimmune—Hashimoto's thyroiditis, Graves' disease.

HYPOTHYROIDISM

Definition

Hypothyroidism is defined as the hypofunction of thyroid gland, characterized by decreased secretion of thyroxine (T4) and triiodothyronine (T3).

It is of 2 types:

- Primary hypothyroidism—means cause in the thyroid gland. It is usually associated with myxoedema.
- Secondary hypothyroidism—means cause in the pituitary (or rarely hypothalamus). In such case, myxoedema is rare. There are other features of hypopituitarism also.

Causes of Primary Hypothyroidism

1. Autoimmune:
   - Spontaneous atrophic hypothyroidism (commonest).
   - Hashimoto's thyroiditis.
   - Graves' disease (associated with TSH receptor blocking antibody).
2. Iatrogenic:
   - Radioiodine therapy for thyrotoxicosis.
   - After surgery (thyroidectomy).
   - Postradiotherapy in the neck.
   - Drugs—such as lithium, amiodarone and antithyroid drug.
3. Others:
   - Endemic iodine deficiency.
   - Postpartum thyroiditis.
   - Rarely, dyshormonogenesis.

Causes of Goitrous Hypothyroidism

- Hashimoto's thyroiditis.
- Graves' disease (there is also exophthalmos and diffuse goitre with dermopathy).
- Endemic iodine deficiency (less common).
- Drugs—lithium, amiodarone, iodide.
- Rarely, dyshormonogenesis.

Nongoitrous Hypothyroidism

- Autoimmune or idiopathic (spontaneous atrophic)—commonest cause.
- Following radio-iodine therapy for thyrotoxicosis.
- Postradiotherapy in the neck.
- After surgery (thyroidectomy).
- Secondary to hypopituitarism, hypothalamic disorders.

Myxoedema

It is the severe form of hypothyroidism due to deposition of mucopolysaccharide substances in subcutaneous tissue.

Clinical Features

Symptoms

- Weight gain and swelling of the whole body.
- Cold intolerance.
- Increased sleepiness, lethargy, anorexia and weakness.
- Constipation.
- Lack of concentration and poor memory.
- In female, menorrhagia.

Signs

- The patient looks apathetic.
- Whole body is swollen. Face is puffy with periorbital swelling, baggy eyelids and loss of outer 1/3rd of the eyebrows.
- Nonpitting oedema (due to deposition of mucopolysaccharide substances).
- Skin is dry, rough, cold and thick.
- Pulse—bradycardia (less than 60/min).
- BP—may be high.

Other Features of Hypothyroidism

1. Haematological—anaemia (may be macrocytic, normocytic normochromic or sometimes microcytic hypochromic due to menorrhagia in female).
2. Cardiovascular features:
   - Sinus bradycardia.
   - Pericardial effusion and pericarditis.
   - Congestive cardiac failure.
   - Atherosclerosis (because of hyperlipidaemia).
   - Ischaemic heart disease.
   - Hypertension.
3. Neurological features—
   - Speech—voice is coarse and husky (or croaky).
   - Memory—may be impaired or dementia.
   - Slow relaxation of ankle jerks.
   - Carpal tunnel syndrome (or tarsal tunnel syndrome).
   - Psychosis (myxoedema madness).
   - Myxoedema coma.
   - Cerebellar syndrome.

Investigations

1. Serum FT3, FT4 and TSH (low FT3, low FT4 and high TSH).
2. Autoantibody (for Hashimoto's thyroiditis—antiperoxidase and antithyroglobulin antibody).
3. Other routine tests—
   - USG of the neck.
   - ECG (low-voltage tracing, sinus bradycardia).
   - X-ray chest (cardiomegaly due to pericardial effusion, heart failure).
   - Serum total cholesterol, LDL and triglyceride (high).

Treatment

Thyroxine—started with low dose (25 μg), increase gradually after 3 weeks. Single dose is preferable, should be taken before breakfast. TSH should be repeated after 6–8 weeks. Once TSH is normal, maintenance dose should be continued.

Treatment of Hypothyroidism in Different Conditions

1. Ischemic heart disease:
   - Thyroxine should be started in low dose (25 μg), to be increased slowly up to the optimum dose.
   - Beta-blocker (propranolol) should be added.
   - Coronary dilator, calcium antagonist may be added.
2. In elderly patient with hypothyroidism: Treatment is same. But care should be taken in IHD. Following thyroxine, it may precipitate angina and myocardial infarction.
3. Hypothyroidism in pregnancy:
   - Most sensitive investigation is TSH, which is high. Also, FT3 and FT4 should be done (total T3 and T4 may be high in normal pregnancy due to increased TBG).
   - Treatment—thyroxine should be given (100–150 μg once daily). Requirement of thyroxine is relatively high (40–50%) in pregnancy.

Subclinical Hypothyroidism

In this condition, T3 and T4 are in the lower limit of normal and TSH is slightly high. The patient may be clinically euthyroid. This may persist for many years, though overt hypothyroidism may occur.

Treatment

Thyroxine therapy may be given, if TSH is persistently raised above 10 IU/L or when there are symptoms. If TSH is marginally raised, the test should be repeated after 3–6 months.

Myxoedema Coma

It is characterized by depressed level of consciousness or even coma. Convulsion may occur. It is rare, may occur in severe hypothyroidism, usually in elderly. CSF studies show high pressure and protein is also high. There is 50% mortality.

Treatment

It is better to be treated in ICU. Before starting treatment, blood is taken for FT3, FT4, TSH and cortisol.

1. Triiodothyronine (T3) 20 μg, 8 hourly I/V. If T3 is not available, oral thyroxine through Ryle's tube should be given.
2. I/V Hydrocortisone—100 mg 8 hourly.
3. Other treatment -
   - Slow rewarming.
   - High-flow O_2 therapy.
   - I/V fluid and glucose.
   - Antibiotic.
   - Assisted ventilation may be necessary.

Cretinism

Definition

It is defined as hypothyroidism due to congenital deficiency of thyroid hormone, also called congenital myxoedema.

Clinical Features

1. Features in neonate:
   - Prolonged physiological jaundice.
   - Hoarse cry.
   - Lethargy.
   - Constipation.
   - Feeding problem.
   - Hypotonia.
2. Features in older baby:
   - Characteristic facies—dull, idiotic look, wrinkling of forehead, large head, sparse hair, broad flat nose with big nostrils, widely set eyes, thick everted lips with macroglossia, protruded tongue. Fontanelles close later.
   - Pot-belly with umbilical hernia.
   - Skin is dry, scaly, rough, cold and pale yellow. Hair is sparse, coarse and brittle.
   - Delayed developmental milestones, such as delayed dentition, delayed crawling, etc.
   - Mental development is retarded, imbecile.
   - Hoarse voice.
   - Short stature.
   - Thick and short neck with presence of supraclavicular pad of fat.
   - Genitalia are poorly developed.
   - Lethargy and hypotonia.
3. In older children—typical features of hypothyroidism are present. Also called juvenile myxoedema. In addition, there is epiphyseal dysgenesis seen in X-ray of femoral head.

Investigations

Routine screening of neonates using blood spot for TSH.

Treatment

Thyroxine should be started immediately. If treatment is delayed, permanent neurological and intellectual damage may occur.

Hashimoto's Thyroiditis

Definition

It is an auto-immune thyroiditis characterized by destructive lymphoid infiltration of thyroid leading to atrophic change with regeneration and goitre formation. It is common in middle aged woman. Goitre is usually diffuse, moderately enlarged and firm or rubbery. It is usually associated with hypothyroidism.

Investigation

Antithyroid antibody (very high)—antimicrosomal (anti-peroxidase) in 90% and anti-thyroglobulin antibodies.

Treatment

Thyroxine (it reduces the size of goitre also).

THYROTOXICOSIS

Definition

It is defined as hyperfunction of thyroid gland due to excess production of thyroid hormones. It is common in female.

Causes

1. Graves' disease—commonest cause (76%).
2. Toxic multinodular goitre (14%).
3. Toxic nodular goitre (5%, toxic adenoma or hot nodule called Plummer's disease).
4. Thyroiditis (subacute thyroiditis, also called de Quervain's thyroiditis and postpartum thyroiditis. All are transient).
5. Hashimoto's thyroiditis, also called Hashitoxicosis (later, hypothyroidism develops).
6. Factitious thyrotoxicosis (self intake of thyroxine).
7. Iodine induced (Jod-Basedow's phenomenon) and drug (Amiodarone).
8. Others (rare):
   - Carcinoma of thyroid (follicular).
   - Struma ovarii (secretes thyroid hormone).
   - Hydatidiform mole and choriocarcinoma (both secrete thyroid-stimulating hormone).

Symptoms

- General features—excessive sweating, heat intolerance, increased appetite, weight loss (inspite of good appetite), insomnia, restlessness.
- Cardiovascular—palpitation, angina pain, breathlessness on exertion.
- Neurological—irritability, insomnia, nervousness, tremor.
- Gastrointestinal—increased appetite, diarrhoea.
- Reproductive—in female, amenorrhoea or oligomenorrhoea, infertility.

Signs

- Pulse >100/min (tachycardia).
- BP—systolic BP may be high.
- In hand—warm and sweaty palm, tremor of outstretched hand.
- CVS—atrial fibrillation, heart failure.
- Neurological—exaggerated reflex.
- Others—goitre, exophthalmos.

Investigations

1. To confirm thyrotoxicosis:
   - FT3, FT4 and TSH (low TSH, high T3 and T4).
   - Radioiodine uptake test (RAIU) and thyroid scanning. RAIU shows rapid uptake and rapid turnover (there is high uptake in 2 or 4 and 24 hours, but rapid fall after 48 hours).
2. To find out causes:
   - Ultrasonography of neck (to see single, multinodular and diffuse goitre).
   - Thyroid autoantibody (in Graves' disease)—TRAb (thyroid receptor antibody).

- Anti-peroxidase and anti-thyroglobulin antibody—slightly high.
- Other tests—ECG, chest X-ray, blood sugar.

Treatment

Three modes of treatment—drugs, radioiodine therapy and sugery.

1. Drugs: carbimazole or propylthiouracil.
   - Carbimazole—45-60 mg daily. When the patient is euthyroid, reduce the dose, then 5-20 mg daily for 18-24 months. Periodic complete blood count is necessary, as there may be agranulocytosis. Also, FT4 and TSH should be measured.
   - Propylthiouracil—400-600 mg daily. Dose is reduced when the patient becomes euthyroid.
   - β-blocker—propranolol (up to 160 mg/day).
2. Radioiodine therapy: Indications are—
   - Usually, above 40 years of age (however, may be used in young).
   - Recurrence after surgery or drugs, irrespective of age.
   - Toxic multinodular goitre or toxic adenoma or hot nodule.
   - In early age, with major serious other illness.
   - Some cases of carcinoma thyroid (follicular, papillary after surgery).
   - Ablative therapy with severe atrial fibrillation, also in heart failure.
   - Psychosis.
   - Poor drug compliance.
   - Hypersensitivity to the drug.

   Contraindications of radioiodine therapy—
   - Pregnancy or planned pregnancy within 6 months of treatment.
   - During lactation.
   - Active or malignant Graves' ophthalmopathy.
3. Surgery (subtotal thyroidectomy): Indications of surgery—
   - Large goitre or multinodular goitre.
   - Relapse or no response to drug.
   - Drug hypersensitivity.
   - Noncompliance with drug.
   - Suspicion of malignancy.
   - Pressure effect.
   - Cosmetic purpose.

   Complications of surgery:
   - Hypothyroidism in 25%
   - Transient hypocalcaemia (10%)
   - Permanent hypoparathyroidism (1%)
   - Recurrent laryngeal nerve palsy causing hoarseness of voice due to vocal cord palsy (1%).

NB: Treatment of different toxic nodular goitre:

- Toxic solitary nodule or hot nodule—radioiodine therapy or surgery.
- Toxic multinodular goitre—radioiodine therapy or surgery.

Thyrotoxic Crisis

It is characterized by life threatening increase of signs and symptoms of thyrotoxicosis (also called thyroid storm). Features are:

- High fever.

- Restlessness, agitation and irritability.
- Nausea, vomiting, diarrhoea and abdominal pain.
- Tachycardia, AF and in elderly cardiac failure.
- Confusion, delirium and coma.

Precipitating Factors

- Infection.
- Stress.
- Surgery in unprepared patient.
- Following radioiodine therapy (due to radiation thyroiditis).

Diagnosis

Mostly clinical and high degree of suspicion is vital. FT3, FT4 and TSH should be done immediately.

Treatment of Thyrotoxic Crisis

- The patient should be treated in ICU.
- Propranolol 80 mg 6 hourly (or 1–5 mg IV 6 hourly).
- IV fluid (normal saline and glucose).
- Carbimazole 40–60 mg daily. Or propylthiouracil 150 mg 6 hourly (if needed, through Ryle's tube).
- Other therapy—sodium ipodate, a radiographical contrast media, 500 mg daily is rapidly effective. Or potassium iodide or Lugol's iodine may be given. Dexamethasone 2 mg 6 hourly and amiodarone are also effective.
- Broad-spectrum antibiotic.
- General measures—control of temperature and O_2 therapy.
- After 10–14 days, carbimazole is continued.

Treatment of Thyrotoxicosis in other Situations

Thyrotoxicosis with AF:

- β-blocker—propranolol. Verapamil or amiodarone may be used, if β-blocker is contraindicated.
- Antithyroid drug, followed by radioiodine therapy.

Thyrotoxicosis in pregnancy:

- Propylthiouracil is preferred (carbimazole can cross placenta, causing foetal goitre). Propylthiouracil is given in lowest dose, less than 150 mg daily to prevent foetal hypothyroidism and goitre. If it is not high, the drug can be stopped 4 weeks before delivery (to prevent neonatal hypothyroidism).
- If needed, propylthiouracil can be given after delivery and breast feeding should be continued, as little is excreted in breast milk.
- If surgery is necessary, it should be done in middle trimester.

GRAVES' DISEASE

Definition

It is an autoimmune thyroid disease due to stimulating antibody against TSH receptor (thyroid stimulating immunoglubulin- TSI), characterized by triad of—

1. Exophthalmos.
2. Diffuse goitre.
3. Dermopathy (pretibial myxoedema).

It is common in female, M:F = 1:5.

Cause of Graves' Disease

Autoimmune due to IgG antibody against TSH receptor, producing excess thyroid hormones. TRAb antibody acts similar to TSH. TRAb is of 2 types:

- TSI, with 80–95% causing thyrotoxicosis.
- TSH receptor blocking antibody, causing hypothyroidism.

Natural History of Graves' Disease

It may be hyperthyroid, euthyroid followed by hypothyroidism.

1. Hyperthyroidism with Graves' disease—when it is associated with features of thyrotoxicosis, such as intolerance to heat, weight loss inspite of good appetite, excessive sweating.
2. Euthyroid Graves' disease—The patient is clinically and biochemically euthyroid, but there is ophthalmopathy.
3. Hypothyroid Graves' disease—In this condition, the patient has Graves' disease with the features of hypothyroidism, such as—coarse puffy face, periorbital puffiness with baggy eyelids, dry, cold and scaly skin, nonpitting oedema, slow relaxation of the ankle jerk, croaky voice.

Investigations

As in thyrotoxicosis.

Treatment

- If there is thyrotoxicosis—treat accordingly.
- In euthyroid case—treatment is only symptomatic and supportive.
- In hypothyroid—thyroxine therapy.

GOITRE

Definition

It is the enlargement of thyroid gland. It is more common in women, may be simple or toxic, single nodular, multinodular, diffuse.

Classification

1. Nodular goitre—single noular or multinodular.
2. Diffuse Goitre.
3. Neoplastic:
   - Benign adenoma.
   - Malignant—papillary, follicular, anaplastic, medullary carcinoma of thyroid, lymphoma (Non-Hodgkin's lymphoma).

Also according to the presence of features of toxicity, goitre may be—

- Simple goitre—absence of features of toxicosis.
- Toxic goitre—presence of features of toxicosis, such as resting tachycardia, tremor of outstretched hand, warm and sweaty palm.

Investigations of Goitre

- Radioactive iodine uptake (RAIU) test.
- Thyroid scan.
- USG of thyroid gland.
- FT_3, FT_4 and TSH (all normal. TSH may be high, due to iodine deficiency).
- Fine needle aspiration cytology (FNAC) of thyroid nodule.

Multinodular Goitre

Common in middle aged and elderly, usually benign, chance of malignancy is rare.

Simple Multinodular Goitre

Causes are:

- Iodine deficiency (commonest cause).
- Drugs—lithium, amiodarone and paraaminosalicylate (PAS).
- Thiocyanate in diet.

Complications of Multinodular Goitre

- May develop thyrotoxicosis (toxic multinodular goitre).
- Compression—such as dysphagia, hoarseness (due to involvement of recurrent laryngeal nerve), stridor and superior vena cava obstruction.
- Severe pain due to haemorrhage in nodule.

Investigations

As in goitre (above)

Treatment

- If small—reassurance. Follow-up annually.
- If large or mediastinal compression or cosmetic reason—partial thyroidectomy.

Toxic Multinodular Goitre

When associated with features of toxicosis, it is called toxic multinodular goitre.

Treatment

- β-Blocker (to reduce heart rate).
- Radioiodine therapy is the treatment of choice. If severe toxicosis, antithyroid drug is given, followed by radioiodine therapy.
- Occasionally, surgery may be necessary, if there is large goitre.

Diffuse Goitre

Simple Diffuse Goiter

It is common in the second and third decade, 15–25 years, more in female.

Causes of Diffuse Goitre

- Physiological—puberty and pregnancy.
- Iodine deficiency (endemic goitre).
- Autoimmune—Hashimoto's thyroiditis, Graves' disease and postpartum thyroiditis.
- Goitrogens—drugs (amiodarone, lithium, PAS). Thiocyanate in diet (cabbage, cauliflower, turnips, soya beans, brussels sprouts).
- Iodide in large doses.
- Subacute thyroiditis (de Quervain's thyroiditis).
- Dyshormonogenesis.
- Riedel's thyroiditis.
- Suppurative thyroiditis.
- Infiltrative disease—amyloidosis, sarcoidosis.

Treatment of Simple Diffuse Goitre

- Mild to moderate—no treatment. Reassurance and follow-up.
- Treatment of primary cause.
- If large goitre associated with pressure effect or cosmetic reason, surgery may be done.

Solitary Thyroid Nodule

Causes of Solitary Thyroid Nodule

- Simple nodular goitre.
- Palpable nodule on diffuse or multinodular goitre.
- Thyroid cyst.
- Thyroid adenoma or toxic adenoma.
- Malignancy (carcinoma and lymphoma).

Nature of Solitary Nodule

Majority benign (80–90%) and may be malignant (5–10%).

Investigations

- USG (to see whether cystic or solid).
- RAIU and thyroid scan.
- FT_3, FT_4 and TSH.
- FNAC and open biopsy (if suspected malignancy).

Fate of Untreated Thyroid Nodule

- May persist for long time.
- Spontaneous regression in 30%.
- Malignancy (5–10%).
- Cystic changes due to haemorrhage within the nodule.
- Secondary infection.

Suspicion of Malignancy in a Single Thyroid Nodule

- History of recent and rapid growth.
- Hoarseness of voice.
- History of radiation therapy in childhood (in head and in neck).
- Family history (medullary carcinoma of thyroid, MCT).
- Gland is solitary, hard, irregular and fixed to the underlying structures.
- Associated palpable lymph node.

Treatment of Solitary Thyroid Nodule

1. 80% of thyroid nodules are solid, cold, nontoxic and colloid. Treatment is—
   - Reassurance and follow-up.
   - Surgery for cosmetic purpose or if suspicion of malignancy.
   - Thyroxine may be given in some cases.
2. 5–10% of the thyroid nodules are hot nodules. Treatment is:
   - Surgery or radioiodine therapy.
   - Ethanol injection into the nodule may be given.
3. Cystic nodule is usually benign. Aspiration is effective in 50% cases. Ethanol injection into the nodule is helpful. If cyst is large, surgical excision should be considered.

Tumours of Thyroid Gland

Tumours of the thyroid gland may be benign or malignant.

Benign

Usually, it is adenoma. Three types—follicular, papillary, Hurthle's cell type.

Treatment

- If nonfunctioning—reassurance and follow-up.
- Thyroxine may be given. Dose 2–3 μg/kg/day for 6 months. If no response, stop the therapy.
- Surgery—for cosmetic purpose or suspicion of malignancy.

Toxic Adenoma

Thyrotoxicosis due to thyroid adenoma , called Plummer's disease (no eye sign and no pretibial myxoedema). Thyroid scan shows hot nodule. It occurs in 5% cases of hyperthyroidism, common in females >40 years.

Treatment

Radioiodine therapy or surgery.

THYROID CARCINOMA

Thyroid carcinoma is less common, 1% of the malignancies. All are common in females except medullary carcinoma of thyroid (MCT), which occurs in both sexes equally. Types of thyroid carcinoma are as follows—

- Papillary—70-80% (commonest).
- Follicular—10%.
- Anaplastic or undifferentiated—5%.
- MCT—5-10%.
- Others—5% (lymphoma and secondary in thyroid).

Papillary Carcinoma

- Commonest type, usually in young, 20-40 years.
- It is slow growing and multifocal.
- Local lymph node metastasis is common, haematogenous spread is less common.
- Usually presents with thyroid nodule, but patient may present with cervical lymphadenopathy without thyroid enlargement.
- FNAC should be done for the diagnosis.

Treatment and Prognosis

- Total thyroidectomy followed by high-dose radioiodine therapy.
- Life-long thyroxine.
- Prognosis is good, survival is almost same as in normal person.
- If distant metastasis, 40% survival up to 10 years.

Follow up (following tests are done periodically):

- Serum thyroglobulin. If rises, indicates recurrence or metastasis.
- Periodic whole body scanning is done to see any metastasis.
- If recurrence, high-dose radio-ablation should be done.

Follicular Carcinoma

- Common in middle aged, 40-60 years of age.
- Usually, a single encapsulated lesion.
- Blood borne metastasis is common (to lung, brain and bone). Lymph node metastasis is rare.
- Diagnosis is done by open biopsy (FNAC is less specific).
- Treatment and follow up—like papillary. Prognosis is good.

Anaplastic or Undifferentiated Carcinoma

- Usually in elderly, >60 years, more in women and highly malignant.
- Rapid thyroid enlargement, over 2-3 months. Goitre is hard, irregular.
- There may be hoarseness of voice due to recurrent laryngeal nerve palsy and stridor due to tracheal compression.
- If possible—total thyroidectomy followed by thyroxine therapy.
- Radiotherapy may be given.
- Median survival is 7 months, if surgery is not possible.

Medullary Carcinoma of Thyroid

- Arises from parafollicular C cells, usually multifocal. May be inherited as autosomal dominant disease.
- Common in middle aged and elderly, may occur in young if there is family history.
- Patient usually presents with firm thyroid mass, cervical lymph node involvement is common but distant metastasis is rare initially.
- Associated with multiple endocrine neoplasia (MEN) type IIa (phaeochromocytoma and hyperparathyroidism) and IIb (as in type IIa plus multiple neuroma and Marfanoid body). May be sporadic too.
- Serum calcitonin is high, it is useful in monitoring response to therapy.

Treatment

Total thyroidectomy with removal of affected lymph nodes followed by thyroxine therapy. External radiotherapy may be given after surgery. Does not take radioiodine, chemotherapy is not effective.

Prognosis

Relatively good. Some may survive up to 20 years, but some <1 year.

Lymphoma of Thyroid

- Rarely may occur as primary or as a part of generalized lymphoma.
- Generally, occurs in thyroid gland affected by Hashimoto's thyroiditis. A rapidly enlarging mass in thyroid in patient with Hashimoto's thyroiditis should arouse suspicion of lymphoma.
- Treatment—external irradiation plus chemotherapy.

PARATHYROID GLAND

Diseases of parathyroid glands:

Hormone excess

- Primary hyperparathyroidism (due to adenoma, hyperplasia).
- Secondary hyperparathyroidism (occurs in CKD, vit-D deficiency).
- Tertiary hyperparathyroidism.

Hormone deficiency: Hypoparathyroidism (due to postsurgical, autoimmune).
Hormone resistance: Pseudohypoparathyroidism, pseudo-pseudo hypoparathyroidism.

Hyperparathyroidism

Definition

It is defined as hyperfunction of parathyroid gland associated with excess parathormone (PTH) secretion.

Types

Three types

1. Primary—Execss secretion of PTH from parathyroid gland. Causes—adenoma (90%), hyperplasia or carcinoma of parathyroid. There is high calcium, low phosphate and high PTH.
2. Secondary—It occurs as a compensatory hyperplasia of parathyroid gland secondary to hypocalcaemia. Causes—CKD, malabsorption, vitamin D deficiency (ricket or osteomalacia). Parathormone is high. However in CKD, calcium is low but phosphate is high. But in ricket or osteomalacia, both calcium and phosphate are low but alkaline phosphatase is high.
3. Tertiary—Continuous stimulation of parathyroid for prolonged period from secondary hyperparathyroidism results in adenoma, which becomes autonomous. Features are like primary.

Primary Hyperparathyroidism

Symptoms

Common in female, above 50. Patient may remain asymptomatic in majority of cases. Most symptoms are due to hypercalcemia.

- General—anorexia, nausea, vomiting, weakness, tiredness, drowsiness.
- Abdominal—abdominal pain, constipation, features of pancreatitis, peptic ulcer, reflux oesophagitis.
- Renal—renal colic (due to stone or nephrocalcinosis), polyuria.
- Musculoskeletal—bone pain, spontaneous fracture, features of gout, pseudogout.
- Neurological—headache, depression, impaired memory, psychosis.
- Ocular—cataract, band keratopathy.
- Cardiovascular—hypertension.

NB: Remember the formula regarding symptoms of hypercalcaemia—"Bones, stones, abdominal groans and psychic moans".

Investigations

- Serum Ca, PO4 and alkaline phosphatase.
- Parathormone assay.

- Hydrocortisone suppression test—hydrocortisone 100 mg 6–8 hourly is given for 10 days, there is failure of suppression of calcium (in other causes, there is fall of calcium).
- X-ray of hand—shows subperiosteal erosion in the medial side of phalanges and resoption of terminal phalanx.
- X-ray of skull—shows 'pepper pot' appearance.
- USG or CT scan of neck.
- Other tests—Thallium/technetium substraction scan of thyroid and parathyroid.

Treatment of Hyperparathyroidism

- Mild and asymptomatic case—follow-up.
- In symptomatic case—total parathyroidectomy followed by transplantation of a small amount of parathyroid in the forearm muscles. After surgery, calcium may fall rapidly and tetany may occur. Hypocalcaemia may persist for several months. So, it is necessary to continue Vit. D and calcium supplement. Treatment of hypercalcaemia should be given.
- Secondary hyperparathyroidism—causes should be treated.
- Tertiary hyperparathyroidism—surgery.

Hypercalcaemia

Causes of Hypercalcaemia

1. Endocrine:
   - Hyperparathyroidism (primary and tertiary).
   - Multiple endocrine neoplasia (MEN- type I and II).
   - Addison's disease.
2. Malignancy:
   - Multiple myeloma.
   - Secondary deposit in bone.
   - Carcinoma of breast, kidney, lung, thyroid.
3. Others:
   - Sarcoidosis.
   - Hypervitaminosis D.
   - Prolonged immobilisation.
   - Drugs (thiazide, lithium).
   - Hypervitaminosis A.
   - Milk alkali syndrome.
   - Paget's disease with prolonged immobilisation.
   - Idiopathic hypercalcaemia in infancy.

Clinical Features

- May be asymptomatic.
- Anorexia, nausea, vomiting, dyspepsia.
- Weakness, lethargy.
- Constipation.
- Polyuria, polydipsia.
- Poor concentration, drowsiness, dizziness, depression.
- Peptic ulcer.
- Renal colic.

Treatment

1. Rehydration—Infusion of normal saline, 4–6 L daily for 2–3 days.
2. Calcium lowering drugs:
   - IV bisphosphonate—disodium pamidronate (90 mg IV over 4 hours with 0.9% saline infusion) or zolendronic acid 4 mg IV.
   - Calcitonin—100 unit 8 hourly IM or SC for 24–48 hours in severe case.
   - Prednisolone (30–60 mg daily. Helpful in hypercalcaemia caused by sarcoidosis, hypervitaminosis D and multiple myeloma).
3. Forced diuresis by IV frusemide along with saline.
4. If all fail, then haemodialysis.
5. Treatment of primary cause.

Hypoparathyroidism

Definition

It is due to decreased secretion of parathormone from parathyroid gland.

Causes

- Postoperative (commonest cause, during thyroid surgery).
- Rarely, infiltration due to haemochromatosis, Wilson's disease.
- Idiopathic.

Clinical Features

1. May be asymptomatic.
2. Features of hypocalcaemia:
   - Tetany.
   - Tingling in hands, feet and around the mouth.
   - Convulsion, epilepsy.

Treatment

- Oral calcium.
- Vit. D analogue—1 alpha hydroxycholecalciferol (alfacalcidiol) or 1,25 dihydroxycholecalciferol (calcitriol).
- Recombinant PTH subcutaneously may be used.

Hypocalcaemia

Causes

- Hypoalbuminaemia.
- Hypoparathyroidism.
- Psedohypoparathyroidism.
- Chronic kidney disease.
- Vitamin D deficiency.
- Acute pancreatitis.
- Alkalosis (metabolic, respiratory).

Clinical Features

- May be asymptomatic.
- Tetany—triad of carpo-pedal spasm, stridor and convulsion. Common in children.
- In adult, carpo-pedal spasm may occur in association with tingling in hands, feet and around mouth. Stridor and convulsion are rare.
- Other features—papilloedema, calcification of basal ganglia, grand mal epilepsy, psychosis, cataract.
- If hypocalcaemia due to Vit. D deficiency—ricket in children and osteomalacia in adult.
- ECG shows prolongation of QT interval, may cause ventricular arrhythmia.

Treatment

1. In acute case—IV 10-20 mL of 10% calcium gluconate slowly over 10 minutes. IV infusion may be required for several hours. Magnesium deficiency should be corrected also.
2. In chronic case:
   - Oral calcium.
   - Vitamin D analogue—1 alpha hydroxycholecalciferol (alfacalcidiol) or 1,25 dihydroxy-cholecalciferol (calcitriol).
3. Treatment of primary cause.

Tetany

Definition

It is characterized by muscle spasm due to increased excitability of peripheral nerves.

Causes

- Hypocalcaemia due to any cause (low serum ionized calcium).
- Alkalosis—due to repeated vomiting, hyperventilation, primary hyperaldosteronism.

Clinical Features

- Triad of carpopedal spasm, stridor and convulsion. Common in children. Carpopedal spasm is characterized by flexion of metacarpophalangeal joints of fingers and adduction of thumb.
- In adult, carpopedal spasm may occur in association with tingling in hands, feet and around mouth. Stridor and convulsion are rare.
- Latent tetany may be detected by following 2 signs—

Trousseau's sign—inflation of sphygmomanometer cuff on the upper arm to more than systolic BP is followed by carpal spasm within 3 minutes.

Chvostek's sign—tapping over the branches of facial nerve over the parotid produces twitching of facial muscles.

Treatment

- IV 10-20 mL of 10% calcium gluconate slowly over 10 minutes. May be required for several hours. Magnesium deficiency should also be corrected.
- In hyperventilation—reassurance and rebreathing in a paper bag.
- Correction of alkalosis—by IV normal saline.
- Treatment of primary cause (e.g.primary hyperaldosteronism) if any.

ADRENAL GLANDS

Disease of adrenal cortex:

Hyperfunction:
- Cushing's syndrome (non ACTH dependent).
- Primary hyperaldosteronism (Conn's syndrome).

Hypofunction:
- Addison's disease.
- Congenital adrenal hyperplasia.

Disease of adrenal medulla: Phaeochromocytoma.

Cushing's Syndrome

Definition

It is a syndrome caused by excess glucocorticoid for long duration that leads to constellation of symptoms and signs.

Causes of Cushing's Syndrome

Commonest cause is prolonged use of steroid.
Other causes:
1. ACTH dependent—
   - Pituitary microadenoma <10 mm, called Cushing's disease (in 80% cases). Common in women.
   - Ectopic ACTH syndrome—due to oat cell carcinoma of bronchus, bronchial adenoma, bronchial carcinoid and carcinoma of pancreas.
   - ACTH therapy.
2. Non-ACTH dependent—
   - Prolonged steroid therapy—commonest cause.
   - Adrenaled adenoma and adrenal carcinoma (common in women).
3. Others—Pseudo Cushing's syndrome (due to alcohol, depression, obesity).

Clinical Features

Symptoms:
- Weight gain but weakness.
- Proximal muscular weakness (characterized by difficulty in combing, raising the hands above the head, standing from squatting).
- In females—hirsutism, amenorrhoea or oligomenorrhoea.
- Loss of libido.
- Backache, pathological fracture (due to osteoporosis), collapse of the vertebra with reduction of height.
- Easy bruising,
- Frequent infection, especially fungal infection, slow wound healing.
- Mood disturbance—depression, insomnia, irritability, lethargy.

Signs
- Moon face, buffalo hump and increased fat above the supraclavicular fossa.
- Hirsutism with puffy and plethoric face, frontal baldness and acne.

- Striae in the skin (pink or purple coloured).
- Growth retardation in children.
- Truncal obesity with thin limbs (called 'lemon on a match stick' appearance).
- Skin is thin, with multiple purpura and bruise.
- Proximal myopathy, more marked in the lower limbs than upper limbs.
- Spine tenderness (due to osteoporosis).
- Hypertension, diabetes mellitus (DM) (30%) or IGT.

Difference between Cushing's Disease and Cushing's Syndrome

- Cushing's disease—there is increased production of ACTH from pituitary that stimulates adrenals.
- Cushing's syndrome is caused by excess glucocorticoid due to any cause.

Investigations

Initial tests are done to confirm the diagnosis and further tests are done to find out the cause.

Tests to Confirm Cushing's Syndrome

1. **First line screening test**
   - 24 hours urinary free cortisol measurement.
   - Overnight dexamethasone suppression test—1 mg dexamethasone is given orally at 11 p.m. Blood sample is taken at 9 a.m. in the next morning to measure serum cortisol. Normally, almost total suppression of cortisol. Failure of suppression indicates Cushing's syndrome due to any cause.
2. **Second line screening test (if above are abnormal):**
   - Serum cortisol level (8 a.m. and 12 midnight)—shows loss of circadian rhythm. Normally, serum cortisol is high in morning and low in midnight (called circadian rhythm).
   - Low-dose dexamethasone suppression test—0.5 mg 6 hourly for 2 days. Measure serum cortisol at 9 a.m. on days 0 and 2. Failure of suppression of cortisol indicates Cushing's syndrome due to any cause.

Tests to find out the Cause (to localize the site of lesion)

Serum ACTH—

1. If ACTH is low or undetectable, adrenal cause is likely. Then USG, CT or MRI of abdomen is done to find adrenal tumour. If no mass is seen, then adrenal vein sampling or adrenal scintigraphy should be done.
2. If ACTH is high—likely cause is pituitary lesion (Cushing's disease) or ectopic ACTH syndrome. Now high-dose dexamethasone suppression test or corticotrophin releasing hormone test is done to differentiate between these two.
   - If Cushing's disease is present—CT or MRI of skull.
   - If ectopic ACTH syndrome is the cause—chest X-ray, CT scan of chest (to see carcinoma of bronchus or bronchial carcinoid).

Other tests (to see the effect):

- Electrolytes (hypokalaemia).
- Blood sugar.
- Bone mass density to see osteoporosis.

Treatment

Depends on the cause:

1. Cushing's disease:
   - Transsphenoidal removal of microadenoma.
   - If surgery is not possible or unsuccessful, bilateral adrenalectomy should be done. Later the patient may develop Nelson's syndrome (see below).
   - If surgery is not possible, pituitary irradiation may be given.
   - To reduce ACTH production—bromocriptine or cyproheptadine is rarely effective.
   - Drugs, such as metyrapone and ketoconazole may be given.
2. Adrenal tumour:
   - In adrenal adenoma or carcinoma—adrenalectomy is done .
   - Radiotherapy or chemotherapy or adrenolytic drugs like mitotane may be given.
   - Other drugs—metyrapone or ketoconazole may be used (which inhibits biosynthesis of cortisol).
3. Ectopic ACTH:
   - If possible—the primary lesion should be treated.
   - If not possible—medical therapy as above or bilateral adrenalectomy may be considered.

Nelson's Syndrome

After bilateral adrenalectomy in Cushing's disease there may be increased pigmentation of the body due to excess ACTH. It is called Nelson's syndrome. It is due to enlarging pituitary tumour. It can be prevented by pituitary radiotherapy after adrenalectomy.

Treatment

Surgical removal of pituitary tumour may be needed.

ADDISON'S DISEASE

Definition

It is the primary adrenocortical insufficiency in which there is deficiency of glucocorticoid and mineralocorticoid due to destruction of the adrenal cortex.

Causes

1. Common causes—
   - Autoimmune—80% (more in female).
   - Tuberculosis of adrenal gland (in 10% cases).
   - Secondary deposit in adrenals.
   - HIV infection.
   - Bilateral adrenalectomy.
2. Other causes (less common or rare)—
   - Amyloidosis.
   - Sarcoidosis.
   - Haemochromatosis.
   - Bilateral adrenal haemorrhage—following meningococcal septicaemia (Waterhouse-Friedrichsen syndrome) and trauma.
   - Lymphoma.

Clinical Features

Symptoms

- Weakness and weight loss.
- Loss of appetite, nausea, vomiting, dizziness and vertigo.
- Pigmentation in different parts of the body.

Signs

- Hypotension, there may be postural hypotension.
- Patient is usually emaciated.
- Pigmentation—may be generalized. More marked in face, neck, mucous membrane of mouth, palmar crease, knuckles, knees, elbows, recent scar.
- Vitiligo may be present.
- Sparse (or less) axillary and pubic hair.

Diagnostic criteria in Addison's Disease

- Weakness or emaciation (100% cases).
- Pigmentation (90% cases).
- Hypotension (88%).

Investigations

1. Routine tests:
   - CBC (shows high eosinophil, lymphocyte and ESR).
   - Blood glucose (low or lower limit)

- Serum electrolytes (hyponatraemia and hyperkalaemia).
- Other tests—serum renin (increased), aldosterone (low) and serum calcium (may be high).

2. Test to confirm:
   - Plasma ACTH and cortisol (high ACTH and low cortisol).
   - Short synacthen test should be done. If cortisol level rises, it rules out Addison's disease. If does not rise, it indicates primary or secondary adrenocortical deficiency.
3. Test to find out cause:
   - Chest X-ray (to diagnose tuberculosis).
   - Plain X-ray abdomen (to see adrenal calcification in tuberculosis (TB).
   - Adrenal autoantibody.
   - USG or CT scan of adrenals (to look for calcification in TB or malignancy).
4. Other tests:
   - Screening for pernicious anaemia and other autoimmune disorders.
   - Thyroid screening.
   - Other tests according to suspicion of cause (e.g. sarcoidosis, amyloidosis, haemochromatosis, HIV, histoplasmosis, metastatic carcinoma, etc.).

Treatment

1. Replacement of hormones:
   - Glucocorticoid—hydrocortisone 15 mg in morning (after waking) and 5 mg in afternoon (6 p.m). According to some authority, 10 mg after waking, 5 mg at 12 noon and 5 mg at 6 p.m. Or if hydrocortisone is not available, prednisolone 5 mg on waking in morning and 2.5 mg at 6 p.m. in afternoon.
   - Mineralocorticoid—fludrocortisone 0.05–0.15 mg (50–300 μg) daily.
   - Androgen—dehydroepiandrosterone (DHEA) 50 mg/day may be given in female. It increases libido and sense of wellbeing, but complications like acne and hirsutism may occur.
2. Treatment of the cause (e.g. antitubercular therapy in tuberculosis).

General Advice to the Patient

- The patient should always carry a bracelet and steroid card, which should contain informations regarding the diagnosis, dose of steroid and doctor's contact address.
- Good nutrition, regular meal, high carbohydrate and sufficient salt.
- The patient should keep ampoules of hydrocortisone at home. If oral therapy is impossible, the patient should take injection by himself, family members or GP.
- The patient should know how to increase steroid replacement dose for intercurrent illness.
- During intercurrent stress (fever, cold and trauma), the dose should be doubled. If vomiting—parenteral hydrocortisone.

NB: Following points are important during stress—

1. During surgery:
   - Minor surgery—hydrocortisone 100 mg IM or IV premedication.
   - Major surgery—hydrocortisone 100 mg IM or IV 6 hourly for 24 hours, then 50 mg 6 hourly. It should be continued until the patient is capable of taking by mouth.
2. If gastroenteritis—IV or IM hydrocortisone should replace oral therapy.

Addisonian Crisis

It is an acute severe adrenocortical insufficiency, characterized by circulatory shock with severe hypotension. It is often precipitated by intercurrent disease, surgery or infection.

Causes

- Sudden withdrawal of steroid (common cause, if patient on steroid for long time).
- Stress (severe infection and operation).
- Bilateral adrenal haemorrhage (meningococcal septicaemia, injury and anticoagulant).
- Thyroxine therapy in a patient with hypopituitarism without steroid therapy.

Clinical Features

- Nausea, vomiting, diarrhoea, acute abdomen.
- Confusion, collapse or shock, even coma.
- Muscle cramps.
- There may be unexplained fever.

Investigations

- S. electrolytes—hyponatraemia, hyperkalaemia, may be hypercalcaemia.
- Hypoglycaemia.
- S. cortisol—low.

Treatment

- Blood is taken to measure cortisol, glucose and electrolytes.
- Three problems are present—shortage of salt, sugar and steroid (**3S**).
- IV fluid, normal saline rapidly (1 L in 30–60 minutes). Subsequently, several liters of normal saline may be required in 24 hours.
- IV 10% glucose.
- IV hydrocortisone 100 mg stat. Then hydrocortisone 100 mg IV 6 hourly, continued until the patient is stable and can take by mouth. Then oral steroid is started.
- Treatment of cause (e.g. infection, adrenal or pituitary pathology).

PHAEOCHROMOCYTOMA

Definition

It is a rare neuroendocrine tumour of chromaffin tissue that secretes catecholamines. Commonly it occurs in adrenal medulla (90%), but may occur in any part of sympathetic chain. Most tumours release adrenaline and noradrenaline, but extra-adrenal and large tumour release mainly noradrenaline.

Phaeochromocytoma may occur in urinary bladder and micturition can precipitate an attack. Rule of **'10'**—10% malignant, 10% extra-adrenal (in sympathetic chain), 10% familial.

May be associated with MEN Type II (primary hyperparathyroidism, medullary carcinoma of thyroid and pheochromocytoma, also called Sipple's syndrome) or MEN Type II b (above plus Marfanoid habitus, skeletal deformity, neuroma of lip, tongue, conjunctiva, eyelid). 25% may be multiple.

Clinical Features

Symptoms

- Recurrent, paroxysmal attack of hypertension with pallor, fear of death or anxiety or panic attack.
- Acute medical crisis (myocardial infarction, CVA, acute renal failure, paralytic ileus).

NB: Recurrent or paroxysmal attack of hypertension in young is highly suggestive of phaeochromocytoma.

Investigations

- 24 hour urinary VMA.
- Urinary catecholamines and metabolites (metanephrine).
- Serum catecholamines.
- Meta-iodobenzyl-guanidine scan (MIBG) helpful for extra-adrenal tumor.
- Abdominal ultrasound, CT scan or MRI.

Treatment

- Surgical resection.
- For hypertension—α blocker (phenoxy-benzamine 10–20 mg 6–8 hourly).
- If tachycardia—β blocker may be added (only β-blocker should not be given, as it may cause crisis).

PRIMARY HYPERALDOSTERONISM (CONN'S SYNDROME)

Definition

It is an aldosterone secreting tumor that causes excess aldosterone secretion from adrenal gland, also called Conn's syndrome. It may cause HTN in 5-15% of patients.

Causes

Excess aldosterone secretion leads to sodium retention, hypokalemia and hypertension. It is due to adrenal adenoma in 60% (Conn's syndrome) and 30% bilateral adrenal hyperplasia. Adrenal adenoma is usually small, common in young female. Adrenal hyperplasia is common in males, after 40 years.

Clinical Features

Symptoms

- Hypertension in young.
- Due to hypokalaemia—muscular weakness, polyuria, polydipsia.

NB: In any patient with hypokalemic alkalosis and hypertension, in the absence of diuretic use, it is highly suggestive of primary hyperaldosteronism.

Investigations

- S. electrolytes—high sodium, low potassium and high bicarbonate (metabolic alkalosis).
- Urine potassium >30 mmol in 24 hours.
- S. renin and aldosterone assay—low renin, high aldosterone.
- USG of adrenal gland.
- High-resolution CT scan or MRI of suprarenal gland is a very helpful investigation.
- 131 iodo-nor-cholesterol scanning of adrenal may be done.
- Selective venous catheter of adrenal for aldosterone measurement.
- Urine for 18-OH cortisol is increased.

Treatment

- If adenoma—surgery.
- If hyperplasia—aldosterone antagonist, such as spironolactone 100-400 mg daily.
- For hypertension—amiloride and calcium channel blocker may be used.

PITUITARY GLAND

Diseases of pituitary gland:

Hormone excess:

Anterior pituitary:	Prolactinoma. Acromegaly. Cushing's disease,
Hormone deficiency:	Hypopituitarism. Cranial diabetes insipidus (DI). Kallmann's syndrome.
Tumours:	Pituitary adenoma. Craniopharyngioma. Metastatic tumour.

Panhypopituitarism

Definition

It is a syndrome produced by complete or near complete destruction of the pituitary, causing deficiency of all the pituitary hormones.

It is characterized by asthenia, loss of sexual function and loss of target organ functions like thyroid, adrenal gland and gonads.

In panhypopituitarism, first there is loss of growth hormone and gonadotrophin (LH and FSH), followed by ACTH, TSH.

Causes of Hypopituitarism

1. Pituitary cause:
   - Pituitary adenoma, carcinoma (rare), secondaries, pituitary cyst, pituitary granuloma (tuberculosis, syphilitic gumma).
   - Pituitary surgery (resection or removal of tumour).
   - Pituitary irradiation.
   - Pituitary trauma.
   - Pituitary apoplexy.
   - Sheehan's syndrome.
   - Infiltrative disorder—haemochromatosis, lymphocytic hypophysitis, sarcoidosis, amyloidosis.
   - Others—autoimmune hypophysitis, idiopathic, congenital, Langerhans cell histiocytosis, MEN-I.
2. Extrapituitary causes:
   - Craniopharyngioma.
   - Others—meningioma, germinoma, glioma, pinealoma.
3. Secondary to hypothalamic disorder.
   - Commonest cause of hypopituitarism—pituitary tumour, surgery, radiotherapy, head injury, craniopharyngioma, meningioma.

Clinical Features

Symptoms

- Weakness, lassitude, malaise,dizziness and giddiness.
- Loss of libido.
- Absence of secondary sex characters.
- Amenorrhoea.
- Weight loss.
- Cold intolerance and constipation.

Signs

- The patient is pale and emaciated.
- Skin is fine and wrinkled.
- There is loss of axillary and pubic hair.

Investigations

1. Routine—CBC, ESR, S. electrolytes, RBS.
2. Serum hormone measurement—
   - For adrenocortical insufficiency—Serum cortisol (low) and ACTH (low).
   - For thyroid—FT4 (low) and TSH (low).
   - For gonadotrophins—FSH and LH. Also testosterone in male.
   - GH assay is not routinely done. Only considered if growth hormone replacement is possible.
3. MRI of the head to see the pituitary gland.

Treatment

- Hydrocortisone 15 mg in morning and 5 mg in afternoon. Or 10 mg after waking, 5 mg at 12 p.m. and 5 mg at 6 p.m. (If hydrocortisone is not available, prednisolone 5 mg in morning and 2.5 mg in afternoon).
- Thyroxine—50-150 μg in the morning before meal.
- In female—sex hormone replacement (to restore sexual function and to prevent osteoporosis).
- If the patient wishes for fertility—hCG + FSH or pulsatile GnRH may be given.
- In males—testosterone IM, orally, transdermally or implant.
- In child with hypopituitarism—GH should be given.
- Steroid card should be maintained.

Sheehan's Syndrome

It is a syndrome of hypopituitarism due to infarction of the pituitary gland following prolonged postpartum haemorrhage. Postpartum pituitary infarction occurs, because the enlarged pituitary gland in pregnancy is more vulnerable to ischaemia after prolonged and massive postpartum haemorrhage and hypotension.

Symptoms

- Failure of lactation is the earliest symptom.
- Other symptoms, such as breast atrophy, amenorrhoea, loss of libido, reduction of secondary sex characters, weakness, asthenia, etc. appear over months or years.

Investigations

As in hypopituitarism.

Treatment

As in hypopituitarism.

ACROMEGALY

Definition

It is characterized by generalized enlargement of the whole body due to excess growth hormone secretion from pituitary macroadenoma after union of epiphysis. If occurs before the union of epiphysis, it is called gigantism.

It is called acromegaly because of the enlargement of peripheral (acral) parts of body (acral means periphery and megaly means big). Acromegaly and gigantism may exist together. If excess growth hormone starts in adolescence and persists in adult life, the two conditions may be present together.

Causes

Eosinophilic adenoma of pituitary (macroadenoma) causing excessive GH secretion.

Clinical Features

Symptoms

- Progressive increase in size of the body (there may be history of change in size of rings, shoes, hats).
- Weight gain but weakness.
- Visual field defect due to pressure over optic chiasma (the patient gives history of collision with doors, person, car accident).
- Features of raised ICP—headache, vomiting.
- Excessive sweating.
- Features of hypertension, diabetes mellitus.
- Change in voice.
- Joint pain.

Signs

- Large head (bulldog scalp) with coarse facies, prominent supraorbital ridges, increased wrinkling of the forehead and baggy eyelids. Nose, lips and ears are large.
- Hands are large, spade like, warm and sweaty with doughy feeling.
- Feet are large.
- Skin is thick, greasy and sweaty.
- Coarse body hair.
- Voice is hoarse, husky and cavernous.
- Gynaecomastia may be present.
- Thyroid is diffusely enlarged.
- BP—may be high.
- Tongue, lips and jaw are enlarged. Lower jaw is protruded with malocclusion of teeth (prognathism).

In the eyes:

- Visual field defect, usually bitemporal hemianopia.
- Others—optic atrophy, papilloedema.

Cardiovascular system:

- Cardiomegaly.

Musculoskeletal system:
- Joints—may be swollen and tender.
- There may be kyphosis, scoliosis.

Investigations

1. Radiology:
   - X-ray skull—enlarged sella turcica, erosion of clinoid process, enlarged skull, mandible and sinuses, double floor sella.
   - X-ray of hands—large soft tissue, bones, widening of joint spaces, tufting of the terminal phalanges.
   - X-ray of feet—to see heel pad. Other changes like hand.
   - X-ray chest—enlarged heart.
   - Other X-ray—knee joints or other joints, if needed.
2. GH assay (radioimmunoassay)—high.
3. GTT with simultaneous measurement of GH (more diagnostic)—normally during GTT, there is suppression of GH <2 mU. But in acromegaly, there is failure of suppression of GH, occasionally paradoxical rise of GH.
4. Measurement of IGF-1 (also called somatomedin-C)—usually increased.
5. CT scan or MRI of skull.
6. Others:
   - Assessment of other anterior pituitary hormones.
   - Comparison with old photographs.
   - Perimetry (to see bitemporal hemianopia).
   - Blood sugar—DM in 10% cases, IGT in 25% cases.
   - ECG.
   - Serum calcium (increased in MEN-I).

Treatment

1. Surgery:
   - Transsphenoidal removal of the tumour is the treatment of choice.
   - Occasionally, transfrontal surgery is done in large macroadenoma with suprasellar extension.
2. Radiotherapy:
   It is used as a second line therapy. Radiotherapy can be used in combination with somatostatin analogue or dopamine agonist.
3. Drugs—given if surgery is not possible or persistent acromegaly after surgery.
   - Somatostatin analogue (octreotide or lanreotide) may be used as injection, every 2–4 weeks.
   - Bromocriptine or cabergoline or quinagolide may be used.
   - A peptide GH receptor antagonist (pegvisomant) may be used.
4. Other treatment
   Control of hypertension and diabetes mellitus.

Assessment of the response of therapy in acromegaly:
- Clinical improvement (decreased facial puffiness, body size, less sweating, improvement of hypertension, DM).
- Progress can be assessed by GH and IGF-1 measurement.

Hyperprolactinaemia

Definition

It is due to excess secretion of prolactin by anterior pituitary. It stimulates milk secretion but not breast enlargement, also inhibits gonadal activity producing hypogonadism.

Causes

1. Physiological—severe stress, pregnancy, lactation, exercise, coitus, sleep.
2. Drugs:
   - Dopamine antagonist—
     - Antipsychotic (phenothiazine, butyrophenons).
     - Antiemetic (metoclopramide, domperidone).
     - Antidepressant.
   - Dopamine depleting drugs (methyldopa).
   - Oestrogen therapy (e.g. oral contraceptive pill).
3. Pathological:
   - Prolactinoma (usually microadenoma <10 mm).
   - Pituitary macroadenoma.
   - Macroprolactinaemia (high prolactin without features of hyperprolactinaemia).
   - Primary hypothyroidism.
   - Polycystic ovarian syndrome.
   - Rarely—renal failure, liver failure, hypothalamic tumour, ectopic tumour, postictal state, chest wall injury or reflex (e.g. postherpes zoster).
   - Idiopathic.

Clinical Features

Symptoms:
- Galactorrhoea, hypogonadism (commonest symptoms).
- In male—decreased libido, impotence, lethargy.
- In female—amenorrhoea, oligomenorrhoea, menorrhagia, infertility.

Investigations

- Serum prolactin (very high).
- CT or MRI of brain.
- Other investigations according to the suspicion of cause, e.g. thyroid function, renal function.

Treatment

- Treatment of primary cause and responsible drugs should be stopped, if any.
- Dopamine agonist drugs (such as bromocriptine, cabergoline and quinagolide) is given.
- Transsphenoidal surgery.
- Radiotherapy—if macroadenoma fails to shrink following dopamine agonist drugs or total surgical removal is not possible.

DIABETES INSIPIDUS

Definition

Diabetes insipidus (DI) is a disease characterized by persistent excretion of excessive quantities of dilute urine associated with thirst due to deficiency of antidiuretic harmone (ADH) or insensitivity ADH to renal tubules.

Classification: Two types—

1. Cranial DI—decreased production of ADH by posterior pituitary.
2. Nephrogenic DI—renal tubules become insensitive to ADH.

Causes

Cranial DI

1. Structural hypothalamic or high-stalk lesion due to:
   - Craniopharyngioma.
   - Head injury.
   - Histiocytosis X.
   - Sarcoidosis.
   - Pituitary tumour with suorasellar extension.
   - Meningitis.
   - Encephalitis.
   - Postsurgical.
2. Idiopathic.
3. Genetic defect.

Nephrogenic DI

1. Genetic defect.
2. Drugs—lithium, demeclocycline.
3. Poisons—heavy metals.
4. Pyelonephritis.
5. Renal amyloidosis,
6. Multiple myeloma.
7. Sjogren's syndrome.
8. Sickle cell anaemia.
9. Others—polycystic kidney disease, prolong hypokalaemia, hypercalcaemia.

Symptoms

- Polyuria—patient may pass 5–20 L or more urine in 24 hours. Urine is of low specific gravity and osmolality.
- Polydipsia.

NB: If there is associated cortisol deficiency, there may not be any feature of DI until glucocorticoid therapy is given.

Investigations

- Serum ADH—may be undetectable.
- Urine osmolality (low), may be below 600 mOsm/kg and plasma osmolality (high).
- Water deprivation test.
- Hypertonic (5%) saline infusion and measurement of ADH secretion.
- S. electrolytes.
- S. calcium.

Treatment

- Cranial DI—desmopressin, DDAVP intranasally as spray. In very sick patient DDAVP should be given as IM.
- Nephrogenic DI—thiazide diuretic (bandroflumethiazide 5–10 mg daily, amiloride 5–10 mg daily) or indomethacin 15 mg 8 hourly.

DIABETES MELLITUS

Definition

Diabetes mellitus (DM) is a clinical syndrome characterized by persistent hyperglycaemia due to absolute or relative **deficiency** of insulin or **resistance** or both.

Clinical Features: Three p's-

1. **P**olyuria (excessive amount of urine).
2. **P**olydipsia (excessive thirst).
3. **P**olyphagia (excessive hunger).
4. Others—weight loss, weakness, dryness of mouth, pruritus vulvae, balanitis, oral candidiasis.
5. Patient may be asymptomatic, detected during routine examination.
6. Features of complications (see below).

Complications of DM

A. Acute complications:
- Hypoglycaemia.
- Diabetic ketoacidosis.
- Hyperglycaemic hyperosmolar state (previously called hyperosmolar nonketotic diabetic coma).
- Lactic acidosis.

B. Long-term complications:

1. Microvascular:
   - Neuropathy—Peripheral neuropathy (sensory, motor or mixed), mononeuritis multiplex, mononeuropathy, autonomic neuropathy.
   - Nephropathy (CKD).
   - Eye complications (retinopathy, cataract).
   - Foot complications (ulcers, gangrene, arthropathy).
2. Macrovascular:
   - Coronary circulation—myocardial ischaemia, infarction.
   - Cerebral circulation—TIA, CVD.
   - Peripheral circulation—ischaemia, claudication.
   - Foot complications (ulcers, gangrene, arthropathy—Charcoat's joint).

C. Others:

Infections—boil, carbuncle, abscess, cellulitis, tuberculosis.

Investigations

- Urine R/M/E.
- Blood sugar (fasting and 2 hours after breakfast).
- HbA1c.
- CBC, ESR.
- Urea, creatinine, electrolytes.
- Serum lipid profile.
- USG of whole abdomen.

- CXR P/A view.
- Plain X-ray abdomen (to see pancreatic calcification).
- ECG.

Criteria for the Diagnosis of DM

In patient with symptoms of diabetes, diagnosis is made by—

- Fasting plasma venous blood sugar level >7.0 mmol/L (or 2 hour postprandial blood sugar level >11.1 mmol/L).
- Random blood sugar >11.1 mmol/L.
- During oral glucosetolerance test (OGTT) >11.1 mmol/L, 2 hours after 75 g glucose.

NB: In asymptomatic patients, 2 diagnostic tests are required to confirm diabetes.

Glycaemia may be classified into 3 types—

1. Normal.
2. Impaired or prediabetes (which includes IGT and IFG).
3. Diabetes mellitus.

Impaired Glucose Tolerance

When fasting glucose is <7 mmol, but during OGTT, 2 hours after the glucose load is 7.8-11.0 mmol/L, it is called Impaired glucose tolerance (IGT). Patient with IGT may develop frank DM type 2 with time. Macrovascular complications are more (mainly cardiovascular).

Lifestyle modification for type 2 DM and annual checkup for glucose are recommended for this patient. Cardiovascular risk factors, such as hypertension and dyslipidaemia should be treated.

Impaired Fasting Glucose (IFG)

Impaired fasting glucose (IFG) is defined as the fasting glucose level between 6.1–6.9 mmol/L (110–125 mg/dL) according to WHO. However, ADA defines it as fasting glucose level between 5.6–6.9 mmol/L (100–125 mg/dL). Those who have IFG are prone to develop frank diabetes mellitus and cardiovascular disease.

Weight reduction about 5–10% of their body weight, regular exercise and follow-up is advised. Usually no drug is needed.

Latent Diabetes

It means blood glucose is usually normal, but may be high under certain stressful conditions, also called 'stress hyperglycaemia.' Examples are—pregnancy, infection, obesity, stress or drugs like steroid, thiazide diuretics, etc. Glucose is usually normal after the stress is resolved.

Potential Diabetes

It means blood sugar usually is normal, but the patient has increased risk of developing diabetes mellitus in future due to genetic reasons like—

- Both parents are diabetic.
- One parent is diabetic and the other has family history of diabetes.
- Has a diabetic sibling.
- In a twin, if one is diabetic.

Aetiological Classification of DM

Primary

- Type 1—IDDM (Insulin Dependent Diabetes Mellitus).
- Type 2—NIDDM (Non Insulin Dependent Diabetes Mellitus).

Secondary

1. Pancreatic diseases:
   - Chronic pancreatitis.
   - Pancreatectomy.
   - Haemochromatosis.
   - Cystic fibrosis.
2. Endocrine diseases:
   - Acromegaly.
   - Cushing's syndrome.
   - Glucagonoma.
   - Thyrotoxicosis.
   - Phaeochromocytoma.
3. Chronic liver disease.
4. Drug induced (e.g. corticosteroid, thiazide diuretics).
5. Gestational diabetes mellitus—in pregnancy.

Gestational Diabetes Mellitus

Gestational diabetes mellitus (GDM) is defined as any degree of glucose intolerance with the onset or first recognition during pregnancy. It constitutes 90% of women with pregnancy complicated by diabetes. More than 50% women ultimately develop diabetes in next 20 years and this is linked with obesity. Usually they develop type 2 DM.

Oral glucose tolerance test with 75 g glucose is used as screening test for GDM for women between 24 and 28 weeks of gestation. Blood glucose is measured at fasting, 1 hour and 2 hours after glucose load. Gestational diabetes millitus is diagnosed if blood glucose is—

- Fasting >5.1 mmol/L.
- After 1 hour 10 mmol/L.
- After 2 hour 8.5 mmol/L.

Mangement of GDM

- Dietary modification.
- Monitoring of blood glucose regularly—premeal glucose should be <5.5 mmol/L and postmeal glucose <7mmol/L.
- If drug is necessary—metformin or glibenclamide is safe (does not cross placenta). Insulin may be required in later stage.
- After delivery, glucose usually becomes normal. Follow-up is necessary.
- There is risk of type 2 diabetes, 15–55% in 5 years. So, dietary and life style advice are necessary to reduce the risk.

Management of Diabetes in Pregnancy

- Dibetes mellitus must be well controlled before planned pregnancy, otherwise there is more chance of complications of mother and foetus. Ketoacidosis, retinopathy and nephropathy may be more in pregnancy. Risk of foetal anomaly is also more.
- Insulin is given usually. Oral drug should be avoided, however, metformin may be given.
- Mother should measure blood glucose daily.

Complications of Foetus in DM

- Teratogenicity—cardiac, renal and skeletal malformations.
- Foetal macrosomia .
- Neonatal hypoglycaemia.
- Hyaline membrane disease.
- Still birth.

Features of Autonomic Neuropathy in DM

In both type 1and 2 DM, there may be autonomic neuropathy. Features are—

- CVS—postural hypotension, fixed heart rate, resting tachycardia and sometimes, sudden death.
- GIT—gastroparesis, nocturnal diarrhoea, constipation.
- Genitourinary—urinary incontinence, difficulty in micturition, erectile dysfunction, retrograde ejaculation.
- Sudomotor—gustatory sweating, nocturnal sweating without hypoglycaemia, hyperhydrosis of upper extremity and anhydrosis of lower extremity. Anhydrosis of foot can cause cracked skin and ulcer.
- Vasomotor—cold feet, dependent oedema.
- Autonomic neuropathy can reduce counter regulatory hormone release, leading to an inability to sense hypoglycaemia appropriately.
- Pupillary—decreased pupil size, resistance to mydriatic and delayed or no reflex to light (called pseudo-Argyll Robertson pupil).

Types of Neuropathy in DM

- Sensory neuropathy (common).
- Mixed motor and sensory neuropathy.
- Asymmetrical motor neuropathy (diabetic amyotrophy).
- Autonomic neuropathy.
- Mononeuropathy.
- Mononeuritis multiplex.

Causes of Loss of Vision in DM

- Diabetic retinopathy.
- Cataract.
- Age-related macular degeneration.
- Retinal vein occlusion.
- Retinal artery occlusion.

- Nonarteritic ischaemic optic neuropathy.
- Glaucoma.

Diabetic Retinopathy

In diabetic patient, retinopathy occurs after 10–20 years. It is the commonest cause of blindness in middle aged and elderly patients in developed countries.

Clinical Features

- Microaneurysms.
- Retinal haemorrhage.
- Exudates.
- Cotton wool spots.
- Venous changes and neovascularization.
- Vitrious haemorrhage, subhyaloid haemorrhage.
- Fibrosis.

Types of Diabetic Retinopathy

1. Simple or background retinopathy—microaneurysm of capillaries, few haemorrhages (dot and blot), hard exudates (yellowish with clear margin). Disc is normal.
2. Maculopathy—above finding plus haemorrhage and hard exudates encroaching upon the macula.
3. Pre-proliferative retinopathy—multiple cotton wool spots (earliest sign), venous abnormality (irregular, beading, reduplication and loops), multiple haemorrhage and intraretinal microvascular abnormality.
4. Proliferative retinopathy—new vessel formation around the disc which are fragile, may rupture causing vitreous haemorrhage.

Treatment

1. General measures—Good control of diabetes, hypertension. Avoidance of smoking, regular ophthalmoscopic review.
2. Specific:
   - Background and preproliferative retinopathy—no medical treatment.
   - Maculopathy and proliferative retinopathy—retinal photocoagulation (argon laser).

Diabetic Nephropathy

Common cause of chronic kidney disease (CKD). About 30% patients with type 1 diabetes develop diabetic nephropathy 20 years after diagnosis of diabetes, less common in type 2 diabetes (15–20%).

Risk Factors for Developing Diabetic Nephropathy

- Poor glycaemic control.
- Long duration of diabetes.
- Presence of other microvascular complication.
- Preexisting hypertension.
- Family history of diabetic nephropathy, hypertension.
- Asian race.

Stages of Diabetic Nephropathy

- Microalbuminuria (most important indicator of risk of developing overt diabetic nephropathy).
- Overt nephropathy, may progress to nephrotic syndrome.
- Chronic kidney diaease.

Treatment

- Good control of blood glucose, hypertension.
- Salt restriction.
- Drugs—ACE inhibitors or angiotentin II receptor blocker.

Microalbumiuria

It is defined as urinary albumin excretion 30–300 mg/day. Normal albumin excretion is <20 mg/day.

It is an important hallmark of early diabetic nephropathy and an indicator of underlying cardiovascular disease. It is more in NIDDM.

Treatment

- Good control of diabetes.
- Good control of hypertension.
- Restriction of protein—40–60 mg/day.
- Drugs—ACE inhibitors.

Diabetic Foot

There may be ulcer, gangrene, osteomyelitis, arthropathy, sepsis. Causes are:

- Ischaemia.
- Neuropathy.
- Combined ischaemia and neuropathy.
- Secondary infection.

Treatment of Diabetic Ulcer

- Good control of diabetes.
- Local dressing.
- Avoid weight bearing.
- Antibiotic to control secondary infection.
- Avoid barefoot, tight shoes and smoking.
- Consult with chiropodist.
- Surgery may be required (amputation or angioplasty).

Diabetic Ketoacidosis

Diabetic ketoacidosis (DKA) is a metabolic complication of DM in which there is severe hyperglycaemia with metabolic acidosis due to excess ketone bodies. It is common in IDDM (type 1), rare in type 2.

Precipitating Factors

Little or no insulin, intercurrent infections, severe stress like trauma, acute MI.

Clinical Features

Symptoms

- Polyuria, polydipsia, weakness.
- Nausea, vomiting, abdominal pain.
- Acidotic deep sighing breathing (kussmaul's breathing), altered consciousness, coma may occur.

Signs

- Severe dehydration (dry tongue, sunken eyes).
- Pulse—weak, tachycardia.
- BP—low.
- Air hunger, Kussmaul's breathing, acetone breath (sweetish).
- Others—reflexes are reduced, but planter is flexor.

Investigations

- Blood sugar and ketone bodies—high.
- Urine sugar and ketone bodies—present.
- Serum electrolytes (low sodium, potassium) and bicarbonate (low).
- ABG—low pH.
- Others—CXR, ECG, CBC, calcium, magnesium, etc.

NB: Three main problems in DKA are:

- Hyperglycemia,
- Hyperketonaemia and
- Metabolic acidosis.

Marked dehydration is common, average loss of fluid and electrolytes are:

- Water—6 litres,
- Sodium—500 mmol,
- Chloride—400 mmol,
- Potassium—350 mmol.
- Half of the lost fluid is intracellular. If bicarbonate is <12 mmol/L, it indicates severe acidosis.

Treatment

- IV normal saline rapidly:
  - 1L in 30 minutes,
  - 1L in 1 hour,
  - 1L in 2 hours,
  - 1L in 4 hours,
  - 1L in 8 hours,
- IV soluble insulin preferably with pump—0.1 IU/kg/h or 20 units IM stat followed by 6 units IM hourly.
- Potassium correction with infusion depending on the blood report.

- When blood glucose is below 14 mmol/L, 5% glucose is added. Insulin dose is adjusted according to blood report.
- Correction of acidosis by sodibicarb, if arterial pH is <7.
- Others—Control of infection by broad-spectrum antibiotic, catherterization, nasogastric feeding if needed, CV line, subcutaneous LMW heparin.

Complications of DKA

- Cerebral oedema.
- ARDS.
- DIC.
- Thromboembolism.
- Acute circulatory failure.
- Mortality is 5–10%, more in elderly.

Hyperglycaemic Hyperosmolar State (HSS)

Previously it was called hyperosmolar nonketotic diabetic coma (HNDC). There may not be coma.

It is characterized by very-high blood glucose (>30 mmol/L), high plasma osmolality (>320 mOsm/kg) and dehydration without ketosis. Here insulin deficiency is partial and low level of endogenous insulin is present, which is sufficient to inhibit hepatic ketogenesis, but insufficient to control hyperglycemia. It may be the first presentation of diabetes mellitus, common in elderly with type 2 (NIDDM).

Precipitating Factors

- Consumption of glucose-rich diet or fruits.
- Concurrent medication like thiazide or steroid.
- Myocardial infarction.
- Intercurrent illness (pneumonia, UTI).

Symptoms

- Onset is less insidious than DKA. Polyuria, polydipsia, altered consciousness, convulsion.
- Signs of severe dehydration are present.

Investigations

- Blood glucose—very high.
- Serum and urinary ketone body—absent.
- ABG—normal pH.
- Plasma osmolality >320 mOsm/kg.

Treatment

- IV 1/2 strength saline (0.45%) should be given. When osmolality is normal, 0.9% normal saline should be given. However, if hypovolaemia is present as evidenced by hypotension and oliguria, 0.9% saline may be given. Usually 4–6 litres fluid may be required in first 8–10 hours.
- Low-dose soluble insulin preferably with insulin pump, 2–6 units hourly. Insulin dose is adjusted to reduce the glucose level by 50–70 mg/dL/h.

- When glucose is 250 mg/dL, 5% dextrose in either aqua or 0.45% saline or 0.9% saline. Rate of glucose infusion should be adjusted to maintain glucose level between 250–300 mg/dL in order to reduce the risk of cerebral oedema. When the urinary output is 50 mL/h or more, IV fluid may be stopped.
- Other treatment—NG tube feeding, catheter if needed, antibiotic if infection, correction of electrolytes, low-dose heparin (as thrombosis is common).

Clinical Features of Hypoglycaemia and Hyperglycaemia

Typical features of hypoglycaemia are:
- Excessive sweating.
- Tachycardia.
- Tremor.
- Other—Jerks may be brisk, but planter response is extensor bilaterally.

Typical features of hyperglycaemia are:
- Severe dehydration.
- Pulse—weak.
- BP—low.
- Air-hunger is present—Kussmaul's breathing and acetone breath.
- Others—Reflexes are reduced, planter is flexor.

Management of Diabetes Mellitus

It comprises general management and management of complications. In a newly diagnosed DM, adequate glucose control by diet and lifestyle changes are the key points. If DM is not controlled with these, oral antidiabetic drugs or insulin may be needed or combination of both may be given depending on blood glucose levels, severity of symptoms and comorbid conditions.

3 modes of treatment:
- Diet control and lifestyle modification.
- Diet control and oral antidiabetic.
- Diet control and insulin (plus occasional oral antidiabetic).

Diet: 50–60% cases, DM can be controlled by diet control alone. Balanced diet comprising carbohydrate, fat and protein as follows:
- Carbohydrate—45–60% (sucrose up to 10%).
- Total fat <35% (saturated <10%, monounsaturated 10–20%).
- Protein—10–15% (not to be exceeded 1 g/kg body weight/day).
- Fruits and vegetables.

Lifestyle
- If obese—reduction of weight.
- Physical activity—aerobic exercise at least 30–45 minutes 5 times per week (walking, swimming, cycling). Rest period should not exceed more than 2 days.
- Smoking should be stopped.
- Alcohol in moderate dose.
- Low-calorie, sugar-free drinks may be given.

Drugs: Oral antidiabetics and insulin.

Oral Antidiabetics

Biguanides

Metformin in type-2 DM if no contraindications (such as—hepatic dysfunction, severe renal failure). It acts by increasing insulin sensitivity and peripheral glucose uptake, also reduceds absorption of glucose from GI tract and inhibits hepatic gluconeogenesis.

Side Effects
Anorexia, nausea, diarrhoea, abdominal cramps, bloating, increased susceptibility to lactic acidosis.

Sulphonylureas

Gliclazide, glibenclamide, glimepiride, glipizide. They promote pancreatic beta cell insulin secretion. Usually added with metformin when DM is not well controlled with metformin alone. It can be used in lean patient with type-2 DM.

Side Effects
Weight gain, hypoglycaemia.

Meglitinide

Repaglinides and nateglinides. They are also insulin secretogogues.

Side Effects
Same as sulphonylurea but less chance of hypoglycemia.

Alpha-glucosidase Inhibitors

Acarbose and miglitols. They control postprandial glucose, delay carbohydrate absorption from the gut. This drug can be used with sulphonylurea.

Side Effects
Flatulence, abdominal bloating, diarrhoea.

Thiazolidinediones

Pioglitazone, rosiglitazone. Pioglitazone can aggravate cardiac failure, risk of bone fracture and possibly bladder cancer. Rosiglitazone increases the risk of myocardial infarction. So, these are less used due to serious adverse effects.

Incretin-based Drugs

- Dipeptidyl Peptidase-4-inhibitors (DPP-4)—sitagliptin, vildagliptin, linagliptin.
- Glucose like peptide -1 (GLP-1) inhibitors—liraglutide, exenatide.
  Used in obese patient and can be used with metformin, sulphonylurea or insulin.

Side effects
GIT upset, nasopharyngitis, rarely pancreatitis.

Insulin

Insulin is used mainly for type1 DM. In type 2 DM, it is used from the beginning if blood glucose is very high or patient is symptomatic.

Human Insulin

- Short acting—Soluble, regular insulin.
- Intermediate acting—Isophane (NPH).
- Premix formulations—30/70 (30% short acting and 70% intermediate acting), 50/50 (50% of each type).

Insulin Analogues

- Rapid acting—lispro, aspart, glulisine. They are ultra short-acting bolus insulin to control postmeal hyperglycemia.
- Premix formulations of rapid acting plus intermediate acting (e.g. aspart 30% plus aspart-protamin 70% (e.g. Novo-mix).
- Long acting—glargine, detemir. They are used as basal insulin to control premeal hyperglycemia.
- Ultra long-acting—degludec.

Absolute Indications of Insulin Therapy

- Diabetic ketoacidosis, hyperosmolar nonketotic diabetic coma and lactic acidosis.
- Surgery.
- Pregnancy.
- Severe infection.
- Hepatic failure.
- Severe renal failure.

Complications of Insulin Therapy

- Hypoglycaemia.
- Weight gain.
- Lipodystrophy at injection sites—lipoatrohy, lipohypertrophy.
- Development of insulin antibody (specially in animal insulin).

Treatment Goal for DM

- Treatment goal and plan should be individualized.
- Preprandial capillary plasma glucose (FBG): <7.0 mmol/L.
- Postprandial capillary plasma glucose: <10 mmol/L.
- HbA1C: <7%.
- BP: <140/80 mmHg.
- Total cholesterol: <200 mg/dL.
- Triglyceride: <150 mg/dL
- LDL: <100 mg/dL and <70 mg/dL if overt CVD.
- HDL: >40 mg/dL for men and >50 mg/dL for women.

HYPOGLYCAEMIA

Definition

Hypoglycemia is defined as when blood glucose level is <3.5 mmol/L (63 mg/dL).

Causes of Hypoglycaemia in Diabetic Patient

- Missed, delayed or inadequate meal.
- Unusual exercise.
- Error in dose or schedule or administration.
- Gastroparesis in autonomic neuropathy.
- Malabsorption.
- Lipoatrophy at injection site.
- Comorbid conditions—Addison's disease.
- Renal impairment.
- Factitious.
- Breastfeeding.
- Others—strict glycaemic control.

Causes of Hypoglycaemia in Nondiabetic Patient

- Endocrine cause—Addison's disease, pituitary insufficiency.
- Neoplastic cause—Insulinoma, hepatoma, retroperitoneal sarcoma, fibroma, mesothelioma.
- Hepatic cause (specially in fulminant hepatic failure)
- Renal—CKD.
- Alcohol.
- Severe falciparum malaria (cerebral malaria), specially during quinine therapy.
- Factitious.
- Postprandial—usually develops 2–5 hours after meal, never during fasting. May occur after alcohol intake, after gastric surgery, e.g partial gastrectomy, gastrojejunostomy, pyroloplasty, etc. (dumping syndrome). Others—may be hypoglycaemia in childhood, e.g. galactossaemia, glycogen storage disease type I.

Symptoms of Hypoglycaemia

Symptoms usually develop when blood glucose level is <2.5 mmol/L, but in diabetic patient, symptoms may appear at a higher level.

- Adrenergic—palpitation, sweating, tremor, hunger, anxiety.
- Neuroglycopenic—confusion, inability to concentrate, drowsiness, dizziness, speech difficulty, irritability, fits, even coma if untreated. Persistent and prolong hypoglycaemia may cause irreversible brain damage (cerebral atrophy, dementia).

Management of Hypoglycaemia

- If the patient is conscious—should take oral glucose or sugar or any sweet.
- If patient is semiconscious or unconscious—I/V 75 mL 20% dextrose is given. I/M glucagon (1 mg) may be given. This is followed by glucose infusion till the patient can take by mouth.

Prevention of Hypoglycaemia:

- Patient's education is important. Should know the features of hypoglycaemia. Should keep glucose or any sweet, so that if any symptoms, patient should take this immediately.
- Those who take insulin, food should be kept ready before taking insulin.
- Undue heavy exercise should be avoided. Alcohol excess is also avoided.
- Risk factors of hypoglycemia should be sorted and managed accordingly.
- Relatives and friends of the patient should also be educated on the topic.

OBESITY

Definition

It is defined as excessive accumulation of body fat, classically when the BMI is >30 kg/m^2. It is associated with higher risk of morbidity and mortality.

Obesity is diagnosed by the following:
- Measuring weight.
- BMI.
- Skin-fold thickness over the middle of triceps. Normal values are 20 mm in male and 30 mm in female.
- Waist or hip circumference ratio >1.0 in male and >0.9 in females indicates obesity.

Causes of Obesity

Multiple factors may be responsible:
1. Genetic.
2. Physical inactivity.
3. Excessive food intake.
4. Psychological factors.
5. Drugs—steroid, oral contraceptive pill, sodium valproate, TCA.
6. Secondary disease:
   - Endocrine causes—hypothyroidism, Cushing's syndrome, insulinoma.
   - PCOS in female.
   - Hypothalamic disorder (tumours, injury). This causes polyphagia and obesity.
   - Metabolic syndrome.
   - Genetic syndrome—Laurence Moon Biedle syndrome, Prader-Willi syndrome.
   - Others—Pickwickian syndrome, Alstrom syndrome.

Link between Obesity and Diabetes Mellitus

Fat cells release free fatty acids and also TNF α which are responsible for insulin resistance. A new protein called resistin secreted by the fat cells also causes insulin resistance.

Complications of Obesity

- Psychological—low self esteem, depression.
- Mechanical—osteoarthrosis of knee and hips, back strain, varicose veins, urinary incontinence, hiatus hernia, abdominal hernia, flat foot.
- Hepatobiliary—nonalcoholic fatty liver disease, cirrhosis, gallstones.
- Respiratory—exertional dyspnoea, obstructive sleep apnoea, Pickwickian syndrome.
- Cardiovascular—hypertension, atherosclerosis, IHD, heart failure, thromboembolism.
- CVD.
- Metabolic—diabetes mellitus type 2, hyperlipidaemia, atherosclerosis, hyperuricaemia and gout.
- Increased cancer risk—breast, uterus, colorectal, prostate, ovary.
- Skin infection—groin and submammary candidiasis.
- Menstrual abnormalities.
- Increased morbidity and mortality.

- Postoperative problems.
- Accident proneness.

Investigations

Detailed history of patient, specially dietary history, history of physical activity or sedentary work, any drug, alcohol should be taken. Whether the weight gain is recent or rapid (to exclude secondary disease like Cushing's syndrome or hypothyroidism) should be noted.
Then following routine investigations should be done -

- Fasting blood sugar.
- Lipid profile.
- Thyroid function test (FT3, FT4, TSH).
- Investigations for Cushing's syndrome.
- Liver function test.
- USG of hepatobiliary system to see fatty liver.
- X-ray chest, ECG, echocardiography—to see cardiac status.
- Lung function test for sleep apnoea.
- X-ray of the individual joints in osteoarthrosis.
- In female, if PCOS is suspected, investigations to be done accordingly (e.g. USG of ovary, serum FSH and LH).

Treatment

Multidisciplinary approach including -

1. Low-calorie diet.
2. Exercise.
3. Social support.
4. Avoidance of offending drug, smoking, alcohol.
5. Treatment of secondary cause.
6. Drug treatment—
   - Sibutramine (it blocks serotonergic pathways).
   - Orlistat (pancreatic and gastric lipase inhibitor). It inhibits dietary fat absorption.
   - Incretins (glucagon like peptide -1).
   - Biguanide—metformin.

   (Other drugs like phenfluramine, amphetamine, phentarmine, etc are not recommended).
7. Surgical management:
   - Bariatric surgery—to reduce the size of stomach (stappling of the stomach).
   - Cosmetic surgery (liposuction).

Indication of Surgery

In some cases of morbid obesity (BMI >40 kg/m^2) or BMI >35 kg/m^2 and obesity related complications, after conventional treatment have failed.

SHORT STATURE

Causes of Short Stature

1. Constitutional (commonest cause).
2. Familial or genetic.
3. Physiological growth delay.
4. Emotional deprivation and psychological factors.
5. Chronic systemic disease—
   - Cardiac—congenital cyanotic heart disease like Fallot's tetralogy.
   - Renal—renal failure, renal tubular acidosis.
   - Respiratory—bronchiectasis, bronchial asthma.
   - GIT—small bowel disease like coeliac disease, Hirschsprung's disease.
   - Cystic fibrosis.
6. Endocrine diseases:
   - Hypopituitarism (pituitary dwarfism).
   - Isolated GH deficiency.
   - Cretinism (hypothyroidism).
   - Cushing's syndrome.
   - Pseudohypoparathyroidism (characterized by short stature, round face, mental retardation, epileptic attack, basal ganglia and subcutaneous calcification, short metacarpal. Hypoparathyroidism is due to defect in end organ resistance to parathormone).
   - Pseudo-pseudohypoparathyroidism.
   - Uncontrolled Juvenile diabetes mellitus.
7. Nutritional:
   - Protein energy malnutrition—marasmus and kwashiorkor.
   - Ricket.
8. Chromosomal or genetic abnormalities:
   - Down's syndrome.
   - Turner's syndrome.
   - Noonan's syndrome (male Turner).
   - Prader-Willi syndrome.
   - Laurence-Moon-Biedl syndrome.
9. Skeletal dysplasia:
   - If there is short limb and normal trunk, may be due to achondroplasia.
   - If there is short limb and short spine, may be due to mucopolysaccharidoses (Hurler's syndrome or Gargoylism).
10. Gross kyphoscoliosis.
11. Drugs like steroid.

Investigations

A detailed history should be taken and the patient should be examined to exclude systemic diseases. It should be done as follows:

1. History to be taken:
   - Family history (parents and relatives).
   - Pregnancy record (growth retardation and weight at birth, and any congenital disease).

- Rate of growth.
- Comparison with peers at school and siblings.
- Systemic disease (respiratory, cardiac, GIT and renal).
- Nutrition (less intake and malabsorption).
- Age of appearance of secondary sexual characters (pubic hair, breast, menarche).
- Use of steroid during childhood.
- Psychosocial deprivation.

2. Physical examination:
   - Height and weight chart (if height is below third percentile, it is considered as short stature).
   - Arm span and height (achondroplasia).
   - Short limbs compared to trunk (achondroplasia).
   - Reduction of weight and height (malnutrition and systemic disease).
   - More weight but short height indicates endocrine disease (hypothyroidism, Cushing's syndrome), and genetic syndrome (Prader–Willi syndrome, Laurence-Moon-Biedl syndrome).
   - Grading of secondary sexual characteristics.
   - Look for evidence of systemic disease (heart, kidney and respiratory).
   - Others (Turner's syndrome, Noonan's syndrome and pseudohypoparathyroidism).

After exclusion of systemic disease, proceed as follows:

1. Thyroid function test—Serum TSH and FT4 to exclude hypothyroidism.
2. GH status:
   - GH response to insulin is the gold standard.
   - Blood level of insulin like growth factor 1 (IGF-1) and insulin like growth factor binding protein 3 (IGF-BP3) may provide evidence of GH under secretion.
   - Basal growth hormone level is of little value. Urinary growth hormone level may be used as a screening.
3. Bone age—nondominant hand and wrist X-rays for the assessment of bone age by comparison with standard charts.
4. Lateral skull X-ray (may show calcification—in craniopharyngioma).
5. Karyotyping in females—to exclude Turner's syndrome.
7. Other tests according to suspicion of causes.

DWARFISM

Definition

It is defined as a condition where the height of a person is much below than the normal according to the chronological age.

Causes

As like short stature.

Cause According to Body Ratio in Dwarfism

1. If upper and lower segments are equal, the causes are:
   - Hereditary.
   - Constitutional.
   - Pituitary dwarfism.

2. If upper segment is bigger than lower segment, the causes are:
   - Achondroplasia.
   - Cretinism.
   - Juvenile myxoedema.
3. If upper segment is smaller than lower segment, the causes are:
   - Spinal deformity.

Treatment

- Any systemic disease should be treated accordingly.
- Nutritional supplementation.
- Psychological support.
- In growth hormone deficiency—recombinant growth hormone (somatropin) is given.

MULTIPLE ENDOCRINE NEOPLASIA

Definition

Multiple endocrine neoplasia (MEN) is a group of genetic syndromes, transmitted as autosomal dominant, characterized by neoplasm of two or more different hormonal tissue of the body.

Types

MEN-1 (Wermer's syndrome)

It comprises primary hyperparathyroidism, pituitary adenoma and pancreatic tumor.
- Primary hyperparathyroidism—most common feature and earliest manifestation of MEN-1. There are four gland hyperplasia.
- Pancreatic neuroendocrine tumor—gastrinoma (40–60%), insulinoma (20%).
- Pituitary adenomas—mainly secrete prolactin.

MEN-2a (Sipple's syndrome)

It comprises:
- Medullary carcinoma of thyroid.
- Primary hyperparathyroidism (usually hyperplasia).
- Phaeochromocytoma.

MEN-2b

- MEN-2a when associated with:
- Marfanoid body habitus.
- Abnormal dental enamel .
- Multiple mucosal neuromas.
- Skeletal abnormalities.

REPRODUCTIVE SYSTEM

Diseases of Reproductive System

Hormone Excess

- Polycystic ovarian syndrome.
- Estrogen secreting tumor.
- Androgen secreting tumour.

Hormone Eeficiency

- Menopause.
- Hypogonadism (gonadotropin deficiency, primary gonadal failure).
- Kallmann's syndrome (GnRH deficiency).
- Anorexia nervosa.

Nonfunctioning Tumour

- Ovarian cyst.
- Carcinoma.
- Teratoma.
- Seminoma.

Delayed Puberty

Puberty is considered to be delayed if onset of signs of puberty are not present by chronological age.

In boys, it is said to be delayed if onset does not occur by the age of 14 years and in girls the age is 13 years.

AMENORRHOEA

Definition

It is defined as failure of menstruation. It may be primary or secondary.

Primary Amenorrhoea

It means menstruation has never occurred or absence of menarche by the age of 16.

Causes

Gonadal dysgenesis (e.g. Turner's syndrome), endometrial hypoplasia, vaginal agenesis, etc.

Secondary Amenorrhoea

It means no menstruation for more than 3 cycles in an individual who has previously had normal menstruation. In nonpregnant women, secondary amenorrhoea results from ovarian, pituitary or hypothalamic dysfunction.

Causes

1. Physiological—pregnancy, menopause.
2. Pathological:
   - Hypogonadotrophic hypogonadism (due to disease of pituitary or hypothalamus).
   - Ovarian dysfunction—PCOS, androgen secreting tumour, premature ovarian failure.
   - Others—any systemic disease like severe anaemia, renal failure, hyperthyroidism.

Investigations

Detailed history, physical examination should be done and then investigations to be done according to suspicion of cause.

- Pregnancy should be excluded first.
- Measurement of serum LH, FSH, estradiol, testosterone, prolactin, T_4 and TSH.
- Karyotype should be performed in suspected case of Turner's syndrome.
- USG of abdomen—to see uterus, ovary, adrenal glands, etc.

Management

Treatment should be given according to aetiology.

TURNER'S SYNDROME

Definition

It is a sex chromosomal abnormality characterized by absence of one of X chromosomes (45, XO). It only affects females and all or part of one X chromosome is deleted, leading to failure of ovarian development. Externally, patient appears female, but does not produce female sex hormones. Hence, the patient remains sexually immature.

Clinical Features

Usually presents with amenorrhoea, underdeveloped secondary sexual characters. Features are:
- Short stature.
- Short, webbed neck, low hairline, redundant skinfold on the back of neck.
- Face—small lower jaw (micrognathia), small, fish-like mouth, high-arched palate, low-set deformed ears.
- Chest—broad, wide apart nipples (shield-like chest).
- Hand—short fourth metacarpal (other metacarpals may be short), lymphoedema of hands (also feet) and hypoplastic nails.
- Elbow—increased carrying angles (cubitus valgus).

Investigations

- Karyotyping from buccal smear—45 (XO) is classical, occasionally 46 (XX) mosaics.
- USG of abdomen—small uterus, fallopian tube and streak gonad.
- Hormone assay—low oestrogen, high LH and FSH.

Treatment

- Oestrogen therapy at puberty.
- Growth hormone may accelerate height but it is not yet established whether there is any effect on final height.
- Gonadal tumour may occur rarely, especially in mosaic involving 'Y' chromosome. Hence, it should be removed.

Associations or Diseases that Occur in Turner's Syndrome

- Heart—coarctation of aorta, ASD, VSD, aortic stenosis, hypertension.
- Kidney—'horse-shoe' kidney, hydronephrosis.
- Endocrine—diabetes mellitus, Hashimoto's thyroiditis, hypothyroidism.
- Lymphoedema in infancy.
- Red and green colour blindness.
- Strabismus and ptosis.
- Premature osteoporosis.
- Pigmented nevi.
- Mental retardation (rare).

Noonan's Syndrome

It is also called male Turner. It is characterized by:

- Short stature.
- Mental retardation (common).
- Downward slanting and wide spaced eyes.
- Low-set ear.
- Webbing of the neck.
- Low posterior hairline.
- Pulmonary stenosis.

It may affect both male and female equally. Female patients have Turner's phenotype but with normal 46, XX. They have normal ovarian function and normal fertility. Cardiac lesion is present more on right side, such as pulmonary stenosis. But left sided cardiac lesion is more in Turner's syndrome.

POLYCYSTIC OVARIAN SYNDROME

Definition

- Polycystic ovarian syndrome (PCOS) is syndrome in which there are multiple cysts in the ovary and hyperandrogenaemia, characterized by:
- Amenorrhoea or oligomenorrhoea.
- Obesity.
- Hirsutism.
- Infertility (due to anovulation).
- Virilisation (in severe cases).

Polycystic ovarian syndrome (previously called Stein-Leventhal syndrome) is associated with increased LH due to abnormality of pulsatile GnRH secretion. There is chronic anovulation without specific underlying disease of adrenal, pituitary or ovary.

Diagnostic Criteria of PCOS

Two of the following 3 features are required to diagnose PCOS:

- Menstrual irregularities (oligomenorrhoea or amenorrhoea).
- Clinical or biochemical evidence of androgen excess.
- Multiple cysts in the ovaries (detected by transvaginal ultrasonography).

Investigations

1. USG of abdomen to see ovaries.
2. Biochemical tests:
   - Serum testosterone (usually high).
   - LH (increased).
   - FSH (normal or low, in a ratio of LH:FSH >2 or 3).
   - Androgens—androstenedione and dehydroepiandrosterone are increased.
   - SHBG—decreased.
   - Prolactin—slightly increased, rarely greater than 1500 mU/L.
   - Oestrogen (oestradiol is usually normal).
3. To exclude other cause, investigations should be done according to suspicion:
   - Serum 17-OH progesterone—high in late onset congenital adrenal hyperplasia (CAH).
   - CT or MRI of adrenal (in suspected tumour).
   - Dexamethasone suppression test.
   - Short ACTH stimulation test with measurement of 17-hydroxyprogesterone is done to diagnose CAH.

Treatment

1. General measures:
   - Reduction of weight.
   - Regular exercise and diet control.
2. For hirsutism:
   - Local therapy—plucking, bleaching, electrolysis, depilatory cream, shaving.
   - Drugs—cyproterone acetate, spironolactone, finasteride, flutamide.

3. For fertility:
   - Metformin—may improve ovulation and achieve conception.
   - Clomiphene 50–100 mg/day, from days 2–6 of cycle. Dexamethasone 0.5 mg at bedtime with clomiphene may increase the likelihood of ovulation by suppressing ACTH.
   - If no response to clomiphene, metformin may be added, 500 mg three times daily. It may enhance ovulation.
4. For menstrual disturbance:
   - Metformin 500 mg three times daily improves menstrual cycle and ovulation. Also may improve hirsutism and obesity.
   - Cyclical low-dose oestrogen or progesterone administration.
   - Patient who does not desire pregnancy should get medroxyprogesterone 10 mg daily orally for first 10 days of each month. It ensures regular shedding of endometrium.
   - Wedge resection or laser surgery of ovary or laparoscopy ovarian drilling may be done in some cases.
   - Menstrual irregularity can be improved by oral contraceptives.
5. For obesity—metformin may be used.

Complications in PCOS

- Hyperinsulinaemia and insulin resistance.
- Glucose intolerance.
- Type 2 DM.
- Hypertension, dyslipidemia and cardiovascular risk.

MALE HYPOGONADISM

Male hypogonadism may be primary (due to disease in the testes) or secondary (due to disease in the pituitary or hypothalamus).

Causes

1. Primary or hypergonadotrophic hypogonadism:
   - Testicular damage—trauma, surgery, chemo- or radiotherapy to testes, mumps orchitis, tuberculosis, haemochromatosis, leprosy.
   - Developmental abnormality—Klinefelter's syndrome, cryptorchidism.
2. Secondary or hypogonadotrophic hypogonadism:
   - Hypopituitarism due to any cause.
   - Prolactinoma.
   - Kallmann's syndrome.

Clinical Features

1. If hypogonadism develops before puberty—presents with features of delayed puberty.
2. If it starts after puberty:
   - Loss of libido.
   - Lethargy with muscle weakness.
   - Decreased frequency of shaving.
   - Infertility and osteoporosis.

Investigations

- Serum testosterone—low.
- Serum LH and FSH—high in primary and low in secondary.
- Other investigations—according to suspicion of cause (e.g. chromosomal analysis in Klinefelter's syndrome).

Treatment

- Testosterone should be given. It does not induce fertility.
- Treatment of secondary cause, if any.

CHAPTER

8

Infectious Disease and Tropical Medicine

CHAPTER CONTENTS

- Mumps
- Measles
- Rubella (German measles)
- Dengue fever
- Herpes simplex virus (HSV)
- Herpes simplex encephalitis
- Rabies
- Enteric fever
  - Typhoid fever
  - Paratyphoid fever
- Typhus fever
- Q fever
- Bacillary dysentery (shigellosis)
- Amoebiasis (amoebic dysentery)
- Cholera
- Diphtheria
- Whooping cough
- Tetanus
- Chickenpox
- Smallpox
- Brucellosis
- Malaria
- Kala-azar (leishmaniasis)
- Post-kala-azar dermal leishmaniasis (PKDL)
- Filariasis
- Ancylostomiasis (hook-worm infestation)
- Ascariasis (roundworm infestation)
- Enterobius vermicularis (thread worm)
- Taeniasis
- Strongyloidiasis
- Giardiasis
- Anthrax
- Leprosy (hansen's disease)
- Leptospirosis (weil's disease)
- Poliomyelitis
- Sepsis
- Hydatid disease (cyst)
- Infectious mononucleosis
- Toxoplasmosis
- Food poisoning

MUMPS

Definition

It is an infection of the parotid gland by mumps virus, common in children.

Incubation Period

2–3 weeks.

Symptoms

- Fever, headache, malaise, myalgia, anorexia, sore throat.
- Ear ache on chewing and swallowing.
- Painful swelling of the parotid gland (unilateral or bilateral).
- Swelling of parotid gland, reaches its maximum on 3rd day, remains for 2 days and then subsides.

Signs

- Parotid glands are enlarged, tender. Submandibular glands may be involved.
- Skin over the parotid gland is red, shiny.

Investigations

Diagnosis is clinical. Investigations are unnecessary.

- CBC—may show leucopenia.
- Serology—IgM antibody to mumps virus indicates recent infection.
- Virus can be isolated from saliva, throat swab, urine and CSF.

Complications

- Orchitis, may be atrophy and sterility if both testes are involved.
- Pancreatitis.
- Epididymitis.
- Oophoritis (in female).
- Otitis media.
- Myocarditis.
- Aseptic meningitis.
- Encephalitis.

Treatment

- Rest and isolation in bed for 10 days.
- Maintenance of hydration, nutrition and oral hygiene.
- Paracetamol for fever or pain.
- If orchitis or oophoritis- prednisolone 40 mg daily for 4 days.

Prevention

Live attenuated MMR vaccine.

MEASLES

Definition

It is a systemic viral disease caused by measles virus (RNA virus), transmitted by infected droplet.

Incubation Period

10–14 days.

Clinical Features

- Prodromal symptoms or catarrhal phase: Fever, headache, sneezing, running nose, dry cough, redness of eyes. At this stage, the patient looks miserable and irritable. Koplik spots are present at this stage, which are small, irregular, greyish white spots surrounded by erythema on the buccal mucosa around the opening of parotid duct at the level of upper second molar teeth. They appear 2 days before the appearance of skin rash, disappear 1–2 days after the development of rash. Koplik spots are pathognomonic for measles.
- Exanthematous stage: Red maculopapular skin rash develops after 3–4 days of prodromal phase. Fever rises abruptly but subsides after eruption of rash. Initially, rashes are pin-head papules and coalesce to form red morbiliform rash, which fade after 4 days. Lymph nodes may be enlarged.

Investigations

Diagnosis is clinical. Investigations are unnecessary.

- CBC may show leucopenia.
- Serology—IgM antibody to measles virus indicates recent infection.
- Isolation of the virus from pharyngeal washing, blood or urine culture.

Complications

- Bronchitis, broncheolitis, bronchopneumonia.
- Conjunctivitis, keratitis, retrobulbar neuritis.
- Otitis media.
- Myocarditis.
- Thrombocytopenia.
- Subacute Sclerosing Panencephalitis (SSPE).

Treatment

- Bed rest and isolation until 5 days after the rash has appeared.
- Adequate fluid, nutrition, oral hygiene, care of eyes.
- Paracetamol for fever.
- Gammaglobulin 0.25 mL/kg can modify the course of disease in immunocompromised patient.

Prevention

Live attenuated measles vaccine.

RUBELLA (GERMAN MEASLES)

Definition

It is an infection caused by rubella virus (RNA virus), transmitted by infected droplet.

Incubation Period

2–3 weeks.

Symptoms

- Fever, malaise, headache, anorexia.
- Running nose, sneezing, cough.
- Arthralgia.

Signs

- Maculopapular rash appears first on the forehead, spreads to the trunk and limbs. Fades after three days. Petechial rash may appear on the soft palate.
- Lymphadenopathy—postauricular, suboccipital and posterior cervical.
- Conjunctivitis.

Complications

- Thrombocytopenia.
- Hepatitis.
- Encephalitis.
- Spontaneous abortion.
- Congenital Rubella Syndrome—if maternal rubella infection occurs in first trimester, there may be transplacental transfer of virus into the foetus causing congenital diseases, such as cataract, microcephaly, mental retardation, deafness, congenital heart defects (PDA, PS).

Investigations

Diagnosis is clinical

- CBC may show leucopenia.
- Serology—IgM antibody to rubella virus indicates recent infection.

Treatment

- Bed rest.
- Adequate fluid and nutrition.
- Paracetamol for fever and arthralgia.

Prevention

MMR vaccine.

DENGUE FEVER

Definition

It is a viral illness caused by dengue virus. Four of the virus that cause dengue are serotypes, Den-1, Den-2, Den-3 and Den-4. It is transmitted by bite of *Ades aegyptei* mosquito.

Manifestations of Dengue Viral Infection

1. Asymptomatic.
2. Symptomatic—
   - Undifferentiated fever.
   - Dengue fever with or without haemorrhage.
   - Dengue hemorrhagic fever.
   - Dengue shock syndrome.

Dengue Fever with or without Haemorrhage

It is an acute febrile illness due to dengue virus. The features are as follows:

- Fever-high, continuous, persists for 2–7 days. After somedays, fever may subside, may reappear after 2–3 days called biphasis or saddleback fever.
- When the fever subsides, platelet may fall, bleeding maneifestations and shock may occur. This is called the 'critical period'.
- Severe headache, retro-orbital pain, nausea, vomiting.
- Acute abdominal pain, may be confused with appendicitis, pancreatitis, etc.
- Severe bodyache, myalgia, arthralgia. So, it is called breakbone fever.
- After 5 days fever may subside, then develops of haemorrhagic skin rash like petechiae, ecchymosis, purpura.
- Hemorrhagic manifestations—epistaxis, gum bleeding, haematemesis, melaena, menorrhagia in female.

Dengue Haemorrhagic Fever

When associated with bleeding manifestations, such as—

- Positive tourniquet test.
- Petechiae or ecchymosis or purpura.
- Epistaxis, gum bleeding.
- Bleeding from injection site.
- Haematemesis, melena, haematuria.
- In female—menorrhagia or early onset of menstrual bleeding with fever.

Investigations

- CBC with platelet and PCV shows leucopenia, thrombocytopenia occurs after 5th day, raised PCV.
- Antidengue antibody (IgG and IgM).
- Other tests—chest X-ray (may be right-sided pleural effusion), USG of abdomen (shows ascites), serum protein (hypoproteinemia).
- Liver function tests—SGOT, SGPT (usually high).

Dengue Shock Syndrome

It is a presentation of dengue fever characterised by circulatory failure with one or more of the following features:

- Hypotension for age.
- Cold clammy skin, restlessness, rapid weak pulse.
- Narrow pulse pressure (20 mm of Hg).
- Profound shock.

Treatment

- Rest.
- For fever—antipyretic (paracetamol), tapid sponging.
- Aspirin should be avoided specially in children, may cause Reye's syndrome. Other NSAID's should be avoided.
- Maintenece of fluid and electrolyte balance through oral rehydration therapy, plenty of fluid, fruit juice, etc.
- If the patient take by mouth—IV infusion (normal saline, Ringer's lactate, etc).
- Antibiotic is not necessary. However, secondary infection may occur specially in children. In such case, antibiotic should be given accordingly.

HERPES SIMPLEX VIRUS (HSV)

Types

Herpes simplex virus is charactised into type 1 and type 2. It is a DNA virus.

Infection may be primary or recurrent. Primary infection is followed by episodes of reactivation throughout life.

Clinical Features

- Primary HSV-1 causes recurrent mucocutaneous infection commonly involving the mucocutaneous surfaces of the head and neck. Causes gingivostomatitis, pharyngitis, herpes labialis (cold sore), keratocunjunctivitis, finger infection (herpetic whitlow), encephalitis. Also stomatitis, genital infection. The primary attack may be associated with fever and regional lymphadenopathy.
- HSV-2 usually causes genital infection, more likely to be symptomatic later in life or painful genital tract lesions.

Recurrence

Occurs most often in association with concomitant medical illness, menstruation, mechanical trauma, immunosuppression, psychological stress. Prodromal hyperaesthesia is followed by vesicle, pastule, painful ulcer and crusting. Recurrent HSV genital disease is a common cause of recurrent painful ulceration.

Complications

- Disseminated cutaneous lesions, such as eczema (eczema herpeticum).
- Herpetic keratitis, dendritic ulcers, corneal scarring and permanent visual impairment.
- Primary HSV-2 can cause meningitis, transverse myelitis.
- Encephalitis usually with HSV-1.
- A haemorrhagic necrotising temporal lobe cerebritis produces temporal lobe epilepsy and altered consciousness.
- Bell's palsy with a lower motor neuron VII nerve palsy.
- Neonatal HSV disease is associated with primary infection during delivery.
- Oesophagitis, hepatitis, pneumonitis, encephalitis or retinitis in immunocompromised person.

Investigations

Diagnosis is usually clinical.

- Anti-HSV antibody 1 and 2.
- Isolation of virus from vesicular fluid by direct immunofluorescence or PCR.
- HSV encephalitis—PCR for HSV in CSF, MRI or CT scan, electroencephalogram (EEG).

Treatment

- Aciclovir is the treatment of choice.
- Oral lesions in an immunocompetent individual may be treated with topical aciclovir.
- Suspicion of HSV encephalopathy is an indication for immediate empirical antiviral therapy.
- Aciclovir resistance is encountered occasionally in immunocompromised hosts, in which case foscarnet is the treatment of choice.

HERPES SIMPLEX ENCEPHALITIS

Herpes simplex type 1 may cause encephalitis, type 2 may cause benign recurrent lymphocytic meningitis. The virus usually affects the inferior aspect of frontal lobes and medial aspect of temporal lobe.

Clinical Features

Herpes simplex encephalitis is characterised by the following:

- Flu-like illness, followed by fever, severe headache, altered consciousness, behaviour abnormality and speech disturbance.
- There may be focal neurological deficit, such as dysphasia, hemiparesis, focal or generalised seizure, commonly temporal lobe seizure.
- Olfactory and gustatory hallucinations and impairment of memory are recognised.
- There may be multiple cranial nerve palsy and ataxia. Untreated patient develop convulsion and laps into comatose state. Mortality is high.

Investigations

- Serum anti-HSV antibody.
- Lumbar puncture and CSF study shows lymphocytic leukocytosis, normal protein and sugar. HSV-DNA, PCR is highly sensitive for rapid diagnosis.
- EEG shows distinctive periodic pattern in some cases.
- CT scan shows low density lesion in temporal lobes, that enhance with contrast. MRI shows orbitofrontal and medial temporal lobe involvement (not found in other virus).

Treatment

- Acyclovir 10 mg/kg 8 hourly IV for 10 days.
- Anticonvulsant may be necessary.
- Dexamethasone for raised intracranial pressure.

RABIES

Definition

Rabies is caused by a rhabdovirus which infects the central nervous system and salivary glands of mammals.

Man is usually infected by saliva through bites of infected dog. Also by licks on abrasions or on intact mucous membranes.

Other mammals infected by rabies are—bat, fox, cat.

Incubation Period

Varies in humans from 9 days to many months, usually 4 to 8 weeks. Depends on site. Severe bites, especially if on the head or neck, are associated with shorter incubation period.

Clinical Features

- Initially, fever and paraesthesia at the site of the bite.
- After 1–10 days, the patient becomes anxious, develops 'hydrophobia', the patient is thirsty but attempts at drinking provoke violent contractions of muscles of diglutition, diaphragm and other inspiratory muscles. Even site or sound of water may cause spasm.
- Delusions and hallucinations may develop, Cranial nerve lesions develop and terminal hyperpyrexia.
- Spitting, biting and mania. Secretion of large amount of thick saliva is common.
- There is lucid intervals in which the patient is more anxious.
- Death ensues, usually within a week of the onset of symptoms.

Investigations

Diagnosis is usually clinical.

- Rapid immunofluorescent techniques can detect antigen in corneal impression smears or skin biopsies.
- Infected animal is killed and brain is examined to see Negri bodies.
- Isolation of virus by saliva or CSF.

Treatment

Postexposure prophylaxis—

- Wound should be thoroughly cleaned with running tap water, and soap. Damaged tissues should be excised, no suturing of the wound.
- Rabies can be prevented, if treatment is started within a day or two of biting.
- Hyperimmune serum and vaccine should be given—human rabies immunoglobulin 20 U/kg body weight, half is infiltrated around the bite and half is given intramuscularly at a different site.
- Hyperimmune animal serum may be used but hypersensitivity reactions, including anaphylaxis are common.
- Human diploid cell strain vaccine—1.0 mL I/M on days 0, 3, 7, 14, 30 and 90.
- Where human products are not available and when the risk of rabies is slight (licks on the skin, or minor bites of covered arms or legs), treatment may be delayed. Biting animal is observed or await examination of its brain, rather than using the older vaccine.

- Biting animal is observed for at least 10 days. If the animal dies within 10 days, then brain is examined for 'Negri bodies'. If it is normal after 10 days, probably there is no rabies.

Established Disease

- Should be treated in ICU. Only palliative treatment is given once symptoms have appeared.
- Sedation with diazepam, supplemented by chlorpromazine if needed.
- Maintenance of fluid balance and nutrition.

Pre-exposure Prophylaxis

This is given to individuals with a high risk of contracting rabies, such as laboratory workers, animal handlers and veterinarians. Three doses (1.0 mL) of human diploid (HDCV) or chick embryo cell vaccine given by deep subcutaneous or intramuscular injection on days 0, 7 and 28. Booster dose is given after 1-year and every 3–5 years depending on the risk of exposure.

ENTERIC FEVER (TYPHOID AND PARATYPHOID)

Definition

Typhoid: It is an enteric infection caused by gram negative bacteria Salmonella typhi and paratyphi A, B, C. It is transmitted by faeco-oral route through contamination of food, milk or water.

Clinical Features

First week

- Fever, more in the evening, called step-ladder pattern.
- Headache, malaise, lassitude, weakness, body ache.
- Constipation.
- Cough, epistaxis.

Second week

- Fever is continuous.
- At the end of first week, rash may appear on the upper abdomen and back as sparse, slightly-raised, pink called rose spots, fade on pressure. It persists for 2–3 days, then disappear.
- Diarrhoea (pea soup stool).
- Hepatosplenomegaly.

At the end of second weak, patient becomes very weak. There may be muttering delirium, coma vigil, with picking at bed clothes or imaginary object which is called 'typhoid state'.

Third to fourth weak: If not treated properly, there may be—

- Melaena.
- Perforation (at the terminal ileum).

Signs

- Coated tongue.
- Relative bradycardia (pulse rate is not proportionally raised with the rise of temperature).
- Spleen is enlarged (after 7–10 days), hepatomegaly.
- Caecal gurgling.

Complications

- Bowel perforation.
- Haemorrhage.
- Others - Meningitis, pericarditis, myocarditis, endocarditis, bronchitis, cholecystitis , glomerulonephritis.

Investigations

- CBC—may be leucopenia.
- Blood culture.
- Widal test, usually after 1st week.
- Stool and urine culture in third week.

Treatment

General measures should be taken:
- Rest, hydration, adequate nutrition.
- For fever—paracetamol, tepid sponging.
- Correction of fluid and electrolytes imbalance.

Specific Treatment
- Ciprofloxacin (500 mg 12 hourly) or Ofloxacin (400 mg 12 hourly) or Pefloxacin (400 mg 12 hourly) or Cefixime (400 mg 12 hourly) or Azithromycin (500 mg 12 hourly) for 2 weeks.
- Ceftriaxone (75 mg/kg/day) is an alternative.
- Azithromycin 500 mg b.d for 7–10 days.
- In pregnancy-Ceftriaxone or Amoxicillin 750 mg–1000 mg 6 hourly.
- In severely ill patient, dexamethasone (3 mg/kg for initial doses, followed by 1 mg/kg every 6 hours for 48 hours).
- Surgical intervention is required in case of intestinal perforation.

Carrier State

After clinical recovery, 5–10% patients will continue to excrete *S. typhi* through stool for several months. This is called 'convalescent carrier'. 1–4% patients will carry the organism for years, which is called 'chronic carrier'. Chronic carrier state is common in people of age > 50 years, more in females. Usual site is gallbladder and may be associated with gallstones. Chronic carrier cases should be treated with Ciprofloxacin 750 mg 12 hourly for 4 weeks or Norfloxacin 400 mg 12 hourly for 4 weeks. Cholecystectomy may be needed.

Paratyphoid Fever

The course is shorter and milder than that of typhoid fever and the onset is more abrupt with acute enteritis. The rash may be more abundant and the intestinal complications less frequent.

Treatment

Same as in typhoid fever.

Prevention of Enteric Fever

Good sanitation and living conditions reduce the incidence of typhoid. Prevention of faecal contamination of food and milk. Hand wash is important. Travellers to the countries where enteric infections are endemic, should take typhoid vaccines.

TYPHUS FEVER

Scrub Typhus Fever

It is caused by *Orientia tsutsugamushi* (Rickettsia tsutsugamushi), transmitted by infected mites.

Clinical Features

Incubation period is 10–12 days.

- Mild or subclinical cases are common.
- Initial lesion is eschar, surrounded by an area of cellulitis and enlargement of regional lymph nodes.
- Onset is sudden, with headache, usually retro-orbital, fever, malaise, weakness and cough.
- There is high fever, remittent type with sweating, falls on the 12th to18th day.
- In severe illness, the general symptoms increase, withapathy and prostration.
- Erythematous maculopapular rash appears on about the 5th to7th day and spreads to the trunk, face and limbs, including the palms and soles. The rash fades by the 14th day.
- There is generalised painless lymphadenopathy.
- In severe infection, there is prostration, cough, pneumonia, confusion and deafness.
- Cardiac failure, renal failure and haemorrhage may develop.
- Convalescence is often slow and tachycardia may persist for some weeks.

Epidemic (Louse-borne) Typhus

It is caused by *R. prowazekii*, transmitted by infected faeces of human body louse, usually through scratching the skin.

Clinical Features

Incubation period is usually 12–14 days.

- Onset is sudden with fever, rigors, frontal headaches, pains in the back and limbs, constipation and bronchitis.
- The face is flushed and cyanotic, the eyes are congested and the patient becomes confused.
- The rash appears on the 4th to 6th day. In its early stages, it disappears on pressure but soon becomes petechial with subcutaneous mottling. It appears first on the anterior folds of the axillae, sides of the abdomen or backs of hands, then on the trunk and forearms. The neck and face are seldom affected.
- During the second week, symptoms increase in severity.
- Sores develop on the lips. The tongue becomes dry, brown, shrunken and tremulous.
- The spleen is palpable, the pulse feeble and the patient stuporous and delirious.
- The temperature falls rapidly at the end of the second week and the patient recovers gradually. In fatal cases, the patient usually dies in the second week from toxaemia, cardiac or renal failure, or pneumonia.

Endemic (Flea-borne) Typhus

Flea-borne or 'endemic' typhus caused by *R. typhi* is endemic worldwide. Humans are infected when the faeces or contents of a crushed flea, which has fed on an infected rat, are introduced into the skin. The incubation period is 8–14 days. The symptoms resemble those of mild louse-borne typhus. The rash may be scanty and transient.

Investigation of Rickettsial Infection

- Routine blood investigations are not diagnostic but malaria must be excluded by blood film examination in most cases, and there is usually hepatitis and thrombocytopenia.
- Diagnosis is made on clinical grounds and response to treatment.
- May be confirmed by antibody detection or PCR in specialised laboratories. Differential diagnoses include malaria, typhoid, meningococcal sepsis and leptospirosis.

Management of Rickettsial Fevers

The different rickettsial fevers vary greatly in severity but all respond to:

- Tetracycline 500 mg 4 times daily, doxycycline 200 mg daily or chloramphenicol 500 mg 4 times daily for 7 days.
- Louse-borne typhus and scrub typhus can be treated with a single dose of 200 mg doxycycline, repeated for 2–3 days to prevent relapse.
- Chloramphenicol and doxycycline-resistant strains of *O. tsutsugamushi* have been reported from Thailand and patients here may need treatment with rifampicin.
- Nursing care is important, especially in epidemic typhus.
- Sedation may be required for delirium and blood transfusion for haemorrhage.
- Relapsing fever and typhoid are common intercurrent infections in epidemic typhus, and pneumonia in scrub typhus. They must be sought and treated.
- Convalescence is usually protracted, especially in older people. To prevent rickettsial infection, lice, fleas, ticks and mites need to be controlled with insecticides.

Q FEVER

Q fever is caused by the rickettsia like organism *Coxiella burnetii*, an obligate intracellular organism that can survive in the extracellular environment. Cattle, sheep and goats are important reservoirs and the organism is transmitted by inhalation of aerosolised particles. An important characteristic of *C. burnetii* is its antigenic variation, called phase variation, due to a change of lipopolysaccharide (LPS). When isolated from animals or humans, *C. burnetii* expresses phase I antigen and is very infectious (a single bacterium is sufficient to infect a human). In culture, there is an antigenic shift to the phase II form, which is not infectious. This antigenic shift can be measured and is valuable for the differentiation of acute and chronic Q fever.

Clinical Features

The incubation period is 3–4 weeks.

- The initial symptoms are nonspecific with fever, headache and chills.
- In 20% of cases, a maculopapular rash occurs.
- Others—pneumonia and hepatitis.
- Chronic Q fever may present with osteomyelitis, encephalitis and endocarditis.

Investigations

Diagnosis is usually serological and the stage of the infection can be distinguished by isotype tests and phase-specific antigens. Phase I and II IgM titres peak at 4–6 weeks. In chronic infections, IgG titres to phase I and II antigens may be raised.

Treatment

Prompt treatment of acute Q fever with doxycycline reduces fever duration. Treatment of Q fever endocarditisis problematic, requiring prolonged therapy with doxycycline and rifampicin or ciprofloxacin with hydroxychloroquine; even then, organisms are not always eradicated. Valve surgery is often required.

BACILLARY DYSENTERY (SHIGELLOSIS)

Definition

It is an enteric infection caused by Gram negative rod *Shigella* that invade the colonic mucosa. It is transmitted by faeco-oral route through contamination of food, milk or water.

Incubation Period

1–7 days.

Organisms

There are four groups:

- Shigellae dysenteriae.
- Shigellae flexneri (common in tropical country).
- Shigellae boydii.
- Shigellae sonnei.

Symptoms

Features develop due to release of endotoxin:

- Diarrhoea mixed with fresh blood and mucous.
- Colicky abdominal pain and tenesmus.
- Nausea, vomiting.
- Fever, malaise, and weakness.
- Increased thirst, dryness of mouth.
- Generalised bodyache.

Signs

- Patient may be toxic.
- Tenderness over left iliac fossa.
- Signs of dehydration- dry tongue, shunken eyes, hypotension.

Complications

- Meningism.
- Arthritis.
- Iritis.
- Haemolytic uraemic syndrome (HUS).
- Reiter's syndrome.

Investigations

- Stool for R/M/E and C/S.
- CBC.
- Serum electrolytes.
- Serum creatinine.

Treatment

General measures:
- Correction of dehydration—Oral rehydration therapy (ORS) or, if diarrhoea is severe, IV fluid.
- Maintenance of nutrition.

Specific Treatment
- Ciprofloxacin 500 mg 12 hourly or Norfloxacin 500 mg 12 hourly or Azithromycin 500 mg 12 hourly for 5–7 days.

Prevention

Faecal contamination of food, milk or drink should be avoided. Frequent hand washing is important.

AMOEBIASIS (AMOEBIC DYSENTERY)

Definition

It is an enteric infection caused by protozoa *Entamoeba histolytica* that invade the intestinal mucosa. It is transmitted by faecal-oral route (ingestion of *E. histolytica* cysts) through contamination of uncooked food, milk or water.

Incubation Period

Up to 2 weeks.

Symptoms

- Diarrhoea mixed with mucous and occasionally blood.
- Colicky abdominal pain.
- Nausea, vomiting.
- Fever, malaise, and weakness.

Signs

- Abdominal tenderness mostly in the right lower quadrant.

Investigations

- Stool for R/M/E may reveal motile trophozoites with red blood cells.
- CBC shows leukocytosis and raised ESR.
- USG (if amoebic liver abscess is suspected).
- CXR (raised right dome of diaphragm in liver abscess).
- Serum electrolytes.
- Serum creatinine.
- Sigmoidoscopy reveal typical flask-shaped ulcers in the intestinal wall.
- Serological tests may detect antiamoeba antibody.

Treatment

General Measures

- Correction of dehydration.
- Maintenance of nutrition.

Specific Treatment

- Oral metronidazole 400 mg 8 hourly for 5–7 days or tinidazole 1gm 12 hourly daily for 3–5 days or secnidazole 1 gm 12 hourly daily for 3–5 days or nitazoxanide 500 mg 12 hourly for 3 days.
- Diloxanide furoate 500 mg orally 8 hourly for 10 days after the above treatment to eliminate luminal cysts.

Complications

- Amoebic hepatitis.
- Amoebic liver abscess.
- Chronic amoebiasis. It may cause granulomatous lesion with in the colonic wall called 'Amoeboma' (seen as a mass in right iliac fossa).

Prevention

Avoid eating uncooked vegetables or drinking unboiled water.

CHOLERA

Definition

It is an acute diarrhoeal illness caused by colonisation of the small intestine by *Vibrio cholerae.* Another serotype *El tor* is also responsible. New serotype 0139 in Bangladesh is becoming a pandemic.

The disease is transmitted by the faeco-oral route by contaminated water, food, shellfish.

Incubation Period

From few hours to 5 days.

Clinical Features

The bacteria produces a specific enterotoxin, responsible for the clinical manifestations. The toxin activate adenylate cyclase in the intestinal epithelium, inducing secretion of chloride and water.

- Profuse painless watery diarrhea known as 'rice water stool,' vomiting.
- Fatigue, muscle cramps.
- Signs of severe dehydration including pinched face, sunken eyes, poor skin turgor, dry tongue, tachycardia, thready pulse and hypotension, shock.
- Oliguria.
- Death from acute circulatory failure, if not properly treated.

Complications

- Hypovolaemic shock.
- Electrolyte imbalance.
- Acute tubular necrosis.
- Renal failure.

Investigations

Diagnosis is clinical

- Serum electrolytes and creatinine.
- Stool RME shows the typical shooting star motility of *V. cholerae.*
- Stool C/S or rectal swab for *V. cholerae.*

Treatment

- Rest.
- Oral or I/V replacement of water and electrolytes (ORS or Cholera Saline). Ringer's lactate may be given.
- Oral broad spectrum antibiotics. Tetracycline 250 mg 6 hourly for 3 days. Or doxycycline 300 mg single dose or ciprofloxacin 1gm single dose.
- Zinc supplement.

DIPHTHERIA

Definition

It is an acute infection in the upper respirary tract caused by *Corynebacterium diphtheriae.* It usually spreads by droplet infection from infected cases or carriers.

Incubation Period

2–4 days.

Sites

- Tonsillar.
- Pharyngeal.
- Nasal.
- Others—Skin, genitalia.

Symptoms

Organism is localised at the site of infection but the features are due to absorption of exotoxin, which typically damage heart muscle and nervous system.

- Sore throat.
- Fever, malaise, lethargy.
- Running nose which may be blood-stained, sneezing (if nasal involvement).
- Croupy voice.
- In laryngeal diphtheria—husky voice high pitched brassy cough, even respiratory obstruction requiring tracheostomy.
- Dysphagia.
- Excessive salivation.
- Neck swelling (bull neck).

Signs

- Patient may be very toxic.
- Tachypnoea.
- Wash lather, elevated, greyish green membrane on the tonsils and pharynx, which is thick, glistening, firmly adherent with well-defined erythematous edge. It is called 'pseudomembrane'.
- In severe case, there may be cervical tender lymphadenopathy and marked oedema of the submandibular space giving rise to 'bull neck appearance'. It is also called 'malignant diphtheria'.

Complications

Effects due to diphtheria exotoxin:

- Myocarditis—in first or second week, causing arrhythmia and cardiac failure. Death may occur due to acute circulatory failure within the first 10 days. Most complications recover with no permanent damage.
- Neurological involvement—paralysis of soft palate and posterior pharyngeal wall causing bulbar and pseudobulbar palsy (nasal voice, nasal regurgitation), peripheral neuropathy,

paralysis of accommodation which is manifested by difficulty in reading small print. Also cranial nerve palsy, rarely encephalitis.

Effects due to Pseudomembrane

- Laryngeal obstruction or paralysis.

Investigations

Diagnosis is clinical, therapy should be started if suspicion.

- CBC may show leucocytosis.
- Throat swab smear for Albert's stain.
- Throat swab culture in Loeffler's serum.

Treatment

- Rest and isolation of patient.
- Maintenance of adequate hydration and nutrition.
- Diphtheria antitoxin, should be given immediately (it has no role once the toxin is fixed to the tissue). It neutralizes the circulatory toxin.
- I/V Benzyl Penicillin, 1200 mg 6 hourly daily or Amoxicillin 500 mg 8 hourly daily for 2 weeks. If the patient allergic to penicillin, erythromycin can be given.
- In case of myocarditis or severe neck swelling—corticosteroid.
- In case of laryngeal obstruction emergency tracheostomy.

Prevention

Active immunisation should be given to all children. If diphtheria occurs in a closed community, contacts should be given erythromycin. All contacts should also be immunised or given a booster dose of toxoid.

WHOOPING COUGH

Definition

It is an infectious disease caused by Bordetella pertussis, which is a gram negative coccobacillus. Transmission is through contaminated droplets.

Incubation Period

7–16 days.

Clinical Features

There are three stages:

1. Catarrhal stage: Infectivity is greatest during this stage.
   - Cough, running nose, congested eyes, lacrimation, fever, malaise.
2. Paroxysmal stage:
   - Paroxysm of cough, ending with a high-pitched deep inspiratory "whoop". Vomiting, cyanosis may occur, 'Whoop' may not always be present in infants. Episodes of chocking and apnoea may occur. There may be engorged conjunctiva, periorbital oedema and petechial haemorrhage.
3. Convalescent stage:
   - Patient's symptoms improve, cough becomes less.

Complications

- Convulsion, subconjunctival haemorrhage.
- Pneumonia, bronchopneumonia, bronchiectasis.
- Rectal prolapse.

Investigations

- CBC-lymphocytosis
- Culture of nasopharyngeal swab or sputum in Bordet–Gangou media.
- X-ray chest may show enlarged mediastinal nodes and patchy atelectasis.
- PCR, Direct fluorescent antibody test may be done.

Treatment

- Erythromycin 50 mg/kg/d in 6 hourly for 14 days, or clarithromycin 10 mg/kg/d 12 hourly for 7 days, or azithromycin 10 mg/kg/d once daily for 5 days.
- A short course of steroid may shorten the clinical course.
- Antispasmotics, antitussives, sedatives are of no proven value.
- Close contacts should be treated with erythromycin for 14 days. Children should be isolated for 5 days after initiation of erythromycin therapy.

Prevention

Prevention includes active immunisation with triple vaccine (DPT).

TETANUS

Definition

It is an infection caused by *Clostridium tetani,* an anaerobic gram positive bacilli. This bacteria produces exotoxin 'tetanospasmin', responsible for the clinical manifestations. The toxin involves the anterior horn cells and causes rigidity and convulsion.

Mode of Transmission

Organism is found in soil and the disease is due to contamination of cuts, wounds or umbilical stump.

Incubation Period

7–8 days.

Clinical Features

- Fever, malaise, irritability.
- Lockjaw or Trismus—due to spasms and stiffness of masseter muscles. It is painless.
- Risus sardonicus—due to sustained contraction of facial muscles (occipito-frontalis).
- Opisthotonos—due to contraction of neck muscles along with contraction of back muscles produces an arched back.
- Difficulty swallowing due to oesophageal spasm.
- Abdominal rigidity, may be board-like.
- In severe case, there may be generalised muscular spasm.
- Spasms may be spontaneous lasting for several minutes, triggered by loud noise, light, or handling the patient. Patient remains conscious and experiences severe pain during the spasm.
- Autonomic dysfunction—hypertension or hypotension, tachycardia or bradycardia, hyperpyrexia, profuse sweating, peripheral vasoconstriction.
- Retention of urine due to urethral spasm.

Complications

- Spine or bone fracture due to spasm.
- Laryngeal spasm causing obstruction of upper airway and apnoea.

Treatment

- Patient should be admitted in an isolated, quiet, well-ventilated dark room or ICU.
- Wound debridement.
- Adequate ventilation, hydration and nutrition.
- Diazepam 5 mg I/V or I/V infusion. Alternative drugs are midazolam and propofol infusion. Sometimes, Inj. magnesium sulphate may also be beneficial.
- Injection benzyl penicillin or cephalosporine or erythromycin or clindamycin for 10 days. I/V Metronidazole is also effective.
- Human tetanus immunoglobuline—Inj. TIG 500 IU I/M.
- Inj. tetanus toxoid I/M at a different site.
- If airway is obstructed, intubation and mechanical ventilation may be necessary.
- Treatment of secondary infection.

Prevention

By active immunisation with triple vaccine (DPT vaccine).

Neonatal Tetanus

It occurs due to infection of umbilical stump with clostridium tetani.

Features

- Failure to thrive.
- Poor sucking.
- Irritability.
- Grimacing, rigidity and spasm.

Investigations

Diagnosis is clinical.

CHICKENPOX

Definition

It is an infectious disease caused by varicella zoster virus and transmission is through contaminated respiratory droplets.

Incubation Period

10–21 days.

Clinical Features

- Fever, malaise, generalised bodyache, headache.
- Loss of appetite, nausea, vomiting.
- Oral sores.
- Rash—itchy rash develops in crops at first on back then chest, abdomen, face, and limbs. Distribution is centripetal, more on upper arms and thighs, upper part of face. Initially macule, then become pink papule, then multiple vesicles develop. Vesicle turns into pustules in 24 hours. Scabs in 2–5 days.

Investigations

Diagnosis is clinical. Investigation is rarely necessary.

Treatment

- Rest and isolation of patient.
- Maintenance of adequate hydration and nutrition.
- Oral therapy with aciclovir (20 mg/kg/dose, maximum 800 mg/dose) given as 4 doses/day for 5 days.
- Antihistamin for itching, also calamine lotion.
- For severe cases or immunocompromised patient, I/V aciclovir 250 mg/m^2 8 hourly over 1 hour for 10 days.

Complications

- Pneumonia.
- Postvaricella encephalitis.
- Secondary skin infections
- Herpes zoster or shingles due to reactivation of dormant varicella virus.

Prevention

Active immunisation with varicella vaccine and passive immunisation with varicella immunoglobulin.

SMALLPOX

It was an infectious disease caused by Smallpox virus. The virus had two variants, Variola major and Variola minor. Clinical features include high fever and development of characteristic rash. The disease is now eradicated.

BRUCELLOSIS

Definition

It is a zoonotic infectious disease caused by Brucella, a gram-negative bacillus, contacted from cows, goats, pigs or sheep. Person to person transmission is rare.

Brucellosis is caused by 3 species-

- *B. abortus* (cattle).
- *B. melitensis* (goat or sheep).
- *B. suis* (pigs).

Infection occurs usually through gastrointestinal tract, due to consuming unpasteurised milk. From gastrointestinal tract, bacilli travel to the lymphatics and infect lymph nodes, and eventually there is haematogenous spread to other organs.

Incubation Period

2–4 weeks.

Symptoms

- Onset is insidious. Malaise, headache, myalgia, arthralgia, weakness and night sweats are common. There is an undulant high fever.
- Back pain.
- Lymphadenopathy is common. Hepatosplenomegaly may be present, splenomegaly usually indicates severe infection. Tenderness is relatively common.
- There may be arthritis, orchitis, endocarditis, osteomyelitis and meningoencephalitis.
- Brucellosis may be chronic, associated with fatigue, myalgia, depression, occasionally fever. Splenomegaly is characteristic. Infection may be localised to specific organs, such as the bone, heart or central nervous system. In such cases, systemic features are absent in 60% cases and antibody titers are low.

Investigations

- CBC may reveal pancytopenia.
- Blood culture.
- Serological tests—Brucella agglutination test is positive within 4 weeks of the onset of illness.
- Serum IgG—it may be raised.
- Species specific PCR test.

Treatment

1. Nonlocalised disease—Doxycycline 100 mg orally twice daily for 6 weeks plus gentamicin 5 mg/kg for 7 days or Doxycycline 100 mg orally twice daily plus rifampin 600–900 mg orally once daily for 6 weeks.
2. Localised disease
   - Bone disease—Doxycycline 100 mg orally twice daily plus rifampin 600–900 mg orally once daily for 6 weeks plus gentamicin 5 mg/kg for 7 days. Or Ciprofloxacin 750 mg twice daily plus rifampin 600–900 mg orally once daily for 3 months.

- Neurobrucellosis—Doxycycline 100 mg orally twice daily plus rifampin 600–900 mg orally once daily for 6 weeks plus Injection ceftriaxone 2 g twice daily until CSF is clear.
- Endocarditis—Doxycycline 100 mg orally twice daily plus rifampin 600–900 mg orally once daily for six weeks plus trimethoprim 5 mg/kg for 6 month plus gentamicin 5 mg/kg IV for 2–4 weeks.

Complications

- Uveitis.
- Retinal thrombophlebitis.
- Cranial nerve palsies.
- Pneumonia or abscess.
- Pravertebral or psoas abscess.
- Osteomyelitis.
- Meningitis.
- Stroke, intracranial or subarachnoid haemorrhage.
- Myocarditis, endocarditis
- Splenic abscess.

Prevention

- Careful handling of infected animals.
- Vaccination of animals.
- Pasteurisation of milk.

MALARIA

Definition

It is a protozoal disease caused by plasmodium species.

Organisms: Four species of plasmodium are—

- *P. vivax*
- *P. falciparum*
- *P. malariae*
- *P. ovale*

Mode of Transmission

- Bite by infected female anopheles mosquito.
- Blood transfusion (rare).

Symptoms

In *P. vivax and ovale* (benign tertian malaria)—

1. Typical paroxysm of fever has three stages—
   - Cold stage—patient feels severe chill and rigor, whole body shivers vigorously, teeth chatter. The patient needs warm bed cloths or blanket. This stage last for 20–30 minutes.
   - Hot stage—temperature is very high, with headache, flushing, tachycardia. Patient feels very hot, throws blanket. It last for 1–4 hours.
   - Wet or sweating stage—there is profuse sweating, temperature falls, patient feels comfortable. This stage last for 2–4 hours.

   In benign tertian malaria, classical fever is repeated on alternate day in vivax (tertian). In *P. malariae,* fever is mild, occurs in 2 days interval (quartan fever).
2. Other features—headache, fatigue, weakness, nausea and vomiting.

   Falciparum malaria (malignant tertian malaria)—Incubation period 5–10 days. Infected RBC develop knob like surface projection, which causes adhesion of RBC to the endothelium of blood vessel resulting in vascular occlusion. As a result, there is severe organ damage.
   - Fever. No particular pattern, may be continuous, typhoid like, sometimes prolonged and irregular. No typical three stages.
   - Headache, malaise, vomiting, cough, diarrhoea.
   - In cerebral type—headache, confusion, seizure even coma.
   - Other features—hypoglycaemia, pulmonary oedema, renal failure, severe anaemia, DIC, GIT features like diarrhoea, bleeding, jaundice.

Signs

Appears after some days.

- Anaemia.
- Jaundice.
- Hepatomegaly.
- Splenomegaly.

Complications of Falciparum Malaria

- CNS—cerebral malaria.
- Haematological—severe haemolytic anaemia, DIC.
- Renal—oliguria, acute renal failure, immune complex glomerulonephritis.
- Respiratory—pulmonary oedema.
- GIT—diarrhoea, jaundice.
- Metabolic—hypoglycaemia, metabolic acidosis.
- Others—shock.

Causes of Anaemia in Malaria

- Haemolysis of infected and uninfected red cells.
- Dyserythropoiesis.
- Splenomegaly (causing sequestration and haemodilution).
- Reduction of folate store.

Benign Malaria and Malignant Malaria

- Benign malaria—it is mainly due to *P. vivax,* less frequently by P. ovale and malariae. Less serious.
- Malignant malaria—it is due to *P. falciparum* associated with widespread organ damage due to capillary blockage. It is more serious.

Investigations of Malaria

- CBC.
- Peripheral blood film for malarial parasite (both thick and thin).
- Serology (for *P. falciparum* antigen, ICT).

Thick and thin Film

- In thick film, erythrocytes are lysed releasing all blood stages of parasite, helpful to detect the parasite, even with low level of parasitaemia.
- Thin film is necessary to detect the species and also to quantify the parasite load in Plasmodium falciparum.

Treatment

For *P. vivax, P. ovale and P. malariae*

- Chloroquine: 1st day 600 mg (4 tablets), then 300 mg (2 tablets) after 6 hours. From next day, 150 mg (1 tablet) BD for 2 days.
- For radical cure—primaquine from 4th day, 15 mg daily for 14 days.

For *P. falciparum*

1. Mild or uncomplicated case:
   - In many cases, there is chloroquine resistance. Coartemether (artemether plus lumefantrine)— 4 tablets stat, then 4 tablets after 8 hours, then 4 tablets 12 hourly for 2 days. Total 24 tablets to be given in 60 hours.

   - Or single dose of sulfadoxine 1.5 g plus pyrimethamine 75 mg (Fansidar 3 tablets).
   - Or quinine 600 mg (10 mg/kg) 8 hourly for 5–7 days orally. After quinine therapy, doxycycline 200 mg daily for 7 days or clindamycin 450mg 8 hourly for 7 days. Or Malarone (proguanil plus atovaquone)—4 tablets once daily for 3 days.
2. Complicated or severe falciparum infection or cerebral malaria:
   - Quinine IV, initially 20 mg/kg (maximum 1.4 g), with 5% DA 500 cc for 4 hours, then 10 mg/kg 8 hourly (maximum 700 mg) for 7 days, until patient can take orally.
   - Injection artemether is a suitable alternative. Dose is 80 mg IM twice daily for 1 day, then 80 mg daily for 4 days or 80 mg IM twice daily for 3 days (should be avoided during pregnancy, unless strongly indicated).
   - Other treatment—If coma persists, lumbar puncture and CSF study to exclude other diseases, such as meningitis or encephalitis. Water and electrolyte balance, renal failure, hepatic failure, if present. Quinine may cause hypoglycaemia.

Radical Cure

It is the eradication of hypnozoite form of malarial parasite from the liver. *P. vivax* and *P. ovale* persist in liver cell as dormant form called hypnozoite, may develop into merozoite months or years later, causing relapse of malaria.

For this, after treatment of malaria, primaquine 15 mg daily for 14 days is given to eradicate exoerythrocytic cycle. *P. falciparum* and *P. malariae* have no exoerythrocytic cycle.

NB: Remember the following points:

- Before giving primaquine, glucose-6-phosphate dehydrogenase (G-6-PD) should be measured in blood, as primaquine can cause haemolysis in patient with G-6-PD deficiency. However, in such a case, primaquine 30 mg weekly for 8 weeks may be given without harmful effect.
- Primaquine can also cause cyanosis due to formation of methaemoglobin in red cells.

Treatment During Pregnancy

- Chloroquine should be given as usual dose. In vivax and ovale infection, no primaquine until delivery. Chloroquine 600 mg weekly should be given and continued until delivery. If no response to chloroquine, quinine 600 mg 8 hourly for 1 week.
- In falciparum malaria, quinine 600 mg 8 hourly for 1 week.

Complications of Malaria in Pregnancy

- In foetus—still birth, low birth weight, foetal distress. High foetal death in falciparum malaria, especially in the last trimester.
- In mother—maternal death, abortion, premature labour, anaemia, hypoglycaemia and acute pulmonary oedema. Congenital malaria may occur in 5% cases.

KALA-AZAR (LEISHMANIASIS)

Organisms: *Leishmania Donovani* complex.
- *L. donovani* (India and South East Asia).
- *L. infantum* (Middle East, Mediterranean area).
- *L. chagasi* (South, Central America).

Source or Reservoir

Human (Indian kala-azar).

Incubation Period

1–2 months (may be months to years, even 10 years).

Modes of Transmission

- Bite by infected female sandfly (common).
- Congenital—transplacental.
- Blood transfusion.

NB: Following points are important:
- Man is the only reservoir in Indian subcontinent.
- Other reservoirs are dog, jackal, fox and wild rodents in other countries.
- Leishmania has two forms—amastigote and promastigote.
- Amastigote form (oval) is found in human, LD body is found in monocyte/macrophage system.

Symptoms

- Fever—usually intermittent, double or triple rise. May be continuous.
- Loss of weight but good appetite.
- Heaviness in left upper abdomen.
- Blackening of skin.

Signs

- Cachexia.
- Anaemia.
- Abdominal distension (due to hepatosplenomegaly).
- Lymphadenopathy—common in African and Chinese kala-azar, rare in Indian Kala-azar.
- Skin pigmented.
- Bleeding spots may be found.

Complications

- Secondary infection (pneumonia, tuberculosis).
- Anaemia.
- Bleeding.
- Gastroenteritis, bacillary dysentery.
- Liver disease (cirrhosis of liver).

- PKDL.
- Rarely, cancrum oris.

Causes of Death

If no treatment is given, patient may die within 1-2 years due to
- Secondary infection.
- Bleeding.

Investigations

1. CBC—leucopenia, high lymphocyte and monocyte, neutropenia, thrombocytopenia and high ESR. If CBC is repeated after some days, there is 'progressive leucopenia'.
2. Immunological tests, based on antibody—
   - Direct agglutination test (DAT) - May be positive after 2 weeks (usually within month). It remains positive years after cure (so it does not indicate active infection).
   - Immunochromatographic test (ICT)—also called rapid dipstick rk-39 test.
   - Indirect haemagglutination assay (IHA).
   - Indirect fluorescent antibody test (IFAT).
   - ELISA.
   - Complement fixation test (CFT)—it is nonspecific, positive after 3 weeks.
   - Aldehyde test—still helpful where there is no facility.
3. Detection of antigen—done by latex agglutination test (Katex) for detecting leishmanial antigen in urine. This test is very simple, more specific than antibody-based test, highly sensitive (96%) and also specific (100%).
4. Definitive diagnosis—by isolation of LD body from bone marrow and spleen puncture, also from liver, lymph node and skin lesion. Culture is done in NNN media (Nicolle-Nove-Mc-Neal).
5. PCR (from lymph node or bone marrow aspiration).
6. Blood for total protein and A/G ratio (high total protein, low albumin and high globulin).

Treatment

- Sodium stibogluconate—20 mg/kg for 28 days IV or IM. Can be given in infusion with normal saline. IM injection is very painful, may be given, if ECG abnormality (arrhythmia or long QT interval).
- Meglumine antimoniate—50 mg/kg is an alternative drug.
- Liposomal amphotericin B—drug of choice, 3-4 mg/kg daily, given on days 1-5, 14 and 21. Safe in pregnancy.
- Conventional amphotericin B—1 mg/kg for 20 days, given in slow infusion for 4-6 hours. It is more protein bound and nephrotoxic.
- Oral drug—miltefosine, a cytotoxic drug. Also helpful in resistant kala-azar. Dose is 50-100 mg or 2.5 mg/kg daily orally for 28 days (50 mg, if <25 kg body weight and 100 mg, if >25 kg body weight). It has more foetal toxicity, so not used in pregnancy.
- Paromomycin—11 mg/kg/day intramuscularly for 21 days.

NB: Following points are important while treating with sodium stibogluconate:

- Before starting the therapy, perform renal and hepatic function tests, ECG (to see dysrhythmia, prolonged QT and ischaemia) and chest X-ray (latent TB, pneumonia).

- During IV injection, if the patient complains of chest pain or cough, stop the drug immediately.
- Monitor ECG, FBC including platelet, hepatic and renal functions.
- The drug should be stopped, if there is bleeding, ECG change.
- No limitation of dose (previously it was thought that dose should not exceed 1 g/day).

Response to Therapy

- Clinical improvement—improvement of fever, feeling of well-being.
- Reduction in the size of spleen (may take months).
- Weight gain.
- Laboratory findings include increased Hb%, total count of WBC and increased albumin.

Treatment in Relapse

Same therapy with sodium stibogluconate for 60 days (double the duration).

Treatment of Resistant Kala-azar

- Pentamidine isethionate—3 to 4 mg/kg, 3 times per week for 5–25 weeks (at least 5 weeks and 15 injections should be given). Then, sodium stibogluconate 20 mg/kg for 30 days. Pentamidine may cause hypoglycaemia, hyperglycaemia and shock. It is not used as a first drug, because of more side effects and development of quick resistance.
- Amphotericin B, preferably liposomal amphotericin B.
- Plus adjuvant therapy—γ interferon, allopurinol, ketoconazole.

Treatment Kala-azar in Pregnancy

Same treatment with sodium stibogluconate.

Kala-azar Treatment Failure (KATF)

When kala-azar does not respond to usual therapy with sodium stibogluconate, it is called KATF. It is usually due to inappropriate or suboptimal dose or irregular therapy. Treatment is same as in resistant kala-azar.

POST-KALA-AZAR DERMAL LEISHMANIASIS (PKDL)

Definition

It is a nonulcerative cutaneous lesion that occurs after treatment and apparent recovery from visceral leishmaniasis.

Initially, there is macules, then erythematous lesion followed by wart like nodular lesions. Mainly involves the face, around the chin and ear lobules. May be butterfly distribution. Hypopigmented macules can occur in all parts of the body.

Types

Type are characterised as two types:

African form (Sudanese form)—

- About 50% patients with visceral leishmaniasis develop PKDL. In Sudan, children are more affected than Indian subcontinent.

- May develop with visceral leishmaniasis or within 6 months afterwards.
- Lesions are discrete papules on the cheeks, chin, ears, extensor surfaces of forearms, buttocks and lower legs.
- Maculopapular rash may develop all over the body.
- Improves spontaneously in 3/4th cases within 1 year.

Indian Type

- This type occur in few patients, within 6 months to 3 years.
- Involves the face, trunk, extremities (may be confused with lepromatous leprosy).
- These are progressive and seldom heal spontaneously.
- Histopathology reveals chronic inflammatory cells with parasites in dermal macrophage.

Symptoms

- History of kala azar.
- Several hypopigmented or erythematous lesions all over the body, nodules on the face, nose, cheeks.

Investigations

- Biopsy from nodular lesions shows amastigote form of LD bodies.
- PCR detects parasites in 80% cases.

Treatment

- Inj. sodium stibogluconate (given in cycle), 20 mg/kg daily for 20 days. After 10 days interval, the injection is repeated. Total 6 cycles are given.
- If second course is required, it is given after 2 months.
- In Sudan, sodium stibogluconate is given for 2 months.
- Amphotericin B infusion may also be given.
- Miltefosine may also be effective in PKDL.

Complications

Apart from disfigurement, PKDL patients are important source of infection. Treatment should be given for the benefit of the community.

FILARIASIS

Definition

Filariasis is a parasitic infection caused by thread like nematode filariae. The disease is transmitted by bite of infected culex and anopheles mosquito.

Organisms

- *Wuchereria bancrofti.*
- *Brugia malayi.*

Clinical Features

Acute lymphangitis—
- Fever, pain, redness along the inflamed lymphatic vessels.
- Lymphadenitis of regional lymph nodes (axillary or inguinal) with retrograde lymphangitis.
- Local oedema.
- Epididymitis, orchitis.

Chronic lymphatic disease
- Skin of the affected area becomes coarse, corrugated and fissured.
- Subcutaneous oedema and thickening.
- Hydrocele and massive scrotal enlargement.
- Chyluria and chylous effusion.
- Progressive enlargement of skin and subcutaneous tissue gives rise to 'Elephantiasis.' It is due to lymphatic obstruction.

Investigations

- CBC shows eosinophilia.
- Serum IgE—high.
- ICT for filaria.
- Indirect fluorescence and ELISA.
- Blood film at night, to see microfilarae.
- Microfilarae can be detected from chylous urine or scrotal swelling.
- PCR.

Treatment

- Diethylcarbamazine (DEC)—6 mg/kg in three divided doses for 2 weeks.
- Single dose of ivermectin 200 mg/kg.
- Or single dose of albendazole 400 mg with DEC (300 mg) is also effective.
- Other treatment—crepe bandage, elastic stockings, elevation of the limbs may be helpful. Plastic surgery, surgical removal of tissues of elephantiasis may be done in some cases.

Tropical Pulmonary Eosinophilia

In this condition, microfilariae may become trapped in the pulmonary capillaries and destroyed by allergic inflammation. The patient usually complains of cough, wheeze, fever. It is associated with a high peripheral eosinophil count. If untreated, may progress chronic interstitial lung disease.

Serological test is strongly positive and serum IgE level is very high. CXR shows miliary mottling.

Treatment

DEC 6mg/kg in three divided doses for 14 days.

ANCYLOSTOMIASIS (HOOKWORM INFESTATION)

Definition

It is an infestation caused by *Ancylostoma duodenale or Necator americanus*. The infection usually occurs to the persons by walking barefoot over contaminated soil by the filariform larva that penetrates through the skin.

Symptoms

- By the larva—creeping eruption usually on the feet (ground itch).
- By the adult worm—upper abdominal pain, anorexia, nausea, vomiting, diarrhea, features of anaemia, etc.

Signs

No specific sign except anaemia.

Investigations

- Stool RME—ovum may be found.
- CBC—may show anaemia and eosinophilia.

Complications

- Iron deficiency anaemia.
- Protein losing enteropathy and hypoproteinaemia in the undernourished.
- Mental and physical retardation in children.

Treatment

- Mebendazole 100 mg 12 hourly for 3 days.
- Or albendazole 400 mg or pyrantel pamoate 11mg/kg, maximum 1gm as a single dose orally.
- For anaemia - oral iron therapy.

Prevention

- Personal hygiene, regular washing of hands.
- All members of the family should be treated simultaneously.
- Night clothes and bed linens of the patient should be washed thoroughly.

ASCARIASIS (ROUNDWORM INFESTATION)

Definition

It is an infestation caused by *Ascaris lumbricoides*. Infection occurs by eating food contaminated with mature ova.

Clinical Features

- May be asymptomatic.
- Abdominal pain.
- Intestinal obstruction in children.
- Loeffler's syndrome—during migration of larva to the lungs, there may be cough, wheeze, and breathlessness. It is called Loeffler's syndrome (also called ascaris pneumonia).

Investigations

- Stool for RME—ova may be found.
- CBC—may show eosinophilia.

Treatment

- Mebendazole 100 mg orally 12 hourly for 3 days or albendazole 400 mg orally as a single dose or pyrantel pamoate 11mg/kg, maximum 1gm as a single dose orally.

Complications

- Intestinal obstruction.
- Intussusception.
- Volvulus, haemorrhagic infarction or perforation.
- Obstruction of the common bile duct causing obstructive jaundice.
- Acute appendicitis.

Prevention

- Personal hygiene, regular washing of hands.
- All members of the family should be treated accordingly.
- Night clothes and bed linens of the patient should be washed thoroughly.

ENTEROBIUS VERMICULARIS (THREAD WORM)

Definition

It is an infestation caused by *Enterobius vermicularis*. Infection occurs by eating food contaminated with mature ova.

Clinical Features

- Itching around the anus, especially at night. The ova are often carried to the mouth on the fingers and so re-infection takes place.
- In females, the genitalia may be involved. The adult worms may be seen moving on the buttocks or in the stool.

Investigation

Ova can easily be detected. Investigation is rarely necessary.

Treatment

A single dose of mebendazole 100 mg or albendazole 400 mg orally. May be repeated after 2 weeks to control autoinfection.

Prevention

- Personal hygiene, regular washing of hands.
- All members of the family should be treated accordingly.
- Night clothes and bed linens of the patient should be washed thoroughly.

TAENIASIS

Definition

It is an infestation caused by Taenia species.

Causative Organisms

- *Taenia saginata.*
- *Taenia solium.*
- *Taenia asiatica.*

Mode of Infection

- *T. solium* infection occurs by eating undercooked beef contaminated with larva.
- *T. saginata* and *T. asiatica* infection occurs by eating undercooked pork contaminated with larva.

Clinical Features

- Usually asymptomatic.
- Upper abdominal pain, anorexia, nausea and diarrhoea.
- Weakness, lassitude, hunger, giddiness.
- Subcutaneous nodules may develop over lips, neck, chest, masseter muscles, back and groin.

Investigations

- Stool RME—ova or adult segments may be found.
- CBC shows eosinophilia.
- X-ray of muscles and soft tissue shows calcification.
- CT/ or MRI of brain may show circular or ring-shaped shadow of calcified larva.

Treatment

- *T. saginata*—Praziquantel 5–10 mg/kg or Niclosamide 2 gm both as a single dose or Nitazoxanide 500 mg twice daily for 3 days.
- *T. solium*—Niclosamide followed by laxative.

Complications

Cysticercosis

It is caused by the larval stage of *T. solium.* The larvae penetrate the intestinal mucosa, carried to many parts of the body, where they develop and form cysticerci, 0.5–1 cm cysts that contain the head of the young worm. Common locations are subcutaneous tissue, skeletal muscles and brain (neurocysticercosis). Neurocysticercosis may cause epileptic seizures, personality changes, staggering gait and signs of hydrocephalus.

Investigations

- CBC shows eosinophilia.
- X-ray shows calcification.
- CT or MRI of the brain.

Treatment

- Albendazole 15 mg/kg daily for 8 days or praziquantel 50 mg/kg in three divided doses for 10 days.
- Prednisolone 10 mg 8 hourly, started 1 day before starting above drugs for 14 days.
- Antiepileptic, if brain is involved.

STRONGYLOIDIASIS

Definition

It is an infestation caused by *Strongyloides stercoralis.*

Mode of Infection

Penetration of human skin by filariform larva. Sometimes, the larval form can penetrate directly the perianal skin and reinfect the host (autoinfection).

Clinical Features

- Itchy rash at the site of penetration.
- Upper abdominal pain, anorexia, nausea, diarrhoea, weight loss.
- Migration of larva through the lungs may cause cough, wheezing, respiratory distress, pneumonia.
- Urticarial plaques and papules due to allergic reaction. Migratory linear wheel around the buttock and lower abdomen called 'Cutaneous Larva Currens' may also occur.

Complication

- Meningoencephalitis.

Investigations

- Stool RME—motile larvae may be found. Excretion is intermittent, so repeated examination is required.
- CBC shows eosinophilia.
- Serology—ELISA.

Treatment

Two doses of ivermectin 200 microgram/kg on successive days. Alternatively, albendazole orally 15 mg/kg twice daily for 3 days.

GIARDIASIS

Definition

It is the infection caused by *Giardia lamblia.*

Mode of Infection

Ingestion of contaminated water by the cyst which remain viable up to 3 months in water.

Incubation Period

1–3 weeks.

Symptoms

- Diarrhoea.
- Abdominal pain, distention, bloating.
- Weakness, anorexia, nausea and vomiting.

Signs

- Abdominal distension and tenderness.

Investigations

- Stools RME shows cyst.
- Duodenal or jejunal aspiration by endoscopy shows trophozoite form.
- Jejunal biopsy specimens may show *G. lamblia* on the epithelial surface.

Treatment

- Single dose of tinidazole 2 g or metronidazole 400 mg 3 times daily for 10 days or nitazoxanide 500 mg orally twice daily for 3 days.

ANTHRAX

Definition

It is a zoonotic disease caused by *Bacillus anthracis.* The bacteria produces number of toxins which are responsible for the clinical manifestation of the disease.

Anthrax is a disease of sheep, goat, cattle. Infectious form is spore, which is transmitted to the human from contaminated animal, animal products or soil by inhalation or rarely by ingestion of spores.

Types of Infection

3 types of infection—

- Cutaneous anthrax.
- Gastrointestinal anthrax.
- Pulmonary anthrax.

Clinical Features

- Cutaneous anthrax: There is single skin lesion which is associated with occupational exposure to anthrax spores during processing of hides and bone products, or with bioterrorism. Lesion is single papule on a haemorrhagic oedematous base, which progress to a depressed black eschar.
- Gastrointestinal anthrax: It develops after ingestion of contaminated or incompletely cooked meat. There is nausea, vomiting, anorexia and fever followed by severe abdominal pain and bloody diarrhoea. Death may occur.
- Inhalational pulmonary anthrax: Fever, dyspnoea, cough, headache and septicaemia may develop 3–4 days following exposure. Chest X-ray may show widening of the mediastinum and pleural effusion.

Complications

- Meningitis.
- Septicaemia.
- Respiratory failure.

Investigations

- CBC.
- Culture from skin swab.
- Chest X-ray.

Treatment

- Ciprofloxacin 500 mg daily 12 hourly. Alternative regimen is benzylpenicillin 2.4 g IV 4 hourly or phenoxymethylpenicillin 500–1000 mg 6 hourly for 10 days. Aminoglycoside can also be used in severe disease.
- Ventilatory assistance may be needed in inhalational disease.

Prevention

Prophylaxis with ciprofloxacin (500 mg 12 hourly) is recommended for anyone at high-risk of exposure to anthrax spores.

LEPROSY (HANSEN'S DISEASE)

Definition

Leprosy is a chronic granulomatous disabling disease caused by *Mycobacterium leprae*. It involves the peripheral nerves, skin, mucous membrane, bone and viscera.

M. leprae is a Gram positive, acid fast and alcohol fast bacillus, also called Hansen's bacillus. Man is the only reservoir of infection.

Route of Transmission

By droplet infection from nasal mucosa of leprosy patient, sometimes skin contact (if ulcerated).

Types (or Classification) of Leprosy

Leprosy is classified into following types (Flowchart):

- Tuberculoid leprosy (TT).
- Borderline tuberculoid (BT).
- Borderline leprosy (BB).
- Borderline lepromatous leprosy (BL).
- Lepromatous leprosy (LL).

Depending on the cell mediated immunity (CMI), leprosy is divided into two—polar forms and a borderline form.

Also classified into 2 types:

- Paucibacillary—Few organisms in tissue. Skin smear for *M. leprae* bacilli is negative or few (found in TT and BT).
- Multibacillary—Large number of organisms in tissue. Skin smear for *M. leprae* bacilli is positive (found in BT, all BB, BL and LL).

Symptoms

Lepromatous Type

- Initially, hypopigmented erythematous macules. Later, multiple nodular lesions on ear lobe, face, forearm and legs. In the face, it is called 'Leonine facies'.
- No loss of sensation.
- Hypopigmented lesions.

Flowchart

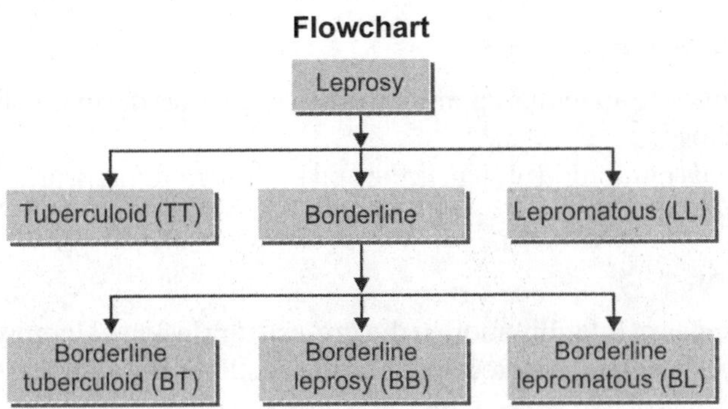

Tuberculoid Type

- Hypopigmented small macules in differents parts of the body with loss of sensation.
- Skin lesions are dry, scaly with anhydrosis.
- Supraorbital, great auricular, median, ulnar, radial, lateral popliteal and posterior tibial nerves are thickened bilaterally, but nontender.

Investigations

- Slit skin smear, nasal scraping or biopsy material from skin or thickened nerve—shows acid fast bacilli
- Skin biopsy for histopathology.

Histological Findings

- In tuberculoid type—epithelioid granuloma may be found.
- In lepromatous leprosy—*M. leprae* may be found in skin macrophage (also Schwann cells and perineurium).

Nerves Commonly Involved in Leprosy

- Facial nerve—Crossing the zygomatic arch.
- Great auricular nerve—Posterior triangle of the neck.
- Radial nerve—In the radial groove of humerus at the insertion of deltoid muscle.
- Radial cutaneous nerve—In the wrist.
- Ulnar nerve—In elbow, in between the medial epicondyle and olecranon process.
- Median nerve—Middle of the front of wrist.
- Lateral popliteal or common peroneal nerve—Around the neck of fibula.
- Posterior tibial nerve—Ankle, a little below and posterior to medial malleoli.

Treatment: WHO Recommended Protocol

- Paucibacillary (3–5 skin lesions, skin smear negative or few, tuberculoid and BT)—Rifampicin 600 mg monthly (supervised) plus dapsone 100 mg daily (self administered) for 6 months.
- Paucibacillary single lesion—Rifampicin 600 mg plus ofloxacin 400 mg plus minocycline 100 mg, in single dose (ROM therapy).
- Multibacillary (>5 lesions, skin smear positive, BT, all BB, BL and LL)—Rifampicin 600 mg and clofazimine 300 mg monthly (supervised) plus dapsone 100 mg and clofazimine 50 mg daily (self-administered) for 12 months or until smear negative (may be up to 24 months).

Common Side Effects

- Dapsone—Haemolytic anaemia, agranulocytosis, exfoliative dermatitis, hepatitis, hypoproteinaemia, psychosis.
- Clofazimine—Red colouration of skin, urine and body secretions, pruritus, anorexia, nausea, vomiting, abdominal pain.

Lepra Reaction

It is defined as episodes of inflammation in the pre-existing lesion of leprosy. It may be the first manifestation of the disease. Lepra reaction may be insidious or rapid, destroying the affected tissue within hours. It is of two types: type 1 and type 2.

Type 1 Lepra Reaction

It is a delayed hypersensitivity reaction (type IV) that occurs in 30% borderline patients. It occurs spontaneously or by treatment. There is rapid swelling of one or more nerves with pain and tenderness. Nerve function is lost rapidly. Foot drop, claw hand and facial palsy may occur. Skin lesions become erythematous, swollen and new lesion may appear. There may be oedema of hands, feet and face. Improves after starting treatment and also after completion of therapy.

Treatment

- In mild case, aspirin 600 mg 6 hourly.
- In severe case, prednisolone 40–60 mg daily, should be reduced by 5 mg/day each month,tapered over 3–6 months.
- Clofazamine can be added upto 300 mg daily. If fails, ciclosporin 5–10 mg/kg may be given.
- Treatment of leprosy should be continued.

Type 2 Lepra Reaction (Erythema Nodosum Leprosum, ENL)

It is due to immune-complex deposition (type 3 hypersensitivity reaction). Occurs in BL and LL patient.

It is characterised by fever, arthralgia and crops of small pink painful nodules on the face and limbs. Iritis, iridocyclitis, keratitis, conjunctivitis and episcleritis are common. Other signs are neuritis, orchitis, myositis, nephritis, epistaxis, pleurisy, bone pain, arthritis, lymphadenitis and hepatomegaly. ENL may be the first manifestation of leprosy in 50% lepromatous and 25% borderline lepromatous leprosy, either during the course of the disease or more commonly in the second year of treatment.

Treatment

- In mild cases—aspirin 600 mg 6 hourly.
- In severe case—thalidomide 100 mg 6 hourly. When symptoms improve, dose should be reduced slowly over weeks or months, maintenance dose is 50–100 mg daily.
- Or prednisolone 40–60 mg is given, taper the dose over 1–6 months.
- Clofazimine is given with increase dose.
- Antileprosy therapy must be continued.

LEPTOSPIROSIS (WEIL'S DISEASE)

Definition

Leptospirosis is caused by the spirochaete *Leptospira interrogans*. The main types occurring in human are *Leptospira icterohaemorrhagica* (from rodents), *Leptospira canicola* (dogs and pigs), Leptospira hardjo (cattle) and *Leptospira pomona* (pigs and cattle).

Rodents, particularly rats, are the most important reservoir of infection. The organism is excreted in the urine and may survive in the soil for several weeks. Entry into the human host is through cuts and abrasions on the skin, or through intact mucous membranes or contaminated water.

People Prone to Leptospirosis

Sewerage workers, fishermen, vets and farmers.

Pathology

Replication occurs in the blood, tissue and multisystem involvement may occur. Kidney and liver are commonly affected. In kidney, there may be acute interstitial nephritis and tubular necrosis. In liver, centrilobular necrosis in severe case.

Incubation Period

1–2 weeks.

Clinical Features

- Initial or septicaemic phase—Persists for 4–7 days, characterised by fever, headache, myalgia, abdominal pain, vomiting, skin rash (macular, maculopapular or haemorrhagic), conjunctival ingestion (blood-shot eyes). Proteinuria and haematuria may be present, renal failure may occur in 50% cases. 90% cases are anicteric, jaundice and impairment of liver function are present in severe cases. Hepatosplenomegaly is present in 20% cases. Lung involvement is common, there is dry cough, haemoptysis and confluent shadow in chest X-ray.
- Second or immune phase—Lasts for 4–30 days. No fever. Antibody to leptospira rises. Deterioration in liver and renal function may continue. Meningism, uveitis and rash's are common. Thrombocytopenia, haemolytic uremic syndrome may occur. Endothelial injury may cause blood loss from gastrointestinal tract and lungs. Pulmonary syndrome may occur characterised by haemoptysis, patchy lung infiltrate on CXR and respiratory failure. Bilateral lung consolidation and ARDS with multiorgan dysfunction may occur.

Investigations

- CBC shows leucocytosis, thrombocytopenia.
- Blood culture in special media is positive in first 10 days.
- Urine culture is positive in second week.
- Antileptospira antibody (or microscopic agglutination test- MAT).
- Liver function tests—high SGPT, PT may be prolonged.
- CPK—high.
- PCR—Leptospiral DNA by PCR is also helpful in blood and urine.

Treatment

- IV benzyl penicillin (1.5 mega unit 6 hourly) for one week. IV ceftriaxone 1 g daily is equally effective.
- Doxycycline 100 mg 12 hourly for one week is also helpful.
- Renal failure may require dialysis. Doxycycline prophylaxis may be used in highly endemic area.
- Blood transfusion, if bleeding.

Complications

- DIC.
- Fulminating hepatic failure.
- Carditis.

NB: Combination of hepatitis, renal failure and carditis is highly suggestive of leptospirosis.

POLIOMYELITIS

It is caused by RNA virus which replicates in GI tract. There are three serotypes - 1, 2 and 3. Spread by faeco-oral route as the virus is excreted in the faeces.

The virus particularly involves nervous system, mainly anterior horn cells of spinal cord and cranial nerve neurons. Also, causes lymphocytic meningitis and infects grey matter of spinal cord, brain stem and cortex.

Clinical Features

Incubation period is 7–14 days. May be inapparent in 90–95% cases. Common in childhood, may occur in adult also. Three types of clinical features are discussed below:

1. Abortive poliomyelitis (4–5%)—mild fever, headache, sore throat, myalgia, weakness. It persists for 24–48 hours, with spontaneous cure.
2. Nonparalytic poliomyelitis (1–2%)—after a week of well being, there is recurrence of fever, headache, myalgia and meningism. This stage may persist for 24–48 hours, recovery is complete.
3. Paralytic poliomyelitis (0.5–1%)—
   - Spinal form—in some cases, paralytic form of the disease may occur 4–5 days of initial illness. Meningeal irritation and muscle pain recur, followed by asymmetrical flaccid paralysis without sensory loss, commonly involving the lower limbs below 5 years of age and upper limb in older children. In adult, there may be paraplegia or quadriplegia.
   - Bulbar poliomyelitis—characterised by cranial nerve (IX, X) involvement and respiratory muscle paralysis. Soft palate, pharyngeal and laryngeal muscle palsies are common. The patient complains of facial weakness, dysphagia, dysphonia, nasal voice, nasal regurgitation.

Stage of Residual Disability

Muscular wasting leads to persistent contracture, deformity and shortening of limb may occur usually in one limb.

Investigation: Diagnosis is Clinical

- CSF shows high lymphocytic, high protein and normal sugar. Virus may be cultured from CSF and stool.

Treatment

- Complete bed rest.
- If respiratory paralysis—ventilatory support, tracheostomy may be needed.
- After recovery—physiotherapy, occupational therapy, orthopaedic measures.
- Prevention—by live (Sabin) vaccine.

SEPSIS

Definition

It is defined as the systemic inflammatory response caused by documented infection with or without localising signs and development of shock.

Risk Factors

- Diabetes mellitus.
- Immunodeficiency (cytotoxic drug, chemotherapy, radiotherapy).
- Trauma.
- Burn.
- Alcohol and substance abuse.
- Chronic illness (heart, lung, kidney, liver).
- Haematological disease.
- Recent surgery or invasive procedure.
- Invasive line—IV lines, urinary catheter, nasogastric tube.

Causes

- Bacteria—*Staph. aureus, Neisseria meningitides, E. coli* and other Gram-negative organisms, Pseudomonas aeruginosa, *Mycobacterium tuberculosis, Mycobacterium avium complex* (MAC).
- Fungal—*Histoplasma capsulatum, Candida.*
- Parasitic—*Falciparum malaria.*

Clinical Features

1. Evidence of severe infection plus signs of systemic inflammatory response syndrome (SIRS), which is defined by the presence of 2 or more of the following:
   - Temperature >38°C or <36°C.
   - Pulse rate >90/min.
   - Respiratory rate >20/min.
   - WBC >12/cmm or <4/cmm.
   - $PaCO_2$ <32.5 mmHg.
2. Features of septic shock-sepsis with unexplained hypotension unresponsive to fluids, along with organ dysfunction.
3. Others—
   - Generalised erythroderma (toxic shock syndrome by *S. aureus*) and petechial or haemorrhagic rash (*N. meningitides*).
   - Damage to different organs (multiorgan failure).
   - Confusion, delirium and coma.
   - Acute respiratory distress syndrome (ARDS) may occur.
   - Acute renal failure due to prolonged hypotension and/or toxic injury.
   - Hepatic dysfunction—high bilirubin and enzymes.
   - Features of disseminated intravascular coagulation (DIC).

Investigations

- CBC, ESR shows polymorphonuclear leucocytosis.
- Culture of blood, urine, sputum, wound secretion, IV line, tracheal aspirate.
- Urea, creatinine and electrolytes.
- LFT (bilirubin and SGPT).
- Coagulation profile (prothrombin time, APTT, D-dimer, FDP).
- ABG analysis.
- CXR (to see consolidation, ARDS).
- USG of abdomen (to see any abdominal pathology, e.g. abscess).
- Other investigation according to suspicion of cause.

Treatment

- IV fluid and correction of electrolytes.
- Maintenance of adequate nutrition.
- High-flow oxygen.
- Broad spectrum antibiotic covering both Gram-negative and Gram-positive organisms.
- Ventilatory support, if needed.
- Vasopressor agents in hypotension—noradrenaline, dopamine or dobutamine.
- IV corticosteroid may be given (hydrocortisone or methylprednisolone).

HYDATID DISEASE (CYST)

Definition

Hydatid disease is a parasitic infestation due to echinococcus species mainly echinococcus granulosus.

Cyst has 3 layers—outer derived from host (pericyst), intermediate laminated layer (ectocyst) and inner germinal layer (endocyst) that buds off brood capsule to form daughter cyst. May be single or multiple cyst, may calcify.

Definitive Host

Dog, also fox and jackel.

Intermediate Host

Human.

Mode of Infection

Close contact with infected dogs or eating undercooked vegetables or drinking water contaminated with faeces of infected dog.

Organisms

- *Echinococcus granulosus* of dogs.
- *Echinococcus multilocularis*—life cycle between fox and vole. Man is infected accidentally.

Sites of Hydatid Cyst

- Liver—60%, usually right lobe.
- Lungs—30%.
- Kidneys—3%.
- Brain—1%.
- Other organs (spleen, heart, muscles and biliary tree).

Clinical Features

Infection occurs in childhood, grows slowly.

- Usually asymptomatic.
- Mass in right hypochondrium (due to hepatomegaly). Occasionally, jaundice due to obstruction in bile duct.
- Rarely, rupture into the abdominal cavity, pleural cavity or biliary tree may occur. If rupture into the biliary tree, there may be intermittent jaundice, abdominal pain and fever. Cyst rupturing into the bronchus may cause expectoration and spontaneous cure.
- Features of cyst in other organs—cyst in the lung, which may be infected causing lung abscess. Cyst in the brain may cause seizure. Renal cyst may cause haematuria.
- Calcification of cyst occurs in 40% cases.

Complications of Hydatid Cyst

- Pressure effect to the surrounding tissue.
- Rupture may cause anaphylactic shock.
- Secondary infection.

Investigations

- CBC shows high eosinophil.
- USG and CT scan shows cyst and daughter cysts within the parent cyst.
- Serology—CFT (positive in 70 to 80%), haemagglutination test (positive in 85%), flocculation test, indirect fluorescent antibody test, immunoelectrophoresis (Arc 5-test) and ELISA (positive in 70 to 90%).
- Plain X-ray of abdomen—calcification may be seen.
- Casoni's test (nonspecific)—it is done by intradermal injection of 0.2 mL hydatid fluid in forearm (control with normal saline in other arm). In positive cases, there is formation of wheal with pseudopodia in 20–30 minutes (it disappears in 1 hour).

Treatment

- Surgical treatment—cyst should be removed if possible after sterilizing the cyst with alcohol, 2.7% NaCl or 0.5% silver nitrate. Praziquantel 20 mg/kg for 14 days kills protoscolices perioperatively.
- Medical treatment—Albendazole 15 mg/kg in two divided doses for 12 weeks to 6 months. May be repeated (cure in 30%, symptomatic relief in 50%) or mebendazole 400 mg twice daily for 12 weeks to 6 months, may be repeated.
- PAIR therapy (puncture, aspiration, injection and re-aspiration)—percutaneous aspiration of cyst, followed by injection of 100% ethanol into the cyst, then reaspiration of cyst contents. Mebendazole may be combined with PAIR.
- Calcified cyst may be left untreated.

INFECTIOUS MONONUCLEOSIS

Definition

Infectious mononucleosis is a clinical syndrome caused by Epstein-Barr virus, characterised by pharyngitis, lymphadenopathy, fever and lymphocytosis.

Mode of Transmission

Oral contact via saliva, either by droplet infection or environmental contamination in childhood or by kissing among adolescents and adults.

Clinical Features

Incubation period may be 7–10 days.

- Fever, headache and malaise.
- Sore throat or tonsillitis.
- Lymphadenopathy,which are mostly cervical, nontender, usually involves the anterior and posterior chain. May be generalized.
- Palatal petechiae, periorbital oedema. Macular, petechial or erythema multiforme rashes may occur. Rash aggravates by taking 'ampicillin'.
- Hepatitis with or without jaundice.
- Splenomegaly.
- Fever resolves over 2 weeks, fatigue and other abnormalities settle over a further few weeks.

Complications

- Chronic fatigue syndrome.
- Hepatitis.
- Haematological—haemolytic anaemia, thrombocytopenia.
- Myocarditis, pericarditis.
- Neurolgical—cranial nerve palsy, transverse myelitis, meningoencephalitis.
- Renal—glomerulonephritis.
- Rupture of spleen.

Investigations

- CBC—leucopenia, high lymphocytes, also atypical lymphocytes.
- Paul-Bunnell or 'Monospot' test.
- Specific EBV serology—IgM antibody.
- CNS infections may be diagnosed by detection of viral DNA in cerebrospinal fluid.

Treatment: Usually Symptomatic

- Rest.
- Paracetamol for fever.
- Ampicillin or amoxicillin should be avoided.
- When pharyngeal oedema is severe-short course of prednisolone 30 mg daily for 5 days may help.
- Current antiviral drugs are not effective against EBV.

Diseases Caused by EBV Virus

- Infectious mononucleosis.
- Lymphoma in immunocompromised and some forms of Hodgkin's disease are EBV associated.
- Burkitt's lymphoma.
- Nasopharyngeal carcinoma.
- Hairy leukoplakia in AIDS.
- X-linked lymphoproliferative (Duncan's) syndrome is a familial lymphoproliferative disorder that follows primary EBV infection in boys without any other history of immunodeficiency.

TOXOPLASMOSIS

Causative Organism

Toxoplasma gondii, an intracellular parasite.

Mode of Infection

- Oöcyst contaminated with soil, salads and vegetables.
- Ingestion of raw or undercooked meats containing tissue cysts. Sheep, pigs and rabbits are the most common meat sources.
- Transplacental transfer from mother to the foetus.
- Blood transfusion.
- Outbreaks of toxoplasmosis may occur due to consumption of unfiltered water.

Clinical Features

Toxoplasmosis may be congenital or acquired. Most acquired primary infections are subclinical. In HIV-1 infection, toxoplasmosis occurs as opportunistic infection.

- Common presenting feature is painless lymphadenopathy, local or generalised. Cervical nodes are commonly involved, but mediastinal, mesenteric or retroperitoneal groups may be affected.
- Spleen may be palpable.
- Most patients have no systemic symptoms, some may have malaise, fever, fatigue, muscle pain, sore throat and headache.
- Some may develop encephalitis, myocarditis, polymyositis, pneumonitis or hepatitis.

Congenital Toxoplasmosis

Seropositive females infected 6 months before pregnancy have no risk of foetal transmission. Congenital disease affects foetus in early gestation. Many foetal infections are subclinical at birth, but central nervous system is mainly affected. If the infant survives, parasites disappear from all organs except brain. Long-term sequelae are choroido-retinitis, microcephaly, hydrocephalus.

Investigations

- Indirect fluorescent antibody test (Sabin-Feldman dye test)—detects IgG antibody. Fourfold or greater increased titre indicates recent infection.
- Toxoplasma specific IgM antibody indicates acute infection.
- Isolation of toxoplasma organisms in lymph node biopsy.
- PCR to detect toxoplasma specific DNA.
- X-ray of skull may show calcification.
- MRI of brain shows single or multiple ring enhancing lesions.

Treatment

- In immunocompetent asymptomatic case—no treatment is necessary.
- In symptomatic case or progressive disease or in immunocompromised patient—pyrimethamine or sulfadiazine and folinic acid.
- Pregnant woman with recent infection—spiramycin (3 g daily in divided doses) should be given until term. If foetal infection is present, sulfadiazine and pyrimethamine plus calcium folinate is given (spiramycin does not cross placental barrier).

FOOD POISONING

Definition

Food poisoning is defined as gastroenteritis caused by consumption of food or water contaminated with bacteria or their toxins or chemical.

Diagnosis is likely when more persons are ill after eating the same food.

Causes

1. Infective:
   - Toxin producing—*Staph. aureus, Bacillus cereus, E.coli* (ETEC), *E.coli* 0157:H7, *Clostridium perfringens, Clostridium difficile, Vibrio parahaemolyticus.*
   - Invasion of mucosa—*Campylobacter jejuni, Yersinia enterocolitica,* Salmonella, Shigella, *Bacillus anthracis.*Others - without invasion such as rota virus, novo virus (nor walk virus).
2. Noninfective: shellfish, strawberries, phallotoxin, amatoxin, scrombotoxin (fish), ciguatoxin (tropical fish).

Clinical Features

- Vomiting, diarrhoea—bloody or mucous if invasion of intestinal or colonic mucosa, profuse rice watery if cholera.
- Cramping abdominal pain.
- Headache, fever.
- Features of dehydration—dry tongue, low BP, low volume pulse, cold and clammy extremities, scanty urine, pinched face, shrunken eyes, etc.
- More serious cases can result in life threatening neurologic, hepatic and renal dysfunction, leading to permanent disability or death.

Investigations

- CBC may show leucocytosis.
- Serum electrolyte, BUN and creatinine.
- Stool for RME and C/S.
- Blood culture.

Treatment

- Correction of dehydration and electrolyte imbalance. ORS should be given.
- If the patient has vomiting—IV fluid (e.g. normal saline, cholera saline, Ringer's lactate).
- Patient should avoid milk, dairy products and other lactose containing foods during episodes of acute diarrhoea.
- Antibiotic—ciprofloxacin, norfloxacin, rifaximin, etc.

Prevention

- Maintenance of strict personal hygiene.
- Food should be cooked adequately.
- Avoid cross-contamination of raw and cooked foods.
- Keep all foods at appropriate temperature.

CHAPTER

9 Nephrology

CHAPTER CONTENTS

INVESTIGATIONS IN RENAL DISEASES

Following investigations are done in renal diseases:
- Examination of urine—RME and C/S.
- Blood for biochemistry.
- Imaging of renal system.
- Radionuclide study.
- Renal biopsy.

Examination of urine: Physical, chemical and microscopic.

Physical examination: To see quantity, colour, appearance, presence of sediment and specific gravity.

Quantity: To see polyuria, anuria, oliguria.

Colour: Normally straw colour due to presence of urochrome and urobilinogen.Changes in colour may occur in:
- Yellow—due to presence of bilirubin or excess urobilinogen.
- Red—due to presence of haemoglobin, RBC, myoglobin.
- Milky—due to chyluria.
- Dark brown—due to presence of methaemoglobin.
- Orange—due to rifampicin.

Specific gravity: Normal specific gravity is 1.010 to 1.020.
- Low specific gravity (<1.003)—Diabetes insipidus, renal failure.
- High specific gravity (>1.025)—Diabetes mellitus , acute water loss, heart failure, liver disease.

Chemical Examinations

1. **Reaction**—normal urine is acidic (pH 4.6–6.3).
2. **Proteins**—normal urine may contain up to 150 mg proteins in 24 hours. Presence of excess protein in urine is called proteinuria.
3. **Sugar**—it is present in DM.
4. **Ketone bodies** (acetone, acetoacetate, beta hydroxy butyric acid)—appear in urine in ketosis due to diabetic ketoacidosis, persistent vomiting, prolong starvation.
5. **Bilirubin**—normally no bilirubin. Conjugated bilirubin may be found in obstructive and some cases of hepatocellular jaundice.
6. **Bile salt**—absent in normal urine. May be present in obstructive jaundice.
7. **Blood**—
   - Haematuria—presence of RBC in urine.
   - Haemoglobinuria—presence of haemoglobin in urine. It indicates intravascular haemolysis.
   - Myoglobinuria—presence of myoglobin in urine. It indicates rhabdomyolysis.
8. **Chyle**—milky urine due to fat particles in urine. Causes are—filariasis, fistula between urinary tract and lymphatic system due to malignancy.

Microscopic Examination

1. **Epithelial cells**—found in normal urine.
2. **Red cells**—>2/mm^3 in urine is abnormal. It indicates bleeding from urogenital tract. Presence of dysmorphic red cells suggests nephritis.
3. **Pus cells**—>10/mm^3 is abnormal, called pyuria. It indicates urinary tract infection (UTI).
4. **Casts**—formed in kidney tubules by coagulation of proteins. Common casts are:
   - Epithelial casts—found in AGN, degeneration of renal tubules.
   - RBC casts—found in AGN. It indicates glomerular lesion.
   - WBC casts—suggestive of pyelonephritis. Also found in interstitial nephritis.
   - Granular casts—found in inflammation and degeneration of renal tubules. Most often it indicates chronic renal disease.
   - Hyaline casts—may be present in normal urine. Also found in chronic glomerulonephritis, hypertension, fever, after exercise, due to loop diuretics.
   - Tubular cell casts—it is found in acute tubular necrosis.
5. **Crystals**—may not be pathological. But it is important in stone formers.
   - Cystine crystals—found in cystinuria.
   - Oxalate crystals—indicates predisposition to form calculi.
   - Calcium oxalate crystals—may be present in renal stone.
   - Triple phosphate crystal—may be present in phosphate stone.

Blood Tests

1. **CBC, ESR and PBF:**
   - Normocytic normochromic anaemia—may be due to CKD.
   - Haemolytic anaemia and presence of fragmented RBCs in urine—in haemolytic uraemic syndrome (HUS), thrombotic thrombocytopenic purpura (TTP).
2. **Biochemistry:**
   - Serum urea and creatinine.
   - Serum calcium.
   - Serum phosphate.
   - Serum alkaline phosphate.
   - Serum uric acid.
   - Creatinine clearance test.
   - Serum parathyroid hormone (PTH).
3. **Immunology:**
   - **ANCA**—in glomerulonephritis due to systemic vasculitis.
   - **Anti-GBM antibody**—found in Goodpasture's syndrome.
   - **Low serum complement (C3 and C4)**—in postinfectious glomerulonephritis, subacute bacterial endocarditis, SLE, HUS, mesangiocapillary glomerulonephritis, cryoglobulinaemia.

Renal Imaging

- **Plain X-ray of abdomen**—to see renal calcification or nephrocalcinosis.
- **Ultrasonography.**

- **Doppler ultrasound**—to diagnose renal artery stenosis.
- **CT urography (CTU)**—it is used to evaluate cysts, mass lesion in the kidney or filling defect within the collecting systems.
- **CT scan.**
- **CT angiography**—helpful in renal artery stenosis, renal trauma, haemorrhage from renal tract, vascular aneurysm.
- **MRI**—useful for staging of prostate, bladder and penile cancers.
- **Magnetic resonance angiography (MRA)**—alternative to CT angiography for imaging renal vessels.
- **Renal arteriography**—in renal artery stenosis.
- **Intravenous urography (IVU).**
- **Retrograde pyelography**
- **Micturating cystourethrography (MCU)**—to see vesico-ureteric reflux. It is used in children with recurrent infection.

Radionuclide Studies

- **99^{m} T_c DPTA**—done to study the renal blood flow, evidence of obstruction, measurement of GFR.
- **$99^{m}$$T_c$ DMSA**—done for demonstrating cortical scarring in reflux nephropathy, assessing individual function of each kidney.

Renal biopsy: Done to detect types of glomerulonephritis, malignancy.

PRESENTING PROBLEMS AND SYMPTOMS OF RENAL DISEASE

- Frequency.
- Dysuria.
- Urgency, hesitency.
- Incontinence.
- Polyuria, oliguria, anuria.
- Nocturia.
- Loin pain.
- Haematuria.
- Proteinuria.
- Oedema.
- Hypertension.
- Anaemia.

Causes of Red Urine

- Ingestion of beet root, senna, some dyes used to colour sweets.
- Haematuria.
- Haemoglobinuria (indicates intravascular haemolysis).
- Myoglobinuria (indicates rhabdomyolysis).
- Drugs—rifampicin (usually orange colour), clofazimine, phenindione, purgative like phenolphthaline.

Causes of Black Urine

(Fresh urine is normal, but when kept for hours, it turns dark)

- Acute intermittent porphyria.
- Alkaptonuria.

Haematuria: Passage of blood in urine.

Types of Haematuria

- Initial haematuria—presence of blood at the beginning of micturition, usually due to penile urethral cause.
- Terminal haematuria—presence of blood at the end of micturition, usually due to bladder neck or prostatic urethral cause.
- Total haematuria—presence of blood throughout micturition, usually due to bladder or urinary tract disease (such as renal cell carcinoma, papilloma of urinary bladder, UTI, renal stone) or blood dyscrasias or excess anticoagulant.

Causes of Haematuria

Prerenal

- Bleeding disorders—haemophilia, Christmas disease, ITP.
- Anticoagulant or antiplatelet drug therapy.
- Malignant hypertension.
- Infective endocarditis.

Renal

- Glomerulonephritis, commonly IgA nephropathy.
- Renal tuberculosis.
- Trauma.
- Renal calculi.
- Polycystic kidney disease (clot colic).
- Renal cell carcinoma.
- Interstitial nephritis.

Postrenal

- Ureter—stone, neoplasm.
- Urinary bladder—cystitis, papilloma, transitional cell carcinoma, stone, bilharziasis (schistosomiasis).
- Urethra—urethritis.
- Prostate—benign enlargement of postate (BEP), carcinoma of prostate.
- Trauma.
- Haemorrhagic cystitis due to cyclophosphamide.

Causes of Painless Haematuria

- Glomerulonephritis, commonly IgA nephropathy.
- Renal tuberculosis.
- Polycystic kidney disease.
- Renal cell carcinoma or hypernephroma.
- Papilloma of the urinary bladder.

- BEP.
- Bilharziasis (schistosomiasis).
- Interstitial nephritis.
- Anticoagulant or antiplatelet drug therapy.
- Bleeding disorder (haemophilia, Christmas disease, ITP).

Causes of Painful Haematuria

- Urethritis, cystitis.
- Renal calculi.
- Trauma.
- Polycystic kidney disease (clot colic).
- Renal papillary necrosis.
- Loin pain haematuria syndrome.
- Haemorrhagic cystitis due to cyclophosphamide.

Proteinuria: Presence of protein in urine above normal limit (normally <150 mg in 24 hours). Causes are:

- Physiological—orthostatic or postural proteinuria.
- Nephrotic proteinuria (>3.5 g/24 hours)—nephrotic syndrome due to any cause.
- Nonnephrotic proteinuria (<3.5 g/24 hours)—glomerunephritis due to any cause.
- Nonrenal cause—toxaemia of pregnancy (eclampsia and pre- eclampsia), malignant hypertension, high fever, severe exercise.

Orthostatic proteinuria: Presence of proteinuria that occurs in a person with prolonged upright position (e.g. traffic police). It is absent in the morning specimen of urine after getting up from sleep.

MICROALBUMINURIA

Urinary albumin excretion 30–300 mg in 24 hours or 20–200 μg/min is called microalbuminuria. It is not detected by routine urine dipstick test.

Significance: It is a predictor of early diabetic nephropathy. Occurs both in IDDM and NIDDM, but more common in NIDDM, also more in male. 30–40% develop irreversible nephropathy. Patient with microalbuminuria has 20 times greater incidence of nephropathy than normal people. It is associated with atherosclerosis, peripheral vascular disease, hypertension and IHD, also proliferative diabetic retinopathy and increased incidence of blindness.

Treatment

- Good control of diabetes.
- Control of hypertension—by ACE inhibitor or calcium antagonist.
- Restriction of protein—intake should be 40–90 g/day.

Few Common Definitions

- **Anuria**—Failure to pass urine more than 50 mL in 24 hours.
- **Oliguria**—Failure to pass less than 400 mL of urine in 24 hours.
- **Polyuria**—Passing of large volume (>3 L of urine) in 24 hours.

- **Nocturia**—Need to get up during the night to pass urine.
- **Frequency of micturition** - Repeated scanty urination without increase in volume.
- **Dysuria**—Pain or discomfort during micturition.
- **Pyuria**—presence of pus in urine.

Incontinence of Urine

Involuntary passage of urine. four types:

1. **Stress incontinence**—leakage of urine with activity, such as coughing, sneezing, lifting any object, exercise. Found in women after child birth and in man after prostate operation.
2. **Urge incontinence**—uncontrolled leakage of urine preceded by strong urge to void urine. It is due to UTI, enlargement of prostate, stone in urinary bladder.
3. **Overflow incontinence**—it occurs when the bladder is chronically over distended. Found in benign prostatic enlargement, pelvic surgery leading to pelvic nerve damage.
4. **Continual incontinence**—patient voids urine at any time, at any position due to loss of sphincter efficacy. Found in vesicovaginal fistula, ureterovaginal fistula.

Different Urinary Casts Present in Different Diseases

- RBC cast—AGN.
- WBC cast—Pyelonephritis.
- Granular cast—GN.
- Hyaline cast—Normal finding.

Causes of oliguria or anuria: Any cause of acute renal failure.

Prerenal Cause

- Fluid loss due to diarrhoea, vomiting, dehydration, etc.
- Blood loss due to haemorrhage.
- Plasma loss in burn.
- Hypotension due to myocardial infarction, shock, vasodilator drugs, heart failure.
- Other causes of acute renal failure—rhabdomyolysis, haemolytic uraemic syndrome, hepatorenal syndrome, renal artery stenosis.

Renal (Intrinsic Renal Disease)

- Acute tubular necrosis or toxic or septic renal failure (85%)
- RPGN due to—Primary GN (e.g. MCGN, IG nephropathy).
- Systemic disease, such as SLE, rheumatoid arthritis, systemic sclerosis, multiple myeloma, vasculitis.
- Tubulointerstitial disease (10%) due to drugs (NSAID, ciprofloxacin, allopurinol, sulfonamide, ciclosporin).

Postrenal

- Urethral—phimosis, paraphimosis, stricture, stone, blood clot, sloughed papilla.
- Bladder neck—prostatic hypertrophy, malignancy, stone.
- Bilateral ureteric—calculus, following surgery, pelvic tumour, uterine prolapse, retroperitoneal fibrosis (due to radiation, idiopathic).

Cause of Polyuria

1. Physiological—excess intake of fluid, alcohol, tea, coffee.
2. Pathological
   - Diabetes mellitus.
   - Diabetes insipidus.
   - Hypercalcaemia due to any cause.
   - CKD.
3. Psychogenic polydipsia.
4. Drug—diuretic.

Causes of Nocturia

- CKD.
- CCF.
- Insomnia.

Causes of Frequency of Micturition

- Excessive fluid intake.
- Diabetes mellitus.
- Diabetes insipidus.
- Cystitis.
- BEP.
- Stone and tumour of urinary bladder.

NEPHROTIC SYNDROME

Definition

Nephrotic syndrome is characterized by generalized oedema, massive proteinuria (>3.5 g/day) and hypoalbuminaemia, with or without hyperlipidaemia.

Causes

Primary renal disease: Glomerulonephritis due to any cause:

- Minimal change glomerular disease (common in children).
- Membranous GN (common in adult).
- Mesangiocapillary and proliferative glomerulonephritis.
- Focal and segmental glomerulosclerosis.
- IgA nephropathy.

Secondary to Other Disease

- Diabetic nephropathy.
- Collagen disease—SLE, rheumatoid arthritis (by amyloidosis).
- Amyloidosis.
- Drugs—penicillamine (common), captopril, gold, mercury.
- Neoplastic—carcinoma (bronchial carcinoma), lymphoma.
- Infection—malaria (quartan malaria), bacterial endocarditis, HBV, HCV, HIV, secondary syphilis, leprosy.
- Hereditary—congenital nephrotic syndrome, Alport syndrome
- Allergies—bee stings, snake bite, anti-snake venom, pollens.

NB: Commonest cause in children is minimal change and in adult membranous glomerulonephritis.

Clinical Features

Symptoms

- Generalized body swelling. At first there is periorbital oedema, then become generalized and massive (anasarca).
- Scanty urine, which may be frothy.

Signs

- Bilateral pitting leg oedema.
- Whole body is swollen.
- May be ascites, bilateral pleural effusion.

History to be Taken in Nephrotic Syndrome

- Diabetes mellitus.
- Malignancy (lymphoma, leukaemia).
- Drugs, eg captopril, NSAIDs, penicillamine, gold.
- Skin rash, arthritis, arthralgia, alopecia (SLE).
- History of other diseases like malaria, leprosy, syphilis, HBV, HCV, amyloidosis, vasculitis.
- Family history of sickle cell disease, Alport syndrome, nail patella syndrome.

Investigations

Routine

- Urine R/E—shows gross proteinuria.
- Urine for sugar (to exclude diabetic nephropathy).
- 24 hours urinary total protein (more than 3.5 g/ 24 hours is suggestive of nephritic syndrome).
- Serum total protein, serum albumin and A:G ratio (hypoalbuminaemia).
- Serum lipid profile (high cholesterol and TG).
- Blood sugar.
- Blood urea, serum creatinine, serum electrolytes.
- USG of whole abdomen to look for renal pathology.

To Find Out Causes

- Blood sugar (to exclude diabetic nephropathy).
- Chest X-ray (to exclude bronchial carcinoma, lymphoma. Also to see bilateral pleural effusion, pericardial effusion).
- ANA, anti-ds DNA (if suggestive of SLE).
- p-ANCA and c-ANCA (if suspicion of vasculitis).
- HBsAg and anti HCV screening.
- Complement C3 and C4.
- Renal biopsy (to see type of GN, whether minimal, membranous or membranoproliferative).

Complications of Nephrotic Syndrome

- Hypercoagulability leading to venous thrombosis (renal vein thrombosis, DVT) and pulmonary embolism.
- Infection —pneumococcal infection, cellulitis, streptococcal infection.
- Hyperlipidaemia causing atherosclerosis.
- Oliguric renal failure.
- Bilateral pleural effusion, pericardial effusion.
- Loss of vitamin D binding protein causing osteomalacia.

Treatment

General Treatment

- Fluid restriction—depending on previous day's output and patient's oedema status (average—500-1000 mL/day).
- Salt restriction.
- High-protein diet (2 g/kg/day). In severe case, intravenous salt poor albumin may be given.
- Diuretic—Loop diuretic (frusemide, bumetanide). If needed, potassium sparing diuretic (spironolactone) may be added.

Specific Treatment

- In minimal change disease:
  - Prednisolone 60 mg/m^2 body surface (maximum 80 mg/day) for 4–6 weeks, then 40 mg/m^2 every alternate day for 4–6 weeks.
  - Or, prednisolone 1mg/kg/day up to response (urine protein free), then tapering the dose in next three months.

- If relapse after withdrawal of steroid, it should be given again with gradual withdrawal. Some patients may require low-dose maintenance dose (5–10 mg/day) for 3–6 months.
- If frequent relapse or need high-dose steroid or incomplete response to steroid—cyclophosphamide (2.0 mg/kg/day for 8–12 weeks) and mycophenolate mofetil with low-dose steroid.

- In membranous glomerulopathy:
  - Inj. methylprednisolone—500–1000 mg IV for 3 days, then oral prednisolone 0.5 mg /kg/ day for 27 days in 1st, 3rd and 5th month and Tab. cyclophosphamide 2 mg/kg/day or chlorambucil 0.2 mg/kg/day for 30 days in 2nd, 4th and 6th month.
  - Ciclosporin and mycophenolate mofetil with oral steroid may be used.
  - Anti CD20 antibody (rituximab) may be given. It improves renal function, reduce proteinuria and increase serum albumin.
- In focal and segmental glomerulosclerosis:
  - Symptomatic and supportive treatment.
  - Tab prednisolone 1 mg /kg /day for 3 months, then taper. Total duration of treatment is at least about 6 months to 1 year.
- In mesangiocapillary or membranoproliferative GN—only symptomatic and supportive treatment.

Treatment of Underlying Cause if Any

Treatment of complications:

- If infection—antibiotic. Pneumococcal vaccine is recommended.
- To prevent venous thrombosis, prolong bed rest should be avoided. Prophylactic heparin if immobile (enoxaparin) may be given, followed by oral anticoagulant.
- For hyperlipidaemia—statin may be added.

GLOMERULONEPHRITIS

Definition

It means inflammation of the glomeruli.

Causes

Mostly immunologically mediated and there is deposition of antibodies in the glomerulus.

Types: 2 types

1. Primary glomerulopahty.
2. Secondary to systemic diseases.

Primary: On the basis of histology, it is divided into:

- Minimal change disease.
- Focal segmental glomerulosclerosis (FSGS).
- Focal segmental glomerulonephritis (FSGN).
- Membranous glomerulonephritis.
- IgA nephropathy.
- Mesangiocapillary glomerulonephritis (MCGN).
- Postinfectious glomerulonephritis.

Secondary: Due to diferrent systemic diseases.

- SLE.
- Goodpasture's syndrome
- Polyarteritis nodosa.
- Wegener's granulomatosis.
- Microscopic polyangitis
- Amyloidosis
- Bacterial endocarditis
- Diabetes mellitus
- Mixed essential cryoglobulinaemia.

Minimal Change Disease

- Common cause of nephrotic syndrome in children, but may occur in all ages.
- On light microscopy, there is no abnormality. On electron microscopy, there is fusion of podocyte foot process.
- No immune deposit. Progression to renal failure is rare.
- Good response to steroid and cytotoxic drugs.

Focal Segmental Glomerulosclerosis (FSGS)

- There is segmental scar in glomeruli, no acute inflammation, podocyte foot process fusion may be found. There is C3 and IgM deposition in the affected portions of glomerulus.
- Cause is unknown but may be related to HIV, heroin misuse, morbid obesity, reflux nephropathy, secondary to other GN.
- Mostly present as idiopathic NS. There is massive proteinuria, haematuria, hypertension.
- May progress to renal failure.
- Often resistant to steroid therapy, recurs after renal transplantation.

Focal Segmental Glomerulonephritis (FSGN)

- There is segmental inflammation and/or necrosis in some glomeruli with or without crescent formation.
- Small-vessel vasculitis is present. ANCA, ANA should be checked.
- Causes—occurs in systemic disease, e.g SLE, polyarteritis nodosa.
- Treatment—steroid and immunosuppressant

Membranous Glomerulopathy

- Common cause of NS in adult, predominantly in male.
- Causes—Idiopathic. May be secondary to SLE, bronchial carcinoma, drugs (penicillamine), heavy metals like mercury, HBV, HCV.
- Renal vein thrombosis is a common complication.
- May progress to CKD.
- Renal biopsy shows thickening of glomerular basement membrane, increased matrix deposition and glomerulosclerosis.
- There is granular subepithelial IgG deposit.
- Treatment—High-dose steroid and cyclophosphamide.

IgA Nephropathy

- It is a nephropathy of unknown cause characterized by mesangial IgA deposition. Also there is increased mesangial matrix and cells.
- There may be underlying liver disease.
- Usually presents with recurrent macroscopic haematuria and hypertension.

Mesangiocapillary Glomerulonephritis (MCGN)

- Also known as membranoproliferative glomerulonephritis (MPGN), characterized by an increase in mesangial cells, thickening of glomerular capillary walls and subendothelial deposition of immune complex and complement.
- Causes—infection (hepatitis C), autoimmunity, subacute bacterial endocarditis, cryoglobulinaemia
- Usual presentations are proteinuria and haematuria.
- 3 subtypes:
  1. **Type 1** (immunoglobulin type)—Characterized by deposition of immunoglobulins within the glomeruli. It is associated with chronic infections, autoimmune diseases and monoclonal gammopathy.
  2. **Type 2** (Complement type)—Characterized by deposition of complement in the glomeruli, associated with inherited or acquired abnormalities in the complement pathway. It is also called '**dense deposit disease**', in which there is deposition of electron-dense deposits within the GBM. This type is associated with partial lipodystrophy (loss of subcutaneous fat on face and upper trunk).
  3. **Type 3**—in which neither immunoglobulins nor complement are deposited in the glomeruli. This is associated with healing in HUS and TTP.
- Treatment—primary cause should be treated. Mycophenolate mofetil or cyclophosphamide may be used in immunoglobulin deposits. No specific treatment in complement deposition type.

Rapidly Progressing Glomerulonephritis (RPGN)

- Also known as 'crescentic glomerulonephritis' characterized by rapid loss of renal function over days to weeks.
- Causes:
  - Goodpasture's disease (due to anti-GBM antibody),
  - Small vessel vasculitis.
  - Also SLE, IgA and other nephropathies.
- Rapid-onset disease may be associated with relatively little proteinuria.
- Renal biopsy shows crescentic, necrotising lesions within the glomerulus.
- Treatment—depends on the underlying cause:
  - In Goodpasture's disease, plasma exchange with steroid and immunosuppressant.
  - In ANCA associated vasculitis and SLE, treated with corticosteroid and immunosuppressant.

Post-infectious Glomnerulonephritis

- Usually due to poststreptococcal infection, may be due to other infections.
- There is diffuse proliferation of endothelial and mesangial cells, infiltration of neutrophils and macrophages with or without crescent formation.
- Patient usually presents with severe sodium and fluid retention, hypertension, haematuria, oliguria.
- Usually resolves spontaneously.

ACUTE GLOMERULONEPHRITIS (ACUTE NEPHRITIC SYNDROME)

Definition

Acute glomerulonephritis (AGN) is the acute inflammation of the glomeruli characterized by haematuria, hypertension, oedema (periorbital, leg or sacral) and oliguria. Urine shows proteinuria and red cell cast.

Pathology: Histological pattern shows cellular proliferation (mesangial and endothelial) with inflammatory cell infiltration (neutrophils, macrophages).

Causes

- Infection—poststreptococcal (commonest). Other infections—infective endocarditis, infectious mononucleosis, HBV.
- Primary glomerular disease—diffuse proliferative GN, IgA nephropathy, membranous GN, focal segmental GN.
- Systemic disease—SLE, Henoch-Schonlein purpura, Goodpasture syndrome, vusculitis, cryoglobulinaemia.
- Shunt nephritis.

Clinical Features

Symptoms

- Puffiness of face.
- Scanty urination.
- High coloured, smoky or red urine.
- Anorexia, nausea, vomiting.
- Fever, lethargy and weakness.
- Features of hypertension.
- Features of complication—breathlessness and cough (due to LVF).

Signs

- Periorbital swelling, puffy face.
- Oedema.
- High BP.
- Evidence of skin infection (healing skin lesion).

Investigations

Routine

- Urine R/E—looks smoky, mild to moderate proteinuria, RBC, RBC cast and granular cast (RBC cast is suggestive of AGN).
- 24 hours urinary total protein (increases, but less than 3 g/litre) and volume is less.
- Blood urea, serum creatinine and serum electrolytes.
- CBC (leucocytosis may be present).
- ASO titre (high in poststreptococcal glomerulonephritis).
- Throat swab for C/S to find streptococcal infection.
- USG of whole abdomen (to look for renal pathology).

- CXR (cardiomegaly or pulmonary oedema, if LVF).
- Serum C3—reduced.

Other investigations—according to suspicion of cause—
- ANA, Anti-ds DNA (in SLE).
- P-ANCA, c-ANCA (in vasculitis).
- HbsAg, Anti HCV.
- Renal biopsy may be done in some cases.

Complications

- Acute renal failure.
- Hypertension and its complications, such as acute LVF, CVD, hypertensive encephalopathy.
- Fluid and electrolyte imbalance.
- Nephrotic syndrome.
- May lead to chronic glomerulonephritis.

Treatment

- Rest.
- Fluid restriction (total intake 500–1000 mL/day).
- Salt restriction.
- Protein restriction (if urea and creatinine are high).
- Diuretic (frusemide)—to relieve oedema.
- If hypertension—antihypertensive.
- Antibiotic—oral phenoxymethyl penicillin or erythromycin for 7–10 days, especially in PSGN.
- Management of complication—pulmonary oedema, hypertensive encephalopathy, ARF (dialysis may be needed).
- If recovery is slow—corticosteroid may be given.

POST-STREPTOCOCCAL GLOMERULONEPHRITIS

Posts treptococcal glomerulonephritis (PSGN) is a common cause of acute nephritic illness caused by group A beta haemolytic streptococci, can occur due to other infection.

Common in children than adult. There is a latent period of about 10 days (1–3 weeks) after a throat infection or longer after skin infection (such as infected scabies, impetigo, furunculosis), suggesting an immune mechanism. Even streptococcal otitis media or cellulitis can lead to PSGN.

It is common with poor personal hygiene, overcrowding and skin infection like scabies.

Clinical Features

- Periorbital puffiness.
- Reduced urinary volume.
- Anorexia, nausea, vomiting, fever, malaise.
- Hypertension.

Investigations

- Urine R/E—red or smoky, proteinuria, haematuria, etc.
- Blood urea and serum creatinine.

- Serum electrolytes.
- Evidence of streptococcal infection (high ASO, culture of throat swab).
- Low serum C3 and C4.
- USG of renal system.

Treatment

- Complete rest.
- Salt and fluid restriction.
- Diuretic (frusemide).
- Antibiotic—oral phenoxymethyl penicillin for 7-10 days.
- Spontaneous cure may occur in 7-10 days.

IgA NEPHROPATHY

Symptoms

Common in children and young male, 20-35 years of age:

- Most patients are asymptomatic, presents with recurrent microscopic or even gross haematuria following a viral respiratory or GIT infection.
- Haematuria is universal, proteinuria is usual and hypertension is common.
- Five percent may develop nephrotic syndrome.
- In some cases, progressive loss of renal function, leads to end stage renal failure (20%) in 20 years.

Investigations

- Urine RME—shows RBC.
- Urea, creatinine, electrolytes.
- Serum IgA, immune complex estimation
- USG of renal system, plain X-ray KUB.
- CT scan of renal system.
- Kidney biopsy—shows focal proliferative glomerulonephritis. Immune deposits are present diffusely in mesangium of all glomeruli and contain usually IgA.

Treatment

Episodic attack resolves spontaneously:

- Steroid is indicated if-patient has proteinuria over 1-3 g/day, mild glomerular change and good renal function.
- In progressive renal disease—prednisolone plus cyclophosphamide for 3 months, then prednisolone plus azathioprine.
- Combination of ACE inhibitor and ARB should be given to all cases.
- Tonsillectomy may be helpful, if recurrent tonsillitis.

POLYCYSTIC KIDNEY DISEASE

Definition

Polycystic kidney disease (PKD) is an inherited cystic disease of kidney.

Types

Two types

1. Adult polycystic kidney disease (APKD)—It is inherited as autosomal dominant, common type, males and females are equally affected.
2. Infantile polycystic kidney disease (IPKD)—It is inherited as autosomal recessive, rare, associated with cyst in other organs and hepatic fibrosis. Fatal in first year due to hepatic or renal failure.

Clinical Features

- May be asymptomatic (renal mass, detected during routine examination).
- Discomfort, pain or heaviness in the loin.
- Recurrent painful haematuria (due to rupture of cyst in renal pelvis or infection).
- Recurrent UTI.
- Acute loin pain or renal colic.
- Features of hypertension (usually after 20 years of age) and its complications.
- Features of renal failure.
- CVA (usually subarachnoid haemorrhage, due to rupture of berry aneurysm. Sometimes, may be cerebral haemorrhage as a complication of hypertension).

Other Features of PKD

- Cystic liver—30%, but hepatic dysfunction is rare. There may be cyst in spleen, ovary and pancreas.
- Berry aneurysm in circle of Willis—10% (may rupture causing subarachnoid haemorrhage).
- Polycythaemia (due to increased erythropoietin secretion).
- Renal stone—10% cases (usually calcium oxalate, urate).
- Renal neoplasm—rarely.

Investigations

- USG of whole abdomen.
- Urine RME—haematuria, proteinuria.
- CBC—polycythaemia.
- Renal function—urea, creatinine, electrolytes.
- IVU.
- CT scan.

Causes of Death in PKD

- Chronic renal failure (in 1/3rd cases).
- Intracerebral haemorrhage (subarachnoid haemorrhage).
- Myocardial infarction.

Treatment of PKD

- Control of hypertension.
- Control of UTI.
- Plenty of fluid.
- Salt (there may be salt looser in some cases).
- For renal pain or if large cyst—ultrasonic guided aspiration or laparoscopic cystectomy may be done.
- Treatment of renal failure. Dialysis and even renal transplantation may be done.
- Genetic counseling.
- Family screening—USG of the abdomen should be done in all members of the family over 20 years of age to detect cysts.
- MR angiogram to detect berry aneurysm may be considered in some cases, where other members have history of subarachnoid haemorrhage.

Cystic Diseases of Kidney

- Simple cyst, usually congenital.
- Acquired cyst, after dialysis (in chronic renal failure).
- Polycystic kidney disease.
- Medullary sponge kidney—cause is unknown, but not genetic. Cyst is confined to the papillary collecting ducts. Age 40–60 years, prognosis is good. Usually no hypertension or no renal failure.
- Medullary cystic disease—small cysts in cortical area or corticomedullary junction. Renal failure is common, hypertension may occur. Patients usually have polyuria and increased thirst and are salt loser.

ALPORT'S SYNDROME

It is hereditary disease of kidney inherited as X-linked dominant, autosomal dominant and rarely autosomal recessive.

Pathology

There is thickening of GBM with splitting of lamina densa.

Clinical Features

- Haematuria.
- Sensory neural deafness.
- Ocular abnormality.
- May cause renal failure at early age.

Treatment

- Symptomatic and supportive.
- Control of hypertension, if present—with ACE inhibitor.
- Management of renal failure.
- May need renal transplant.

ACUTE RENAL FAILURE

Definition

It is characterized by sudden deterioration of renal function occurring within days or weeks, associated with reduced urine volume, biochemically detected by high urea and creatinine level. It is usually reversible. It is also called acute kidney injury (AKI).

Causes

Prerenal

- Fluid loss—due to diarrhoea, vomiting, excessive sweating, etc.
- Blood loss—due to haemorrhage.
- Plasma loss in burn.
- Hypotension or decreased cardiac output—due to myocardial infarction, shock, vasodilator drug, heart failure.
- Rhabdomyolysis.
- Haemolytic uraemic syndrome.
- Hepatorenal syndrome.
- Renal artery occlusion or stenosis.
- Disease affecting arterioles.

Renal (Intrinsic Renal Disease)

- Acute tubular necrosis—due to toxin (contrast material) or septic renal failure (85%).
- Glomerular disease—MCGN, IgA nephropathy.
- Systemic disease—SLE, rheumatoid arthritis, systemic sclerosis, multiple myeloma, vasculitis.
- Tubulointerstitial disease (10%) due to drugs (NSAID, ciprofloxacin, allopurinol, sulfonamide, ciclosporin).

Postrenal

- Urethral—phimosis, paraphimosis, stricture, stone, blood clot, sloughed papilla.
- Bladder neck obstruction—prostatic hypertrophy, malignancy, stone.
- Bilateral ureteric calculus, following surgery, pelvic tumour, uterine prolapse, retroperitoneal fibrosis (due to radiation, idiopathic).

Clinical Features

- Scanty or no urination (oliguria or anuria).
- Features of water and electrolyte imbalance (hyperkalaemia, hyponatraemia).
- Features of metabolic acidosis.
- General—anorexia, nausea, vomiting.
- Neurological—drowsiness, confusion, hiccough, fit or convulsion, coma.

Investigations

- Urine RME.
- CBC, ESR.

- Serum urea, creatinine and electrolytes.
- Plain X-ray KUB.
- Chest X-ray.
- USG of abdomen.
- Complement—C3, C4.
- Others—according to suspicion of cause.

Treatment

- Restriction of fluid and salt.
- Restriction of protein.
- Maintenance of nutrition by carbohydrate and fat.
- Correction electrolytes (specially hyperkalaemia).
- Correction of acidosis (IV sodiumbicarbonate).
- Treatment of primary cause.
- Dialysis, if necessary.

CHRONIC KIDNEY DISEASE/CHRONIC RENAL FAILURE

Definition

Chronic kidney disease (CKD)/chronic renal failure (CRF) is the irreversible deterioration of renal function classically developing over months to years.

End stage renal disease or failure (ESRD): It is the stage when renal replacement therapy is compulsory either dialysis or renal transplantation, without which death is likely.

Causes of CKD

- Chronic glomerulonephritis (30–40%).
- Diabetes mellitus (20–40%).
- Hypertension (5–20%).
- Obstructive uropathy.
- Chronic pyelonephritis.
- Tubulointerstitial diseases (5–10%).
- Systemic diseases (5–10%), e.g. SLE, vasculitis.
- Renal artery stenosis (5%).
- Congenital and inherited (5%), e.g. polycystic kidney disease, Alport syndrome.
- Unknown (5–20%).

Clinical Features

- May be asymptomatic, until GFR falls below 30 mL/min/1.73 m^2 of body surface area. High urea and creatinine may be found on routine investigation.
- There may be hypertension, anaemia, proteinuria on routine urine examination.
- General features—early features may be nocturia, polyuria, anorexia, nausea, vomiting, diarrhoea, weakness, malaise, insomnia, breathlessness on exertion, paraesthesia, bone pain, oedema, amenorrhoea in woman, sexual dysfunction in man.
- In ESRD—general features are more severe and CNS symptoms may be more. Features like hiccough, pruritus, deep respiration (Kussmaul's respiration), muscular twitching, fit, drowsiness, even coma may occur.
- Other features—due to involvement of different systems of the body described below.

Bone Diseases (Renal Osteodystrophy)

- Osteomalacia (or ricket called renal ricket).
- Osteoporosis.
- Osteosclerosis (in vertebral body, giving rise to **Rugger- Jersey spine**).
- Osteitis fibrosa cystica.

Skin Disease

- Dryness, hyperpigmentation, ecchymosis.
- Pruritus—due to retention of nitrogenous waste products. Patient on dialysis, inadequate dialysis may have pruritus.

Gastrointestinal

- Anorexia, nausea, vomiting.
- Decreased gastric emptying, increased risk of reflux oesophagitis, peptic ulceration, acute pancreatitis and constipation.

Metabolic Abnormalities

- Hyponatraemia, hyperkalaemia, hypokalaemia.
- Metabolic acidosis.
- Hyperuricaemia and gout.
- Hypocalcaemia and hyperphosphataemia.
- Ipid abnormalities (hypercholesterolaemia, hypertriglyceridaemia).

Endocrine Abnormalities

- Secondary hyperparathyroidism, may be tertiary.
- Insulin—half life is prolonged. Insulin requirement in a diabetic patient decreases. But in advanced CKD, insulin resistance may occur.
- Hyperprolactinamia.
- Others—increased LH, decreased testosterone, oligo or amenorrhoea (in female), growth retardation in children, abnormal thyroid hormone levels (hypothyroidism).

Muscle Dysfunction

- Generalized myopathy (due to poor nutrition, vitamin D deficiency, electrolyte imbalance, hyperparathyroidism).
- Muscle cramps.
- Restless leg syndrome.

Nervous System

Peripheral nervous system

- Polyneuropathy—both motor and sensory.
- Median nerve compression in the carpal tunnel due to beta 2 microglobulin related amyloidosis.

CNS

- Clouding of consciousness, convulsion, coma.
- Asterixis (flapping tremor), myoclonus.
- Dialysis disequlibrium syndrome, dialysis dementia.
- Psychiatric problems—anxiety, depression, phobia, phychosis.

Autonomic Dysfunction

- Postural hypotension, fixed heart rate.
- Urinary retention or incontinence.
- Constipation.
- Impotence.

- Pupillary constriction.
- Gustatory sweating.
- Anhydrosis.

Cardiovascular

- Hypertension.
- Cardiac failure.
- Pericarditis, pericardial effusion, constrictive pericarditis.
- Uraemic cardiomyopathy.
- Increased atherosclerosis.
- Coronary artery calcification.

Respiratory: Pulmonary oedema (uraemic lung) due to fluid overload.

Malignancy: Incidence of renal cell carcinoma is increased.

Calciphylaxis (calcific uraemic arteriolopathy): Rare but life threatening.

Stages of CKD

Stage	*Features*	*GFR (mL/min/1.73m²)*
1	Kidney damage with normal or ↑ GFR	≥90
2	Kidney damage with mildly ↓ GFR	60–89
3	Moderately ↓ GFR A&B	30–59 (A: 45–59, B: 30 –44)
4	Severely ↓ GFR	15–29
5	Kidney failure	<15 (or dialysis)

Causes of Anaemia in CKD

- Erythropoietin deficiency.
- Diminished erythropoiesis due to toxic effects of uraemia on bone marrow.
- Reduced dietary intake and absorption of haematinics (iron, vitamin B12, folic acid).
- Reduced red cell survival.
- Increased blood loss due to capillary fragility, poor platelet function, occult gastrointestinal bleeding and blood loss during haemodialysis.
- Erythropoietin therapy may cause anaemia (by pure red cell aplasia).

Investigations in CKD

- Urine R/E—(to see pus cells, RBC or WBC cast, proteinuria, haematuria).
- CBC and PBF—shows normocytic, normochromic anaemia.
- Renal function tests (blood urea, serum creatinine—high).
- Creatinine clearance.
- Serum electrolytes.
- Serum calcium (low) and phosphate (high).
- Serum uric acid (high).
- Plain X-ray abdomen (renal stone, kidney size).
- USG of the KUB (shows shrunken kidneys. Kidneys may be large in size in diabetic glomerulosclerosis, amyloidosis, polycystic kidney diseases and bilateral hydronephrosis).

- CT scan of abdomen.
- IVU (rarely needed).
- Isotope renogram.
- Renal biopsy—to find out the cause.
- Other investigation according to suspicion of cause—ANA and anti-ds DNA for SLE, screening for hepatitis B and C, HIV.

Treatment of CKD

General measures

- Fluid restriction.
- Salt restriction.
- Protein restriction (0.5 g/kg body weight/day). Severe protein restriction is avoided.
- Smoking should be stopped.
- Social and psychological support.

Symptomatic and Supportive

1. Hypertension—Target control of BP is 130/80 mmHg (if UTP <1 g/day) and 125/75 mm Hg (if UTP >1 g/day).
2. ACE inhibitor or ARB and diuretics may be added.
3. Calcium channel blocker (verapamil or diltiazem) is added, if goal is not achieved.
4. Dyslipidaemia—statin.
5. Hyperkalaemia:
   - Dietary restriction of potassium intake (fruits like banana, orange, coconut).
   - Drugs causing potassium retention should be stopped (eg. spironolactone).
   - Injection 10% calcium gluconate 10 cc over 5 minutes, may be repeated.
   - Glucose and insulin (50 mL of 50% glucose I/V plus injection insulin 10 units), may be repeated.
   - Correction of acidosis.
   - Occasionally, ion exchange resins may be needed (calcium resonium powder 15 g in 1 cup water to be taken orally.
   - If all measures fail or hyperkalaemia is severe, haemodialysis or peritoneal dialysis may be needed.
6. Acidosis—sodium bicarbonate (1.26% IV) or calcium carbonate (up to 3 g/day). Bicarbonate should be maintained above 22 mmol/L.
7. Calcium and phosphate control and suppression of PTH
8. For hypocalcaemia—calcitriol or alpha-calcidol and calcium supplementation.
9. For hyperphosphataemia—dietary restriction of phosphate containing food (milk, cheese, eggs) and phosphate binding drugs like calcium carbonate, aluminium hydroxide and lanthanum carbonate may be used with food to prevent phosphate absorption.
10. Anaemia:
    - Erythropoietin. Side effects are hypertension and thrombosis.
    - Blood transfusion may be given in severe anaemia.
11. Male erectile dysfunction:
    - Testosterone deficiency should be corrected.
    - Phosphodiesterase inhibitors like sildenafil may be used.

12. Treatment renal osteodystrophy:
    - Calcium supplement.
    - 1-α hydroxylated synthetic analogue of vitamin D.
13. Treatment of primary cause, if any—diabetis mellitus, hypertension, APKD, removal of obstruction in obstructive uropathy.

Definitive treatment: Renal replacement therapy, such as:
- Hemodialysis.
- Hemofiltraiton.
- Peritoneal dialysis.
- Renal transplantation.

Indications of Renal Replacement Therapy

- Serum creatinine >600–800 μmol/L (7–9 mg/dL).
- Hyperkalaemia (plasma potassium >6 mmol/L despite medical treatment).
- Metabolic acidosis pH <7.25, HCO_3 <10 mmol/L.
- Fluid overload and pulmonary oedema.
- Uraemic pericarditis or encephalopathy.

Reversible Factors in CKD

- Hypertension.
- Reduced renal perfusion, such as renal artery stenosis.
- Hypotension due to drug treatment, sodium and water depletion, poor cardiac function.
- Urinary tract infection.
- Urinary tract obstruction.
- Other systemic infections that causes increased catabolism and urea production.
- Nephrotoxic drugs.

Indications of Urgent Dialysis

- Severe hyperkalaemia.
- Pulmonary oedema or severe fluid overload.
- Severe metabolic acidosis.
- Uraemic pericarditis.
- Uraemic encephalopathy.
- Toxicity with a dialyzable poison (methanol, barbiturate, etc.).
- Recurrent vomiting due to uraemia.

Haemodialysis

Complications

- Hypotension during dialysis due to fluid removal and hypovolaemia. There may be chest pain and leg cramps.
- Cardiac arrhythmia due to potassium and acid base shift.
- Haemorrhage due to anticoagulation. Also venous needle disconnection may lead to haemorrhage.
- Anaphylactic reaction.

- Sepsis, usually involving vascular access devices.
- Pulmonary oedema due to fluid overload.
- Haemolytic reactions.
- Air embolism.
- Hard water syndrome.
- Dialysis disequilibrium due to over rapid correction of uraemia.

Contraindication of HD

- CCF with low ejection fraction.
- Generalized atherosclerosis with poor vascular access for AVF.
- These cases are treated by peritoneal dialyses.

Peritoneal Dialysis

Complications

- Peritonitis due to infection.
- Infection around the catheter site.
- Constipation.
- Massive pleural effusion (dialysate leak through a diaphragmatic defect into the thoracic cavity). Dialysate may leak into the scrotum down through a patent processus vaginalis.
- Failure of peritoneal membrane function due to long-term CAPD.
- Sclerosing peritonitis (potentially fatal).

Contraindications

- Previous peritonitis causing peritoneal adhesions.
- Presence of a stoma (e.g. colostomy).
- Active intra-abdominal sepsis (absolute contraindication).
- Abdominal hernia.
- Comorbidities like coronary artery disease, congestive cardiac failure.

Complications of Long-term Dialysis

- Cardiovascular disease
- Sepses are the leading cause of death in long-term dialysis patient.
- Dialysis associated ascites.
- Dialysis amyloidosis.
- Dialysis associated arthropathy.

Contraindications of Renal Transplantation

Absolute

- Active malignancy—a period of at least 2 years of complete remission recommended for most tumours.
- Active vasculitis or recent anti-GBM disease.
- Severe heart disease or any severe comorbid condition.
- Severe occlusive aortoiliac vascular disease.

Relative

- Age—while practice varies, transplants are not routinely offered to very young children (<1 year) or older people (>75 years).
- High risk of disease recurrence in the transplant kidney.
- Disease of the lower urinary tract—in patients with impaired bladder function, stricture urethra. (An ileal conduit may be considered.)
- Significant comorbidity.

To prevent rejection: Combination of—

- Ciclosporin or tacrolimus
- Azathioprine or mycophenolate mofetil/ sirulumus or evanolimuas.
- Prednisolone.

Complications after Renal Transplantation

- Acute rejection—characterized by rising of creatinine, fever, loin pain, hypertension, swelling of the graft. Urine shows protein, lymphocyte, and renal tubular cells. Occurs in 10-30% cases within 6 months. Graft biopsy shows immune cell infiltrate and tubular damage. Treatment—high-dose methylprednisolone, resistant cases may require antithymocyte globulin or ALG or OKT3 may be used.
- Chronic rejection—after 6 months. The patient presents with gradual rise of creatinine and proteinuria. Graft biopsy shows vascular change, fibrosis and tubular atrophy. It is not responsive to increased immunosuppression.
- Infection—CMV, pneumocystis jiroveci, oral candidiasis, polioma virus. Bacterial infection is common in first few months.
- Complication of immunosuppressive drugs including steroid.
- Acute tubular necrosis (ATN)—it is the commonest cause of cadaveric graft dysfunction (40—50%). It is associated with a worse long-term outcome and predisposes to rejection.
- Technical failures—occlusion or stenosis of the arterial anastomosis, occlusion of the venous anastomosis and urinary leaks.
- Posttransplantation lymphoproliferative disorder—EBV associated malignancies (such as lymphoma) are common in patients who received biological agents and in children.
- Chronic allograft nephropathy—most common cause of late graft failure.
- Malignancy—skin tumour (including basal and squamous cell carcinoma), renal, cervical and vaginal.
- Hypertension.
- Atherosclerosis.
- Recurrence of renal disease.

For complication of renal transplantation (remember the formula - 'TROPICAL') -

T—Thrombosis of graft kidney artery and vein.
R—Rejection of graft kidney.
O—Obstruction of graft ureter with perinephric hematoma, seroma, urinoma, or lymphocele.
P—Primary disease recurrence. Common recurrence is MCGN type II (80–100%).
I— Infection. Bacterial (any, TB), viral (CMV, chicken pox, polioma virus), fungal (*Cryptococcus neoformans*), parasite (*Pneumocystis jeroveci, Isopspora cycloporium*, Microspora, Giardia).
C—Ciclosporin toxicity and other imunosupressive drugs toxicities.
A—Acute tubular necrosis.
L—Leakage of graft ureter due to error or ischaemia.

ACUTE INTERSTITIAL NEPHRITIS

Definition

It is an acute inflammation of tubulointerstitium of the kidney commonly due to drugs, but may be also systemic infection and toxin.

Causes

1. Drugs (70%):
   - Penicillin and NSAID (commonest).
   - Sulfonamide, allopurinol, cephalosporin, rifampicin, phenytoin, diuretic (frusemide).
2. Others:
   - Autoimmune.
   - Infection (acute bacterial pyelonephritis, tuberculosis, CMV and hanta virus, leptospirosis).
   - Multiple myeloma.
   - Idiopathic.

Symptoms

- Fever, arthralgia, skin rash, bodyache.
- Oliguria, anuria.
- Features of renal failure.

Investigations

- Urine RME—RBC, proteinuria, leucocyte. Eosinophil count is also very high in 70% cases.
- CBC—very-high eosinophil.
- Urea, creatinine, electrolytes.
- USG of KUB.
- IVU.
- CT scan.
- Renal biopsy—shows infiltration of eosinophil, polymorph and lymphocyte surrounding the tubules and blood vessels. Tubular necrosis may be seen.

Treatment

- Offending drug should be stopped.
- Prednisolone 1 mg/kg/day. Taper the dose when clinical improvement.
- Correction of electrolytes.
- Dialysis may be required if renal failure.

ANALGESIC NEPHROPATHY

Definition

It is the chronic tubulointerstitial nephritis with papillary necrosis following prolonged use of NSAID.

Symptoms

It is twice as common in women and is an important cause of chronic renal failure.

- Hypertension—60% of patients are hypertensive at presentation.

- Sloughing of renal papillae can cause urinary tract obstruction, which may precipitate acute renal failure.
- Recurrent UTI are common.
- There may be sterile pyuria.
- Also, occasionally a salt-losing nephropathy.

Diagnosis can be made by the history and characteristic appearances on intravenous urography. There is risk of tumors of uroepithelium. Total recovery of renal function occur in 25% patients.

Investigations

- Urine RME.
- Blood urea, creatinine and electrolytes.
- USG of KUB.
- CT scan of abdomen.
- IVU.
- Renal biopsy is sometimes performed, which shows interstitial fibrosis and tubular atrophy.

Treatment

- Withdrawal of offending drug.
- Maintain a fluid intake of 2–3 liter per day.
- Control of hypertension and biochemical correction.

RENAL TUBERCULOSIS

Genitourinary TB develops in approximately 5% cases after pulmonary TB. It is usually due to haematogenous spread to the renal cortex during the primary infection.

Symptoms

- General features of TB—fever, malaise, night sweat, weight loss.
- Haematuria, frequency of micturition, burning, urgency.
- Features of complication—retention of urine due to urethral stricture.
- Features of CKD.

Investigations

- Urine RME—pus cells, RBC.
- Urine for routine C/S—shows sterile pyuria.
- Urine for AFB, mycobacterial C/S.
- MT.
- Chest X-ray.
- USG of KUB.
- CT scan of renal system.
- IVU.

Treatment

- Standard anti Koch's therapy, to be continued for 9 months to 1 year.
- Steroid may be added.
- Surgery—if obstructive uropathy or if kidney is severely damaged.

URINARY TRACT INFECTION

Definition

Urinary tract infection (UTI) is the infection involving the urinary tract.

Types

- Upper UTI—involving the pelvis called pyelonephritis.
- Lower UTI—acute urethritis and cystitis.

Causative Organisms

- Bacteria—*E. coli, Proteus, Pseudomonas,* streptococci, *Staphylococcus epidermidis, Klebsiella.*

Some Common Definitions

- Cystitis—infection of the urinary bladder,
- Urethritis—infection of the urethra.
- Prostatitis—infection of the prostate.
- Pyelonephritis—infection of the renal pelvis.
- Sterile pyuria—presence of pus cell in the urine but no organism is detected in routine culture.
- Asymptomatic bateriuria—presence of organism in urine on culture, but no symptom.
- Significant bacteriuria—presence of bacteria in urine >1,00,000/mL.

Spectrum of Presentations of UTI

- Asymptomatic bacteriuria
- Symptomatic acute urethritis and cystitis
- Acute pyelonephritis.
- Acute prostatitis.
- Septicaemia (usually Gram-negative bacteria).

Predisposing Factors for UTI

1. Incomplete bladder emptying:
   - Bladder outflow obstruction due to—benign prostatic enlargement, prostate cancer, urethral stricture.
   - Vesicoureteric reflux.
   - Uterine prolapse.
   - Neurological problems—multiple sclerosis, spina bifida, diabetic neuropathy.
2. Foreign body:
   - Urethral catheter or ureteric stent.
   - Urolithiasis.
3. Loss of host defense:
   - Atrophic urethritis and vaginitis in postmenopausal women.
   - Diabetes mellitus.
4. Instrumentation of the bladder may also introduce organisms.

Clinical Features

Features of lower UTI (cystitis and urethritis):

- Frequency of micturition.

- Urgency and scalding pain in the urethra during micturition (dysuria).
- Suprapubic pain during and after voiding.
- Intense desire to pass more urine after micturition, due to spasm of the inflamed bladder wall (strangury)
- Urine that may appear cloudy and have an unpleasant odour.
- Haematuria, microscopic or visible.
- Systemic symptoms are usually slight or absent.
- Prostatitis is suggested by perineal or suprapubic pain, pain on ejaculation and prostatic tenderness on rectal examination.

Investigations

- Urine RME and C/S (midstream urine).
- CBC, ESR.
- Blood sugar.
- Serum urea, creatinine and electrolytes.
- USG of KUB.
- In some cases—CT scan or MRI, IVU, micturating cystourethrogram may be needed.

Management

1. Antibiotic should be given. Ideally urine for C/S should be sent and then empirically antibiotic can be started while awaiting for the result. May be changed after the report.
2. Antibiotic:
   - Trimethoprim 200 mg 12 hourly or
   - Nitrofurantoin 100 mg 6 hourly or
   - Ciprofloxacin 500 mg 12 hourly or
   - Cephalexin 250 mg 6 hourly or
   - Co-amoxiclav 625 mg 8 hourly or amoxicillin 500 mg 8 hourly.
   - Penicillin and cephalosporin are safe in pregnancy, but trimethoprim, sulfonamide, quinolone and tetracycline should be avoided.
   - Antibiotic should be continued for 7–14 days.
3. Seriously ill patients may require intravenous therapy with cephalosporin, quinolone or gentamicin or amikacin.
4. General measures:
   - Plenty of fluid of at least 2 L/day.
   - Regular complete emptying of bladder.
   - Good personal hygiene.
   - Emptying of bladder before and after sexual intercourse.
   - Cranberry juice may be effective.

Asymptomatic Bacteriuria

This is defined as >1,00,000 organisms/mL of urine of apparently healthy asymptomatic patients. Approximately 1% of children under 1 year age, 1% of schoolgirls, 0.03% of schoolboys and men, 3% of nonpregnant women and 5% of pregnant women have asymptomatic bacteriuria. It is increasingly common in those over 65 years.

Usually no treatment is necessary. 30% will develop infection in 1 year. Treatment is required in infants, pregnant woman and those with urinary tract abnormality. Antibiotic should be given as described in UTI.

Urethral Syndrome

In some patients, commonly female, there are symptoms of urethritis and cystitis, but no bacteria is found in culture. It is called urethral syndrome.

It may occur in postcoital bladder trauma, vaginitis, atrophic vaginitis or urethritis in elderly. If there is sterile pyuria, chlamydia and tuberculosis should be excluded.

Persistent or Recurrent UTI

If the causative organism persists on repeated culture despite antibiotic, or if there is reinfection with any organism after an interval, then an underlying cause is more likely to be present (see predisposing factors of UTI written above) and more detailed investigation should be done. In women, recurrent infections are common. Recurrent UTI may cause permanent renal damage.

Treatment

- Underlying cause should be treated.
- Suppressive antibiotic therapy should be given continuously for several months—trimethoprim 100 mg at night or nitrofurantoin 50 mg at night or co-amoxyclav (250/125 mg) at night.

Sterile Pyuria

It means presence of pus cells in urine but no organism on routine culture. Causes:

- Renal tuberculosis.
- Partially treated UTI with antibiotic.
- Nongonococcal urethritis.
- Schistosomiasis.
- Tubulointerstitial nephritis.
- Papillary necrosis.
- Renal calculi.

ACUTE PYELONEPHRITIS

Definition

It is the infection of renal pelvis and surrounding parenchyma. Small abscesses are often evident in the renal parenchyma.

Predisposing Factors

- Diabetes mellitus.
- Chronic urinary tract obstruction.
- Analgesic nephropathy.
- Sickle cell disease.
- Renal cyst or scarring.
- A necrotising form of pyelonephritis with gas formation, 'emphysematous pyelonephritis', is occasionally seen in patients with diabetes mellitus.

Causes

Usually ascending infection from urinary bladder. Organisms are same as lower UTI (see above).

Clinical Features

- Classic **triad** of loin pain, fever and tenderness over the kidneys.
- Systemic symptoms—fever with chill and rigor, nausea, vomiting, hypotension.
- Associated symptoms of cystitis or urethritis—dysuria, frequency, urgency.

Investigations

- Urine RME and C/S (midstream urine).
- CBC, ESR.
- Blood sugar.
- Serum urea, creatinine and electrolytes.
- USG of KUB.
- In some cases—CT scan or MRI, IVU, micturating cysto-urethrogram may be needed.

Treatment

- Antibiotic (as in UTI).
- Plenty of fluid, if needed, IV infusion.
- Treatment of primary cause.
- If obstruction is present—percutaneous nephrostomy or ureteric stenting may be done.

Complications

- Pyeonephrosis or abscess formation.
- Emphysematous pyelonephritis.
- Chronic pyelonephritis.
- Septic shock.

Differential Diagnoses

- Acute appendicitis.
- Diverticulitis.
- Cholecystitis.
- Salpingitis.
- Ruptured ovarian cyst or ectopic pregnancy.

CHRONIC PYELONEPHRITIS

It is occurs from recurrent urinary infection due to vesico-ureteric reflux and infection acquired in infancy or early childhood. It is called **reflux nephropathy.**

Vesicoureteric reflux: Normally vesicouereteric junction acts as a one way valve. No urine enters during voiding as the urinary bladder contracts. If the valve is incompetent, there is reflux of urine into the ureter during voiding of urine. As a result, there is infection and reflux of infected urine that leads to kidney infection and damage.

In kidney, there is gross scarring, reduction of size, narrowing of cortex and medulla, atrophy with impaired kidney function.

Investigations

- Urine RME and C/S.
- Serum urea, creatinine and electrolytes.
- USG of KUB.
- IVU
- Micturating cystourethrogram.
- CT scan—shows irregular renal outline, clubbed calyces and reduction of renal size.

Treatment

- Antibiotic according to C/S for prolong period (3–6 months).
- Removal of any obstruction.
- If pyeonephrosis in one kidney—nephrectomy may be needed.

RENAL ARTERY STENOSIS

Renal artery stenosis is a rare disorder, in which the patient usually presents with hypertension.

Causes

- Atherosclerosis in elderly.
- Fibromuscular dysplasia in young, aged 15–30 years. Commonly presents with hypertension, more in women.
- Rare causes–vasculitis, thromboembolism, aneurysm of renal artery.

Pathophysiology: Renal artery stenosis causes reduction in renal perfusion, which activates the renin-angiotensin system, leading to increased circulating levels of angiotensin II. This causes vasoconstriction and increases aldosterone secretion from the adrenals, which causes sodium retention by the renal tubules.

- In atherosclerosis, there is small vessel disease which affects the kidneys. As the stenosis becomes more severe, global renal ischaemia leads to shrinkage of the affected kidney and may cause renal failure. Patients with peripheral vascular disease, coronary artery disease, congestive cardiac failure and aortic aneurysm are at high risk of developing renal artery stenosis.
- In fibromuscular dysplasia, there is hypertrophy of the media (medial fibroplasia), which narrows the artery but rarely leads to total occlusion. Irregular narrowing (beading) may occur in the distal renal artery and also intrarenal branch.
- Rarely, may occur as a complication of large-vessel vasculitis, such as Takayasu's arteritis, polyarteritis nodosa.

Clinical Features

- May be asymptomatic.
- Hypertension.
- Renal failure, if there is bilateral disease.
- Deterioration in renal function when ACE inhibitors or ARBs are used or acute pulmonary oedema.

Signs

- Renal bruit present on auscultation.

NB: Renal artery stenosis is more likely if:

- Hypertension is severe, of recent onset or difficult to control.
- Kidneys are asymmetrical in size
- There is peripheral vascular disease of the lower limbs
- There is renal impairment (with bilateral disease).
- Renal function has deteriorated on ACE inhibitors or angiotensin II receptor blockers
- Flash pulmonary oedema (It means pulmonary oedema without any underlying cardiopulmonary disease) occurs repeatedly.

Investigations

- Doppler ultrasonography—shows asymmetrical size (>1.5 cm) of two kidneys.
- CT angiography.

- MR angiography (gadolinium enhanced) reveals a characteristic string of beads appearance in fibroplasia.
- Serum urea, creatinine and electrolytes (hypokalaemia due to hyperaldosteronism).
- Elevated plasma renin activity.
- Previously, rapid sequence IVU was done—shows delayed entry and delayed clearance of dye of the affected kidney.

Treatment

1. If due to fibromuscular dysplasia—angioplasty, sometimes with stenting plus antihypertensive.
2. If due to atherosclerosis:
   - Antihypertensive drug, supplemented with statins and low-dose aspirin.
   - Angioplasty and stenting may be tried in atherosclerotic disease.

NB: Interventions to correct the vessel narrowing is done:

- In young patients (age below 40), those in whom blood pressure cannot easily be controlled with antihypertensive agents;
- Those who have a history of 'flash' pulmonary oedema or
- Accelerated phase (malignant) hypertension.
- Those in whom renal function is deteriorating.

NEPHROCALCINOSIS

Definition

It is the diffuse deposition of calcium within the renal parenchyma. Commonly, it involves the medulla and rarely the cortex.

Causes

- Distal renal tubular acidosis.
- Chronic pyelonephritis.
- Hypercalcaemia (due to hyperparathyroidism, multiple myeloma, sarcoidosis, hypervitaminosis D).
- Medullary sponge kidney.
- Healed renal tuberculosis.
- Milk alkali syndrome.

Clinical Features

- May be asymptomatic.
- Frequency of micturition.
- Haematuria.
- Polyuria.
- Recurrent renal colic or pain in the loin.
- Recurrent UTI.

Investigations

- Urine R/E and C/S.
- Renal function tests (blood urea, creatinine, creatinine clearance).
- Plain X-ray KUB.
- USG of KUB.
- IVU.
- Serum calcium, phosphate, uric acid.
- Other investigations according to the suspicion of causes.

Treatment

- Treatment of primary cause.
- Plenty of fluid.

RENAL CALCULUS

It may occur in any part on urinary tract like kidney, ureter and bladder.

Causes

- Dehydration (in hot environment).
- Hypercalcaemia due to any cause.
- Hypocalciuria.
- Hyperoxaluria.
- Hyperuricaemia and hyperuricosuria.
- Infection—by *Proteus mirabillis* (causes magnesium ammonium phosphate stone).
- Cystinuria.
- Renal tubular acidosis.
- Primary renal disease (APKD, medullary sponge kidney).
- Drugs—some drugs may promote stone formation. Calcium stone (by loop diuretic, antacid, vitamin C and D), uric acid stone (by thiazide, salicylate).
- Bladder stone—usually due to bladder outflow obstruction e.g. urethral stricture, BEP, presence of foreign body (e.g. catheter, nonabsorbable suture).

Types

- Oxalate stone.
- Phosphate stone.
- Mixed.
- Magnesium ammonium phosphate.
- Rarely, cystine, uric acid, xanthine stone.

Clinical Features

1. Renal stone:
   - May be asymptomatic.
   - Renal colic.
   - Haematuria.
   - UTI.
2. Ureteric stone:
   - Severe pain radiating from loin to groin (towards right iliac fossa or testes in male or labia in female.
   - Sweating, vomiting and pallor.
   - Patient is restless.
3. Vesical calculus:
   - Frequency, dysuria, haematuria.
   - Anuria and painful bladder distension, if bladder outflow obstruction.

Stag horn calculus: It is so called because calculi fill all or most of the collecting system, giving it a stag horn-like appearance. It is a phosphate stone, formed in alkaline urine.

Investigations

- Urine RME and C/S.
- Serum urea, creatinine and electrolytes.
- Serum uric acid, calcium, phosphate.
- Plain X-ray KUB.
- USG of KUB.
- CT KUB.
- IVU.
- Sometimes retrograde pyelography.

Radiolucent stones: Radiolucent stones are uric acid stone and xanthine stone. All other stones are radioopaque.

NB:
- In alkaline urine—formation of calcium, phosphate stone is more.
- In acidic urine—formation of uric acid and cysteine stone is more.

Treatment

1. During pain—diclofenac 75 mg IM or pethidine IM.
2. Plenty of fluid, if needed IV infusion.
3. Small stone <0.5 cm may pass out spontaneously.
4. Stone >1 cm—surgical interference.
   - Either ESWL (extracorporal shock wave lithotripsy).
   - Ureteroscopy with YAG laser can be used for large stone.
   - Percutaneous nephrolithotomy may be used.
   - Pyelolithotomy—for pelvic stone.
   - Ureterolithotomy—for ureteric stone.
   - Open surgery is rarely needed.
5. Treatment of primary cause.

RENAL CELL CARCINOMA

The tumor is adenocarcinoma, arising from proximal tubular epithelial cells. Common in elderly, 65–75 years. Males affected twice more than females.

Symptoms

- Commonly presents with **triad** of painless hematuria, loin pain or heaviness and palpable mass in loin.
- In 10% cases, tumour may be bilateral.
- In 20% cases, PUO may be the only manifestation, due to secretion of pyrogen by the tumour.
- Hypertension.
- Features of metastasis—By lymphatic to the para-aortic lymph node. By blood borne metastasis to lung, brain and bone.
- General features—malaise, anorexia, weight loss, features of polycythaemia.

Investigations

- Urine for RME—shows RBC.
- Urine for malignant cells.
- CBC—normocytic and normochromic anaemia, polycythaemia due to excess erythropoietin.
- Urea, creatinine, electrolytes—hypokalaemia may occur,
- S. calcium—hypercalcaemia due to bony metastasis or secretion of parathormone like substance.
- USG of renal system—investigation of choice.
- IVU, CT scan.
- Biopsy—USG or CT guided.

Treatment

1. Nephrectomy:
   - Radical—that includes perirenal fascial envelope and ipsilateral paraaortic lymph nodes is done, if possible.
   - Partial—may be done if tumour is small (<4 cm).
3. Radiotherapy is not helpful.
4. Chemotherapy—interferon and interlukin-2 may be used in metastasis. Two new drugs—sunitinib and pazopanib (tyrosine kinase inhibitor). Also, temsirolimus and evarolimus may be used.

WILMS' TUMOUR (NEPHROBLASTOMA)

It is the malignant tumour of kidney that occurs in childhood. Mainly occurs within the first 3 years of life, usually unilateral, but may be bilateral.

Clinical features: May be asymptomatic.

- Abdominal mass.
- Rarely, haematuria.

Investigations

- Ultrasonography.
- CT or MRI.

Treatment: A combination of nephrectomy, radiotherapy and chemotherapy. Overall, the 5-year survival rate is 90%.

TUMOURS OF URINARY BLADDER

Two types
- Benign—papilloma.
- Malignant—carcinoma, usually transitional cell.

Papilloma of Urinary Bladder

Patient usually presents with painless haematuria. Diagnosis is confirmed by cystoscopy. Treatment is also cystoscopic removal.

Carcinoma of Urinary Bladder

The tumour usually arises from the transitional epithelium causing transitional cell carcinoma. It is rare under the age of 40, common in males.

Causes

- Exposure to industrial carcinogens like aromatic amines, aniline dyes and aldehydes.
- Cigarette smoking.
- Chronic inflammation or irritation due to stones or schistosomiasis.

Clinical Features

- Painless, macroscopic haematuria.
- Symptoms of obstruction, depending on the site of involvement.
- Dysuria, urinary frequency, urgency.
- Features of metastasis.

Investigations

- Urine for RME—shows RBC.
- USG.
- Cystoscopy (usually flexible cystoscopy under a local anaesthetic) is mandatory.
- CT urogram is the gold standard.
- IVU.
- CT scan of the abdomen, pelvis and chest for staging.

Treatment

- Transurethral resection of tumour by endoscope.
- Intravesical chemotherapy with mitomycin C is usually administered postresection to prevent tumour recurrence, or may be given as a prolonged course to treat multiple low-grade bladder tumours.
- Patient with carcinoma *in situ* have a high risk of progression to invasive cancer. This responds well to intravesical Bacille Calmette Guérin (BCG) treatment, but more radical treatment may also be needed if this is unsuccessful.
- Regular check cystoscopies are required to look for evidence of recurrence.
- If recurrences with superficial disease—usually treated with further resection and diathermy, but if unsuccessful, a cystectomy may be needed.
- In invasive bladder tumour—radical cystectomy with urinary diversion into an incontinent ileal conduit or a continent catheterisable bowel pouch.

BENIGN ENLARGEMENT OF PROSTATE

Benign enlargement of prostate (BEP) is common in men over the age of 60 years, cause is unknown.

Microscopically, hyperplasia affects the glandular and connective tissue elements of the prostate. Enlargement of the gland stretches and distorts the urethra, obstructing bladder outflow.

Clinical Features

- Frequency of urination, usually first noted as nocturia.
- Urgency of micturition and urge incontinence.
- Difficulty in voiding urine due to obstruction of the urethra by the prostate, postvoid dribbling.
- Hesitancy, poor urinary flow, reduction of flow after straining and sensation of incomplete emptying.
- Sometimes acute urinary retention with painful distended bladder.
- Occasionally, severe haematuria due to rupture of prostatic veins.
- Per rectal examination—shows gland is smooth, soft in consistency with prominent median sulcus.

Investigations

- USG is the simplest test with PVRV (postvoidal residual volume).

Treatment

1. Patients with moderate prostatic symptoms can be treated medically.
2. Drugs:
   - Alpha-blocker—tamsulosin 0.4 mg daily at night.
   - Finasteride or dutastaride—it is a competitive inhibitor of 5 α-reductase, which causes conversion of testosterone to dihydrotestosterone. This androgen is responsible for prostatic growth and enlargement. Finasteride decreases prostatic volume with an increase in urine flow.
3. Surgery—if deterioration in renal function or upper tract dilatation.
   - Transurethral resection of prostate (TURP).
   - Other therapy—Holmium laser enucleation.
   - Open prostatectomy, if suspicion of malignancy.

PROSTATIC CARCINOMA

It is common in elderly, accounts for 7% of all cancers in men and is the sixth most common cancer in the world.

Histologically, the tumour is an adenocarcinoma. Hormonal factors may be responsible for developing the cancer.

Clinical Features

- May be asymptomatic.
- Frequency of micturition, nocturia, haematuria.
- Features of metastasis—back pain, weight loss or anaemia.
- PRE—shows stony hard irregular gland with loss of median sulcus.
- Incidental histological finding after prostatectomy.

Investigations

- USG, preferably TRUS (transrectal ultrasound scan).
- Serum prostate specific antigen (PSA)—PSA >4 ng/mL is abnormal, but between 4 and 10 ng/mL can be due to benign hypertrophy and cancer.
- If PSA is >10 ng/mL, prostatic biopsy shows cancer in >50% cases.
- Other investigations to see metastasis—isotope bone scan, CT or MRI scan of the involved organ.
- Endorectal coil MRI helps detect extraprostatic extension.

Treatment

1. If the disease is confined to the gland—radical prostatectomy, radical radiotherapy or brachytherapy (implantation of small radioactive particles into the prostate).
2. Locally extensive disease—radiotherapy with or without androgen ablation therapy.
3. Metastatic disease:
   - Orchidectomy.
   - Luteinizing hormone-releasing hormone (LHRH) analogues, such as buserelin or goserelin are equally effective.
   - Abiraterone inhibits CYP17A1, an enzyme necessary for androgen production and has been used for aggressive prostate cancer.
   - Androgen receptor blockers—bicalutamide or cyproterone acetate, may also prevent tumour cell growth.
4. Nonhormonal chemotherapy is usually unhelpful.

RENAL TUBULAR ACIDOSIS

Definition

Renal tubular acidosis (RTA) is characterized by severe metabolic acidosis associated with failure to acidify urine either due to defect in excretion of hydrogen ion by distal tubule or due to failure of absorption of bicarbonate by proximal tubule. There is failure of acidification of urine despite severe metabolic acidosis.

Types: 4 types

Type-1 or distal tubular acidosis (DTA): It is due to failure of hydrogen ion excretion in the distal tubule. There is acidosis, hypokalemia and inability to lower urine pH<5.3, despite severe acidosis.

Causes

- Congenital (AD, AR or sex linked).
- Autoimmune disease—Sjogren's syndrome, chronic active hepatitis, primary biliary cirrhosis, SLE.
- Drugs—amphotericin B, lithium, NSAID, lead.
- Others—amyloidosis, cryoglobulinaemia, obstructive uropathy, renal transplant rejection.

Treatment: Sodium bicarbonate, potassium supplement and treatment of underlying cause.

Type-2 or proximal tubular acidosis (PTA): It is due to failure of sodium bicarbonate reabsorption in the proximal tubule. Common in children.

Causes

- Congenital (AD).
- Cystinosis.
- Wilson's disease.
- Tyrosinaemia.
- Glycogen storage disease type 1.
- Multiple myeloma.
- Hyperparathyroidism.
- Drugs (degraded tetracycline, carbonic anhydrase inhibitor).

In PTA, there is proximal tubular defect resulting in aminoaciduria, glycosuria, phosphaturia, called "Fanconi syndrome".

Treatment: Sodium bicarbonate in high dose, potassium supplement and treatment of underlying cause.

Type-3: Combined proximal and distal tubular acidosis (rare).

Type-4: It is also called hyporeninaemic hypoaldosteronism. Main features are hyperkalaemia and acidosis in a patient with mild chronic kidney disease usually caused by tubulointerstitial disease and diabetes mellitus. Plasma renin and aldosterone are low.

Treatment

- Fludrocotisone—0.1 mg daily.
- Sodium bicarbonate.
- Diuretic or ion exchange resin to remove potassium.

Clinical Features of RTA

1. Distal RTA: May present at any age.
   - In children, the patient presents with failure to thrive.
   - Adult presents with renal colic, muscular weakness due to hypokalaemia, osteomalacia.
2. Proximal RTA:
   - Features of acidosis.
   - Polydipsia, polyuria.
   - Hypokalaemia, myopathy.
   - Ricket or osteomalacia.

NB: Diagnosis is suspected in any patient with hyperchloraemic acidosis and can be confirmed by early morning urinary pH >5.3. In patient in whom the diagnosis is suspected, but no acidosis is present, an acid load test using ammonium chloride is done. Following this test, if urinary pH remains >5.3 despite a plasma bicarbonate of 21 mmol/L, diagnosis is confirmed.

CHAPTER

10 Rheumatology

CHAPTER CONTENTS

INTRODUCTION

- Arthralgia means painful joint without swelling.
- Arthritis means painful joint with swelling.
- Seropositive arthritis—means RA test is positive (e.g. rheumatoid arthritis).
- Seronegative arthritis—means RA test is negative (e.g. ankylosing spondylitis, psoriatic arthritis, Reiter's syndrome, enteropathic arthritis).
- Monoarticular—single joint involved.
- Oligoarticular or pauciarticular—2-4 joints involved.
- Polyarticular—5 or more joints involved.
- Migratory or fleeting—arthritis involving one joint then involving another.
- Acute arthritis means <6 weeks duration and chronic means >6 weeks duration.
- Features of inflammatory arthritis are pain at rest, morning stiffness, joint inflammation and loss of function.
- Noninflammatory (mechanical) arthritis is more painful with activity and improves on rest.

Causes of Monoarthritis

As follows (remember the mnemonic: **GRASP-TH**)—

- **G:** Gout.
- **RA:** Reactive arthritis.
- **S:** Septic arthritis (pyogenic).
- **P:** Pseudogout.
- **T:** Trauma, tuberculous.
- **H:** Haemophilia (in early age).

NB: In children, septic arthritis and JIA are the common causes. Also, haemophilic arthritis, leukaemia and osteomyelitis may occur.

Causes of Polyarthritis

1. Infective (bacterial and viral).
2. Inflammatory:
   - Rheumatic fever.
   - RA and its variants.
   - Seronegative arthritis (ankylosing spondylitis, Reiter syndrome, enteropathic arthritis and psoriatic arthritis).
   - JIA (<16 years).
   - Collagen disease (SLE, dermatomyositis, systemic sclerosis and polyarteritis nodosa).
3. Degenerative (osteoarthrosis).
4. Metabolic (gout, pseudogout).
5. Neuropathic arthropathy (Charcot joint).
6. Haematological—haemophilic arthritis, Henoch-Schönlein purpura.
7. Others—polymyalgia rheumatica, sarcoidosis, haemochromatosis, acromegaly and hypertrophic.

Spondyloarthropathy or Spondarthritis: It is a group of inflammatory arthritis characterized by:
1. Seronegative rheumatoid factor (RA test is negative).
2. Sacroiliitis and inflammatory spondylitis.
3. Asymmetrical inflammatory oligoarthritis (lower>upper limbs, bigger joints are involved).
4. Inflammatory enthesitis.
5. Absence of nodules and other extra-articular features of rheumatoid arthritis.
6. Typical overlapping extra-articular features:
   - Mucosal inflammation—conjunctivitis, buccal ulceration, urethritis, prostatitis, bowel ulceration.
   - Pustular skin lesions and nail dystrophy.
   - Anterior uveitis.
   - Aortic root fibrosis (AR, conduction defects).
   - Erythema nodosum.
7. Familial association (high in HLA-B27).

Diseases in Spondyloarthropathy
- Ankylosing spondylitis.
- Reiter's syndrome or reactive arthritis.
- Enteropathic arthritis (Crohn's disease and ulcerative colitis).
- Psoriatic arthritis.

ANKYLOSING SPONDYLITIS

Definition

It is a chronic inflammatory arthritis characterized by progressive stiffening and fusion of axial skeleton. Common in young adult, 20–40 years, Male:Female = 3:1.

Causes

Unknown, probably autoimmune.

Symptoms

- Low back pain with morning stiffness, worse in the morning and with inactivity. Pain improves after exercise.
- Peripheral arthritis occurs in 10% cases.

Signs

- There is loss of lumbar lordosis, thoracic kyphosis and compensatory hyperextension of neck (in advanced stage, question mark "?" or stoped posture).
- The patient is unable to look up and unable to turn to any side without movement of whole body.
- Restricted movement of spine in all directions.
- Standing against the wall, the patient is unable to make contact between the occiput of head and the wall.
- Sacroiliitis, Achilles tendinitis and plantar fasciitis are present.

Extra-articular Manifestations of Ankylosing Spondylitis

- Eyes—Anterior uveitis (iritis), conjunctivitis.
- Heart—Aortic regurgitation, mitral regurgitation, conduction defect.
- Lungs—Upper lobe fibrosis, cavitation, chest pain (pleuritic), reduced chest expansion, pulmonary hypertension and cor pulmonale.
- Prostatitis (80%), usually asymptomatic.
- Neurological—cauda equina syndrome (weakness of lower limb, loss of sphincter and rectal control with saddle sensory loss).
- Others—plantar fasciitis, Achilles' tendinitis, amyloidosis and osteoporosis.

Investigations

- X-ray of SI joints and spine (lumbosacral, dorsal and cervical).
- CBC with ESR (may be high).
- CRP (may be high).
- Rheumatoid factor is negative.
- HLA-B27 is positive in 90% cases.

X-ray Shows

- Sacroiliitis—irregularities, marginal sclerosis, later on fusion of SI joint.
- In lumbodorsal spine—squaring of vertebrae, syndesmophyte formation, ossification of anterior longitudinal ligament, bamboo spine appearance.

Treatment

- Exercise is the mainstay. Swimming is the best.
- Prolong sitting or inactivity should be avoided.
- NSAID to relieve pain.
- Physiotherapy.
- DMARD—sulphasalazine or methotrexate (MTX)
- In persistent active inflammation, anti-TNF drug therapy (e.g. etanercept, infliximab).
- Local steroid injection may be given for persistent plantar fasciitis, other enthesopathies and peripheral arthritis.
- High-dose steroid may be needed for acute uveitis.
- Orthopedic measures—may be needed for severe hip, knee or shoulder restriction.

RHEUMATOID ARTHRITIS

Definition

It is a chronic inflammatory arthritis characterized by bilateral symmetrical involvement of small peripheral joints, with recurrence and remission. Common in young, more in females, in 30–40 years.

Cause

It is an autoimmune disease.

Diagnostic Criteria

ARA (American Rheumatism Association) criteria:
1. Morning stiffness (>1 hour).
2. Arthritis of three or more joint areas.
3. Arthritis of hand joints and wrist.
4. Symmetrical arthritis.
5. Rheumatoid nodule.
6. Positive RA factor.
7. Typical radiological changes (erosion or periarticular osteopenia).

NB: When four or more criteria are present, there is 93% sensitivity and 90% specificity. Duration is 6 weeks or more.

Symptoms

- Polyarthritis involving small joints of hands and feet.
- Morning stiffness lasting >1 hour, improves with activity.
- There may be extra-articular manifestations.

Signs in Hand

- Spindle-shaped swelling of proximal interphalangeal (PIP) joints of both hands.
- Swan-neck deformity, boutonniere deformity, Z-deformity of thumb, ulnar deviation and dorsal subluxation of ulnar styloid.
- Wrist joints may be swollen with synovial thickening.
- Generalised wasting of small muscles of hands with dorsal guttering.

Signs in Other Joints

- In foot—loss of arch causing flat foot, dorsal subluxation of metatarsophalangeal joints.
- In knee—there may be synovitis, swelling, tenderness, Baker's cyst in popliteal fossa.

NB: Distal interphalangeal joint (DIP) is not involved

Extra-articular Manifestations in RA

1. Eye—episcleritis, scleritis, scleromalacia, scleromalacia perforans, keratoconjunctivitis sicca.
2. Respiratory—pleurisy, pleural effusion , fibrosing alveolitis, nodules in the lungs (Caplan's syndrome).
3. Cardiac—pericarditis (30%), pericardial effusion (rare), chronic constrictive pericarditis (rare).

4. Vasculitis—digital arteritis, nail fold infarct, Raynaud's phenomenon, visceral arteritis, mononeuritis multiplex, myoderma gangrenosum.
5. Neurological—entrapment neuropathy, commonly carpal tunnel syndrome (compression of median nerve) and tarsal tunnel syndrome (compression of posterior tibial nerve), peripheral neuropathy, mononeuritis multiplex, cervical cord compression (due to atlantoaxial subluxation).
6. Haematological— anaemia, thrombocytosis, pancytopenia (due to hypersplenism in Felty's syndrome).
7. Others—lymphadenopathy, splenomegaly, osteoporosis, general features (malaise, fever, weakness, loss of weight, wasting), amyloidosis.

Investigations

- CBC with ESR (ESR is high, pancytopenia occurs in Felty's syndrome).
- RA test and RW test.
- Anti-CCP antibody (cyclic citrullinated peptide).
- X-ray of hands and other involved joints, chest X-ray.
- Others—CRP (high).

Objective of the Treatment

- Relief of symptoms by rest, NSAID and physiotherapy.
- Suppression of activity and progression of disease by disease modifying antirheumatic drug (DMARD).
- Restoration of function of affected joint.

Treatment

- Relief of symptoms—rest and NSAID.
- Suppression of activity and progression—by disease modifying antirheumatic drug (DMARD).
- Physiotherapy.
- Patient's education.
- Surgical treatment may be needed.

DMARDs

- First choices are methotrexate or sulphasalazine.
- Other drugs—chloroquine, hydroxychloroquine, leflunomide, azathioprine and ciclosporin.
- Biological agents—These are highly expensive, used only when there is failure of 2 DMARDs.
- DMARD should be started from the beginning, if no effect in 6–12 weeks, combination with methotrexate and sulphasalazine may be given. Prednisolone 7.5–10 mg may be added.

Methotrexate—7.5–10 mg, in a fixed day weekly (up to 25 mg). Folic acid 5 mg/day should be given on the next day. Folinic acid is more preferable.
Side effects—anorexia, nausea, vomiting (prevented by using antiemetic before starting the drug). Periodic check up—CBC, liver function test (SGPT) and renal function test (creatinine) should be done.

Sulphasalazine—started with low dose, increase the dose every weekly. Initially, 250 mg (½ tablet) twice daily for 1 week. Then 500 mg (1 tablet) twice daily for 1 week. Then 1,000 mg (2 tablets) twice daily to be continued (maximum dose 2–3 g daily).

Side effects—GIT upset (anorexia, nausea, vomiting, diarrhoea), skin rash, Stevens Johnson syndrome, reversible sterility in males, blood dyscrasia (agranulocytosis, megaloblastic anaemia and haemolytic anaemia). Periodic check up—FBC, liver function test (SGPT) and renal function test (creatinine), every 1-3 months.

Chloroquine—250 mg daily as a single dose.
Side effects—Anorexia, nausea, vomiting, skin rash. Prolonged use may cause neuromyopathy and ocular toxicity. To reduce ocular toxicity, the drug can be given for 10 months in a year.

Hydroxychloroquine—200-400 mg daily. Used alone in mild disease or as an adjuvant with other DMARD.

Leflunomide—100 mg daily for 3 days, then 10-20 mg daily.
Side effects—Skin rash, diarrhoea, reversible alopecia, hepatotoxicity, carcinogenic and teratogenic. Periodic blood checkup is mandatory.

SJÖGREN SYNDROME

Definition

It is an autoimmune disorder characterized by dryness of eye (keratoconjunctivitis sicca) and dryness of mouth (xerostomia) with nonerosive arthritis. Fibrosis and atrophy of the salivary glands occur. There is infiltration of lymphocytes and plasma cells in lacrimal and salivary glands.

Types: 2 Types

1. Primary—Not associated with collagen disease (sicca syndrome).
2. Secondary—Associated with collagen disease (commonly RA).

Clinical Features

Common in females, F:M = 9:1, 40–50 years.

- Dryness of mouth and eyes.
- Arthralgia and nonprogressive arthritis.
- Raynaud phenomenon.
- Dysphagia.
- In lung—pulmonary diffusion defect and fibrosis.
- Renal (renal tubular acidosis, nephrogenic diabetes insipidus).
- Vasculitis.
- Others (fever, weakness, lymphadenopathy and neuropathy, fit, depression).
- Lymphoma—increased incidence of non-Hodgkin
- B cell lymphoma. (It is associated with 40-fold risk).
- May be associated with other autoimmune disease like thyroid disease, myasthenia gravis, PBC, autoimmune hepatitis.

Investigations

1. CBC (high ESR).
2. Schirmer test (a strip of filter paper is placed inside lower eyelid. In normal people, at least 6 mm is wet in 5 minutes. In Sjögren syndrome <5 mm).
3. Biopsy of lip or salivary gland (lymphocytic and plasma cell infiltration).
4. Rose Bengal staining of eyes shows punctate or filamentary keratitis.
5. Antibody test:
   - RA test (positive in 90%).
   - ANA (positive in 60–70%).
   - Anti-Ro (SS-A, positive in 70%. It can cross placenta causing congenital complete heart block).
   - Anti-La (SS-B).

Treatment

- Artificial tear (hypromellose), contact lens, oral hygiene, artificial saliva, oral gel and chewing gum.
- Stimulation of saliva flow by sugar-free chewing gum or lozenges may be helpful.
- Oral candidiasis should be treated promptly.

- Vaginal dryness is treated with lubricants, such as K-Y jelly.
- Hydroxychloroquine (2–3 mg/kg daily, may improve the flow of tear).
- Treat the primary cause.
- Extraglandular and MSK manifestations may respond to steroid. Immunosuppressive drugs can be added.

SYSTEMIC SCLEROSIS (SCLERODERMA)

Definition

It is a connective tissue disease characterized by fibrosis and degenerative changes in skin, blood vessels and internal organs.

Types: 2 Types

1. Diffuse cutaneous systemic sclerosis (DCSS, 30%)—Skin involvement of trunk and extremities above the knee and elbow. Fibrosing alveolitis and renal involvement are more in DCSS who have topoisomarase 1 antibody.
2. Limited cutaneous systemic sclerosis (LCSS, 70%)—Skin involvement only at the extremities, hands, feet or forearm may be involved. CREST is a localized type of systemic sclerosis. Pulmonary hypertension is more common in limited disease.

Other Varieties (Localized)

- Scleroderma sine scleroderma—involves internal organ without skin lesion.
- Morphoea—localized, well-demarcated plaque with central hypopigmentation and tethering of skin, usually in extremities and face.
- Linear—skin involvement usually in lower limbs.

Pathology or Pathogenesis

- Vascular change—There is intimal proliferation, vessel wall inflammation and endothelial damage.
- Fibrotic change—Fibrosis in dermis and internal organs.

Clinical Features

Common in female (F:M = 4:1), age 30–50 years.

- Raynaud's phenomenon—90–97% cases. May occur before other symptoms.
- Tightening and thickening of skin of hands and other parts of the body.
- Arthralgia and arthritis (nonerosive inflammatory).
- Heartburn (reflux oesophagitis), dysphagia, odynophagia.
- Occasional diarrhoea and constipation (blind-loop syndrome).
- Shortness of breath, cough (DPLD).

Investigations

Diagnosis is usually clinical:

1. CBC and ESR (high).
2. Serology:
   - RA test (positive in 20–30% cases).
   - ANA (positive in 70% cases).
   - Anti-topoisomerase 1 or anti-Scl-70 (positive in 30% in diffuse type).
   - Anti-centromere antibody (positive 60% in CREST and 10% in diffuse systemic sclerosis).
3. Skin biopsy for histopathology.

4. Others—according to the organ involvement.
   - Urine R/E (may be proteinuria).
   - X-ray of hands (deposition of calcium around the fingers, erosion, resorption of phalanges and disorganization of joints).
   - Chest X-ray (DPLD and honeycomb lung).
   - CT scan of the chest (to detect DPLD).
   - Lung function tests (restrictive lung disease).
   - Barium swallow (reduction of peristalsis, narrowing and dilatation. Hiatus hernia may be present).
   - Barium follow through.
   - Motility study may be done.
   - ECG.

Histological Findings of Skin Biopsy

- Thinning or absence of epidermis.
- Excess collagen and fibrosis of dermis, loss of appendages in dermis.
- Chronic inflammatory cells infiltration.

Systemic Features

1. Skin changes:
   - Hands—initially nonpitting oedema of fingers, then skin becomes shiny, thick and tight, distal skin creases disappear. Erythema and tortuous dilatation of capillary loops in nail bed.
   - Face and neck—thinning of lips, radial furrowing, microstomia.
   - Skin in other parts of the body (thick, tight, hyper or hypopigmented and vitiligo).
   - Skin of chest is tight and thick (looks like Roman breast plate).
2. Raynaud's phenomenon, cause tissue ischaemia, skin ulceration, infarction and pulp atrophy at fingertips.
3. Joints and muscles—arthralgia, morning stiffness, flexor tenosynovitis, flexion contracture or deformity. Proximal or distal muscle weakness and wasting.
4. Gastrointestinal:
   - Oesophagus—50% involvement. Dysphagia and odynophagia due to reflux oesophagitis, sliding hiatus hernia, constriction or secondary achalasia, dysmotility.
   - Stomach—early satiety, gastric outlet obstruction and recurrent occult upper GIT bleeding causing "watermelon stomach".
   - Intestine—hypomotility, bloating, distension, intestinal obstruction or pseudoobstruction, blind-loop syndrome, diarrhoea and wide-mouth diverticula in colon. Rarely, a serious disorder called pneumatosis cystoides intestinalis, in which there is radiolucent cyst or streaks in the wall of small intestine due to air in the intestinal wall (detected by plain X-ray abdomen) can occur. The patient presents with severe abdominal pain.
5. Liver—primary biliary cirrhosis may be associated.
6. Respiratory:
   - DPLD, pulmonary hypertension and cor pulmonale. Pulmonary hypertension is more common in limited type.
   - Others—pneumonitis, rarely pleural effusion, alveolar cell carcinoma.

7. Heart—dysrrhythmia, conduction defect, heart failure, cardiomyopathy, myocardial fibrosis and pericardial effusion.
8. Kidneys (20% involvement):
   - Renal failure in advanced stage.
   - Malignant hypertension.
9. Endocrine:
   - Hypothyroidism (thyroid gland fibrosis).
   - Impotence.
10. Neurological:
   - Entrapment neuropathy.
   - Facial nerve palsy.
   - Autonomic dysfunction.

Treatment

1. General measures for Raynaud's phenomenon:
   - Avoidance of cold (use of gloves or mittens), smoking should be stopped.
   - Regular exercise, cleanliness of digital ulcer.
   - Drugs to be avoided—beta-blocker, ergotamine, oral contraceptive.
   - Antiplatelet—aspirin or clopidogrel.
   - Calcium antagonist (nifedipine), ACE inhibitor, ARB (valsartan) may be effective.
   - If no response or severe—prostacycline analogue epoprostenol infusion intermittently.
   - If still no response—surgical treatment. If gangrene—amputation of fingers or toes.
2. For arthritis—NSAID's, physiotherapy.
3. Other treatment:
   - Penicillamine—reduces cross-linking of collagen.
   - Methotrexate (weekly—7.5–15 mg).
   - Ciclosporin or interferon-γ, recombinant human relaxin.
4. Treatment of complications:
   - DPLD—cyclophosphamide or azathioprine with steroid.
   - Hypertension—ACE inhibitor.
   - Pulmonary hypertension—oral vasodilator, warfarin. In advanced case—prostacycline or oral endothelin receptor antagonist (bosentan, sitaxentan) should be given.
   - CCF—diuretic, digoxin. In selected case, heart-lung or single lung transplantation.
   - Reflux oesophagitis—proton pump inhibitor, prokinetic drug.
   - Blind-loop syndrome—broad-spectrum antibiotic.
   - If renal involvement—ACE inhibitor may be helpful.
   - Myositis—corticosteroid and cytotoxic drugs may be needed.

Prognosis

Depends on type, age, sex, involvement of internal organ and extent of skin involvement. Bad prognostic factors are:

- Diffuse cutaneous systemic sclerosis.
- Elderly patient.
- Male sex.
- Involvement of internal organs (especially kidney, lung and heart). Proteinuria, high ESR, low gas transfer of carbon monoxide and pulmonary hypertension.

Limited Cutaneous Systemic Sclerosis (CRST or CREST)

- Prognosis is relatively better
- Usually mild.
- Seventy percent show 10-year survival.
- Pulmonary hypertension may develop later on.

Diffuse Type

- Seventy percent show 5-year survival.
- Death due to cardiac, renal and pulmonary involvement.

MIXED CONNECTIVE TISSUE DISEASE

Definition

Mixed connective tissue disease (MCTD) is a group or combination of features of systemic sclerosis, SLE and polymyositis (or other collagen disease, e.g. rheumatoid arthritis). It is better to be called overlap syndrome.

Clinical Features

Common in females, third to fourth decade, rare in children and elderly.

- Patients usually present with Raynaud's phenomenon, muscular pain or weakness, swollen, oedematous hands and fingers.
- Later, features like sclerodactyly, calcinosis, cutaneous telangiectasia.
- Skin rash of SLE or dermatomyositis.
- Pulmonary fibrosis, pulmonary hypertension, Sjogren's syndrome, may develop later. Synovitis.
- Lung involvement occurs in 85% cases, but frequently asymptomatic. Carbon monoxide (CO) transfer is diminished. Pleurisy is common. Pulmonary hypertension is the common cause of death.
- In 25% cases—renal disease usually membranous glomerulonephritis may occur.
- Gastrointestinal involvement occurs in 70% cases.
- In heart, pericarditis (30%), myocarditis, arrhythmia, mitral valve prolapse may occur.

Investigations

1. Anti-RNP antibody—high.
2. ANA—positive with a speckled nucleolar pattern.
3. Anti-scl 70—may be positive.
4. CPK may be high.
5. Other investigations:
   - CBC and ESR (high).
   - X-ray chest—shows reticulonodular shadow.
   - Barium swallow.
   - Skin biopsy.

Treatment

- Prednisolone, which responds quickly. 10-years survival in 80% cases.

GOUTY ARTHRITIS

Definition

Gout is a disorder of purine metabolism characterised by hyperuricaemia associated with deposition of monosodium urate monohydrate (MSUM) crystals giving rise to arthritis, tenosynovitis, bursitis and tophaceous deposit.

Types

- **Primary**—cause is unknown.
- **Secondary**—due to some underlying disease.

Secondary Causes of Gout

1. Defect in renal excretion:
   - Renal failure.
   - Drugs include diuretic (thiazides), low-dose aspirin, pyrazinamide, ethambutol, nicotinic acid, ethanol, cytotoxic drug and cyclosporine.
   - Hyperparathyroidism.
   - Myxoedema.
   - Chronic lead poisoning.
   - Down syndrome.
   - Lactic acidosis (alcohol, starvation, toxaemia of pregnancy and type I glycogen storage disease).
2. Excess production of uric acid:
   - Myeloproliferative disease.
   - Lymphoproliferative disease.
   - Psoriasis.
   - Excess purine synthesis (hypoxanthineguanine phosphoribosyltransferase [HGPT] deficiency, glucose-6-phosphatase deficiency).
   - Idiopathic (common)

Symptoms (In Typical Acute Attack)

Severe pain mainly metatarsophalangeal (MTP) joint of great toe, usually in early morning or late night, awaking the patient from sleep. Other joints are also involved.

Signs

- The joint is red, swollen and tender.
- In advanced or chronic tophaceous gout, repeated attack may cause deformity with swelling of joints commonly DIP joints. There may be tophus.

Investigations

Diagnosis is clinical and investigation should be done to find out any secondary causes.

- CBC, ESR (high) and leukaemia should be excluded.
- CRP (high).
- Urea and creatinine (to exclude CRF).

- Blood sugar and lipid profile.
- To confirm—aspiration of joint fluid to see MSUM crystal. In chronic case, X-ray of joint may be done.

NB: MSUM crystal is needle shaped and negatively birefringence (in pseudogout, calcium pyrophosphate dehydrate—CPPD crystals are rhomboid and positively birefringence).

Treatment

1. **In acute attack**
   - For pain—NSAID (indomethacin, naproxen and diclofenac by oral or suppository).
   - If no response—colchicine 0.5 mg 2–3 times daily till relief of symptoms (side effects—nausea, vomiting, diarrhoea and abdominal pain).
   - In severe arthritis—aspiration and intra-articular steroid may be given.
2. **Other treatment**
   - Dietary restriction—avoid uric acid containing diet (liver, kidney, brain, red meat, cabbage, cauliflower, carrot and spinach). No need of strict dietary restriction.
   - Avoid alcohol and starvation.
   - Reduction of weight in obese patient (slow reduction).
   - Avoid precipitating drugs.
   - Allopurinol—staring dose 100 mg/day, 50 mg in elderly and renal failure. Febuxostat is alternate to allopurinol.

NB: Hypouricaemic drugs should not be given in acute attack, may be started after several weeks of acute attack.

OSTEOARTHRITIS

Definition

It is a degenerative disease of the joint characterized by degeneration of articular cartilage with proliferation of new bone and remodelling of joint contour. Commonly involves weight bearing joints—knee, ankle, etc.

Causes—Two types

1. Primary—unknown cause.
2. Secondary—to some other diseases, usually asymmetrical, commonly involves the weight-bearing joints. Causes are:
   - Trauma.
   - Congenital or developmental.
   - Inflammatory—rheumatoid arthritis, septic arthritis, gout, haemophilic arthritis.
   - Neuropathic joints (Charcot's joint).
   - Endocrine diseases—acromegaly, hyperparathyroidism.
   - Metabolic—haemochromatosis, alkaptonuria, Wilson's disease, chondrocalcinosis.

Symptoms

- Pain of the affected joints. Pain increases with activity and diminishes with rest. Commonly knee and hip joints are involved.
- Limitation of movement.

Signs

- Joints are swollen with restricted movement. Later on joint deformity may occur.
- In hand—bony swelling at the proximal (Bouchard node) and distal (Heberden's node) interphalangeal joints. DIP joints are commonly involved.
- Crepitus on movement of the joints.

Investigation

X-ray of the affected joints—shows joint space narrowing, osteophyte and marginal sclerosis.

Treatment

- Explanation and reassurance.
- Patient's education.
- Regular exercise.
- Weight reduction if obese.
- Reduction of adverse mechanical factors.
- Use of appropriate footwear, walking stick, etc.
- Pain relief—paracetamol, NSAID. Intra-articular corticosteroid may be needed.
- Chondroitin sulphate and glucosamine sulphate may be helpful.
- Intra-articular hyaluronic acid is also helpful.
- Physiotherapy should be given.
- Surgery in some cases—osteotomy and joint replacement.

OSTEOPOROSIS

Definition

It is a metabolic bone disease characterized by reduction of bone mass with an increased risk of fracture. Ratio of osteoid tissue to calcium and phosphate is normal (calcium, phosphate and alkaline phosphatase are normal).

Bony matrix decreases but mineralization is normal.

(**NB:** In osteomalacia, bone matrix is normal but mineralization decreases. Calcium and phosphate are low, but alkaline phosphatase is high)

Causes

1. Postmenopausal.
2. Senile.
3. Secondary:
   - Endocrine—hypogonadism, hyperparathyroidism, hyperthyroidism, Cushing's syndrome.
   - Inflammatory disease—ankylosing spondylitis, rheumatoid arthritis.
   - Drugs—corticosteroid, anticonvulsant, alcohol excess, heparin.
   - GIT—malabsorption, chronic liver disease.
   - Genetic disease—osteogenesis imperfect, homocystinuria, Ehlers-Danlos syndrome.
   - Others—smoking, prolonged immobilization, CKD, multiple myeloma, anorexia nervosa.

Symptoms

- Usually asymptomatic.
- May present with spontaneous fracture (neck of the femur), back pain, collapse of a vertebrae (with loss of height) and kyphoscoliosis.

Signs

- No specific sign.

Investigation

- X-ray of bone—shows reduction of bone density (called osteopenia). X-ray of vertebra may show collapse.
- Serum calcium, phosphate and alkaline phosphatase are normal.
- Serum 25-hydroxy vitamin—low.
- Bone Mineral Density (BMD) by DEXA is the gold standard.

Treatment

General Measures

- Smoking must be stopped.
- Alcohol restriction.
- Weight-bearing exercise, 30 minutes, three times a week.
- Adequate calcium and vitamin D in diet. Calcium 800–1000 mg/day, vitamin D 400–800 IU/day. Calcitriol may be given.
- Physiotherapy.

Drug Therapy

- Bisphosphonate—alendronate (10 mg/day or 70 mg once a week), risedronate (5 mg/day or 30 mg once a week), zoledronic acid (5 mg IV once yearly), ibandronate (150 mg once a month).
- Denosumab (60 mg SC every 6 months).
- Raloxifene (60 mg orally).
- Calcitonin may be used (Nasal spray or S/C).
- Teriparatide (20 μg/day).
- Hormone replacement therapy (HRT) in early menopause, if no contraindication (risk of breast cancer and cardiovascular disease).
- Surgical treatment of osteoporotic fractures.

PSORIATIC ARTHRITIS

Definition

It is a seronegative arthritis associated with psoriasis. It occurs in 7–20% of patients with psoriasis, most commonly with current or previous psoriasis, but may occur before the onset of psoriasis.

Types of Arthritis in Psoriasis—5 types

1. Asymmetrical inflammatory oligoarthritis—40%.
2. Symmetrical seronegative polyarthritis (like rheumatoid) —25%.
3. Sacroiliitis or spondylitis—15%. More among males.
4. Predominant DIP joint arthritis—15% (typical), nail dystrophy is invariable.
5. Arthritis mutilans—5%.

Symptoms

Mainly pain, swelling in the affected joints with history of psoriasis.

Signs

- Patch of psoriatic lesions
- Joint may be swollen, tender.

Extra-articular Features

- Skin lesions (typical psoriatic patch).
- Nail change is present in 85%—nail pitting, horizontal ridging and thickening of nail, onycholysis and subungual hyperkeratosis.
- Eye—conjunctivitis and uveitis.

Investigations

- CBC (ESR may be high).
- CRP (high).
- RA and ANF (negative).
- X-ray of the joint.
- Serum uric acid (may be high), can cause secondary gout.

Treatment

1. For psoriasis—General measures, local therapy and systemic therapy (for details see chapter dermatology).
2. Treatment of arthritis:
   - NSAID.
   - In persistant and progressive—methotrexate, sulphasalazine, azathioprine (these drugs are helpful in both skin lesion and arthritis). Cyclosporin is also helpful.
   - Biological agents—monoclonal antibody (e.g. infliximab and etanarcept may be given when all other drugs fail).

- Acitretin 20 mg daily is effective in both arthritis and skin lesion (avoid in young female as it is teratogenic).
- Prednisolone may be needed (sometimes steroid is given intra articularly).

3. PUVA is mainly for skin lesion.

NB: Drug to be avoided in psoriasis—chloroquine, hydroxychloroquine, beta-bloker, ACE inhibitor, lithium, alcohol.

SYSTEMIC LUPUS ERYTHEMATOSUS

Definition

It is an autoimmune chronic multisystem disease characterized by production of multiple autoantibodies, immune complexes and widespread immune-mediated organ damage.

More in females, F:M = 9:1, second and third decades. Sex ratio is equal in children and elderly.

Diagnostic Criteria of SLE

1. Malar rash.
2. Discoid rash.
3. Photosensitivity (rash on exposure to sunlight).
4. Oral ulcer (oral or nasopharyngeal ulcer, painless).
5. Arthritis (nonerosive arthritis involving two or more peripheral joints).
6. Serositis (pleurisy or pleural effusion, pericarditis or pericardial effusion).
7. Renal involvement—persistent proteinuria >0.5 g per day (in 24 hour urinary protein) or greater than 3+ (if total urinary protein is not performed) or cellular casts (red cell, granular and tubular).
8. Neurological disorder—seizure or psychosis in the absence of offending drug or metabolic derangement (uraemia, ketoacidosis and electrolyte imbalance).
9. Haematological disorders—haemolytic anaemia or leucopenia (<4,000/mm^3 in two or more occasions) or lymphopenia (<1,000/mm^3 in two or more occasions) or thrombocytopenia (<100,000/mm^3 in the absence of offending drug).
10. Immunological disorders—anti-ds DNA antibody or anti-Sm antibody or positive antiphospholipid antibody.
11. **ANA** positive (in the absence of drugs causing lupus syndrome).

NB: Presence of *four or more* criteria at a time or sequential appearance is diagnostic.

Symptoms

Common in young females. Presents with:

- Fever, arthritis and arthralgia, butterfly photosensitive rash, oral ulcer, alopecia.
- In females—history of repeated abortion.
- Other features according to involvement of multiple organs. (see below)

Diferent Systems involved in SLE

- **Heart**—pericarditis, pericardial effusion, myocarditis, mitral regurgitation may occur. Rarely, noninfective endocarditis called Libman—Sacks endocartitis .
- **Vascular**—Raynaud's phenomenon, vasculitis, arterial and venous thrombosis (in antiphospholipid syndrome) and atherosclerosis.
- **Lungs**—pleural effusion (may be bilateral) and pneumonitis. Atelactasis and shrinking lung with elevation of diaphragm (shrinking lung syndrome).
- **Eyes**—episcleritis, scleritis and optic neuritis, secondary Sjogren's syndrome (dry eye and dry mouth).Retinal vasculitis (fundoscopy shows white, hard exudate called cytoid body).
- **GIT**—mouth ulcer, mesenteric vasculitis causing small bowel infarction or perforation.
- **Haematological**—anaemia, Coomb's positive autoimmune haemolytic anaemia, thrombocytopenia, leucopenia and lymphopenia.

- **Neurological**—epilepsy, migraine, cerebrovascular disease, organic psychosis, paralysis, depression, transverse myelitis, lymphocytic meningitis, cerebellar ataxia, cranial nerve palsy and peripheral neuropathy.
- **Kidney**—glomerulonephritis, nephrotic syndrome and renal vein thrombosis.
- **Others**—lymphadenopathy, splenomegaly, hepatomegaly, fever and weight loss.

Drugs Causing SLE

Hydralazine (common (90%), procainamide, anticonvulsant (carbamazepine and phenytoin), phenothiazine, INH, oral contraceptive pill, ACE inhibitor, penicillamine, methyldopa, minocycline.

Features of Drug-induced SLE

- Sex ratio—equal.
- Lung involvement is common, but renal and neurological involvement are rare.
- ANA is usually positive.
- Anti-dsDNA is negative.
- Complements are normal.
- Anti-histone antibody is positive in 95% (characteristic, but not specific).
- Drugs causing SLE-like syndrome usually do not aggravate primary SLE.

Treatment

Withdrawal of drugs. Short course of steroid is necessary.

Investigations in SLE

1. CBC (anaemia,leucopenia,thrombocytopenia, lymphopenia, high ESR).
2. Urine (proteinuria, haematuria and RBC or granular cast).
3. 24-hour urinary protein.
4. CRP—normal (if CRP is high, it indicates infection).
5. ANA is positive in 95% cases.
6. Anti-ds DNA—positive in 30–50% cases.
7. Anti-Sm (Smith) antibody is positve in 10–25% cases.
8. Complements—C3 and C4 (low in active disease).
9. Serum antiphospholipid antibody.
10. Others (indicate presence of antiphospholipid antibody):
    - VDRL (false positive).
    - Platelet (low).
    - Prothrombin time (prolonged).
    - APTT (prolonged, not corrected by addition of normal plasma).
12. Skin biopsy—immunofluorescence test shows deposition of immune complex at dermo-epidermal junction (lupus band).
13. If renal involvement investigate accordingly.
14. If CNS involvement—EEG, CT or MRI.

Treatment

1. General measures—explanation, reassurance, psychological support.
2. Drug therapy:

- Mild case—NSAID (if fever, arthralgia and headache).
- Chloroquine or hydroxychloroquine—effective in cutaneous lesion, arthritis, arthralgia and serositis without organ involvement.
- Mild to moderate with active disease (rash, synovitis or pleuropericarditis)—short-course steroid.
- Acute life-threatening case—high-dose prednisolone (40–60 mg/day) or IV methyl prednisolone (500 mg to 1 g) for 3–5 days, followed by prednisolone.
- Methylprednisolone and pulse cyclophosphamide in renal and cerebral lupus.

Prognosis in SLE

5-year survival >90%.

Pregnancy with SLE

- Pregnancy is not contraindicated.
- Repeated abortion (due to presence of antiphospholipid antibody), stillbirth and intrauterine growth retardation may occur.
- The disease should be in remission and pregnancy should be avoided if there is neurological, renal and cardiac abnormality.
- Relapse may occur in the first trimester and in puerperium.
- If the mother has "anti-Ro antibody" (SSA), there may be congenital complete heart block of the baby due to transplacental transfer of antibody.
- Treatment—Prednisolone should be continued (avoid dexamethasone and betamethasone, which are broken by placental enzymes).

POLYMYOSITIS AND DERMATOMYOSITIS

Definition

Polymyositis is the nonsuppurative, noninfective inflammation of skeletal muscle of unknown cause, characterized by necrosis, fibrosis and regeneration of muscles.

When associated with skin rash, it is called dermatomyositis.

Classification: 5 types

1. Primary idiopathic polymyositis.
2. Primary idiopathic dermatomyositis.
3. Dermatomyositis or polymyositis associated with neoplasia.
4. Childhood dermatomyositis or polymyositis associated with vasculitis.
5. Dermatomyositis or polymyositis associated with collagen vascular disease.

Causes of Dermatomyositis

Unknown. Probable factors are:

- Autoimmune mechanism.
- Viral (coxsackie B, rubella and influenza have been suggested).
- Associated with malignancy (commonest cause is bronchial carcinoma in males and ovarian carcinoma in females).
- Drugs—D-penicillamine and zidovudin.

Clinical Features

Common in female, F:M = 2:1, age 50–60 years.

- Gradual and progressive muscular weakness and wasting, mainly involving the proximal muscles (shoulder and pelvic girdle).
- Skin rash—typically in upper eyelids with erythema called "Heliotrope rash" (photosensitive, erythematous and scaly). Flat, red rash on face and upper trunk, erythematous rash of knuckles with raised violaceous scaly eruption (Gottron's sign). Erythematous rash also may occur in knee, elbow, malleoli, neck and anterior chest (V sign) or back and shoulder (shawl sign).
- Pharyngeal, laryngeal and respiratory muscles involvement may cause dysphagia, dysphonia and respiratory failure.
- Other features—arthralgia, arthritis, myalgia, Raynaud's phenomenon.
- Ocular involvement is rare.
- The patient may present with acute renal failure due to myoglobinuria secondary to rhabdomyolysis.

Investigations

1. CBC, ESR (high).
2. Muscle enzymes:
   - CPK—very high (most sensitive test).
   - Other enzymes (serum aldolase, SGOT, SGPT, LDH may be high).
3. EMG.
4. Muscle biopsy shows:
   - Necrosis, swelling, vacuolation, disruption of muscles.

- Infiltration of lymphocyte, plasma cell, eosinophil, macrophage.
- Fibrosis, perivascular inflammatory cells infiltration and thickening of vessel wall.

5. Other tests:
   - To exclude malignancy (chest X-ray, USG, CT scan, MRI, PET scan, mammogram, gastrointestinal tract imaging).
   - Others—X-ray (limbs or hands) to see soft-tissue calcification.Common in childhood dermatomyositis.
   - RA test and ANF (positive in 50% cases).
   - Anti-Jo1 antibody—more specific. Positive in 30% cases of dermatomyositis and 50% cases of polymyositis (if anti-Jo1 antibody is present, respiratory muscles involvement may occur).
   - MRI of muscles—to detect abnormal muscles.
   - Urine for myoglobin in acute cases.

Causes of Proximal Myopathy

- Myopathy (limb girdle, fascioscapulohumeral) except myotonic dystrophy.
- Dermatomyositis or polymyositis.
- Myasthenia gravis.
- Myasthenic myopathic syndrome (Eaton-Lambert syndrome).
- Thyrotoxicosis, also in hypothyroidism.
- Cushing's syndrome.
- Osteomalacia.
- Diabetic amyotrophy.
- Hyperparathyroidism.
- Drugs—lovastatin, chloroquine, colcichin (all are associated with high CPK). Steroid can cause proximal myopathy (it is not associated with high CPK).

Treatment

- Prednisolone 0.5–1 mg/kg daily to induce remission. Continued for 1 month after myositis is clinically and enzymatically inactive. Then taper the dose slowly. Maintenance dose 5–7.5 mg daily, may be required for months, even years.
- If severe respiratory or pharyngeal weakness—methylprednisolone 1 g daily for 3 days. Then prednisolone therapy.
- If no response to steroid—methotrexate or azathioprine may be given.
- Ciclosporin or cyclophosphamide or mycophenolate mofetil may be tried.
- High-dose IV immunoglobulin may help in some cases.
- Treatment of underlying malignancy may improve the condition.
- Physiotherapy.

Prognosis

- 5 years survival in treated patient is >95%, 10 year survival is 84%.
- Worse if severely affected at presentation, delay of treatment, severe dyspahgia or respiratory difficulty, older patient and if underlying malignancy.
- Dermatomyositis responds better than polymyositis. So better prognosis.

EATON–LAMBERT SYNDROME

It is a paraneoplastic syndrome characterized by proximal muscle weakness and wasting due to defective acetylcholine release at the neuromuscular junction. It commonly involves the lower limb but may involve any muscle.

Cause

- There is defect in acetylcholine release at the neuromuscular junction which is thought to be due to an auto-antibody against prejunctional voltage gated calcium channel on the motor nerve terminal. Small cell carcinoma of the lung may trigger the autoantibody reaction.
- Commonly due to small cell carcinoma of lung, may be associated with or may precede the manifestations of carcinoma.

Features

- Proximal weakness, commonly in lower limbs but any muscle may be involved. Ptosis and diplopia may occur in 70% cases.
- Reflexes are absent or diminished.
- Muscle power may be increased and tendon reflexes may return after repeated activity or sustained contraction of the relevant muscle (reverse of myasthenia gravis).
- Patient may have autonomic dysfunction (dry mouth, constipation, impotence).

Investigations

- EMG shows progressive incremental response (reverse of myasthenia gravis where there is decremental response).
- Antibody to P/Q type voltage gated calcium channel (anti VGLC)—found in 90% cases.

Treatment

- 3, 4 diaminopyridine.
- IV immunoglobulin may be helpful.
- Pyridostigmine is helpful for symptomatic relief.
- Plasmapheresis in some cases.
- Treatment of primary cause.

TUBERCULOSIS OF BONE OR JOINT

Any joint or bone may be involved, commonly knee and hip. Organism is *M. tuberculosis*. In children, it occurs as primary disease. In adult, it is due to haematogenous spread from lung.

Symptoms

- Pain and swelling of the involved joint with eventual deformity.
- General features like fever, night sweating and weight loss may be present.

Signs

- Joint is swollen and tender, may be stiff with deformity and limitation of movement.
- Joint effusion may be present.

Investigations

- FBC (ESR is high usually).
- X-ray chest PA view (primary focus may be seen).
- X-ray of joints shows soft-tissue swelling, reduction of joint space with bony destruction.
- MT.
- CT scan or MRI of joint.
- FNAC (CT or USG guided).
- Arthroscopy and biopsy may be needed
- Sometimes open synovial biopsy—shows caseating necrosis and giant cells.

Treatment

- Standard anti-Koch's therapy comprising four drugs, continued for at least 1 year.
- Prednisolone may be added.

TUBERCULOSIS OF SPINE (POTT'S DISEASE)

Definition

Pott's disease is the tuberculosis of the spine, also called tuberculous spondylitis. It is usually due to reactivation of dormant haematogenous focus. Rarely, spread from local paravertebral lymph node.

Infection starts at the intervertebral disc (discitis), then spread along the spinal ligaments to involve the adjacent margins of vertebral body, causes erosion and destruction of disc and vertebral body. There is collapse of the vertebra, causes anterior wedging of one or more adjacent vertebrae and 'gibbus' formation. Also paravertebral abscess formation.

Symptoms

- Usually chronic back pain, mainly the lower thoracic and lumbar spine. Swelling (due to gibbus), restriction of movement.
- General features of TB, such as fever, malaise, night sweating and loss of weight.
- Features of complications (e.g. paraplegia).

Signs

- Local tenderness over the spine.
- Gibbus (swelling over the spine).
- Paravertebral abscess.
- If spinal cord compression, spastic paraplegia (if the lesion is above L1) or flaccid (if the lesion is below L1).

Investigations

- FBC (ESR is high usually).
- X-ray chest PA view (primary focus may be seen).
- X-ray of spine shows collapse of vertebrae, may be paravertebral shadow.
- MT.
- CT scan or MRI of spine.

- FNAC (CT or USG guided).
- Occasionally, open biopsy may be needed.

Treatment

- Standard anti-Koch's therapy comprising four drugs—rifampicin, INH, ethambutol, pyrazinamide for two months. Then INH and rifampicin continued for another 10 months, even more.
- Prednisolone may be added.
- If spastic paraplegia—Standard anti-Koch's therapy. Neurosurgical intervention (decompression and drainage of abscess).

REITER'S SYNDROME

Definition

Reiter's syndrome is a seronegative arthritis characterized by arthritis, conjunctivitis and urethritis.

Reactive arthritis means when only arthritis follows after an attack of diarrhoea or dysentery or sexual exposure. It is called reactive, because pathology in one site, but affecting the joints. It is a variety of Reiter's syndrome. Organisms are—*Salmonella, Shigella, Campylobacter, Chlamydia* and *Yersinia.*

Reiter's syndrome is common in male (M:F = 15:1), 16–35 years of age.

Triad of Reiter's Syndrome

- Arthritis.
- Conjunctivitis.
- Urethritis (nonspecific).

Symptoms

1. History of urethritis, diarrhoea or dysentry and sexual exposure.
2. After 1–3 weeks—asymmetrical oligoarthritis involving the bigger joints (knee and ankle), conjunctivitis and urethritis.
3. Extra-articular features:
   - Conjunctivitis and iritis.
   - Achilles tendinitis and plantar fascitis.
   - Circinate balanitis.
   - Skin rash (macular, vesicular or pustular).
   - Keratoderma blennorrhagica (in palm, sole or toes).
   - Nail dystrophy and buccal erosion.

Signs

- Eyes—conjunctivitis, usually bilateral, may be iritis.
- Back—evidence of sacroiliitis.
- Foot— Achilles tendinitis and plantar fasciitis
- Circinate balanitis and keratoderma blennorrhagica (in palm, sole and toes).

Investigations

- Hb%, TC, DC and ESR (high).
- Urine—shows pus cells, sterile on routine culture (sterile pyuria).
- CRP (high).
- RA test and ANA (negative).
- X-ray of the joints involved and SI joint.
- If joint effusion is present—aspiration of fluid and analysis.
- HLA-B27 positive in 70% cases.

Treatment

- Rest and NSAID for pain. Sometimes, Intra-articular steroid injection.
- Antibiotic (tetracycline or azithromycin for non-gonococcal urethritis).
- Short-course prednisolone may be given.
- In some cases of recurrent and remitting arthritis, disease modifying drugs, such as sulphasalazine or methotrexate or azathioprine, should be given.
- In severe case, high-dose steroid may be given.
- Anti-TNF may be helpful in severe case.
- Physiotherapy.

ACUTE OSTEOMYELITIS

Definition

Osteomyelitis is the primary site of infection in bone or bone marrow. Any part of a bone may be involved but there is preferential targeting of the juxta-epiphyseal regions of long bones adjacent to joints.

Pathologically, the infection causes localized areas of osteonecrosis (bone death). A separated part of dead is called 'sequestrum'. Perforation of the cortex by pus stimulates local new bone formation ('involucrum') by the subperiosteum and periosteum, often with sinuses that discharge through the skin.

Causes

- Haematogenous, direct infection may complicate a compound fracture, penetrating injury or orthopaedic surgery.
- Organisms are—Staphylococci(90%). Others—Streptococci, *H. influenza* and Salmonella.
- Risk factors—childhood and adolescence, diabetes mellitus, AIDS, sickle cell disease.

Clinical Features

- Metaphysis of long bones in children is involved.
- Pain at the site of infection, swelling and redness. Pain is localized and child may limp.
- High fever with chill and rigor.
- Sinus tract with discharge of pus may be present.
- Chronic infection may be associated with abscess within the bone (Brodie's abscess).

Investigations

- CBC and ESR.
- Blood for C/S.
- X-ray of the involved bone—after 1-2 weeks, X—ray will show radiolucent lesion and periosteal elevation. Reactive sclerosis will be absent.
- CT or MRI.

Treatment

- For pain—NSAID.
- IV broad-spectrum antibiotic for at least 2 weeks, followed by oral antibiotic for at least 4 weeks.
- Surgical decompression and removal of any dead bone
- Rehabilitation.

HAEMOPHILIC ARTHRITIS

In a patient with haemophilia, when plasma level of factor VIII is <1%, arthritis may occur. It may be spontaneous without trauma or may follow even minor trauma.

Symptoms

Commonly knee, elbow, ankle, hip joints are involved.

- Initially—tingling, abnormal sensation, stiffness and instability of the joint.
- Later on—the joint is red, hot, swollen and painful.
- Progression of arthritis may cause ankylosis of joint.

Treatment

- Complete rest, if needed splinting of joint.
- Factor VIII transfusion—20-30 IU/kg. It is repeated after 12 hours, also after 24 and 36 hours.
- For pain—COX 2 inhibitor like celecoxib may be used. Orally opioid may be given.
- Physiotherapy—once bleeding is settled, mobilization and physiotherapy should be started. Usually after 48 hours—isometric exercise, followed by active movement and hydrotherapy or shortwave diathermy.
- Arthrocentesis is rarely necessary, but in some cases with massive bleeding, aspiration of blood from joint followed by factor VIII therapy may be needed.
- To prevent recurrent bleeding into the joint—patient with severe haemophilia are given factor VIII infusions regularly 3 times per week.

JUVENILE IDIOPATHIC ARTHRITIS (JIA)

Definition

Arthritis developing before 16 years of age.

Types

1. Systemic onset (Still's disease)—It is a systemic disorder characterized by fever, skin rash, arthritis, hepatosplenomegaly and serositis.
2. Oligoarthritis (pauciarticular)—four or less joints are affected.
3. Polyarthritis—more than four joints are affected.
4. Others:
   - Enthesitis-related JIA.
   - Psoriatic arthritis.
   - Atypical JIA.

Investigations

- CBC with ESR (leucocytosis in Still's disease, lymphocytosis, thrombocytosis and high ESR).
- CRP (high).
- RA test (usually negative, positive in 10% cases).
- X-ray of the joint involved.
- Other investigations—to exclude other diseases (according to history).

Features of Systemic Onset JIA (Still's disease)

- Arthritis—involving knee, wrist and ankle. Other joints may be involved.
- Fever—high, intermittent, may be continuous.
- Skin rash—appears with fever and disappears when fever subsides. These are macular or maculopapular, salmon- pink colour rashes (salmon rash).
- Extra-articular features—hepatosplenomegaly and lymphadenopathy (common). There may be pericardial effusion, pleural effusion and disseminated intravascular coagulation (DIC).
- In chronic case—micrognathia (small mandible), fusion of cervical spine and retardation of growth.

Treatment

1. General measures:
   - To relieve pain—NSAID. Rest and passive movement of the limb to prevent contracture.
   - Physiotherapy.
   - Explanation and reassurance to the parents.
2. In severe case—prednisolone. Pulse methylprednisolone may be given, followed by methotrexate.
3. Disease modifying drugs should be given in all cases:
   - Methotrexate—5 mg weekly (increase the dose gradually).
   - Sulphasalazine—30-50 mg/kg.
   - If methotrexate fails—anti TNF may be given.
4. Orthopaedic surgery—if needed.

ANTIPHOSPHOLIPID SYNDROME

Definition

Antiphospholipid syndrome is characterized by the presence of antiphospholipid antibody, which causes venous or arterial thrombosis and recurrent miscarriage.

It is due to the effect on platelet membrane, endothelial cell and clotting components, such as prothrombin, protein C and S. Antiphospholipid antibody includes lupus anticoagulant and anticardiolipin antibody. In some patients, only one of these is positive and in others, both are positive.

Causes

1. May be primary.
2. Secondary to other diseases:
   - SLE.
   - Rheumatoid arthritis.
   - Systemic sclerosis.
   - Behcet's syndrome.
   - Temporal arteritis.
   - Sjogren's syndrome.
   - Psoriatic arthropathy.

Clinical Features

Presence of this antibody may be associated with:

- Thrombosis (venous or arterial).
- Recurrent abortion.
- Thrombocytopenia.
- Livedo reticularis.
- Neurological (stroke, TIA, epilepsy, migraine, chorea).
- Sterile endocarditis (Liebmann Sach's).
- Pulmonary hypertension.
- Avascular necrosis of head of femur.
- Renal involvement—proteinuria in 50%, lupus nephritis (membranous).

Investigations

1. Indirect evidence of antiphospholipid antibody:
   - False positive VDRL.
   - Thrombocytopenia.
   - Prolonged prothrombin time.
   - Prolonged APTT (not corrected by normal plasma).
2. ANA.
3. Anti-ds DNA.
4. Serum antiphospholipid or anticardiolipin antibody.

NB. In any young patient, if presents with features like CVA or TIA, antiphospholipid syndrome should be excluded. Clue for the diagnosis is prolonged APTT, which is not corrected by addition of normal plasma.

Treatment

- Low-dose aspirin (in mild to moderate case) or clopidogrel.
- Warfarin in severe case.
- In pregnancy, heparin and low-dose aspirin may be used.

CHAPTER

11 Dermatology

CHAPTER CONTENTS

INTRODUCTION

Layers of Skin

Consists of 3 layers—

1. Epidermis—It has 5 layers from top to bottom, they are:
   - Stratum corneum (horny layer)
   - Stratum lucidum
   - Stratum granulosum (granular layer)
   - Stratum spinosum (prickle cell or Malpighian layer)
   - Stratum basale (basal layer)
2. Dermis
3. Hypodermis or subcutis

Epidermis is an avascular stratified squamous epithelium, attached to dermis by basement membrane. Basal cells move outwards towards superficial horny layer and the time taken is 4 weeks. 95% cells of epidermis are keratinocytes, remaining 5% are Langerhans cells and melanocytes. There are a few Merkel cells.

Dermis contains blood and lymphatic vessels, nerves, muscle, appendages and immune cells, such as mast cells and lymphocytes. It also contains collagen, elastin and ground substance.

Functions of the Skin

- Protection against chemicals, ultraviolet radiation (UVR), antigens and microbes.
- Physical barrier against friction and shearing forces.
- Preservation of a balanced internal environment (by preventing loss of water, electrolytes and macromolecules).
- Sensation (pain, touch and temperature).
- Synthesis of vitamin D and testosterone.
- Temperature regulation.
- Body odour and psychosocial factors.

Appendages of the Skin

- Nail.
- Hair.
- Sebaceous gland.
- Sweat gland.

ITCHING OR PRURITUS

Causes of Itching

May occur due to skin disease and systemic (or medical) disease.

Systemic Disease

1. Liver disease:
   - Obstructive jaundice
   - Primary biliary cirrhosis
2. Renal
   - Chronic renal failure
3. Haematological
   - Polycythaemia rubra vera (after warm bath)
   - Lymphoma (e.g. Hodgkin's disease)
   - Leukaemia
   - Multiple myeloma
   - Iron deficiency anaemia
4. Endrocrine:
   - Hypothyroidism.
   - Thyrotoxicosis.
   - Diabetes mellitus (associated with candidiasis).
5. Any internal malignancy.
6. HIV.
7. Psychogenic
8. Senile pruritus

Skin Diseases

- Eczema
- Scabies
- Dermatitis herpetiformis
- Lichen planus
- Urticaria

Dermatological Manifestations of Internal Malignancy

- Dermatomyositis—bronchial carcinoma, malignancy of GIT, genitourinary.
- Acanthosis nigricans—may be found in malignancies of GIT, lung, liver.
- Paget's disease of nipple—ductal carcinoma of breast.
- Erythroderma—lymphoma, leukaemia.
- Tylosis—oesophageal carcinoma.
- Icthyosis—lymphoma.
- Erythema gyratum repens (concentric rings of erythema)—malignancy of lung, breast.
- Necrolytic migratory erythema (burning, geographic and spreading annular areas of erythema)—glucagonoma.

SCABIES

Causative Organism

Sarcoptes scabiei.

Sites of Scabies

Commonly interdigital area, fingers, ulnar edge of hand, wrist.

Other sites—anticubital fossa, elbow joint, axilla, areola, around umbilicus, lower abdomen, genitalia, buttock, dorsum of foot (face and scalp are never involved except in infants, children and immunocompromized population).

Mode of Transmission

- Direct skin contact from affected individual.
- From bed sheet, clothing.

Symptoms

- Intense itching, mostly at night.
- Presence of same symptoms among family members.
- In women, itching of nipple. In man, itchy papules in scrotum and penis.

Signs

- 'Burrow' which is short, wavy, dirty appearing line found in the edge of fingers, toes or at the sides of hand, foot. Burrow contains female mites, eggs and faeces of the mite.
- Papular lesions, excoriations at the sites of predilection.

Diagnosis

- Usually clinical (hand lens is used to see burrow and mite).
- Microscopical examination by scraping from lesion to see the mites.

Complications

- Secondary bacterial infection.
- Eczematization and lichenification.
- Poststreptococcal glomerulonephritis.

Treatment

Drugs

- Permethrin 5% cream—single application (from neck to toe), may be repeated after 1 week.
- One percent gamma benzene hexachloride lotion.
- Benzyl benzoate 25% lotion (applied for consecutive 3 nights).
- Monosulphirum 5–8% emulsion (applied for consecutive 3 nights).
- Ten percent precipitated sulphur in white petrolatum (applied for consecutive 3 nights).
- Crotamiton 10% lotion or cream.
- Ivermectin may help in immunocompromized, crusted or Norwegian scabies (200 mg/kg in single dose).

General Measures

- Control of secondary infection.
- For itching—antihistamine (e.g. loratidine, desloratidine, fexofenadine).
- Washing of the clothes and bed sheet.
- Simultaneous treatment of the affected family members.

PSORIASIS

Definition

It is a chronic inflammatory disease of skin characterized by well-defined erythematous plaque with silvery white scales, associated with recurrence and remission.

Pathology

Rapid proliferation and abnormal differentiation of epidermis and infiltration of inflammatory cells (polymorph, T-lymphocyte and other inflammatory cells).

Sites of Psoriatic Skin Lesion

- Extensor surfaces of knee, elbow, wrist, extensor surface of limbs.
- Back of ear, scalp, hairline.
- Sacrum.
- Around the umbilicus, submammary fold.
- Intergluteal cleft and flexures (natal cleft, axillary fold) and submammary fold and nails.

Types: 4 types

1. Chronic plaque psoriasis (commonest)—characterized by well-demarcated, red, covered with dry silvery white scale. It commonly involves elbow, knee and lower back but may also involve scalp , nails, flexures and palm.
2. Guttate psoriasis—characterized by raindrop-like red small circular or oval plaques, over the trunk. Occurs about 2 weeks after streptococcal sore throat. Common in children and young adults.
3. Pustular psoriasis—may be localized in palm and sole, rarely generalized.
4. Erythrodermic psoriasis—skin becomes red, scaly, generalized.

Clinical Features

- Skin—red, dry, well demarcated, with silvery scales.
- Nails—pitting, onycholysis (separation of nail plate from its bed), thickening and subungual hyperkeratosis.
- Joints—arthropathy.
- Eye—iritis, keratitis, conjunctivitis.
- Auspitz's sign—when scales are removed, there is bleeding points over the lesion. It is called Auspitz's sign.
- Koebner's phenomenon—appearance of psoriatic skin lesion after scratching over normal skin area.

Types of Arthritis

5 types

- Asymmetrical DIP joint involvement.
- Symmetrical polyarthritis—like rheumatioid arthritis.
- Asymmetrical oligoarthritis involving one or more joints of hand.
- Ankylosing spondylitis.
- Arthritis mutilans.

Investigations

Diagnosis is clinical.

1. Routine:
   - CBC.
   - Liver function tests.
   - Serum creatinine.
   - Lipid profile.
   - X-ray chest.
   - Urine R/E (to see proteinuria).
   - Serum electrolytes.
   - Serum uric acid.
   - Serum IgE.
2. Specific tests:
   - Skin biopsy for histopathology (definitive).
   - ASO titre (high in guttate psoriasis).
   - Throat swab culture and sensitivity (in guttate psoriasis).
   - X-ray of the affected joints.

Factors that Aggravate Psoriasis

1. Trauma.
2. Infections—β haemolytic streptococci (aggravates guttate psoriasis) and HIV infection.
3. Psychological factors—emotion and anxiety.
4. Drugs:
   - β-Blockers.
   - Anti-malarial (chloroquine and hydroxychloroquine).
   - Lithium.
   - Alcohol.
   - ACE inhibitors.
   - NSAID's (e.g. indomethacin).
   - Systemic steroid—aggravated after withdrawal of steroid (rebound phenomenon) and after stopping following prolonged use of local steroid.

Complications

- Psoriatic arthropathy.
- Exfoliative dermatitis.
- Secondary infection.
- Hyperuricaemia and gout.
- Others—amyloidosis, renal failure, hepatic failure, high- output cardiac failure due to erythroderma.

Treatment

1. General measures—explanation and reassurance, avoid trauma, precipitating drugs and anxiety.
2. Specific treatment:
   - Local therapy.

- Systemic therapy.
- Combination therapy.

Local Therapy (topical therapy on the lesion)

- Emollient—petroleum, paraffin, urea (up to 10%), olive oil.
- Salicylic acid (≥5%).
- Crude tar (3–5%).
- Dithranol.
- Calcipotriol (vitamin D3 analogue).
- Tazarotene.
- Topical steroid.
- UVR therapy (narrow band UVB).
- Tacrolimus and pimecrolimus.
- Excimer laser.

Systemic Therapy

- PUVA (psoralen and UVA)—long-term use may cause squamous cell carcinoma, basal cell carcinoma, melanoma.
- Retinoid (acitretin). Avoided in young female (teratogenic).
- Methotrexate.
- Azathioprine.
- Ciclosporin.
- Biologic agents—anti-TNFα (infliximab, etanercept, adalimumab, efalizumab) may be given when all other drugs fail.
  Drugs that cure both psoriasis and arthritis: Methotrexate, azathioprine and acitretin.

EXFOLIATIVE DERMATITIS OR ERYTHRODERMA

Definition

It is a disease characterized by generalized exfoliation, scaling and erythema involving different parts of skin.

Causes

1. Primary or Idiopathic.
2. Secondary to:
   - Skin diseases—psoriasis, atopic dermatitis, dermatomyositis, SLE, pemphigoid, pemphigus foliaceus.
   - Systemic disease or malignancy—leukaemia, lymphoma, carcinoma of the lung, rectum, multiple myeloma, graft versus host disease.
   - Drugs—allopurinol, carbamazepine, sulphonamide, barbiturates.

Clinical Features

More in males.

1. Cutaneous manifestations:
   - Skin exfoliation, scaling, pruritus, widespread erythema.
   - Loss of hair (often).
   - Nails may be dystrophic, brittle, subungual hyperkeratosis, distal onycholysis.
   - Palms and soles are involved.
   - Mucous membranes are usually spared.
2. General features—anorexia, nausea, diarrhoea, anaemia, oedema, tachycardia.

Investigations

1. Routine
   - CBC.
   - Chest X-ray P/A view.
   - Urine R/E (to see proteinuria).
   - Total protein, A:G ratio (hypoproteinaemia, altered A:G ratio).
   - Serum electrolytes (hypokalaemia, hyponatraemia, hypochloraemia).
   - Blood urea and serum creatinine.
   - Serum uric acid.
   - Serum IgE.
2. Definitive—by skin biopsy for histopathology.
3. Others to exclude primary cause -
   - Skin scraping for fungus and fungal culture in dermatophytosis.
   - Anti HIV I and II (if HIV is suspected).
   - USG of whole abdomen.
   - Bone marrow—to exclude leukaemia.
   - CT and MRI—in some cases.

Treatment

1. General measures—
   - Maintenance of fluid and electrolyte balance, good nutrition.
   - Frequent bathing.
   - Offending drug should be stopped.
2. Topical treatment—
   - Lubricant and emollient (e.g. liquid paraffin)—applied two times daily.
   - Mild topical steroid ointment (hydrocortisone).
3. Symptomatic treatment—
   - Antihistamine (cetirizine, loratidine).
   - Antibiotic, if secondary infection is present.
   - Iron, vitamin, folic acid supplement.
4. Treatment of primary causes—such as psoriasis, lymphoma, leukaemia, etc.

Complications

- Secondary bacterial infection.
- Fluid loss, dehydration and electrolyte imbalance.
- Protein loss (hypoalbuminema), leading to oedema.
- Hypothermia.
- High-output cardiac failure.
- Dermatogenic enteropathy.
- Thrombophlebitis.

BULLOUS DISEASES OF SKIN

Causes

1. Congenital:
   - Epidermolysis bullosa.
2. Acquired
   - Pemphigus vulgaris.
   - Bullous pemphigoid.
   - Stevens-Johnson syndrome or erythema multiforme.
   - Toxic epidermal necrolysis or staphyloccal scalded skin syndrome.
   - Others—impetigo, diabetic bullae, herpes gestationalis.

Pemphigus Vulgaris

Definition

It is an autoimmune blistering disease characterized by thin walled, flaccid, easily ruptured bullae occurring in skin and mucous membrane.

Types: 4 types

1. Pempigus vulgaris.
2. Pemphigus foliaceus.
3. Paraneoplastic pemphigus.
4. IgA pemphigus.

Causes

Unknown. Probable factors are:
- Autoimmunity.
- Genetic predisposition.
- Drugs—penicillamine, captopril, rifampicin, cephalosporin.
- UV light, PUVA and ionizing radiation.
- Increased incidence in myasthenia gravis and thymoma.

Clinical Features

Common in middle age, 50-60 years, equal in both sexes.
- Multiple thin walled, flaccid bullae over scalp, face, neck, axilla, groin and genitals. Some bullae may rupture forming denuded areas that enlarge by confluence with crusts.
- Multiple painful, irregular ulcerations in the oral mucous membrane.
- Weakness and weight loss.
- Nikolsky and Asboe-Hansen signs are positive.

Nikolsky Sign

Rubbing of unaffected skin results in separation of epidermis.

Asboe–Hansen Sign

Pressure on the intact bullae gently forces the fluid to wander under the skin away from pressure site.

Investigations

1. Routine—CBC, blood sugar, urine R/E, liver and renal function tests.
2. Specific:
   - Skin biopsy for histopathology and immunofluorescence test.
   - Cytological (Tzanck test)—smears are taken from the base of a bulla and (using Giemsa stain) is used for rapid demonstration of acantholytic cell.
   - Direct immunofluorescence—shows intercellular deposition of IgG throughout epidermis or oral mucosa.

Treatment

1. General measures:
   - Bed rest.
   - Daily bath to remove thick crusts and foul odour.
   - Maintenance of fluid and electrolyte balance and nutrition.
   - Antibiotic and blood transfusion (if necessary).
   - Antiseptic mouth wash.
   - Care of the eye.
2. Topical—1% silver sulfadiazine is applied.
3. Systemic:
   - Prednisolone—100–200 mg/day. Dose is tapered when remission occurs. Maintenance dose is given for longtime (even lifelong). If new blister occurs, dose of prednisolone should be increased.
   - Other treatment—IV methylprednisolone 1 g/day for 5 days, mycophenolate mofetil 1–1.5 g orally is given twice a day, azathioprine, cyclophosphamide, methotrexate, ciclosporin and dapsone.
   - In resistant case—IV immunoglobulin may be tried.
   - Biologic agent (infliximab, rituximab and etanercept).

Complications

- Secondary bacterial infection (pneumonia, septicaemia),
- Hypoproteinaemia,
- Side effects of systemic prednisolone.

Bullous Pemphigoid

Definition

It is characterized by tense bullae with less tendency to rupture, mostly in trunk, limbs and flexures.

Site of Lesion

The lesion is in the basement membrane between epidermis and dermis (subepidermal). So, less tendency to rupture.

Clinical Features

Common in elderly, >60 years.

- Multiple large tense bullae over different parts of body. Intact blisters contain clear fluid.
- Mouth involvement is rare.

Investigations

1. Routine—CBC, blood sugar, urine R/E.
2. Specific:
   - Tzanck test.
   - Skin biopsy—shows subepidermal bullae, absence of acantholysis and superficial dermal infiltration of eosinophils.
   - Direct immunofluorescence—shows deposition of IgG and complement C3 at the basement membrane (in a linear pattern).

Treatment

1. General treatment—bed rest, maintenance of electrolytes, adequate nutrition.
2. Specific:
   - Prednisolone 0.5–0.75 mg/kg/day, should be tapered slowly over few weeks after clinical improvement.
   - Potent topical steroid can be given alone.
   - In severe cases—methylprednisolone 15 mg/kg I/V daily for 3 doses.
3. Tetracycline 500 mg 6 hourly with nicotinamide 500 mg 8 hourly.
4. Other drugs—dapsone, azathioprine, methotrexate, cyclophosphamide, ciclosporin, mycophenolate mofetil.
5. IV immunoglobulin.
6. Antihistamine, if needed.

Erythema Multiforme and Stevens–Johnson Syndrome

Definition

Erythema multiforme is an acute inflammatory reaction in the skin and mucous membrane characterized by multiple erythematous skin lesions, such as macules, papules, vesicles, bullae and target lesions involving the extensor surfaces of limbs.

It is due to circulating immune complex that follows 7–14 days after precipitating factors (infections and drugs). It is usually self-limiting, resolves in 3–6 weeks, may recur.

Stevens–Johnson Syndrome

It is the severe form of erythema multiforme with widespread bullous lesion in skin and mucous membrane of mouth, eyes, and genitalia associated with severe constitutional symptoms.

Causes

1. Infections
   - Herpes simplex virus type 1 (30% cases).
   - Mycoplasma pneumoniae (common).
   - Other infections—Streptococcus and Histoplasma.
2. Drugs—sulfonamides, carbamazepine, thiacetazone, barbiturate, penicillin, phenytoin.
3. Idiopathic (50% cases).
4. Others
   - Malignancy (carcinoma and lymphoma).
   - Collagen disease (SLE and dermatomyositis).

- Wegener's granulomatosis.
- Sensitivity to vaccination (polio and BCG).

Clinical Features

- Multiple erythematous, maculopapular, urticarial, vesicular and bullous lesions involving the skin of whole body with few target lesions.
- Mouth ulcer is present in Stevens–Johnson syndrome (SJS).

NB:

- Typical lesion is target lesion (also called iris lesion or Bull's eye lesion). In this lesion, there is central pallor or dusky purpura with oedema and peripheral redness.
- SJS has <10% body surface area (BSA) involvement.
- If 10–30% BSA involvement, it is called SJS–TEN (toxic epidermal necrolysis) overlap.
- When more than 30% of BSA involved, it is called TEN.

Investigations

- CBC.
- ASO titre.
- Antibody to herpes simplex type 1.
- Anti-mycoplasma antibody.
- Other investigations according to suspicion of causes.

Treatment

- Offending drugs should be stopped.
- Symptomatic (IV fluid, antipyretic and antibiotic).
- Local care of eyes and mouth.
- Treatment of primary cause.
- In severe cases, especially in SJS, IV immunoglobulin can be given.
- Aciclovir (for recurrent herpes simplex infection).
- Steroid—its use is controversial. However, it can be used and should be tapered rapidly because once skin loss occurs, it may aggravate morbidity and mortality of the disorder due to immunosuppression.

ERYTHEMA NODOSUM

Definition

It is an inflammatory disorder characterized by non-suppurative, painful, palpable, tender, erythematous nodular lesion in the skin, common in shin below the knee.

Causes

- Acute sarcoidosis.
- Streptococcal β-haemolyticus infection (in throat).
- Primary pulmonary tuberculosis.
- Drugs—sulphonamide, penicillin, oestrogen containing oral contraceptive pill, salicylates, barbiturates, sulphonylureas, bromides, iodides.
- Inflammatory bowel disease (Crohn's disease, ulcerative colitis).
- Fungal infections (histoplasmosis, coccidioidomycosis, blastomycosis—common in USA).
- Protozoal (toxoplasmosis).
- Leprosy (erythema nodosum leprosum).
- Idiopathic (in 50% cases).
- Physiological—pregnancy (often unilateral).
- Others—brucellosis, chlamydia, rickettsia, lymphoma, cat-scratch disease, Behçet's syndrome.

Clinical Features

Common in adult female.

- Multiple reddish painful lesions over front of both legs associated with fever, malaise and arthralgia.
- Nodules may be 2–6 cm in diameter, occur in crops, over 2 weeks, then resolves slowly over months, leaving bruise stain in the skin. It never ulcerates, may be recurrent.
- Features of primary disease.

Investigations

- CBC, ESR, PBF (leucocytosis in streptococcal infection, high ESR in TB).
- ASO titre, throat swab for C/S, blood for C/S (in streptococcal infection).
- Chest X-ray (TB and sarcoidosis).
- MT and sputum for AFB (in TB).
- Lymph node—FNAC and/or biopsy.
- In inflammatory bowel disease—double-contrast barium enema, sigmoidoscopy or colonoscopy, barium follow through.
- Other investigations—according to suspicion of cause.

Treatment

- Rest.
- For pain—NSAID.
- Treatment of primary cause (e.g. penicillin, if streptococcal infection).
- In severe cases—prednisolone should be given. In some cases, dapsone 100 mg daily, colcichine 500 mg twice daily may be helpful.
- Potassium iodide 400–900 mg daily may be helpful.

ACNE VULGARIS

Definition

It is a disease in which there is excessive sebum secretion associated with obstruction of pilo-sebaceous duct.

Common Sites

Face, nose, back, shoulders, upper chest.

Clinical Features

Common in young, <25 years, often familial and found in oily skin.

- Comedones—It is the primary lesion of acne. It may be open comedones (black heads) and closed comedones (white heads). Also papule, pustules or cyst.
- Seborrhoea (greasy skin) is obvious, often present in face and scalp.
- Scarring may occur on skin if left untreated. May be atrophic, pitted or hypertrophic.

Treatment

General Measures

- Explanation and reassurance.
- Face should be washed with soap and water 2–3 times daily.
- Avoidance of cosmetics.
- Squeezing or scratching the lesion should be avoided.

Local Measures

- Topical benzoyl peroxide 2.5–5%.
- Topical retinoid.
- Isotretinoin 0.5–1 mg/kg.
- Tazarotene—applied once at night or every other night.
- Topical antibiotic—clindamycin 1% or erythromycin.
- Retinoic acid cream applied 2–3 times a week at night for 3–4 months.

Oral Therapy

- Tetracycline—250–500 mg 1–4 times daily with gradual reduction of dose depending on clinical response.
- Doxycycline—50–100 mg once or twice daily.
- Minocycline—50–100 mg once or twice daily.
- Erythromycin—if intolerant to tetracycline or in pregnant women, 250–500 mg 2–4 times a day, reduced gradually after control is achieved.
- Clindamycin—150 mg three times daily, reduced gradually.

Other Measures

- Cryotherapy, chemical cauterization, laser therapy.
- Surgical removal of comedone or pastule or cyst.
- Intralesional Inj. triamcinolone acetonide in inflamed nodules.

Complications

- Scarring, hyperpigmentation.
- Keloid.
- Pyogenic granuloma formation.
- Folliculitis.
- Rhinophyma.

LUPUS VULGARIS

Definition

It is the tuberculosis of skin.

Common Sites

Skin of head, neck, face mainly around the nose, also in arms and legs.

Clinical Features

- Reddish brown plaque (or nodules) or ulcerated area with irregular margin with smooth and glistening fine scaling over it.
- Lesions heal with scarring and new lesions slowly spread out to form chronic solitary erythematous plaque.

Clinical Types

5 types:

1. Plaque form.
2. Ulcerative and mutilating form.
3. Vegetating form.
4. Tumour like form.
5. Papular and nodular form.

Mode of Infection

Commonly occurs at the site of inoculation by direct extension from underlying infected gland or joints, lymphatic or haematogenous spread from other site.

Investigations

- CBC, ESR.
- MT.
- Chest X-ray.
- Skin biopsy for histopathology.

Treatment

- Standard antitubercular therapy—rifampicin, INH, ethambutol, pyrazinamide for 2 months.
- In continuation phase—rifampicin and INH for 4–10 months.

LEG ULCER

Causes

1. Traumatic.
2. Diabetes mellitus.
3. Infection—pyogenic, tuberculosis, leprosy, cutaneous leishmaniasis, fungal infection.
4. Arterial causes—atherosclerosis, peripheral vascular disease (including Buerger's disease, Raynaud's disease, etc.).
5. Venous ulcer—usually due to varicose vein.
6. Neuropathic ulcer—due to diabetes mellitus, tabes dorsalis, syringomyelia, leprosy, polyneuropathy.
7. Collagen disease—SLE, rheumatoid arthritis, Felty's syndrome, cryoglobulinaemia, polyarteritis nodosa.
8. Haematological diseases—sickle cell disease, thalassaemia, hereditary spherocytosis, paroxysmal nocturnal haemoglobinuria.
9. Neoplastic—squamous cell carcinoma, basal cell carcinoma, Kaposi's sarcoma.
10. Others—pyoderma gangrenosum, dermatitis, artefact, drugs.

Investigations

- CBC, ESR and PBF.
- Blood sugar.
- Lipid profile.
- Pus (if any) for C/S, AFB, LD bodies.
- Doppler USG of lower-limb vessels.
- X-ray of leg (calcification in artery).
- Arteriography.
- Biopsy.
- Others—according to suspicion of causes, e.g. ANA, cold agglutinin, RA test.

Treatment

1. General Measures

- Smoking must be stopped.
- Control of DM, hypertension, obesity (if any).
- Treatment of primary cause.
- Local care (cleaning and dressings).

2. Specific Measures

- Antibiotic, if any infection.
- Low-dose aspirin.
- In some cases, surgery (balloon dilatation), amputation, if necessary.
- Consultation with chiropodist.

MYCOSIS FUNGOIDES

Definition

Mycosis fungoides (cutaneous T cell lymphoma) is a rare skin tumour that develops slowly over many years (sometimes 20–30 years), characterized by reddish-brown, scaly and itchy plaques. In early stage, resemble erythematous lesions of psoriasis or eczema.

Treatment

- Early cutaneous disease—Follow-up. Topical steroid or PUVA may be given.
- In advanced case—radiotherapy, chemotherapy (e.g. methotrexate), immunotherapy or electron beam therapy may be used.

SEZARY'S SYNDROME

Definition

- It is an erythrodermic variant of mycosis fungoides characterized by erythroderma, lymphadenopathy and large mononuclear cells (Sezary cells) in the skin and blood.
- It is often resistant to treatment and carries poor prognosis.

LICHEN PLANUS

Definition

It is characterized by flat-topped, pruritic, polygonal violaceous papules on the flexors of wrist, trunk, medial aspect of thighs and shins. Oral mucosa shows reticulated whitish (or violaceous) plaques consisting of pin-head papules on the inner aspect of cheeks.

Clinical Features

- Skin—bilateral symmetrical multiple flat-topped violaceous papules.
- Koebner's phenomenon and Wickham's striae are present.
- Oral mucosa—violaceous reticular lesions on the inner aspect of cheeks with silvery-white papules.
- Nails show grooving, onycholysis, ridging and splitting.

Investigations

1. Routine
   - CBC.
   - Viral marker for hepatitis B and C.
   - Liver and renal function tests.
2. Specific
   - Skin biopsy for histopathology.
   - DIF.

Treatment

1. General Measures

- Protection from trauma.
- Precipitating drugs like diuretic, beta-blocker, antimalarial should be avoided.

2. Specific

- For skin—topical steroid, tacrolimus, pimecrolimus, psoralen and ultraviolet light. Oral prednisolone 30–80 mg/day. Etretinate, acitretin, isotretin may be given. If no response—ciclosporin, dapsone, hydroxychloroquine, azathioprine, mycophenolate mofetil may be given.
- Oral lesion—topical steroid, nystatin with clobetasole, topical tretinoin with steroid, 0.1% topical tacrolimus. Oral hydroxychloroquine 200–400 mg daily for 6 months or thalidomide 150 mg/day.

ARSENICOSIS

Cause

Prolonged ingestion of tube well water contaminated with arsenic produces arsenicosis.

Clinical Features

- Melanosis—hyperpigmentation (generalized or localized) with few scattered hypopigmented areas giving rise to 'raindrop' appearance.
- Hyperkeratosis of palm and sole. May be multiple, punctate, hard, discrete, papule and verrucous plaque.
- Nails—brittle, may show transverse white striae of finger nails (Mees' line).
- Hair—dry, sparse, may falloff.
- Eye—conjunctivitis.
- Nose—rhinitis, epistaxis, nasal obstruction, septal perforation.
- May involve any system of the body (liver, kidney, lung and heart).

Investigations

1. Routine—CBC, urine for R/E, chest X-ray, liver and renal function tests (SGPT, S. creatinine).
2. Specific—measurement of arsenic in hair, nail, urine, serum.
3. Others—according to the organ involved.

Systemic effects of chronic arsenic toxicity:

1. GIT—anorexia, nausea, vomiting.
2. Hepatic—hepatomegaly, cirrhosis of liver, noncirrhotic portal hypertension, hepatoma.
3. Nervous system—peripheral neuropathy (mainly sensory), seizure, confusion, encephalopathy.
4. Haematological—anaemia, leucopenia, thrombocytopenia.
5. Musculoskeletal—myalgia, arthralgia, wrist drop or foot drop.
6. Renal—dysuria, anuria, renal tubular necrosis.
7. Heart—cardiomyopathy, arrhythmia, heart failure.
8. Vascular—peripheral vascular insufficiency causing black foot disease.
9. Endocrine—diabetes mellitus may be precipitated.
10. Malignancy:
    - Skin—squamous cell carcinoma, basal cell carcinoma, Bowen's disease.
    - Carcinoma of lung, kidney, urinary bladder, liver, prostate and colon.

Treatment

1. Drinking of arsenic contaminated water must be stopped.
2. High protein diet.
3. Antioxidant (vitamin A 50,000 IU, vitamin C 500 mg and vitamin E 200 mg daily for 3 months).
4. Other vitamin and mineral supplement.
5. Vegetable and fresh fruit.
6. Spirulina (an algae), rich in high protein, may help clear arsenic.
7. For skin lesion—keratolytic emollients (salicylic acid, urea, retinoic acid), cryotherapy, electrocautery, laser therapy.

8. Drugs (chelating agent may be used):
   - D-penicillamine for 3 months, or
   - Dimercaprol (BAL), dimercaptosuccinic acid (DMSA) and dimercaptopropane sulphonate (DMPS).

Preventive therapy—Drinking water should be safe.

TINEA VERSICOLOR (PITYRIASIS VERSICOLOR)

Definition

It is benign superficial skin infection caused by *Malassezia furfur*.

Clinical Features

Common in warm months, also in immunocompromized. Upper trunk is mostly involved.

- Lesions are small white spots on the trunk, neck, upper arm, face.
- May be velvety, faintly brown macules.
- May fuse together forming bigger area of depigmentation.
- On scratching, fine scales may be separated from the patch.
- No itching.

Diagnosis: Clinical

- Direct microscopic examination of scales with KOH.
- Wood's Lamp—blue-green fluorescence of scales.

Treatment

Local Therapy

- Selenium sulphide (2.5%) lotion may be applied from neck to waist for 5–15 minutes.
- Ketoconazole shampoo over chest and back for 5 minutes.
- Azole creams (ketoconazole, econazole, micronazole, clotrimazole).
- Terbinafine 1% solution.
- General measures—personal hygiene should maintained, inner germants should be boiled and changed daily.

Systemic Therapy

- Oral ketoconazole 200 mg daily for 1 week.
- Ketoconazole—400 mg single dose, may be repeated at monthly intervals.
- Oral itraconazole—200 mg once daily for 7 days.
- Fluconazole—400 mg once may be effective, can be repeated at monthly intervals.

DERMATOPHYTE INFECTION (RING WORM)

Caused by different types of dermatophytes that infect the skin and appendages (e.g. hair and nail). Lesion is ring like, annular.

Clinical Types

According to the site of involvement:
1. Tinea capitis—in scalp and hair.
2. Tinea corporis—in trunk and limbs (body).
3. Tinea cruris—in groin.
4. Tinea pedis—in foot, called athlete's foot.
5. Tinea unguium—in nails.
6. Tinea barbae—in beared hair.

Tinea Capitis

Tinea capitis or scalp ringworm, occurs mainly in children (6–10 years), may be seen at all ages. Boys are affected more.

Incubation Period

2–4 days.

Risk Factors

Debilitation, malnutrition, chronic disease.
Transmission: person-to-person, animal-to-person, via fomites.

Clinical Features

- Broken-off stumps of hair, rounded patches with crusts or pustules and few hair. The broken-off hair are surrounded by or contain fungus. Hair shaft becomes brittle, breaking off at or slightly above scalp.
- May be scaling, diffuse or circumscribed alopecia, occipital or posterior auricular lymphadenopathy.
- If inflammation—pain, tenderness may be present.

Investigations

- Wood's Lamp.
- Direct Microscopy.
- Fungal culture—dermatophytes are usually seen in 10–14 days.
- Bacterial culture to rule out infection, usually *Staph. aureus*.

Treatment

1. Topical agents—imidazoles (clotrimazole, miconazole, ketoconazole, econazole, oxiconazole), allylamines (naftifine, terbinafine).
2. Systemic antifungal—griseofulvin, itraconazole, terbinafin, fluconazole may be given.
   - Terbinafine—3–6 mg/kg/day for 1–4 weeks.

- Itraconazole—5 mg/kg/day for 2-3 weeks.
- Fluconazole—6 mg/kg/ day for 2-3 weeks.

3. Selenium sulfide shampoo or ketoconazole shampoo left on the scalp for 5 minutes 3 times a week. Can be used as adjunctive therapy to oral antifungal agents.
4. Combs, brushes, hats should be cleaned carefully.
5. Prednisolone—1 mg/kg/day for 14 days for children with severe, painful kerion.

Tinea Cruris

Common in adult, more in males, caused by *T. rubrum, T. mentagrophytes.*

Clinical Features

- Large, scaling, well demarcated dull red or tan or brown plaques with central clearing. Papules, pustules may be present at margins.
- Commonly affect in groins and thighs, may extend to buttocks. Scrotum and penis are rarely involved.

Diagnosis

Usually clinical. Skin scrapings for fungus and culture on a suitable medium.

Treatment

1. Localized disease without fungal folliculitis:
   - Topical therapy—miconazole, clotrimazole, econazole, ketoconazole, terbinafine.
2. Extensive disease or fungal folliculitis—requires systemic antifungal treatment.
   - Terbinafine—250 mg/day for 1-2 weeks.
   - Itraconazole—200 mg/day for 1week.
   - Fluconazole—150 mg once a week for 4 weeks.

Tinea Corporis

Caused by *T. rubrum* involving trunk, legs, arms, neck. Common in animal workers.

Clinical Features

- Scaling, sharply marginated plaques.
- Peripheral enlargement and central clearing, produce ring-like or arcuate lesions, fusion of lesions produces gyrate patterns.
- Single or scattered multiple lesions.

Diagnosis: Clinical

Skin scrapings for fungus M/E and culture on a suitable medium.

Treatment

Same as *T. cruris.*

TINEA UNGUIUM (ONYCHOMYCOSIS)

Definition

It is the infection of the nail plate by fungus, mainly caused by *Trychophyton rubrum*.

Clinical Features

- Usually starts at the distal corner of nail and involves the junction of nail and its bed.
- Affected nail becomes rough, friable, discoloured, nail plate is fragmented. Subungual hyperkeratosis may occur.
- Gradually, the entire nail becomes brittle and separated with characteristic branny scaling and erythema.

Diagnosis: Clinical

Fungus can be isolated by microscopic examination and culture.

Treatment

Local Treatment

- Topical agent—ciclopirox and amorolfine nail lacquers are modestly effective.

Systemic Treatment

- Terbinafine—250 mg/day for 6–8 weeks. For toe nails, 12–16 weeks.
- Itraconazole—200 mg twice daily for 1 week of each month, for 2 months when treating fingernails and for 3–4 months when treating toe nails.
- Fluconazole—150–300 mg once a week for 6–12 months.

Tinea Barbae

It is characterized by red inflammatory papules, vesicles or pustules surrounding the hair root of bear. Oozing and crust formation may occur. Involved hairs are usually shed off.

Treatment

Like *T. corporis*. Griseofalvin may be given for about 1 month.

MELASMA (CHLOASMA)

Definition

Melasma is an acquired light- or dark-brown hyperpigmentation that occurs in the exposed areas, most often on the cheeks.

It may be associated with:

- Pregnancy.
- Oral contraceptive pill.
- Sun exposure.
- Certain medications, such as diphenylhydantoin.
- May be idiopathic.

Clinical Features

Common in young.

- Macular hyperpigmentation, sharply defined in the malar and frontal areas of the face. Usually uniform but also blotchy.

Treatment

1. Exposure to sunlight should be avoided and sunblock with broad-spectrum UVA coverage should be used daily.
2. Topical therapy:
   - Hydroquinone cream (2–4%).
   - Tretinoin cream may be added.
   - Combination of hydroquinone, tretinoin and steroid called "Kligman's formula"—can be used once daily.
   - Mequinol, azelaic acid, kojic acid, vitamin E cream may be used.

ECZEMA

Definition

Eczema is defined as pruritic inflammatory disease of skin caused by various external and internal factors.

It is characterized clinically by papules, vesicles and oozing in its acute stage, scaling and crusting in its subacute stage and lichenification in its chronic stage.

Classification

Can be classified into various ways:

On the Basis of Aetiological Factors

Exogenous and endogenous.

Exogenous Eczema

Related to external trigger factors, such as:
- Irritant contact dermatitis.
- Irritant photocontact dermatitis.
- Allergic contact dermatitis.
- Allergic photocontact dermatitis.
- Infective dermatitis.
- Eczematous polymorphic light eruption.
- Posttraumatic eczema.

Endogenous Eczema—due to factors within the body, such as:
- Atopic dermatitis.
- Seborrhoeic dermatitis.
- Asteatotic eczema.
- Discoid or nummular eczema.
- Gravitational eczema.
- Eczema associated with systemic disease.
- Chronic superficial scaly dermatitis.

Clinically

- Acute—there is itching with erythema, papulovesicular eruption, scab formation.
- Subacute—there is scab and crust formation.
- Chronic—scratch mark and fissure, lichenification or hyperpigmentation.

Clinical Features

Depend upon the type of eczema. In case of endogenous eczema, atopic dermatitis and seborrhoeic dermatitis are common.

Diagnostic Tests for Eczema

Diagnosis is clinical. But some tests are helpful to confirm the diagnosis or to differentiate it from other diseases:

- CBC, ESR.
- Serum IgE.
- Skin-scraping microscopy and culture to exclude fungal infection.
- Skin biopsy for histopathology.
- Patch test—may be done in some cases.

ATOPIC DERMATITIS

1. It is divided into 3 stages:
   Infantile (2 months to 2 years)—begins as erythema and scaling in cheek. May involve scalp, neck, forehead, wrist and extensor surface of the extremities. Lesions are exudative with crusts, infiltration and pustules.
2. Childhood (2–10 years)—less exudative. Mainly involve the antecubital and popliteal fossae, flexor surface of wrist, eyelids, face and around the neck.
3. Adolescent and adult (above 10 years)—usually there is childhood disease. In adolescent, involves the antecubital and popliteal fossae, front and sides of neck, forehead and area around eyes. In older adult, mainly involve hand, nipple and eyelid are involved.

Management

General Measures

- Patient's education and psychological support.
- Moisturizing with petrolatum after bath.
- Avoidance of excessive rubbing, vigorous bathing, tight clothings, scratching.
- Avoidance of excessive soap, extreme heat and cold, sweating, stress, external irritants.

Symptomatic Treatment

1. Topical or systemic antibiotic—if any infection.
2. To control pruritus:
   - Antihistamine (e.g. diphenhydramine, hydroxyzine, cetirizine, fexofenadine).

Specific Treatment

1. Topical therapy
   - Topical corticosteroid—in infants, low-potency steroid ointment like 1% or 2.5% hydrocortisone. In older children and adult, medium-potency steroid like triamcinolone is used. In refractory cases and thick plaques, potent steroid like betamethasone, clobetasole or halobetasole are used.
   - Tacrolimus, pimecrolimus are alternatives to steroid.
   - One to five percent crude coal tar in white petrolatum or hydrophilic ointment is sometimes used.

2. Phototherapy—narrow-band UVB therapy when topical therapies fail.
3. Systemic therapy:
   - Systemic steroid—to control acute exacerbation.
   - Ciclosporin is highly effective but response is rarely sustained after the drug is withdrawn.
   - Other agents—azathioprine, mycophenolate mofetil, methotrexate, IV immunoglobulin, biologic agent (omalizumab).

SEBORRHOEIC DERMATITIS

Definition

It is characterized by yellow greasy scale on an erythematous base and occurs in the regions where the sebaceous glands are most active.

Sites

Scalp, eyebrows, eyelids, nasolabial creases, lips, ears, sternal area, axillae, submammary folds, umbilicus, groins and gluteal crease.

Clinical Features

May occur in infancy (within first month), puberty, 20–50 years or older. More common in males.

- In skin—orange-red or greyish-white skin, often with 'greasy' or white dry scaling macules, papules of varying size or patches.
- On the scalp—marked scaling (dandruff), diffuse involvement.
- On the face—lesions are scattered, discrete, nummular, polycyclic and annular on the trunk.

Diagnosis

Usually clinical. Laboratory investigations may be done to isolate dermatophyte.

Management

Topical Therapy

Scalp

- Adults—shampoo containing selenium sulfide, zinc pyrithione and/or tar. 2% ketoconazole shampoo, glucocorticoid solution, lotion, or gels after medicated shampoo (ketoconazole or tar) may be used for severe cases. Pimecrolimus, 1% cream.
- Infants—removal of crusts with warm olive oil, followed by 2% ketoconazole shampoo and 1–2.5% hydrocortisone cream or 2% ketoconazole cream and 1% pimecrolimus cream.

Face and Trunk—ketoconazole shampoo, 2% glucocorticoid cream and lotions. In more resistant cases, clobetasol propionate, 2% ketoconazole cream, 1% pimecrolimus cream and 0.03% or 0.1% tacrolimus ointment.

Eyelids—gentle removal of crusts. Apply 10% sodium sulfacetamide in 0.2% prednisolone and 0.12% phenylephrine. 2% ketoconazole cream, 1% pimecrolimus cream or 0.03% tacrolimus ointment.

Systemic Therapy

- In severe case—13-*cis*-retinoic acid orally, 0.5–1 mg/kg. Contraception should be used in females of childbearing age.
- In mild case—itraconazole 100 mg twice daily for 2 weeks

Maintenance Therapy

- Ketoconazole 2% shampoo, tar shampoo and ketoconazole cream.
- If no response—3% sulfur precipitate and 2% salicylic acid in oil water base or 1–2.5% hydrocortisone cream or 0.03% tacrolimus ointment.

CONTACT DERMATITIS

Definition

It may be defined as acute or chronic inflammatory reactions of the skin that occur following contact with any substance.

Types

- Irritant contact dermatitis—caused by chemical irritant.
- Allergic contact dermatitis—caused by antigen (allergen).

IRRITANT CONTACT DERMATITIS

Common Toxic Agents

- Soap, detergent.
- Acids and alkali—hydrofluoric acid, chromic acid.
- Industrial solvent—coal tar solvent, petroleum, chlorinated hydrocarbon.
- Others—fiberglass, wool, rough synthetic clothing.
- Occupational exposure—housekeeping, hairdressing, food preparation and catering, printing, painting, construction.

Predisposing Factors

Atopy, fare skin, low temperature, low humidity.

ACUTE IRRITANT CONTACT DERMATITIS

Symptoms

- Burning, stinging, smarting.

Signs

- Sharply demarcated erythema, vesicle, superficial oedema.
- In severe case—blisters, erosions, frank necrosis as with acid or alkali.
- Later—crusting, shedding of crusts and scaling, then healing.

CHRONIC IRRITANT CONTACT DERMATITIS

It occurs after repeated exposure to mild irritants (water, soap, detergent, etc.) usually on hands.

Treatment of Contact Dermatitis

Acute

- Removal of causative agent.
- Wet dressings with Burrow's solution, changed every 2–3 hours.
- Larger vesicles may be drained, but tops should not be removed.
- Topical glucocorticoid preparations.
- In severe case—prednisolone 40–60 mg initially, then taper.

Chronic

- Removal of causative agent.
- Potent topical steroid—betamethasone or clobetasol.
- Adequate lubrication. As healing occurs, continue with lubrication.

Systemic Treatment

- Acitretinoin 0.5 mg/kg body weight for 6 months.

OCCUPATIONAL CONTACT DERMATITIS

Treatment

- Avoidance of irritating and sensitizing substances.
- Proper use of all available protective devices.
- Personal protective measures—clothing changes, cleansing showers, protective clothing, protective barrier creams.
- Topical steroid.
- Topical tacrolimus ointment and pimecrolimus cream.

PITYRIASIS RUBRA PILARIS

Definition

Pityriasis rubra pilaris is a chronic skin disease characterized by small follicular papules, disseminated, yellowish pink scaling patches and often solid palmoplantar hyperkeratosis.

Types

As follows:
- Type I—adult onset classical.
- Type II—adult onset atypical.
- Type III—juvenile onset classical.
- Type IV—juvenile onset circumscribed.
- Type V—juvenile onset atypical.
- Type VI—HIV associated.

Cause of PRP

Unknown, usually autosomal dominant trait in juvenile onset, may be due to vitamin deficiency particularly vitamin A. Both sexes are affected equally.

Histopathological and DIF findings

1. Skin biopsy shows (specimen is taken from sites where hair follicles are numerous) -
   - Hyperkeratosis and parakeratosis.
   - Follicular plugging at the follicular orifice.
   - Alternating vertical and horizontal parakeratosis in the interfollicular stratum corneum is characteristic.
2. DIF is negative.

Treatment

- Systemic retinoids are effective.
- Isotretinoin 2–5 mg/kg/day for several months.
- Vitamin A 300,000–500,000 units daily with vitamin E 400 units two or three times daily.
- Systemic steroid—for acute short-term management.
- Methotrexate may be used alone or in combination with isotretinoin or acetretin.
- Azathioprine is also effective.
- In severe case, extracorporeal photochemotherapy with systemic retinoids and ciclosporin.
- Treatment of secondary infection, if present.

Complications

- Exfoliative dermatitis.
- Prolonged erythema.
- Ectropion.
- Peripheral edema.
- High-output cardiac failure.
- Eruptive seborrhoeic keratosis.

DARIER'S DISEASE OR KERATOSIS FOLLICULARIS

Definition

It is inherited as autosomal dominant. New mutations are common. Both sexes are affected equally, usually before 30 years.

Sites of involvement and manifestation:

1. Seborrhoeic area—symmetrical and widespread dirty, wart like, greasy, crusted papules usually over the face, scalp, forehead, nasolabial fold, retroauricular region, lip, front of the chest, back, axilla, anogenital region, natal cleft. Later the lesions fuse to form malodorous, papillomatous and vegetating growths. These are eroded, fissured and covered by purulent exudate. There may be pain, pruritus and bleeding from the lesions.
2. Sites without sebaceous glands—palms and soles in which there are uniform horny thickening, punctate keratosis, minute pits (pathognomonic).
3. Mucous membrane—white cobblestone papules in palate, tongue, buccal mucosa, epiglottis, simulate leucoplakia.
4. Nails—subungual hyperkeratosis, fragility, alternating white and red streaks.
5. Blockage of external auditory meatus and salivary glands.

Types

4 types

1. Classical or seborrhoeic.
2. Unilateral or zosteriform.
3. Hypertrophic—in flexural surface (axilla, groin).
4. Vesicobullous form.

Complications

- Herpes simplex infection.
- Chronic pyogenic infection.
- Kaposis varicelliform eruption.
- Pox virus infection.
- Defect in cell-mediated immunity. No abnormality in humoral immunity.

Diagnosis

Usually clinical. Skin biopsy for confirmation.

Treatment

Mild disease requires no treatment other than simple emollient. Patient should be advised about the effects of sunshine.

1. Topical treatment:
   - Retinoids—tretinoin, 13-cis-retinoic acid, adalpene, tazarotene.
2. Systemic treatment:
   - Isotretinoin, acetretin, ciclosporin can be used to control severe flares.
   - For secondary infection—antibiotic (cloxacillin, fluocloxacillin or cephalosporin).

3. For hypertrophic lesions:
   - Dermabrasion.
   - Laser excision.
   - Excision and grafting.

URTICARIA

Definition

Urticaria is a vascular reaction of the skin characterized by the formation of wheals, surrounded by red halo or flare, associated with severe itching, stinging or pricking sensations. It is secondary to exogenous or endogenous allergen. Wheals are due to localized oedema. Subcutaneous swelling (angioedema) may accompany the wheals.

Causes

- Physical agent—trauma, heat, cold.
- Drugs—sulphonamide, penicillin, NSAID.
- Food allergen—shell fish, crab, egg.
- Other allergens—grass pollen, house dust, mites, feathers, animal dander, cosmetics, aerosols.
- Infection—in upper respiratory tract especially streptococcal, infection in tonsil, tooth, sinuses.
- Parasitic—ascariasis, giardiasis, stronglyloids stercolaris.
- Autoimmune.
- Vasculitis.
- Emotional stress.
- Neoplasm—carcinoma, Hodgkin disease, chronic lymphocytic leukemia.
- Idiopathic.

Pathogenesis

Capillary permeability results from increased release of histamine from the mast cells situated around the capillaries. Other substances that may cause vasodilatation and capillary permeability are serotonin, leukotriens, prostaglandin, proteases and kinins.

Classification

- Acute urticaria—wheals persist for less than 12 hours, complete resolution occurs within 6 weeks.
- Chronic urticaria—daily episodes of urticaria and or angioedema lasting more than 6 weeks. More common in women.

Clinical Features

- Wheals of variable size and shape, blend together forming bigger wheels (called angioedema) that develop within minutes to hours.
- Itching of wheals.
- Angioedema may occur in lips, mouth, tongue. If involves the larynx and trachea, may cause respiratory obstruction.

Investigations

- CBC—eosinophilia.
- Stool for R/E—to exclude parasitic infection.
- Serum IgE—high.
- Others—according to suspicion of cause.

Treatment

Acute Urticaria

- Avoidance of allergen and treatment of primary cause.
- Antihistamine—chlorpheniramine, loratidine, fexofenadine.
- If no response—systemic corticosteroid.
- In angioedema—parenteral dexamethasone and antihistamine. If respiratory obstruction—intubation or tracheostomy may be needed.

Chronic Urticaria

- Antihistamin—cetirizine, levocetirizine, loratidine, acrivastine and azelastine.
- Doxepin, a tricyclic antidepressant may be added.
- Dapsone and colchicine may be helpful in neutrophil-rich urticaria.
- If all fails—systemic corticosteroid.
- Some cases of chronic urticaria have autoantibodies. In such case—immunosuppressive therapy, plasmapharesis or intravenous immunoglobulin.

ALOPECIA

Definition

It is defined as loss of hair.

Types of Alopecia: 3 types:

1. Alopecia areata (localized loss of hair in the scalp).
2. Alopecia totalis (hair loss of entire scalp).
3. Alopecia universalis (total loss of body hair).

Causes of Alopecia

May be nonscarring and scarring or cicatrical.

Nonscarring—Scalp skin looks normal. It may be diffuse and focal hair loss.

1. **Diffuse hair loss**
   - Androgenic alopecia.
   - Endocrine—hypopituitarism, hypothyroidism, hyperthyroidism, hypoparathyroidism,
   - Drugs—cytotoxic drugs, heparin, retinoid, hypervitaminosis A.
   - Abnormality of shedding—telogen effluvium, anagen effluvium.
   - Others—malnutrition, severe prolonged illness, deficiency of protein, iron, zinc and biotin, radiotherapy, postpartum.
2. **Focal hair loss**—tinea capitis, alopecia areata, secondary syphilis, SLE, traction alopecia.

Scarring alopecia: Causes are:

- Physical factors—burn, radiotherapy.
- Infective—furuncle, carbuncle, folliculitis, lupus vulgaris, tertiary syphilis, kerion and favus.
- Chemicals—acid and alkali.
- Autoimmune—DLE, morphea and cicatricial pemphigoid.
- Neoplastic—basal cell carcinoma and squamous cell carcinoma.
- Others—lichen planus, sarcoidosis, lichen sclerosus, follicular mucinosis, pseudopelade.

ALOPECIA AREATA

Definition

It is the localized loss of hair in the scalp.

It may be due to autoimmune mechanism. Found in SLE, associated with other autoimmune diseases, such as Hashimoto's thyroiditis, Graves' disease, pernicious anaemia, diabetes mellitus and vitiligo.

Diagnostic Points of Alopecia Areata

- Usually patches are 1–5 cm in diameter.
- Complete, patchy loss of hair, round or oval in shape.
- At the periphery of bald patches, there are loose hairs that may be broken off leaving short stumps. When they are pulled out, a tapered attenuated bulb is seen called **exclamation point hair**.

- Skin is smooth and shiny without inflammation and scaling.
- There may be nail pitting.

Investigations in Alopecia Areata

- Skin scraping for fungus (to exclude tinea capitis).
- ANA, anti-ds-DNA (SLE).
- Serological test for syphilis.

Treatment Alopecia Areata

1. Topical
   - Topical steroid.
   - One percent anthralin cream.
   - Topical minoxidil (2–5%).
2. Intralesional injection triamcinolone 2–10 mg/mL.
3. Photochemotherapy using topical or systemic methoxsalen and UVA (PUVA).
4. 308 nm xenom chloride excimer LASER helps produce regrowth after 11–12 sessions (9–11 weeks).
5. Analogous hair transplantation.

VITILIGO

Definition

It is the area of localized depigmentation, probably due to autoimmune mechanism due to focal loss of melanocyte. It affects 1% population.

Generalized vitiligo may occur, usually symmetrical involving hand, wrist, knee, neck, around the eyes, mouth, dorsum of feet. The sites at friction or trauma are often affected. Family history may be present in one-third cases. Equally affects both sexes, familial in 30%. Koebner's phenomenon may be present (lesions appear at the site of skin damage).

Diseases Associated in Vitiligo

May be associated with autoimmune diseases, such as systemic sclerosis, Addison's disease, pernicious anaemia, Graves' disease, Hashimoto's thyroiditis, premature ovarian failure, diabetes mellitus and primary biliary cirrhosis.

Types of Vitiligo

- Focal vitiligo—isolated macules or few scattered macules.
- Segmental vitiligo—unilateral macules in a dermatomal distribution. It has stable course, unlikely to be associated with thyroid or other vitiligo associated diseases.
- Generalized vitiligo—common type, characterized by few to many macules.
- Acrofacial vitiligo—involves distal digits and periorificial areas.
- Universal vitiligo—widespread vitiligo with few remaining normal pigmentation.

Differential Diagnoses of Vitiligo

- Tinea versicolor—common in back and chest. It has a fine scale. Yeast and hyphal forms are present (detected with 10% KOH solution).
- Pityriasis alba—associated with fine scale. Lesion is poorly defined.
- Tuberculoid leprosy.
- Morphea and lichen sclerosis—hypopigmented or depigmented area associated with change in skin texture.
- Tuberous sclerosis (ash leaf spot).
- Chemical leucoderma.
- Burn.

Investigations

Diagnosis is clinical.

- Woods light examination shows chalky or ivory-white fluorescence.
- Skin scraping for *Malassezia furfur* (to differentiate from tinea versicolor).
- Others—blood sugar, thyroid function tests and serum cortisol can be done according to the suspicion of causes.

Treatment

1. General measures
   - Reassurance.
   - Use of sunscreen.
   - Use of self-tanning cream containing dihydroxyacetone.

2. Topical
   - Steroid (betamethasone and clobetasol propionate).
   - Topical calcipotriene can be added to topical steroid.
   - 0.1% tacrolimus ointment in facial vitiligo.
3 Phototherapy
   - Narrow band UVB.
   - Topical 8-methoxypsoralen followed by UVA.
4. Surgical
   - Epidermal grafting or autologous minigraft.
   - Transplantation of cultured melanocytes can be applied in patients with segmental vitiligo or with stable vitiligo, not responding to other therapy.

NB: Spontaneous re-pigmentation occurs in 15–25% cases.

CHAPTER

12 Sexually Transmitted Diseases

CHAPTER CONTENTS

- Gonorrhoea
- Lymphogranuloma Venereum
- Chancroid
- Syphilis
  - Congenital syphilis
  - Acquired syphilis
- Nongonococcal Urethritis

GONORRHOEA

Definition

It is a sexually transmitted disease (STD) caused by *Neisseria gonorrhoeae,* a Gram negative diplococcus.

Mode of Transmission

- Sexually from partner.
- Neonate exposed to infected secretions in birth canal.

Clinical Features

In Male

- Dysuria, frequency and burning micturition.
- Urethral discharge—copious, mucopurulent or purulent.
- Lower abdominal pain.
- May cause prostatitis, epididymitis.
- In chronic case—chronic prostatitis, urethral stricture.

In Female

- Dysuria, frequency and burning micturition.
- Urethral discharge—copious, mucopurulent or purulent.
- Lower abdominal pain.
- Vulvovaginitis, cervicitis, salpingitis, salpingo-oophorotis.
- Bartholin abscess.

Other Features

According to site of involvement:
- Anorectum—proctitis with pain and purulent discharge.
- Pharynx—pharyngitis with erythema secondary to oro-genital sexual exposure.
- Disseminated infection—if untreated, disseminated gonococcal infection may occur. Typically affects women with asymptomatic genital infection. There may be arthritis of one or more joints, pustular skin lesions, fever.

In Neonate

- Ophthalmia neonatorum—conjunctivitis, swollen eyelids, severe hyperaemia, chemosis, profuse purulent discharge. Rarely, corneal ulcer and perforation.

Investigations

1. Gram stain - Gram negative diplococci seen on microscopy of smear from infected site.
2. Culture (chocolate agar media, Thayer-Martin media)
   - Men—swab from urethra, rectum, oropharynx.
   - Women—swab from cervix, rectum, oropharynx.

Treatment

- Single dose intramuscular ceftriaxone 500 mg or
- Oral cefixime 400 mg single dose or
- Ciprofloxacin 500 mg orally single dose or
- Ofloxacin 400 mg orally single dose or
- Amoxicillin 3 g plus probenecid 1 gm orally single dose.
- In quinolone resistant case—single dose IM ceftriaxone 500 mg or spectinomycin 2 mg IM stat.
- Disseminated gonococcal infection—IV ceftriaxone 1 gm daily for 5 days.

LYMPHOGRANULOMA VENEREUM

Definition

It is a venereal disease caused by *Chlamydia trachomatis*, an obligate intracellular bacteria.

Mode of Transmission

Through sexual act.

Incubation Period

3 days to 3 weeks.

Clinical Features

1. Within few days after sexual contact, small painless vesicle or ulcer or papule is found in the genitalia, that heals in few days.
2. Infection can spread from primary site to regional lymph nodes through lymphatics.
3. Two syndromes:
   - Inguinal syndrome—painful inguinal lymphadenopathy. Initially, nodes are discrete, but later, nodes are matted, large, suppurative with discharge of yellow pus. Scarring with multiple sinus develop.
   - Genito-anorectal syndrome—common in female and homosexual male. There is perirectal inflammation with discharge of blood, mucous and pus through anus. There may lymphoedema of vulva, penis and scrotum.

Diagnosis

Usually, clinical. Serological test for L1 to L3 serotype. Isolation of organism from swab taken from ulcer or bubo pus for Chlamydia.

Treatment

- Oral tetracycline 500 mg 4 times for 3–6 weeks or
- Oral doxycycline 100 mg twice daily for 21 days or
- Oral erythromycin 500 mg four times daily for 21 days.

CHANCROID

Causative Organism

Haemophilus ducreyi, a Gram negative cocco-bacillus.

Incubation Period

Three to five days.

Mode of Transmission

Sexual contact.

Clinical Features

- Primary lesion—small red papule or pustule on the genitalia and surrounding skin. Within a few days, ulcer develops.
- Ulcer—usually painful with sharp, undermined border. Ulcer may be single or multiple.
- Painful inguinal lymphadenopathy which may suppurate (bubo).

Diagnosis

Painful ulcer with tender lymphadenopathy is suggestive of chancroid. A definitive diagnosis is done by identification of *H. ducreyi* on special culture media.

Treatment

- Azithromycin 1 g in single dose or
- Ciprofloxacin 500 mg twice daily for 3 days or
- Erythromycin 500 mg 3 times daily for 7 days.
- IM ceftriaxone 250 mg in single dose.

SYPHILIS

Causative Organism

Treponema pallidum.

Mode of Transmission

- Sexual contact.
- Congenital infection—transplacental or perinatal transmission.

Classification

- May be congenital and acquired.

Congenital Syphilis

Features develop after four months of gestation when the foetus becomes immune-competent. Its features are as follows:

1. Miscarriage or stillbirth.
2. Premature delivery.
3. Birth of baby with early congenital syphilis (neonatal period), features are:
   - Maculopapular rash
   - Condylomata lata
   - Mucous patches
   - Fissures around the mouth, nose and anus
   - Rhinitis with nasal discharge (snuffles)
   - Hepatosplenomegaly
   - Osteochondritis or periostitis
   - Generalised lymphadenopathy
   - Choroiditis.
   - Meningitis.
   - Anaemia, thrombocytopaenia.
4. Birth of a baby with latent infection who either remains well or shows features of late congenital syphilis:
   - Benign tertiary syphilis
   - Periostitis
   - Paroxysmal cold haemoglobinuria
   - Neurosyphilis
   - 8th nerve deafness
   - Interstitial keratitis
   - Clutton's joints (painless effusion into knee joints).

Stigmata of Congenital Syphilis

- Hutchinson's teeth—notch in incisor teeth
- Mulberry molars—imperfect cusps or deficient dental enamel
- High-arched palate, perforation of palate
- Maxillary hypoplasia

- Saddle nose—depression of nasal bridge
- Rhagades—radiating scars around mouth, nose and anus following rash
- Corneal scars due to interstitial keratitis.
- Sabre tibia due to periostitis
- Bossing of frontal and parietal bones
- Clutton's joints (painless effusion into knee joints)
- 8th nerve damage.

NB: Hutchison's teeth, interstitial keratitis and deafness are called "Hutchison's Triad".

Acquired Syphilis

Types

May be primary, secondary and tertiary.

Primary Syphilis

Incubation Period

Ten to ninety days. Average 21 days.

Clinical Features

- Genital or extragenital lesions at sites of inoculation called 'Chancre,' which is a painless ulcer, usually single with raised border and scanty serous exudate.
- Extragenital chancre occurs at any site of inoculation— anus or rectum, mouth, lips, tongue tonsils, fingers (painful), toes, breast, nipple.
- Chancre heals in 4–6 weeks, even without treatment.

Diagnosis

Clinical suspicion. Confirmed by:

1. Detection of *T. pallidum* by dark ground illumination from chancre.
2. Serological tests:
   - Non-treponemal (nonspecific) tests—
   - Venereal Disease Research Laboratory (VDRL) test
   - Rapid plasma reagin (RPR) test.
   - Treponemal (specific) antibody tests—
   - Treponemal antigen—based on enzyme immunoassay (EIA)
   - Treponemal haemaggutination assay (TPHA)
   - *T. pallidum* particle agglutination assay (TPPA)
   - Fluorescent Treponema antibody absorbtion test (FTA-ABS).

Treatment

- Injection Benzathine penicillin 2.4 million units in single dose IM or
- Oral doxycycline 100 mg twice daily for 14 days.

Secondary Syphilis

Appears 2–6 months after primary infection following healing of chancre.

Clinical Features

1. General features—fever, sore throat, weight loss, malaise, anorexia, headache, meningism.
2. Skin lesions—
   - Maculo-papular rash, copper or roseolar in colour, may be generalized on the trunk, limb, palms and soles
   - Condylomata lata—warty lesion, commonly in ano-genital region, also in moist areas
   - Diffuse hair loss, patchy, moth eaten alopecia on the scalp and beard area. Loss of eyelashes, lateral third of eyebrows.
3. In mucous membrane of mouth—there may be painless greyish ulcer called "snail track ulcer".
4. Generalised lymphadenopathy involving cervical, suboccipital, inguinal, epitrochlear, axillary which are small, discrete and nontender.
5. Other features—periostitis of long bones particularly tibia, arthralgia, iritis, optic neuritis, uveitis, hepatitis, ulcerative colitis, glomerulonephritis and nephrotic syndrome, cystitis, prostatitis.
6. Splenomegaly.

Investigations

- As in primary
- CSF study—abnormal in 40% of patients. Spirochaetes are found in CSF in 30% of cases.

Diagnosis

Clinical suspicion, confirmed by lab tests. Dark ground illumination (DGI) is positive in all secondary syphilis lesions except for macular exanthem.

Treatment

- As in primary syphilis.

Latent Syphilis

In this stage, there is no clinical feature and no organism is detected. Only serological tests are positive. This stage may persist for many years or for life with little or no ill health.

Tertiary or Late Syphilis

This stage can occur at any time after secondary syphilis, even after many years. It may involve any organ. No organism is detected, so this stage is not infective. Typical lesion is formation of "Gumma".

Benign Tertiary Syphilis

Develops between 3 and 10 years after infection. Single or multiple nodular or papulo-squamous plaques (called gumma) that occur at any site of the skin, especially on scalp, face, chest, mucus membranes, bone, muscle and viscera (larynx, liver and stomach) that may ulcerate and form circles.

Neurosyphilis

May be asymptomatic or symptomatic which may present as features of tabes dorsalis or general paresis of insane (GPI). In eye, there is Argyll Robertson pupil.

Meningeal or menigovuscular syphilis

Characterised by headache, nausea, vomiting, neck stiffness, cranial nerve palsy, seizure, change in mental status.

Cardiovascular syphilis

Results from endarteritis obliterans of vasa vasorum. Occurs in 10% of late untreated syphilis, 10–40 years after infection. Aortitis, aortic regurgitation, aortic aneurysm, coronary ostial stenosis may occur.

Diagnosis

Clinical findings, confirmed by STS and lesional skin biopsy. DGI test is always negative.

Treatment

Injection benzathine penicillin 2.4 million units IM once a week for three weeks.

NONGONOCOCCAL URETHRITIS

Definition

Nongonococcal urethritis (NGU) is a sexually transmitted disease caused by organism other than *N. gonorrhoeae*. It is also called nonspecific urethritis.

Causative Organism

- *Chlamydia trachomatis*
- *Ureaplasma urealyticum*
- Others—*Trichomonas vaginalis*, herpes simplex virus, *Candida albicans*

Incubation Period

2–3 weeks.

Clinical Features

- Discomfort or burning during micturition with purulent or mucoid urethral discharge, mainly in the early morning.

Diagnosis

- Routine urine R/E shows pus cell
- Isolation of organism in a special culture media.

Treatment

- Doxycycline 100 mg 12 hourly for 7 days or
- Erythromycin 500 mg 6 hourly for 7 days or
- Azithromycin 1 g single dose orally.

CHAPTER

13 Nervous System

CHAPTER CONTENTS

- Upper motor neuron
- Lower motor neuron
- Extrapyramidal system
- Gait abnormality
- Infection of CNS
- Meningitis
  - Acute bacterial meningitis
  - Viral meningitis
  - Tuberculous meningitis (TBM)
- Encephalitis
- Brain abscess
- Headache
- Migraine
- Cluster headache
- Bell's palsy
- Sixth nerve palsy
- Third nerve palsy
- Ptosis
- Horner syndrome
- Papilloedema
- Optic neuritis
- Optic atrophy
- Multiple cranial nerve palsy
- Pupil
- Trigeminal neuralgia
- Multiple sclerosis
- Syringomyelia
- Polyneuropathy
- Carpal tunnel syndrome (median nerve palsy)
- Ulnar nerve palsy
- Radial nerve palsy
- Subacute combined degeneration
- Parkinsonism
- Involuntary movements
  - Tremor
  - Chorea
  - Athetosis
  - Hemiballismus
  - Myoclonus
  - Tic
  - Torsion dystonia
- Motor neuron disease
- Stroke (CVD or CVA)
- Brief description of different types of CVD
- Coma or unconsciousness
- Myasthenia gravis
- Eaton–Lambert syndrome
- Transverse myelitis
- Cerebellar lesion
- Friedreich's ataxia
- Raised intracranial pressure
- Intracranial space occupying lesion (ICSOL)
- Benign (idiopathic) intracranial hypertension
- Brain tumours
- Wilson's disease
- Paraplegia

- Spastic paraplegia
- Flaccid paraplegia

- Guillain–Barré syndrome
- Chronic inflammatory demyelinating polyneuropathy
- Epilepsy
- Generalised seizures
  - Grandmal and generalised
  - Grandmal and generalised tonic clonic seizure (GTCS)
- Disease of the muscles and myopathy
- Muscular dystrophy
  - Duchenne muscular dystrophy
  - Becker muscular dystrophy
  - Limb girdle myopathy
  - Facioscapulohumeral Dystrophy
  - Myotonia
- Alzheimer's disease
- Creutzfeldt–Jakob disease
- Paraneoplastic syndrome
- Neurofibroma
- Tuberous sclerosis
- Hydrocephalus
- Multi-infarct dementia (MID)
- Dizziness and vertigo
- Syncope
- Funny turn or blackout
- Meniere's disease
- Lateral medullary syndrome (Wallenberg syndrome)
- Central pontine myelinolysis (CPM)
- Nystagmus

UPPER MOTOR NEURON

Upper motor neuron (UMN) includes neurons in the motor area of the cerebral cortex, their axons up to the anterior horn cell of the spinal cord and homologous cells in brain stem.

Signs UMN Lesion

- Weakness or paralysis of limb.
- Hypertonia of muscles (spastic, may be clasp knife).
- Tendon reflex—Exaggerated, clonus may be present (absent abdominal reflex).
- Plantar response—Extensor.
- No wasting (may be due to disuse).
- Normal electrical excitability of muscles.

Sites of UMN Lesion

- Cerebral cortex.
- Internal capsule.
- Brain stem.
- Descending tracts up to the anterior horn cells of spinal cord.

LOWER MOTOR NEURON

Lower motor neuron (LMN) is the motor pathway from anterior horn cells via peripheral nerve to motor end plate of muscle and cranial nerve nuclei in brainstem.

Signs of LMN Lesion

- Weakness or paralysis (flaccid) of limb.
- Hypotonia.
- Loss of all reflexes.
- Wasting of involved muscles.
- Fasciculation of affected muscles.
- Plantar reflex—Normal or absent.

EXTRAPYRAMIDAL SYSTEM

It includes basal ganglia and subthalamic nuclei.

Signs of Extrapyramidal Lesion

- Rigidity (lead pipe or cog wheel).
- Hypokinesia or bradykinesia (poverty of movement) or akinesia (no movement).
- Involuntary movements (tremor, chorea, athetosis, dystonia, hemiballismus).

Causes of Hypotonia

- LMN lesion due to any cause.
- UMN lesion in shock stage.
- Cerebellar lesion (knee jerk may be pendular).
- Dorsal column lesion (e.g. tabes dorsalis).
- Polyneuropathy.
- Chorea (it is the only extrapyramidal lesion with hypotonia).
- Hypokalaemia or hyperkalaemia.
- Down's syndrome.
- Drugs like hypnotics, sedatives, muscle relaxants, anaesthetics.

Causes of Hypertonia

- UMN lesion (spastic, may be clasp knife).
- Extrapyramidal lesion (lead pipe or cogwheel rigidity), except chorea.
- Conversion disorder or HCR (rigidity continues to increase with more and more passive movement).
- Others—tetanus, strychnine poisoning, tetany, catatonic states.
- Myotonia during the contraction phase.
- Decerebrate rigidity (there is marked contraction of all extensor muscles in the body).

Causes of Extensor Plantar Response

- First year of life (due to lack of myelination of pyramidal tract. Myelination occurs in 6–12 months).
- Sleep.
- UMN lesion.
- Deep coma (due to any cause).
- Postepileptic period (after grand mal seizure).

Causes of Absent Ankle Jerk, but Extensor Plantar Response

- Subacute combined degeneration of the spinal cord.
- Friedreich ataxia.
- Multiple sclerosis.
- Taboparesis.
- Diabetes mellitus with cervical myelopathy.

Grading of Muscular Weakness

- Grade 0: Complete paralysis.
- Grade 1: A flicker of contraction only.
- Grade 2: Power detectable, when gravity is excluded by postural adjustment.
- Grade 3: Limb can be held against gravity, but not against examiner's resistance.
- Grade 4: There is some degree of weakness.
- Grade 5: Normal power.

GAIT ABNORMALITY

Types of Gait

- Reeling or drunken gait—Wide-based gait and the arms are held wide. The patient is ataxic and tends to fall to the right or left. It is found in cerebellar lesion.
- Festinate gait—It is characterized by rapid, small, shuffling step, hardly raises the foot from the ground. The patient has difficulty in stopping himself and seems to catch up with his own centre of gravity. There is less swinging of the arms during walking. It is found in Parkinsonism.
- Stamping gait—The patient raises the foot suddenly and tends to throw forward, then both heels and toes slap to the ground with a stamp. It is found in sensory ataxia, which is worse on closing the eye. Commonly found in subacute combined degeneration of spinal cord, tabes dorsalis, cervical myelopathy, Friedreich's ataxia, diabetic pseudotabes.
- High-stepping gait—The patient lifts his foot high to avoid scrapping the toes. It is found in foot drop.
- Hemiplegic gait—The patient's leg is stiff, has difficulty in bending the knee and drags the hemiplegic limb in a semicircle-like motion with the toes scrapping the floor.
- Scissor gait—During walking, one leg crosses in front of the other. It is found in spastic paraplegia, usually due to cerebral palsy.
- Waddling gait—The patient walks on a wide base with trunk moving side to side and pelvis drooping on each side. At each step toes touch the ground before the heel. It is found mostly in myopathy (Duchenne muscular dystrophy), osteomalacia, polymyositis, bilateral hip joint disease. There is increased lumbar lordosis.
- Marche a petit pas—There is slow movement. The patient walks with very short, shuffling and irregular steps with loss of associated movements. The gait is similar to that of Parkinson's disease. It is seen in normal pressure hydrocephalus.

INFECTION OF CNS

Common Definitions

- Meningitis—It means infection of the meninges.
- Encephalitis—It means infection or inflammation of brain parenchyma.
- Meningoencephalitis—It means infection of meninges and brain.
- Myelitis—It means infection or inflammation of spinal cord.
- Myelopathy—It is the disease of the spinal cord.
- Encephalomyelitis—It means infection or inflammation of brain and spinal cord.
- Rediculopathy—It means disease of spinal cord nerve root.

MENINGITIS

Definition

It is the infection or inflammation of the meninges.

Types: 2 types

- Acute meningitis—clinical features lasting less than 4 weeks.
- Chronic meningitis—clinical features lasting for 4 weeks or more.

Causes

1. Bacterial—
   - Pyogenic—*N. meningitides* (meningococcus), *Streptococcus pneumoniae, H. infulenzae* type B (in children), *Listeria monocytogenes, Staphylococcus aureus.*
   - *Mycobacterium tuberculosis.*
2. Viral—coxsackie B, echo, polio, mumps, Epstein-Barr, herpes simplex, HIV.
3. Fungal—*Cryptococcus neoformans, Candida albicans,* Coccidioides, *Histoplasma capsulatum.*
4. Protozoal—toxoplasmosis, cysticercosis.
5. Noninfective—carcinomatous meningitis, SLE, sarcoidosis, Behcet's disease.

ACUTE BACTERIAL MENINGITIS

Causative Organism According to Age

- Neonate—Gram-negative bacillus (*E. coli*, Proteus), *Streptococcus* group B. Also *Listeria monocytogenes.*
- Small child—*H. influenzae, N. meningitidis, S. pneumoniae.*
- Older children and adult—*N. meningitidis, S. pneumoniae,*

NB: *Listeria monocytogenes* infection is common in immunosuppressed, diabetic, alcoholic and pregnant women.

Symptoms

- High fever with chill and rigor.
- Headache, nausea, vomiting, photophobia, drowsiness.
- Impaired consciousness.
- Convulsion.
- Pneumococcal meningitis may be associated with pneumonia, common in elderly and alcoholics.

Signs

- Neck rigidity.
- Positive Kernig's sign (extension of knee with hip joint flexed causes pain due to spasm of hamstring muscles).
- Positive Brudzinski's sign (flexion of the neck causes flexion of hip and knee).
- Petechial or nonspecific blotchy red rashes in skin—in meningococcal meningitis with septicaemia.

Complications of Meningitis

CNS Complications

- Cranial nerve palsy.
- Hydrocephalus.
- Focal neurological deficit.
- Epilepsy.
- Mental retardation and behavioural disturbance.

Other Complications

- DIC.
- Septicaemic shock.
- Renal failure.
- Peripheral gangrene.
- Arthritis.
- Pericarditis.

Investigations

- CBC shows neutrophilic leucocytosis.
- Blood culture.
- Lumbar puncture and CSF study (before doing lumbar puncture, fundoscopy should be done to see papilloedema to exclude raised intracranial pressure).
- CT scan of head.
- Chest X-ray.

Treatment

- Hospitalisation.
- Adequate nutrition and hydration.

1. If *Meningococcus* is suspected:
   - Benzylpenicillin 2.4 g IV 6 hourly or
   - Cefuroxime 1–2 g IV 6 hourly or
   - Ceftriaxone 2 g IV 12 hourly or
   - Cefotaxime 2 g IV 6 hourly.
2. If *S. pneumoniae* or *H. influenzae* is suspected:
   - Ceftriaxone 2 g IV 12 hourly or
   - Cefotaxime 2 g IV 6 hourly for 10–14 days.
3. If *Listeria monocytogenes* is suspected:
   - Ampicillin 2 g IV 4 hourly plus gentamicin IV 5 mg/kg daily.
4. Antibiotic can be changed depending on C/S result.
5. Dexamethasone 0.4 mg/kg every 12 hours can also be used.

Treatment of Pyogenic Meningitis of Unknown Cause

- Adult 18–50 years—Ceftriaxone 2 g IV 12 hourly or cefotaxime 2 g IV 6 hourly. If penicillin resistant *Pneumococcus* or penicillin resistance is suspected—Vancomycin 1 g twice daily should be added.
- Adult >50 years with suspected *Listeria monocytogenes*—as above plus ampicillin 2 g IV 4 hourly.
- Dexamethasone 0.15 mg/kg 6 hourly or 2–4 days.

Prevention of Meningococcal Infection

Close contact with patient should be given oral rifampicin for 2 days. Or single-dose ciprofloxacin.

Meningococcal Septicaemia

It is the fulminant form of septicaemia, may or may not be associated with meningitis.

Features

- Petechial or purpuric skin rash or ecchymosis.
- Features of shock.
- Bilateral adrenal haemorrhage (Waterhouse-Freidrichsen syndrome).
- DIC.

- Renal failure.
- Peripheral gangrene.
- Arthritis.
- Pericarditis.

VIRAL MENINGITIS

Usually it is the common cause of meningitis, commonest organisms are entero virus, echo, Coxsackie and polio virus.

Clinical Features

Common in children or young adult.

- Severe headache, fever.
- Features of meningism.
- Lumbar puncture and CSF study shows high lymphocyte, protein and sugar are usually normal (however, this picture is found if treated with antibiotic).

Treatment

- It is usually benign, self-limiting, improves in 4–10 days.
- Symptomatic and supportive treatment.

TUBERCULOUS MENINGITIS (TBM)

Cause

Commonly occurs after primary infection in childhood or as a complication of military tuberculosis.

Symptoms

Commonly involves base of the brain causing cranial nerve palsy.

- There may be H/O of tuberculosis.
- Low-grade fever, night sweat, weight loss.
- Headache, vomiting, confusion, abnormal behavior.

Signs

- Signs of meningeal irritation (neck rigidity, Kernig's sign).
- Cranial nerve palsy may be present (commonly 3rd and 6th cranial nerve).
- Focal neurological signs.
- Fundoscopy shows choroid tubercle.

Complications of Tuberculous Meningitis

- Cranial nerve palsy.
- Hydrocephalus.
- Focal neurological deficit.
- Epilepsy.
- Mental retardation and behavioral disturbance.

Investigations

- CBC, ESR (high).
- Chest X-ray (to see any tuberculous focus).
- MT.
- CT scan or MRI of brain.
- Lumbar puncture and CSF study—shows increased pressure, straw coloured. When kept for some hours, shows cobweb appearance (Table 1). Biochemistry shows—high protein, low sugar (may be zero). Cytology shows—increased lymphocytes. ADA is high. AFB may be positive. PCR may be done.

Treatment

- Standard antituberculous therapy with INH, rifampicin, pyrazinamide and ethambutol for 2 months. Then INH and rifampicin for 7–10 months depending on clinical response. If eye complication, ethambutol may be replaced by streptomycin.
- Pyridoxine 20 mg/day to prevent INH induced peripheral neuropathy.
- Prednisolone 60 mg for 3 weeks then taper.
- Neurosurgical intervention, if hydrocephalus.

Table 1
CSF findings in different meningitis

Condition	Appearance	Cell type and count	Glucose	Protein	Gram stain and culture
Normal	Clear	Lymphocytes <5/mm^3	>60% of blood sugar (40–80 mg/dL)	<45 mg/dL	
Viral	Clear	Lymphocytes 10–2000/mm^3	Normal	40–80 mg/dL	
Bacterial	Turbid or purulent	Polymorph 1000–5000/mm^3	Very low	50–200 mg/dL	May be positive
Tuberculous	Straw or turbid Cob web formation on standing	Lymphocytes 50–5000/mm^3	Low	50–300 mg/dL (very high)	
Fungal	Clear or turbid	Lymphocytes 50–500/mm^3	Low	Elevated	
Malignant	Clear	Lymphocytes 0–100/mm^3	Low	Normal or elevated	

ENCEPHALITIS

Definition

It is the inflammation of brain parenchyma.

Causes

Mostly by virus, may be bacterial or other infection.

- Herpes simplex type I.
- Enterovirus—polio, Coxsackie, echo virus.
- Mumps virus.
- Influenza virus.
- Japanese B encephalitis.
- Toga virus.
- Rabies virus.
- HIV.
- Lymphocytic choriomeningitis.

Clinical Features

- Fever, headache, nausea, vomiting, photophobia,
- Drowsiness, impaired consciousness even coma.
- Convulsion.
- Focal neurological sign (such as aphasia, hemiplegia, cranial nerve palsy).
- Abnormal behavior, agitation, hallucination.

Investigations

- CT scan or MRI—shows area of oedema, low-density lesion in temporal lobe in herpes simplex encephalitis.
- Lumbar puncture and CSF study—shows clear fluid, high lymphocyte, glucose is normal but protein may be slightly high.
- Viral serology in blood and CSF.
- EEG.

Treatment

- IV acyclovir 10 mg/kg 8 hourly for 2–3 weeks.
- IV dexamethasone—6–8 hourly.
- Others—IV fluid, nutrition, care of eyes, bowel, bladder.

Herpes Simplex Encephalitis

Herpes simplex type 1 may cause encephalitis, type 2 may cause benign recurrent lymphocytic meningitis. The virus usually affects the inferior aspect of frontal lobes and medial aspect of temporal lobe.

It is characterized by flu-like illness followed by fever, severe headache, altered consciousness, behaviour abnormality and speech disturbance. There may be focal neurological deficit, such as dysphasia, hemiparesis, focal or generalized seizure, commonly temporal lobe seizure. Olfactory and gustatory hallucinations and impairment of memory may be present. There may be multiple cranial nerve palsy and ataxia, convulsion and coma. Mortality is high.

Investigations

- Serum anti-HSV antibody.
- CSF study—shows high lymphocyte, normal protein and sugar. PCR is highly sensitive for rapid diagnosis.
- EEG shows distinctive periodic pattern in some cases.
- CT scan shows low-density lesion in temporal lobes that enhance with contrast.
- MRI shows orbitofrontal and medial temporal lobe involvement (not found in other virus).

Treatment

- Acyclovir 10 mg/kg 8 hourly IV for 2–3 weeks.
- Anticonvulsant may be necessary.
- Dexamethasone IV 8 hourly.

BRAIN ABSCESS

Causes

Infection may spread to the brain in the following cases:

1. Direct spread from—
   - Head injury, penetrating injury, trauma.
   - Infection in ear, nose, paranasal sinus and tooth.
2. Haematogenous in septicaemia,
3. Others—HIV infection, immunocompromized case, Fallot's tetralogy.

Causative Organisms

Streptococcus anginosus, Bacteroids, *Staphylococcus*, anaerobes and fungus. Mixed infections are common. Multiple abscess are common in septicaemia, also in HIV.

Clinical Features

- Fever, which may be high with chill and rigor.
- Headache, drowsiness, confusion.
- Nausea, vomiting.
- Convulsion, focal neurosurgical sign (such as hemiparesis, aphasia, hemianopia may occur).
- Signs of meningism.

Investigations

- Full blood count (leucocytosis).
- CT scan or MRI of brain (will show ring-like shadow in the brain).
- Blood for culture and sensitivity.

Treatment

- Broad-spectrum antibiotic—cefotaxime 2 g IV 6 hourly or cefuroxime 1.5 g IV 8 hourly **plus** metronidazole 500mg IV 8 hourly.
- In neurosurgical case—vancomycin should be added.
- Inj. dexamethasone IV 8 hourly.
- Surgery may be necessary, if drug fails (such as burr-hole drainage aspiration or excision).
- Mortality 25%.
- Epilepsy may occur in survivor.

HEADACHE

Causes

- Tension headache—occurs in anxiety, stress, depression, functional.
- Vascular headache—occurs in migraine, cluster headache, transient ischemic attack (TIA), cardiovascular disease (CVD), subarachnoid haemorrhage, temporal arteritis, uncontrolled hypertension.
- Traumatic.
- Infection—meningitis, encephalitis, sinusitis, cerebral abscess.
- Neoplastic—tumour.
- Raised intracranial pressure due to any cause.
- Referred pain from cervical spondylosis, eye, sinus, teeth, temporomandibular joint.
- Cranial neuralgia—trigeminal, glossopharyngeal.
- Drug—nitroglycerine.
- Others—postlumbar puncture headache, any acute febrile illness.

MIGRAINE

Definition

It is characterized by paroxysmal, unilateral headache associated with nausea, vomiting, visual disturbance.

Types

- Classic—with aura.
- Common—without aura.
- Migraine variants—retinal, ophthalmologic, hemiplegic, basilar.

Clinical Features

Three times more common in women, after puberty to middle age. Attacks occur at intervals, persists for hours to days.

- Prodromal symptoms—malaise, irritability, aura, such as silvery zigzag lines, shimmering light, tingling, numbness in one part of the body to other.
- These are followed by unilateral, throbbing headache, associated with nausea, vomiting, visual disturbance.
- Patient prefers to stay in the quiet, dark room.

Precipitating Factors

Stress, food (chocolate, cheese), alcohol, menstruation, OCP, caffeine.

Treatment

During acute attack

- Reassurance, rest in quiet, dark room.
- Analgesic—paracetamol.
- Antiemetic—prochlorperazine, metoclopramide.
- Triptan—sumatriptan, zolmitriptan, rizatriptan.

For prevention

Avoidance of precipitating factors. One or combination of the following drugs can be used:
- Propranolol—80-160 mg daily.
- Amitriptyline—10-50 mg at night. Used alone or in combination.
- Topiramate—80-150 mg daily.
- Pizotifen—1.5-3 mg at night.
- Sodium valproate—300-600 mg per day.
- Verapamil—80-160 mg.
- Flunarizine—5-10 mg.

Pregnancy with migraine: Usually during pregnancy, migraine is improved.

CLUSTER HEADACHE

Definition

It is also called 'migranous neuralgia' characterized by recurrent episodes of unilateral headache usually associated with periorbital pain and autonomic features.

Typically clusters lasts 4-12 weeks, followed by pain free period for month or even 1-2 years before another cluster begins.

Clinical Features

Cluster headache can occur at any age, but common in 30-40 years, more in males. Headache occurs repeatedly in clusters over weeks.
- Severe unilateral headache, usually around one eye, lasts for 15 minutes to 3 hours, radiates to the frontotemporal region down to the jaw, neck or shoulder.
- Autonomic features like lacrimation, facial flushing, nasal or conjunctival congestion, meiosis.
- Ipsilateral eye is red and watery, rhinorrhoea or blocked ipsilateral nostril.
- Typically patient develops these symptoms at a particular period of the day, usually in the early morning or late hours at night, awakening the patient from sleep.

Treatment

During acute attack
- Sumatriptan—subcutaneous or intranasal and high-flow oxygen 100% (10-12 L/min) for 15 minutes.
- Other drugs that are used in migraine are not effective.

For prevention
- Verapamil is the drug of choice.
- In severe case, lithium can be used.

Causes of Unilateral Headache

- Migraine.
- Cluster headache.
- Giant cell or temporal arteritis.
- Intracranial space occupying lesion.
- Unilateral sinusitis.
- Unilateral glaucoma.

Headache of Raised Intracranial Tension

- Headache is diffuse, dull in nature, more on waking from sleep, improves throughout the day, worse on bending forward, cough and straining.
- Associated with morning vomiting without nausea.

BELL'S PALSY

Definition

It is a lower motor neuron type of facial palsy associated with Bell's phenomenon (Table 2).

Cause

Idiopathic in 95% cases, may be due to viral infection.

Site of Lesion

Facial canal, in petrous part of temporal bone

Symptoms (in the affected side)

- Pain around or behind the ear, followed by weakness of face.
- Numbness and stiffness of cheek.
- Dribbling of saliva and liquid.
- Food may accumulate between the cheek and teeth.
- Watering from the eye.
- Loss of taste sensation (if chorda tympani branch is involved) and hyperacusis (if nerve to the stapedius is involved).

Signs (in the affected side)

- Facial asymmetry.
- Inability to wrinkle the forehead.
- Inability to close the eye.
- Eye appears wide and open.
- Affected eye cannot be closed and on attempting to close, there is Bell's phenomenon (eyeball is rolled upwards and outwards).
- Nasolabial fold—less pronounced.
- Drooping of the corner of mouth.
- Weakness of affected side of face on puffing the cheek.
- Failure to whistle and smile.
- If asked to show teeth, affected part of face cannot be opened and face is pushed to the normal side.

Investigation

Diagnosis is clinical. Blood sugar should be done.

Treatment

- Prednisolone 20 mg tds for 07 days.
- Antiviral (acyclovir or valaciclovir) may be given.
- Physiotherapy—facial exercise and electrostimulation.
- Protection of eye during sleep (shut with tape or even tarsorrhaphy), artificial tears or ointment.
- Residual paralysis may occur in 10% cases. Cosmetic surgery may be helpful.

NB: During recovery, aberrant re-innervation may occur producing unwanted facial movement and tear during salivation (called 'crocodile tear').

Ramsay Hunt Syndrome

It is the herpes zoster of geniculate ganglia characterized by ipsilateral 7th cranial nerve palsy (lower motor neuron) with vesicular rash in the external auditory meatus and soft palate.

Ipsilateral loss of taste, buccal ulceration, deafness and 5th nerve lesion may also occur.

Treatment

Antiviral famciclovir plus steroid should be given. However, complete recovery is less likely than Bell palsy.

Causes of Bilateral Facial Palsy

- Guillain-Barré syndrome (GBS).
- Sarcoidosis.
- Bilateral Bell palsy (rare).
- Bilateral parotid disease.
- Lyme disease.
- Any cause of mononeuritis multiplex (rare).

Table 2

Differences between UMN and LMN type of facial palsy:

	UMN type	*LMN type*
Site of lesion	Above the facial nucleus, commonly in internal capsule	In the facial nucleus and distal to the nucleus
Involved area	Lower part of face	Both upper and lower part of face
Bell phenomenon	Absent	May be present
Taste sensation	Not affected	May be affected
Hyperacusis	Absent	May occur, if nerve to the stapedius is involved
Facial wasting or atrophy	Absent	May be present
Associated feature	Usually associated with hemiplegia	Not so, other findings according to site of lesion

SIXTH NERVE PALSY

Causes

- Raised intracranial pressure (commonest cause) due to stretching of the nerve in its long intracranial course (a false localizing sign).
- Brain stem lesion (vascular, neoplastic and multiple sclerosis).
- Cavernous sinus lesion (tumour, thrombosis, infection, aneurysm).
- Trauma.
- Any cause of mononeuritis multiplex.
- Idiopathic (common).
- Subacute meningitis (due to fungal, tuberculous, lymphomatous, carcinomatous).

- Diabetes mellitus.
- Others—sarcoidosis, giant cell arteritis, Lyme disease, acoustic neuroma, nasopharyngeal carcinoma.

Clinical Features

- Convergent squint at rest.
- No lateral movement of affected eye and on attempting to look on that side, there is diplopia (outermost image comes from the affected eye).

Causes of Bilateral 6th Nerve Palsy

- Trauma.
- Wernicke's encephalopathy.
- Mononeuritis multiplex.
- Raised intracranial pressure (6th nerve palsy often associated with 7th nerve lesion also).

THIRD NERVE PALSY

Causes of 3rd Nerve Lesion

1. Nuclear lesion (infarction, haemorrhage, neoplasm, multiple sclerosis).
2. Midbrain CVA (Weber syndrome—ipsilateral 3rd nerve palsy with contralateral hemiplegia due to thrombosis of a branch of posterior cerebral artery).
3. Unruptured aneurysm of posterior communicating artery (painful ophthalmoplegia).
4. Others—
   - Mononeuritis multiplex (causes are—DM, SLE, PAN, sarcoidosis, amyloidosis, leprosy).
   - Subacute meningitis (carcinomatous, lymphomatous, fungal, tuberculous, meningovascular syphilis).
   - Raised intracranial pressure (because the nerve has long tortuous course, so likely to be compressed by any displacement of brain stem).
   - Ophthalmoplegic migraine and Guillain-Barré syndrome.

Signs of 3rd Nerve Lesion

- Ptosis (complete).
- External squint.
- Inability to move the eye upwards, downwards and medially.
- Pupil—dilated, loss of light reflex (direct and consensual).
- Loss of accommodation reflex.

Mechanism of Ptosis and Dilated Pupil in the 3rd Nerve Palsy

- Ptosis is due to paralysis of levator palpebrae superioris (supplied by 3rd nerve).
- Dilated pupil is due to paralysis of constrictor of pupil (supplied by 3rd nerve).
- Dilator of pupil is supplied by sympathetic nerve, which when paralyzed, pupil is constricted as in Horner's syndrome.

Investigations in 3rd Nerve Palsy

- Blood sugar.
- CBC (high ESR in vasculitis).
- CT or MRI of brain.
- Occasionally, cerebral arteriography (if aneurysm is suspected).

PTOSIS

Definition

It means drooping of the upper eyelid.

Causes of Unilateral Ptosis

- Congenital.
- Traumatic.
- Senility.
- 3rd nerve palsy.

- Horner's syndrome (partial ptosis).
- Myasthenia gravis (may cause unilateral or bilateral ptosis).
- Hysterical conversion reaction (HCR).

Causes of Bilateral Ptosis

- Myasthenia gravis.
- Tabes dorsalis (characterized by bilateral ptosis with frontalis overaction, Argyll Robertson pupil, optic atrophy and dorsal column lesion).
- Myopathy (myotonic dystrophy and fascioscapulohumeral myopathy).
- Ocular and oculopharyngeal myopathy.
- Congenital (rare).
- Bilateral Horner syndrome (rare, may occur in syringomyelia).

HORNER SYNDROME

Definition

It is a syndrome due to lesion in the sympathetic pathway characterized by:
- Partial ptosis.
- Miosis (pupillary constriction), reacts to direct and consensual light.
- Enophthalmos.
- Anhydrosis (absence of sweating in affected side of face, whole upper limb and upper part of trunk).

Mechanism of Partial Ptosis, Miosis and Enophthalmos

- Partial ptosis is due to paralysis of upper tarsal muscles.
- Miosis is due to paralysis of the dilator of pupil.
- Enophthalmos is due to paralysis of Muller muscle.

Causes of Horner Syndrome (according to the site of lesion)

1. T_1 lesion:
   - Pancoast tumour.
   - Trauma to brachial plexus.
   - Cervical rib.
2. Neck (sympathetic lesion):
   - Trauma.
   - Neck surgery.
   - Cervical sympathectomy.
   - Lymphoma.
   - Thyroid carcinoma.
3. Brain stem lesion:
   - Vascular (lateral medullary syndrome).
   - Multiple sclerosis.
4. Cervical cord lesion (bilateral Horner syndrome may occur):
   - Syringomyelia.
   - Spinal cord tumour (glioma and ependymoma).
5. Migraine (temporary Horner syndrome may occur).

Investigations

- Chest X-ray.
- X-ray of cervical spine.
- CT scan or MRI of brain.
- Other investigations, according to suspicion of causes.

PAPILLOEDEMA

Definition

It is the swelling of the optic nerve head.

Stages of Papilloedema

- Early sign—absence of spontaneous pulsation of retinal veins and increased pink or red colouration of the disc.
- Blurring of disc margin, first starting in nasal side.
- Filling of physiological cup.
- Fullness of optic disc, then elevation.
- Vessels on the disc become curved over its edge.
- May be haemorrhage surrounding the disc.

Causes

1. Raised intracranial pressure due to any cause:
   - Neoplasm.
   - Abscess.
   - Meningitis, encehalitis.
   - Subarachnoid haemorrhage.
2. Central retinal vein occlusion.
3. Benign intracranial hypertension.
4. Hypertensive retinopathy (stage IV).

OPTIC NEURITIS

Definition

It is the inflammation of optic nerve.

Causes

- Demyelinating disease (e.g. multiple sclerosis).
- Drugs—ethambutol, quinine, chloroquine.
- Toxins—methanol poisoning, lead, arsenic, cyanide poisoning.
- Neurosyphilis.
- Nutritional amblyopia—vitamin B12 deficiency, tobacco, alcohol.

OPTIC ATROPHY

Definition

Optic atrophy (OA) is the degeneration of the optic nerve head, sometimes a sequele to optic neuritis.

Types: 3 types—

1. Primary—due to involvement of optic nerve (as in optic neuritis, compression in optic nerve and glaucoma).
2. Secondary—due to long-standing papilloedema.
3. Consecutive—secondary to the disease of retina (retinitis pigmentosa, choroidoretinitis, Tay-Sach's disease). The term consecutive is controversial, it is actually a secondary OA.

Features of OA

Primary

Disc is pale with clear margin and no change in retina.

Secondary:

- Disc—greyish white.
- Margin—indistinct.
- Some changes in retina may be present (exudate or haemorrhage).

Causes of OA

- Raised intracranial pressure due to intracranial SOL (neoplasm, abscess and cyst).
- Long-standing papilloedema.
- Secondary to optic neuritis.
- Hereditary (Friedreich's ataxia, Leber's OA and DIDMOAD syndrome).
- Ischaemic optic neuropathy (in giant cell arteritis).
- Others—trauma in optic nerve, Paget's disease and retinal artery occlusion.

Investigations

- CBC, PBF—macrocytic anaemia in vitamin B12 deficiency.
- Serological test for syphilis—VDRL, TPHA.
- X-ray of skull.
- CT or MRI of brain.
- Other investigations according to suspicion of causes.

NB: DIDMOAD means—diabetes insipidus, diabetes mellitus, optic atrophy, deafness.

MULTIPLE CRANIAL NERVE PALSY

Causes of 3rd, 4th and 6th Nerve Palsy

1. Raised intracranial pressure due to any cause—
   - Meningitis.
   - Encephalitis.
   - Sarcoidosis.
   - Neoplasm.
   - GBS.
2. Brain stem lesion—
   - Vascular (CVA).
   - Neurosyphilis.
   - Multiple sclerosis.
   - Syringobulbia.
3. Mononeuritis multiplex due to any cause.
4. Cavernous sinus thrombosis or caroticocavernous fistula.

Causes of 3rd and 6th Nerve Palsy

- Raised intracranial pressure due to any cause.
- Mononeuritis multiplex.
- Meningitis.
- Encephalitis.
- Trauma.

Causes of 9, 10, 11 and 12th Cranial Nerve Palsy

According to the site of lesion:

1. Within the brain stem—
   - Infarction.
   - Syringobulbia.
   - MND.
   - Poliomyelitis.
2. Around the skull base—
   - Carcinoma of nasopharynx.
   - Glomus tumour.
   - Neurofibroma.
   - Jugular venous thrombosis.
   - Trauma.
3. Within the neck and nasopharynx—
   - Carcinoma of nasopharynx.
   - Metastasis.
   - Carotid artery dissection.
   - Polyneuropathy.
   - Trauma.
   - Lymph node biopsy in posterior triangle.

4. Others—
   - GBS.
   - Tubercular meningitis.
   - Carcinomatous meningitis.
   - Encephalitis.
   - Brain stem lesion—vascular (CVA) or neoplastic.
   - Bulbar and pseudobulbar palsy.
   - Neurosyphilis.
   - Mononeuritis multiplex.

PUPIL

Causes of Constricted Pupil (Miosis)

- Horner's syndrome.
- Argyll Robertson pupil.
- Pontine haemorrhage.
- Senility (pupil in old age tends to be small and may be irregular).
- Morphine.
- Miotic drugs—pilocarpine, physostigmine.
- Poisoning—organophosphorous, opium.

Causes of Dilated Pupil (Mydriasis)

- 3rd nerve palsy.
- Holmes-Adie pupil.
- Optic nerve lesion—optic neuritis or retrobulbar neuritis.
- Mydriatic drug (anticholinergic)—atropine, homatropine.
- Other drugs—tricyclic antidepressant, amphetamine.
- Datura poisoning.
- Fixed dilated pupil (occurs in brain death, also in deep coma).

TRIGEMINAL NEURALGIA

Definition

It is characterized by lancinating pain along the distribution of trigeminal nerve, commonly along the 2nd and 3rd division territory.

Clinical Features

Usually above 50 years, unilateral.

- Severe, paroxysmal unilateral facial pain of short duration, knife like or electric shock like.
- Precipitated by touching the trigger zone within the trigeminal territory by cold wind, eating, touching, washing, shaving.

Signs

No physical sign. Diagnosis is clinical.

Treatment

- Carbamazepine—200–400 mg 3 times daily (started with low dose, it may cause severe Stevens-Johnson syndrome).
- Phenytoin—200–400 mg daily.
- Gabapentin or pregabalin may be used.
- If no response—Inj. alcohol or phenol into the peripheral branch of the nerve may be given.
- If still no response—radiofrequency lesion in the nerve near the Gasserian ganglion.
- Surgery—decompression of the trigeminal nerve through posterior craniotomy.

MULTIPLE SCLEROSIS

Definition

It is a demyelinating disorder of CNS characterized by multiple plaques of demyelination within the brain and spinal cord, gliosis and varying degree of inflammation.

Presence of two neurological lesions in anatomically unrelated sites or at different times indicates multiple sclerosis. Dissemination in space and time is crucial for diagnosis (also called disseminated sclerosis).

Causes

Unknown, following factors may be associated—

- Environmental factors—more in temperate zone, rare in tropical country. Greater among rural than urban dwellers.
- More frequent in the higher socioeconomic group.
- Genetic—ten times more in first degree relative.
- Immunological.
- Diet—more in those who eat animal fat.
- HLA association—DR_2, DR_3, B_7, A_3.

Sites of Involvement in MS

- Optic nerve.
- Brain stem.
- Cerebellum.
- Periventricular region.
- Spinal cord (posterior column and corticospinal tract).

Symptoms

Twice more common in females 20–45 years of age. It is rare before puberty and after 60 years.

- Weakness of one or more limbs.
- Blurring of vision (due to optic neuritis).
- Features of spastic paraplegia.
- Features of cerebellar signs (ataxia and tremor).
- Features of brainstem dysfunction (vertigo, diplopia, nystagmus, facial numbness or weakness, dysarthria, dysphagia, pyramidal signs in limbs).
- Bladder dysfunction (incontinence, dribbling and hesitancy).
- Sensory disturbance—tingling of the extremities and light banding sensation around the trunk or limbs (due to posterior column involvement).
- Euphoria despite disability.
- Temperature sensitivity—worsening of symptoms or weakness with rise of body temperature, such as after exercise or hot bath.
- Others (rarely)—epilepsy, trigeminal neuralgia, recurrent facial palsy, 6th nerve palsy, dementia, neuropsychiatric dysfunction, depression.

Clinical Courses (or types) of MS

- Relapsing and remitting MS (80–90%)—Episodes of acute attack with recovery and remains stable between relapses.

- Primary progressive MS (10-20%)—Gradual neurological deterioration from the onset. It usually begins after 40 years.
- Secondary progressive MS—Some cases of relapsing and remitting course show gradual neurological deterioration.
- Fulminating MS (<10%).

Signs and Symptoms of MS (remember the formula WATSON)

W—Weakness.
A—Ataxia (cerebellar).
T—Tremor (cerebellar).
S—Speech (scanning).
O—Optic neuritis.
N—Nystagmus.

Investigations

1. MRI of brain and spinal cord—investigation of choice, shows multiple plaques in the periventricular region (CT scan is not sensitive).
2. Lumbar puncture and CSF study—slight increase in lymphocyte, increase in total protein and oligoclonal band mainly IgG on electrophoresis.
3. Evoked potential—mainly VEP (visual evoked potential, usually delayed, if there is optic nerve involvement).
4. To exclude other conditions—
   - Chest X-ray (to exclude bronchial carcinoma).
   - X-ray of spine (to exclude cord compression).
   - Serum angiotensin converting enzyme (to exclude sarcoidosis).
   - Serum B12 (to exclude subacute combined degeneration of spinal cord).
   - ANA (to exclude SLE).
   - Antiphospholipid antibody.

Treatment

1. During acute attack:
   - IV methylprednisolone—1 g for 3-5 days or oral 500 mg for 5 days, then oral prednisolone 40 mg daily for 10 days, then 20 mg for 2 days, then 10 mg for 2 days.
   - Or prednisolone—40-60 mg daily for 10 days, then taper over 2 days (it has no role for long-term use for prevention).
   - Plasmapharesis is helpful in severe, unresponsive to corticosteroid.
2. To prevent relapse (disease-modifying drugs may be given)—
   - Immunosuppressive drug—azathioprine may be helpful.
   - Subcutaneous or intramuscular β interferon (1a or 1b) reduces number of relapse (30%).
   - Glatiramer acetate has similar effect.
   - Monoclonal antibody—natalizumab, alemtuzumab may be helpful in severely affected patient.
   - IV immunoglobulin may be helpful in aggressive cases.
3. Symptomatic treatment for complication and disability—
   - For incontinence or urgency or frequency—intermittent self-catheterization, oxybutynin, tolterodine.

- For spasticity—physiotherapy and baclofen, tizanidine, benzodiazepine or dantrolene may be used. Local intramuscular injection of botulinum toxin or chemical neuronectomy are other options.
- For dysaesthesia—carbamazepine, gabapentin, phenytoin or amitriptyline.
- For ataxia—INH or clonazepam.
- For fatigue—amantadine or amitriptyline.
- For impotence—sildenafil may be used.
- Others—control of infection, prevention of pressure sore, rehabilitation, occupational therapy, walking aids, visual aids, counselling and patient education.

Prognostic Factors in MS

1. Good prognostic factors—
   - Early age of onset.
   - Relapsing and remitting form.
   - Visual or sensory symptoms alone at presentation.
   - Minimum neurological impairment 5 years after onset.
   - More benign course in women than in men.
   - Little residual disability 5 years after onset.
2. Poor prognostic factors—
   - Old age >40 years.
   - Frequent relapse in first 2 years.
   - Short interval between first 2 relapses.
   - Pyramidal, brainstem and cerebellar symptoms.
   - Primary progressive disease.
   - Poor recovery from relapse.
   - MRI shows many lesions.

Uhthoff's Phenomenon

Exaggeration of symptoms after hot bath or exercise is called Uhthoff's phenomenon. The patient feels extreme weakness. It is due to heat induced conduction block of partially demyelinated fibres.

Pregnancy in MS

- Mild protective effect is found during pregnancy.
- Exaggeration may occur in puerperium.

SYRINGOMYELIA

Definition

It is a developmental anomaly in which there are cavities (syrinx) filled with fluid within the spinal cord, mostly originating at C_8 and T_1 segment, but may occur anywhere in the spinal cord.

Expanding cavity in the spinal cord gradually destroys—

- Anterior horn cells of spinal cord.
- Lateral spinothalamic tract.
- Corticospinal tract.
- May extend upwards to involve the brain stem (called syringobulbia).

Causes

- Developmental anomaly at the foramen magnum.
- Obstructions of fourth ventricle by congenital defect of the base of the skull or cervical spine (as in Arnold-Chiari malformation).
- Arachnoiditis in foramina of Magendie and foramina of Luschka.

Symptoms

Usually in 20–40 years, rarely in early age.

- Wasting of muscles of hands, forearms, shoulder girdles.
- Loss of pain and temperature sensation.
- There may be painless burn.
- Difficulty in walking.

Signs

- Scar of painless burn in the upper limbs.
- Dissociated sensory loss in neck, shoulder and arm (loss of pain and temperature, but intact light touch, vibration and position sense).
- LMN lesion signs in the upper limb (wasting of muscles in hand and forearm and loss of reflex).
- UMN lesion signs in lower limbs.

NB: As the syrinx extents into the brain stem (syringobulbia), there may be tongue atrophy and fasciculation, bulbar palsy, Horner's syndrome and impairment of facial sensation.

Investigations

- X-ray of the neck to see congenital anomaly.
- MRI (investigation of choice).
- CSF study—may show high protein.

Treatment

- No specific treatment.
- Surgical decompression may be necessary.
- Supportive—regular activity, physiotherapy, avoid burn, trauma or hot water.

Features of Syringobulbia

- Dissociated sensory loss in the face.
- Horner's syndrome.
- Palatal palsy.
- Dysarthria.
- Nystagmus.
- Cranial nerve involvement (V, VII, IX and X)

POLYNEUROPATHY

Definition

It is a clinical syndrome characterized by disturbance of function of peripheral nerves either motor or sensory or mixed or autonomic. Starts affecting the distal part, then gradually progresses proximally.

Causes

1. Metabolic and endocrine—
   - Diabetes mellitus.
   - CKD.
   - Hepatic failure.
2. Vitamin deficiency—B1, B6, B12, folic acid, nicotinic acid and E.
3. Toxic—
   - Drugs—isoniazid, vincristine, phenytoin, amiodarone, statin, cisplatin, dapsone, nitrofurantoin.
   - Alcoholism.
   - Industrial toxin—lead, arsenic, organophosphate.
4. Paraneoplastic neuropathy (in bronchial carcinoma, lymphoma, multiple myeloma).
5. Infections (leprosy, HIV, diphtheria).
6. Inflammatory—
   - Guillain-Barré syndrome.
   - Chronic inflammatory demyelinating polyneuropathy (CIDP).
   - Vasculitis and connective tissue disease—SLE, polyarteritis nodosa, rheumatoid arthritis.
7. Idiopathic sensory motor neuropathy.
8. Genetic neuropathy (Charcot-Marie-Tooth disease, hereditary sensory and autonomic neuropathy).

NB: Common causes of neuropathy—

- Diabetes mellitus.
- Leprosy.
- Alcohol.
- Guillain-Barre syndrome.
- Chronic kidney disease.
- Drugs—INH, vincristine.
- Deficiency—vitamin B12, B1, nicotinic acid, B6.

Clinical Features

Symptoms

- Sensory—tingling, numbness, burning sensation or pins and needles along the glove and stocking pattern.
- Motor—weakness, heaviness, wasting of muscles (starting in hands or feet). Patient may complain of difficulty in walking.
- Autonomic—vertigo, disturbance of sweating, palpitation, gastrointestinal, bladder and sexual dysfunction.

Signs

1. Sensory system—
   - Both superficial and deep sensation—diminished or lost.
   - Vibration and position sense—absent.
2. Motor system—
   - Wasting of muscle in the affected part.
   - Muscle tone—diminished.
   - Muscle power—diminished.
   - Reflexes—diminished or absent on the affected side.
   - Coordination—impaired.
   - Romberg sign—positive.
   - Gait—high-stepping gait.

Investigations

- CBC, PBF (macrocytosis indicates subacute combined degeneration of the spinal cord due to vitamin B12 deficiency).
- Blood sugar.
- Chest X-ray (to exclude bronchial carcinoma).
- Serum B12 and folate assay.
- Serum urea and creatinine and liver function tests—if needed.
- Bone marrow (if suspicion of B12 deficiency).
- Other investigations according to suspicion of causes (ANA and RA test).
- Nerve conduction studies (axonal or demyelinating).

Pattern of Nerve Involvement in Peripheral Neuropathy

Usually distal part of the limbs is commonly involved, because longer the nerve fibre earlier is the involvement. Since the nerve fibres supplying the distal parts of the limbs are longer, they are first affected.

Causes of Painful Neuropathy

- Diabetes mellitus (diabetic amyotrophy).
- Nutritional (deficiency of vitamins B1 and B12).
- Alcohol.
- GBS.
- Vasculitis and connective tissue disease (SLE, RA).
- HIV.
- Uraemic neuropathy.
- Paraneoplastic sensory neuropathy.
- Porphyria.
- Arsenic or thallium poisoning.

Treatment in Painful Neuropathy

- Tricyclic antidepressant, phenytoin, carbamazepine.
- Topical capsaicin.

Causes of Predominantly Sensory Neuropathy

- Diabetes mellitus.
- Leprosy.
- Deficiency of vitamins B1, B6 and B12
- Chronic renal failure.
- Paraneoplastic neuropathy (in bronchial carcinoma).
- Drugs (INH, vincristine).
- Hereditary sensory neuropathy.
- HIV.
- Multiple myeloma.

Causes of Predominantly Motor Neuropathy

- Guillain–Barré syndrome.
- CIDP.
- Charcot-Marie-Tooth disease.
- Acute intermittent porphyria.
- Chronic lead poisoning.
- Diabetic amyotrophy.
- Diphtheria.
- Paraneoplastic syndrome.

Mononeuritis Multiplex

Involvement of multiple peripheral nerve or cranial nerve by a single disease is called mononeuritis multiplex. Causes are:

- Diabetes mellitus.
- Leprosy.
- Rheumatoid arthritis.
- Vasculitis (SLE, polyarteritis nodosa).
- Amyloidosis.
- Malignancy (carcinomatous neuropathy).
- Sarcoidosis.
- HIV infection.
- Wegener's granulomatosis.
- Acromegaly.
- Paraproteinaemia.
- Lyme disease.
- Idiopathic multifocal motor neuropathy.

Types of Neuropathy in Diabetes Mellitus

- Distal symmetrical sensory neuropathy (common).
- Acute painful sensory neuropathy.
- Mixed motor and sensory neuropathy.
- Asymmetrical motor neuropathy (diabetic amyotrophy).
- Autonomic neuropathy.
- Mononeuropathy.
- Mononeuritis multiplex.

Causes of Autonomic Neuropathy

- Diabetes mellitus (commonest).
- Guillain–Barre syndrome.
- Amyloidosis.
- Toxin (vincristine).
- Paraneoplastic syndrome.
- Porphyria.
- AIDS.
- Shy–Drager syndrome.
- Riley–Day syndrome (familial dysautonomia).
- Hereditary sensory and autonomic neuropathy.

CARPAL TUNNEL SYNDROME (MEDIAN NERVE PALSY)

Definition

It is a type of entrapment neuropathy due to compression of median nerve under flexor retinaculum of wrist.

Causes

- Pregnancy (due to fluid retention, usually in the third trimester).
- Obesity.
- Rheumatoid Arthritis.
- Acromegaly.
- Myxoedema.
- CRF on long-term dialysis (due to deposition of β_2 microglobulin, an amyloid).
- Tuberculous tenosynovitis.
- Primary amyloidosis.
- Tophaceous gout.
- Drug (oral contraceptive pill).
- Osteoarthrosis of carpus (related to old fracture).
- Idiopathic (common in female, middle aged and obese. May occur in male with unaccustomed hand use, e.g. house painting).

Clinical Features

More common in females.

Symptoms

- Tingling, numbness and nocturnal pain and paraesthesia in palm and fingers often occur at night awakening the patient from sleep.
- Pain may be referred to whole arm and shoulder.

Signs

- Wasting, along the distribution of median nerve.
- Sensory loss of radial three and half digits.
- Tinel's sign—percussion over the flexor aspect of the wrist (flexor retinaculum) or tap the

median nerve in forearm, the patient may experience paraesthesia along the distribution of the nerve.
- Phalen's sign—flexion or extension of the wrist for 1 minute produces paraesthesia along the distribution of nerve (lateral three and half fingers).
- Tourniquet test—raise BP above systolic for 2 minutes (produces paraesthesia).
- Durkan's test—direct pressure over carpal tunnel for 30 seconds may produce paraesthesia.
- Closed fist test—flexion of the fingers into a closed fist for 60 seconds produce paraesthesia in the median nerve distribution.

Investigation

Nerve conduction study.

Treatment

- Treatment of primary cause.
- Splint of wrist at night.
- Ultrasound therapy.
- Local steroid injection proximal to the carpal tunnel (not into the tunnel, because it may cause damage to the nerve).
- Diuretic may help.
- In severe cases—surgical decompression of carpal tunnel may be required.

Nerves Involved in Entrapment Neuropathy

- Median nerve (at wrist).
- Ulnar nerve (at elbow or at wrist in Guyon's canal—bounded proximally by pisiform bone and distally by the hook of the hammet).
- Radial nerve (at spiral groove of humerus following fracture).
- Meralgia paraesthetica (at inguinal ligament).
- Common peroneal nerve or lateral popliteal nerve (at the neck of fibula).
- Tarsal tunnel syndrome (at the flexor retinaculum at ankle joint, there is compression of posterior tibial nerve).

Meralgia Paraesthetica

It is a type of entrapment neuropathy due to the compression of lateral cutaneous nerve of thigh. There is pain and paraesthesia over the upper and outer thigh, with reduction of sensation.

It is usually self-limiting. Occasionally, may be treated with corticosteroid and local anaesthetic injection at the anterior superior iliac spine.

Causes

- Obesity.
- Pregnancy.
- DM.
- Idiopathic.
- May be tight jeans.

ULNAR NERVE PALSY

Causes

- Fracture of ulna or dislocation of elbow.
- Injury at the wrist or palm.
- Mononeuritis multiplex due to any cause (DM, PAN, RA, SLE, amyloidosis and leprosy).
- Osteoarthrosis of elbow.
- Occupation—with constant leaning of elbows (clerk) or constant flexion or extension at elbow (carpenter, painter, decorator) and wrist (screw driver, drills).

Clinical Features

- Generalized wasting of small muscles of hands (except thenar) with dorsal guttering.
- Ulnar claw hand (extension of MCP and flexion of IP joint of 5th and 4th fingers).
- Loss of sensation along 5th and half of the 4th finger.
- Weakness of abduction and adduction of fingers.
- Wasting of medial side of forearm (due to involvement of flexor carpi ulnaris and medial half of flexor digitorum profundus).
- Froment sign is positive.

RADIAL NERVE PALSY

Causes

According to the site—
- Axilla—trauma, radiation, compression by improper use of crutch, axillary growth.
- Spiral groove or mid shaft of humerus—trauma, compression (e.g. saturday night palsy).
- Proximal forearm—trauma, subluxation of radius, repetitive forearm supination.
- Wrist—trauma, compression by tight bracelet or handcuff.
- Chronic lead poisoning.
- Mononeuritis multiplex (due to any cause).

Clinically it is detected by wrist drop.

Clinical Features

- Wrist drop.
- Inability to straight the fingers.
- If the wrist is passively extended, the patient is able to straighten the fingers at interphalangeal joint (due to action of interossei and lumbricals).
- There is weakness of extension of wrist and elbow, wrist flexion is normal.
- Triceps reflex—absent.
- Loss of sensation of anatomical snuff box.

Saturday Night Palsy

In this disorder, the patient is heavily sedated with alcohol, sleeps with the arms hanging over the back of chair and radial nerve is compressed at the middle third of the humerus, causing paralysis of the nerve. Brachioradialis, supinator and extensors of forearm are involved. Usually, complete recovery occurs within weeks.

NB: Radial nerve is vulnerable to be involved at 3 sites:
- Axilla (incorrect use of crutch).
- Spiral groove of humerus (mid-shaft fracture and saturday night palsy).
- Damage to the posterior interosseous nerve at proximal forearm where it penetrates the supinator muscle.
- Sensory branch may be compressed at the wrist.

SUBACUTE COMBINED DEGENERATION

Definition

Subacute combined degeneration (SCD) is a clinical syndrome due to B12 deficiency in which there are degeneration of posterior and lateral column of the spinal cord and peripheral nerve.

It is called combined degeneration, because—

- Peripheral neuropathy (due to demyelination of peripheral nerve)
- Posterior column lesion (loss of vibration and position sense).
- Signs of pyramidal lesion (plantar is extensor, knee jerk is brisk and ankle jerk is absent).

Clinical Features

Age 40-60 years, equally involved in both sexes.

- Sensory symptoms—paraesthesia, tingling or numbness, starting in toes and fingers. Lower limbs are more commonly affected than the upper limbs.
- Motor symptoms—weakness, ataxia and loss of all reflexes. May be exaggerated knee reflex with loss of ankle jerk, but extensor plantar.
- Bladder involvement—urinary incontinence and dribbling (usually in late stage).
- Eye—optic atrophy.
- Mental change—dementia, impaired memory, confusion and depression.
- Others—anaemia, glossitis.

Investigations

1. CBC and PBF (macrocytosis and hypersegmented neutrophil).
2. Bone marrow (to see megaloblast).
3. Serum B12 assay.
4. Other investigations according to the suspicion of cause:
   - For Addisonian pernicious anaemia—antiparietal cell and anti-intrinsic factor antibody, endoscopy and biopsy to see gastric atrophy, Schilling test.
   - Investigation for Crohn's disease.

NB: Macrocytosis in blood and megaloblastic marrow are invariable in SCD.

Treatment

- Injection of vitamin B12 1000 μg IM 6 doses 2–3 days apart, then maintenance therapy 1000 μg every 3 months for lifelong in Addisonian pernicious anaemia.
- Following therapy, iron deficiency may occur in the first few weeks. So, oral iron therapy should be given.
- Following B12 therapy, there may be hypokalaemia, which should be corrected.
- B12 orally 2 mg/day may be given. 1–2% is absorbed by diffusion without intrinsic factor. Sublingual B12 may be effective.
- Treatment of primary cause.

NB: Blood transfusion is avoided as it may precipitate heart failure. Before replacing B12, if blood transfusion or packed cell is given, it may aggravate neurological manifestations. However, blood (or packed cell) transfusion may be considered if there is angina, heart failure, cerebral hypoxia (confusion, dizziness, etc.).

If folic acid deficiency is present with B12 deficiency, folic acid should not be given alone without B12, otherwise neurological features are aggravated.

Response of Neurological Lesion to Vitamin B12 Therapy

- Response is variable, may improve, remain unchanged or even deteriorate.
- Sensory abnormality improve more than motor abnormality.
- Peripheral neuropathy responses better than myelopathy.
- Sensory neuropathy may take 6–12 months for recovery.

PARKINSONISM

Definition

It is a syndrome characterized by tremor, rigidity, hypokinesia due to involvement of the basal ganglia.

Parkinson's Disease (Paralysis Agitans)

It is the primary or idiopathic Parkinsonism. There is deficiency of dopamine with relative increase in cholinergic transmission, so imbalance between dopamine and acetylcholine.

Parkinsonian Plus

It is characterized by features of Parkinsonism with other degenerative disease like progressive supranuclear palsy (Steele-Richardson-Olszeweski syndrome), olivopontocerebellar degeneration, nigrostriatal degeneration, primary autonomic failure (Shy-Drager syndrome).

Pathology

In idiopathic parkinsonism:
- Progressive degeneration with depigmention of substantia nigra.
- Formation of eosinophilic cytoplasmic inclusions in neurons (Lewy bodies, which is the pathological hallmark).

Causes of Parkinsonism

Unknown, multiple factors are responsible—
1. Paralytic agitans (idiopathic, also called Parkinson's disease). Usually occurs in middle aged or elderly.
2. Postencephalitic (encephalitis lethargica, Japanese B encephalitis).
3. Drugs—phenothiazines (chlorpromazine, prochlorperazine), butyrophenones (haloperidol), metoclopramide, tetrabenazine.
4. Neurosyphilis.
5. Poisoning—carbon monoxide, manganese and MPTP (methyl-phenyl-tetrahydro-pyridine).
6. Herbicide (paraquat).
7. Trauma (punch drunk syndrome, repeated head injury).
8. Genetic (Wilson's disease, Huntington's disease).
9. Cerebral tumour (involving basal ganglia).
10. Parkinsonian plus (when associated with features of other disease):
    - Shy-Drager syndrome.
    - Steele-Richardson-Olszeweski syndrome (progressive supranuclear palsy, characterised by inability of the movement of eye vertically or laterally and dementia).
    - Olivopontocerebellar degeneration.
11. Creutzfeldt-Jakob disease.
12. Normal pressure hydrocephalus (triad of urinary incontinence, gait apraxia and dementia).
13. Atherosclerotic Parkinsonism (stepwise progressive broad-based gait and pyramidal signs).

Clinical Features

- Prodromal nonmotor symptoms may occur before the typical features of Parkinsonism, such as anosmia, depression or anxiety, sleep disturbance, body pain, constipation, urinary abnormality, restless leg syndrome.
- These may be followed by motor symptoms. Unilateral resting tremor in hand. Initially, it is characterized by pill-rolling movement between thumb and index finger, flexion and extension of fingers, abduction and adduction of thumb and pronation and supination of forearm. Later, tremor may affect arms, legs, feet, jaw and tongue.
- Difficulty in initiating movement, slowness of movement (bradykinesia or hypokinesia), e.g. the patient is unable to fasten button. Inability to touch tip of all fingers with thumb successively, if asked to count, there is slow initiation, unable or can do slowly. If asked to do rapid fine finger movement, it becomes indistinct, slurred and tremulous.
- Micrographia, handwriting is tremulous and untidy.
- Titubation of head.
- Mask like, expressionless face with less blinking of the eyes, staring look and dribbling of saliva.
- Speech—slow initiation, husky, slurred, indistinct, lacking intonation, low volume and monotonous (or mutism).
- Rigidity—lead pipe or cog wheel.
- Glabellar tap—taping in the forehead above the bridge of the nose repeatedly. In normal person, blinking will stop after three to five blinks. But in Parkinsonism, the patient continues to blink. This sign is unreliable.
- Gait—festinate. (see below).

Tremor in Parkinsonism

Tremor is involuntary, coarse (4–6 Hz), present at rest, disappears or reduces during voluntary activity, sleep and holding something and tremor increases with emotion or anxiety.

Types of Rigidity: 2 types—

- Lead pipe—uniform rigidity in flexors and extensors of limbs (better seen in elbow or knee).
- Cog wheel—rigidity is interrupted by tremor (better seen in wrist joint). It is due to exaggerated stretch reflex interrupted by tremor.

Gait in Parkinsonism

- Typically festinate gait, characterized by rapid small shuffling step (hardly raises the foot from the ground), during walking less swinging of the arms with flexed attitude.
- Walking is rapid and the patient has difficulty in stopping himself (rapid short steps in order to avoid falling—festination). The patient seems to catch up with his own centre of gravity.
- He has difficulty in rapid turning (fractionated gait), turns 'en bloc.'
- Obstacles cause the patient to freeze in place.

Other Gaits in Parkinsonism

- Propulsion—if the patient is pushed from behind, he is unable to stop himself and may fall forward.

- Retropulsion—if the patient is pushed from front, he is unable to stop himself and may fall backward.
- Kinesia paradoxa—the patient is unable to initiate a movement, but once started, can complete the whole act (may run down the stairs, but cannot stop at the bottom) or the patient is unable to initiate a movement, but during emotion or fear (e.g. fire in the house), can perform the movement (even run out from the house).

Reflexes and Plantar Response in Parkinsonism

All the reflexes and plantar responses are normal. May be difficult to elicit, because of rigidity. Plantar is flexor, may be extensor if associated with the following disorders:

1. Postencephalitic Parkinsonism.
2. Other diseases (called atypical Parkinsonian syndrome)—
   - Shy-Drager syndrome.
   - Steele-Richardson-Olszeweski syndrome (progressive supranuclear palsy).
   - Olivopontocerebellar atrophy (OPCA)
   - Corticobasal degeneration (CBD).

Investigations

Diagnosis is usually clinical. Investigations are done to find out cause or to exclude other disease:

1. CT scan or MRI (done if pyramidal, cerebellar, autonomic involvement or doubtful diagnosis).
2. In patient <50 years, screening for Wilson's disease:
   - Serum caeruloplasmin (low).
   - Serum copper (high serum free copper).
   - 24 h urinary copper (high). Following penicillamine therapy, 24 h urinary copper >25 mmol is confirmatory.
   - Liver function tests may be done.
   - Liver biopsy with quantitative measurement of copper (less done).

Treatment Modalities in Parkinsonism

- Treatment of the cause and withdrawal of offending drugs, if any.
- Symptomatic treatment of tremor, rigidity and bradykinesia.
- Physiotherapy and speech therapy.
- Surgical treatment.
- Occupational therapy and rehabilitation.

Drug Therapy: Not started in mild case, should be started when the symptoms begin to interfere with work and social life or falling becomes a threat. Combination of levodopa and dopa decarboxylase inhibitor is the treatment of choice. Available combinations are:

- Levodopa and carbidopa (co-careldopa, 110 or 275).
- Levodopa and benserazide (co-beneldopa) 62.5 mg.

Drug should be started with low dose and gradually increased as needed.

- Tremor and rigidity may be controlled by anticholinergic drugs (trihexiphenidyl, benztropine, orphenadrin, benzhexol, biperiden).
- Other drugs—Amantadine, selegilin, catechol-O-methyl transferase (COMT) inhibitors (entacapone, tolcapone), dopamine agonist (pergolide, bromocriptin, lisuride, ropinirole and pramipexole) may be used.

General Measures

- Physiotherapy and speech therapy.
- Occupational therapy and rehabilitation.

Role of surgery in Parkinsonism: Surgery is rarely done. Options are:

- Stereotactic thalamotomy or pallidotomy.
- Deep brain stimulation.
- Foetal midbrain or adrenal tissue implantation in basal ganglia.

After 3–5 years of levodopa therapy, there may be fluctuating response to levodopa in one third to one half of the patients. These include:

- **End of dose deterioration (wearing off effect)**—Due to progression of disease and loss of capacity to store dopamine, duration of action of a dose of levodopa becomes progressively shorter. As a result, the patient complains of freezing and rigidity before the next dose of levodopa. It is called 'end of dose effect'. In such case, levodopa should be divided into smaller but frequent doses, or slow-release preparations or addition of dopamine agonist or addion of amantadine may be used.
- **On-off phenomenon**—After prolonged use, the drug is less effective. There is sudden, unpredictable change in response, in which periods of severe Parkinsonism (freezing and immobility—**off period**), alternate with periods of dopamine induced dyskinesias, agitation, chorea and dystonic movements (**on period**). Adjust L-dopa dose or interdose interval or add COMT inhibitor or add dopamine agonist.

INVOLUNTARY MOVEMENTS

Usual involuntary movements are:
- Tremor.
- Chorea.
- Athetosis.
- Hemiballismus.
- Myoclonus.
- Tic.
- Torsion dystonia.

Tremor

Definition

It is the involuntary, oscillatory, rhythmical movement of one or more parts of the body due to alternate contraction of a group of muscles and their antagonists.

Causes
- Functional—anxiety, nervousness, hysterical conversion reaction.
- Endocrine—thyrotoxicosis, phaeochromocytoma, hypoglycaemia.
- Parkinsonism.
- Cerebellar tremor (also called intention tremor).
- Benign essential tremor.
- Senile tremor.
- Drugs—salbutamol and other beta agonist, phenothiazine, butyrophenone, methyldopa, lithium intoxication, anticonvulsant (phenytoin, carbamazepine, sodium valproate).
- Alcohol (chronic alcoholism and alcohol withdrawal).
- Toxin (mercury, arsenic and lead).
- General paresis of insane (GPI).
- Flapping tremor.

Types: 3 types
- Resting tremor (typical of Parkinsonism).
- Action tremor or postural tremor (present on outstretched hands).
- Intention tremor—it comes on voluntary movement but disappears on rest. It is caused by cerebellar lesion due to any cause.
  According to the amplitude or nature, tremor may be fine or coarse.

Causes of Action Tremor
- Anxiety.
- Thyrotoxicosis.
- Senile tremor.
- Benign essential tremor.
- Cerebellar tremor (increases near the target).
- Familial.
- Idiopathic (in many cases).

Causes of Fine Tremor

- Anxiety or nervousness.
- Thyrotoxicosis.
- Senile tremor.
- Benign essential tremor.
- Drugs (salbutamol, terbutaline).
- Familial.
- GPI

Causes of Coarse Tremor

- Parkinsonism.
- Intention tremor.
- Flapping tremor in hepatic precoma.
- Wilson's disease.
- Sometimes in senile tremor.

Benign Essential Tremor

It is a familial tremor inherited as autosomal dominant, usually present in outstretched hands and also when hands adopt a posture, such as holding a glass or spoon. Occasionally, present at rest. Worse in upper limbs. Often, there is titubation. It is common in elderly (but may occur at any age).

It is slowly progressive, rarely produces severe disability. No rigidity and no hypokinesia. Tremor is not aggravated by movement.

Treatment

- Propranolol is helpful in small dose.
- Alcohol may relieve the tremor, but there is chance of addiction.
- Primidone is sometimes helpful.
- Rarely in severe case, injection botulinum toxin may be helpful.
- Rarely in intractable case, stereotactic thalamotomy.

Chorea

Definition

It is the involuntary, nonrepetitive, quasi-purposive, irregular and jerky movements of one or more parts of the body due to extrapyramidal lesion.

Chorea may be unilateral or generalized. It worsens with anxiety or activity and disappears during sleep (chorea—means dance, a Greek word).

Site of Lesion

Caudate nucleus of the basal ganglia.

Causes

- Rheumatic chorea (poststreptococcal, called Sydenham's chorea or St. Vitus' dance).
- Senile chorea.
- Hereditary—Huntington's chorea, Wilson's disease, benign familial chorea.

- Drug induced—phenothiazine, butyrophenone, OCP.
- Pregnancy (chorea gravidarum).
- Encephalitis lethargica.
- Following stroke.
- Others (rare)—Polycythaemia rubra vera, SLE and anti-phospholipid syndrome, endocrine (thyrotoxicosis, idiopathic hypoparathyroidism and hypoglycaemia), kernicterus.

Treatment

- Reassurance and treatment of primary cause (if any).
- Drugs that may be helpful are phenothiazine, butyrophenones (haloperidol), tetrabenazine and sodium valproate.

Sydenham's Chorea

It is one of the major criteria of rheumatic fever. History of rheumatic fever may be present in one third cases. Common in children and adolescents, more in females, age 5–15 years.

Features

- Chorea is associated with emotional instability, irritability, inattentiveness, confusion and fidgety. Speech is often affected.
- Other evidences of rheumatic fever may be absent when chorea is present.
- Carditis may be first manifestation and rheumatic heart disease may occur.
- Fever is unusual. ESR, ASO titre and CRP are usually normal.
- Usually self-limiting, recovers within weeks or one month. Recurrence may occur in 20% cases. Occasionally, may relapse during pregnancy (called chorea gravidarum) or in those who use OCP.

Treatment

- No treatment in most cases as recovery is spontaneous.
- In severe chorea—benzodiazepine, haloperidol, tetrabenazine or valproate may be given.
- Penicillin prophylaxis as in rheumatic fever.

Huntington's Chorea

It is inherited as autosomal dominant, in which chorea is associated with progressive dementia. Gene responsible is on the short arm of chromosome 4.

Symptoms

Common in adults, during third to fourth decade. Lower limbs are more involved than upper limbs. Occasionally, there is juvenile onset where Parkinsonism is the main feature.

Huntington's Chorea is Diagnosed by

- Family history.
- Chorea followed by progressive dementia
- There may be dancing gait.

Pathological Change

Cerebral atrophy with neuronal loss in caudate nucleus and putamen.

Investigations
- CT scan or MRI—atrophy of caudate nucleus and cerebral atrophy.
- DNA analysis.

Treatment
- Haloperidol or phenothiazine for dyskinesia. Tetrabenazine may be given.
- Psychological support.
- Institutional care for dementia.
- Genetic counselling is essential.

Athetosis

It is the involuntary, slow, coarse, writhing movement of limbs, face or trunk. Causes are—
- Basal ganglia lesion—due to cerebral palsy, kernicterus.
- Drugs—phenothiazine.
- Metabolic—Wilson's disease.

Hamiballismus

It is the involuntary, flinging or swinging movement of limbs. Cause—haemorrhage or infarction of the contralateral subthalamic nucleus.

Myoclonus

It is the sudden, involuntary, jerky movement of a single muscle or group of muscles. Cause—benign essential myoclonus, epilepsy.

Tics

These are repetitive, jerky or twitching movement of face, neck or hands. Examples are—shrugging of shoulder, sniffing, grimacing.

Dystonia

It is the involuntary movement of limb or head with abnormal posture. It may be generalized or localized, such as spasmodic torticollis, writer's cramp, oromandibular dyskinesia, blepharospasm and hemiplegic dystonia. Cause—mostly drugs, such as phenothiazine (e.g. prochlorperazine), metoclopramide.

MOTOR NEURON DISEASE

Definition

Motor neuron disease (MND) is a progressive disease of unknown cause, characterised by the degeneration of motor neurons in the spinal cord, cranial nerve nuclei and pyramidal neurons in the motor cortex.

Causes

Unknown, possible factors are—

- Familial in 5–10%, may be inherited as autosomal dominant.
- May be due to viral infection, trauma, toxin, electric shock.

Pathology

Degeneration of Betz cells, pyramidal tract, cranial nerve nuclei and anterior horn cells. Both UMN and LMN may be involved, but no sensory involvement.

Clinical Features

Common in middle aged and elderly males, rare before 30 years. No remission, fatal within 3–5 years.

Symptoms

- Weakness and inability to walk.
- Weight loss and wasting of the muscles of limb.
- Occasional twitching of the muscles.

Signs

1. Motor system—
   - Wasting of muscles.
   - Muscle tone—may be increased.
   - Muscle power—may be diminished.
   - Reflexes—may be diminished or exaggerated.
   - Patellar and ankle clonus may be present.
   - Coordination may be impaired.
   - Multiple fasciculations may be present.
2. Sensory—intact.

Types of MND

According to the site of lesion:

1. Spinal cord lesion—
   - Lower motor neuron lesion—Progressive muscular atrophy (PMA).
   - Combined upper motor neuron and lower motor neuron lesion (LMN lesion in upper limbs and UMN lesion in lower limbs)—Amyotrophic lateral sclerosis (ALS).
   - Pure upper motor neuron lesion (rare)—Primary lateral sclerosis (PLS).
2. Cerebral lesion—
   - Medullary lesion—progressive bulbar palsy.
   - Cortical lesion—pseudobulbar palsy.

According to the type of lesion:
1. Pure UMN lesion—PLS, pseudobulbar palsy.
2. Pure LMN lesion—PMA, bulbar palsy.
3. Mixed lesion—ALS.

Progressive Muscular Atrophy

- Weakness, wasting and fasciculation of distal limb muscles, usually starts in small muscles of one or both hands.
- Tendon reflex is lost (due to involvement of anterior horn cell).

Amyotrophic Lateral Sclerosis

- Weakness, wasting, fasciculation and loss of all reflexes (LMN lesion) in upper limb **plus** spastic weakness with exaggerated reflexes and extensor plantar response in lower limbs (UMN lesion) or commonly there is generalized hyperreflexia.
- Bulbar and pseudobulbar palsy may follow eventually.

Primary Lateral Sclerosis

- Only UMN lesion (both in upper and lower limbs).
- Progressive tetraparesis with terminal pseudobulbar palsy occur.

Progressive Bulbar Palsy

Site of lesion—Nucleus of lower cranial nerves in medulla (IX, X, XI and XII). Lesion is bilateral and LMN type.

Common Causes of Bulbar Palsy

- Motor neuron disease.
- Guillain-Barré syndrome.
- Syringobulbia.
- Brain stem infarction.
- Poliomyelitis.
- Neurosyphilis.
- Neurosarcoid.

Clinical Features

- The patient presents with **3 "D"s**—dysarthria, dysphonia and dysphagia. There is nasal regurgitation, dribbling of saliva.
- Speech is nasal, indistinct and slurred.
- Tongue—wasted, wrinkled and fasciculating.
- There is palatal palsy.
- Gag reflex is absent.

Pseudobulbar Palsy

Site of lesion—Bilateral UMN lesion (supranuclear) involving the pyramidal tract (supranuclear lesion of lower cranial nerves—IX, X, XI, XII).

Causes of Pseudobulbar Palsy

- Bilateral repeated CVA involving internal capsule (multi-infarct dementia).

- Demyelinating disease (multiple sclerosis).
- Motor neuron disease.

Clinical Features

More common in women.

- Speech—nasal, slurred, indistinct and high pitched (so called **Donald Duck** or **hot potato** dysarthria due to tight immobile tongue).
- Tongue—small and tight, spastic, unable to protrude, but no wasting or fasciculation.
- Jaw jerk is exaggerated.
- Palatal movement is absent.
- Gag reflex is present.
- The patient is emotionally labile (crying and laughing).

Investigations in MND

No specific test, diagnosis is usually clinical. Investigations are done to exclude other disease:

- Blood sugar (to exclude diabetic amyotrophy).
- VDRL or TPHA (to exclude neurosyphilis).
- Chest X-ray (to exclude bronchial carcinoma).
- X-ray of cervical spine.
- Ultrasonogram of whole abdomen (to see any neoplasm).
- EMG (to confirm fasciculation and denervation).
- NCV (normal motor and sensory conduction).
- Lumbar puncture and CSF study (no abnormality).
- CT or MRI (brain and spinal cord).

There are some 'No's in MND:

- No sphincter disturbance (rarely involved in late case).
- No sensory involvement.
- No loss of awareness till death.
- No dementia.
- No ocular involvement.
- No cerebellar or extrapyramidal lesion.
- No abnormality of CSF usually.

Treatment of MND

No curative treatment. Only symptomatic and supportive treatment:

- Psychological support.
- Nutritional care—if needed, enteral feeding, percutaneous endoscopic gastrostomy (PEG).
- Speech and communication therapy.
- Respiratory therapy.
- Palliative care.
- Physical rehabilitation and occupational rehabilitation
- Neuroprotective agents—riluzole, vit E, Co-enzyme Q-10. Riluzole is a glutamate antagonist, may retard progression and prolong the survival.

Prognosis of MND

Motor neuron disease (MND) is a progressive disorder, remission is unknown, fatal within 3–5 years. Younger patient with early bulbar syndrome tend to show a more rapid course.

STROKE (CVD OR CVA)

Definition

Stroke may be defined as sudden development of focal neurological deficit due to nontraumatic vascular cause.

Subvarities

- Transient ischaemic attack (TIA)—sudden neurological dysfunction due to cerebral ischaemia lasting less than 24 hours, the patient recovers completely within 24 hours.
- Stroke in evolution—symptoms worsen gradually or in a stepwise pattern over hours or days, neurological deficit persists for more than 24 hours.
- Completed stroke—clinical signs of neurological deficit are persistent.
- Reversible ischaemic neurological deficit (RIND)—neurodeficit persists for more than 24 hours, but recovers within 3 weeks.
- Partial nonprogressive stroke (PNS)—neurodeficit persists for more than 3 weeks, but is either partial or ends up with minimal residual deficit.

Diseases included in CVA

- Cerebral haemorrhage.
- Cerebral thrombosis.
- Cerebral embolism.
- Subarachnoid haemorrhage.
- Hypertensive encephalopathy.
- Cerebellar haemorrhage.
- Cerebellar infarction.

Risk Factors in CVD

1. Nonmodifiable:
   - Age.
   - Gender (more in males).
   - Ethnicity or race.
   - Genetics.
   - Family history.
2. Modifiable:

- Hypertension
- Diabetes mellitus
- Smoking, alcohol.
- Lifestyle.
- Obesity.
- Heart disease (atrial fibrillation, ischaemic heart disease, cardiomyopathy).
- Dyslipidaemia.
- Oral contraceptive pill.
- Carotid vessel atherosclerosis and atheromatous aortic arch.

Clinical Features

Symptoms

- Weakness of one side of the body.
- Difficulty in speech and swallowing.
- Urinary incontinence.
- Semi or unconsciousness.

Signs

1. Patient may be semi or unconscious.
2. Slurring of speech may be present.
3. Motor system (signs of upper motor neurone lesion)—usually hemiplegia.
   - Muscle tone may be increased in one half of body.
   - Muscle power may be reduced in one half of body.
   - Reflexes—exaggerated on the affected side.
   - Patellar and ankle clonus may be present.
   - Coordination—impaired.
   - Gait—hemiplegic gait.
4. Sensory system—may be intact.

Investigations

1. CT scan of the head (first investigation to be done).
2. Routine:
   - CBC with ESR, blood sugar, urea and serum creatinine, electrolytes.
   - Serum lipid profile.
   - Chest X-ray P/A view.
   - ECG.
3. To find source of event:
   - Doppler study of carotid vessels.
   - Echocardiography.
   - Magnetic resonance angiography (MRA) of cerebral vessels.
   - Digital substraction angiography (DSA) of the cerebral vessels.
4. Other tests according to suspicion of cause—
   - For collagen vascular disease—ANA, anti-ds DNA, anticardiolipin and antiphospholipid antibody.
   - p-ANCA, c-ANCA.
   - Coagulation screening, serum antithrombin III, protein C and protein S.
   - Others—red cell mass (in PRV), chromatographic test in serum and urinary level of homocystine or methionine (in homocystinuria), TPHA and VDRL (in syphilis).

Treatment

1. General measures:
   - Oropharyngeal suction.
   - I/V channel.
   - NG tube feeding.
   - Maintenance of nutritional status.

- Regular change of posture (2 hourly) to prevent bed sore.
- Care of bowel, bladder (catheterization), mouth, eyes.

2. Control of risk factors—hypertension, diabetes mellitus, hyperlipidaemia.
3. If cerebral oedema—dexamethasone or mannitol.
4. Specific treatment according to the type of stroke (after CT scan)—
   - Cerebral infarction—antiplatelet drugs (e.g. aspirin, clopidogrel). Cerebral vasodilator like vinpocetin. If atrial fibrillation, heparin followed by warfarin should be considered.
   - Cerebral haemorrhage—for massive haemorrhage, neurosurgical intervention may be required. Other treatment is symptomatic and supportive.
   - Subarachnoid haemorrhage—nimodipine. Neurosurgical intervention is essential.
5. Others (to improve quality of life):
   - Physiotherapy.
   - Speech therapy.
   - Occupational therapy.

Prevention of Stroke

- Risk factors like hypertension, diabetes mellitus, obesity, etc. should be identified and controlled.
- Smoking and alcohol should be stopped.
- Antiplatelet drug (e.g. aspirin) in ischaemic stroke.
- Lifestyle modification—regular physical exercise, dietary modification.
- Statin should be given to all patients.
- Treatment of primary cause.

Causes of CVD in Young Patient

- Mitral stenosis with atrial fibrillation. Other cardiac cause—Patent foramen ovale (PFO), VSD, TOF.
- Antiphospholipid syndrome.
- SLE.
- Haematological disease—sickle cell anaemia, polycythemia rubra vera, inherited deficiency of naturally occurring anticoagulant (Protein C, Protein S, antithrombin III, factor V Leiden).
- Vasculitis.
- Behcet's disease.
- Vascular malformation—AVM, berry aneurysm causing SAH.
- In females—OCP, eclampsia.
- Homocystinuria.
- Premature atherosclerosis may occur in familial hyperlipidaemia.

Investigations in Young Patient with Stroke

- Chest X ray, ECG and echocardiography (to exclude cardiac cause like MS with AF, PFO, TOF).
- CBC, ESR—to exclude polycythaemia rubra vera.
- Serum lipid profile—in juvenile hyperlipidaemia.
- For collagen disease—ANA, anti-ds DNA, anticardiolipin and antiphospholipid antibody.
- Coagulation screening, serum antithrombin III, protein C and protein S level.
- Others—red cell mass (in PRV), chromatographic test in serum and urinary level of homocystine or methionine (homocystinuria), TPHA and VDRL (syphilis).

BRIEF DESCRIPTION OF DIFFERENT TYPES OF CVD

Cerebral Infarction or Ischaemic Stroke

- Commonest cause of CVA in middle aged or elderly (85%).
- Commonest site is internal capsule and commonest vessel involvement is middle cerebral artery.
- Risk factors—atherosclerosis, systemic hypertension, diabetes mellitus, polycythaemia rubra vera, collagen vascular disease, dyslipidaemia, smoking, obesity, oral contraceptive pill, alcohol, obesity, carotid artery occlusion.
- Onset is insidious with stepwise progression. Commonly occurs during sleep or soon after waking.
- Loss of consciousness is rare, but there may be headache, convulsion.

Cerebral Embolism

- Onset—very acute or stormy (develops quickly in seconds), during exertion or activity, no warning signs of TIA.
- Site—left-sided vascular lesion is common as left common carotid artery arises directly from the aorta. Left middle cerebral artery is commonly involved.
- There is usually a source of embolus or vulvular heart disease with atrial fibrillation.
- Sometimes, features may be diminished or disappear due to dislodgement of the embolus. Shifting hemiplegia may occur.
- Recovery—may be rapid.
- Cause—atherosclerosis, mitral stenosis with atrial fibrillation, infective endocarditis, paradoxical embolism, myocardial infarction.

Cerebral Haemorrhage

- Usually occurs in elderly, cause of CVD in 15% cases.
- Site—internal capsule. Other sites—pons, thalamus, cerebellum and cerebral white mater.
- Common vessel involved—lenticulostriate branch of middle cerebral artery.
- Onset—usually sudden.
- Causes—common in uncontrolled hypertension. Ruptured intracerebral aneurysm, blood dyscrasia, vascular anomaly like arteriovenous malformation, haemorrhage in a cerebral neoplasm.

Subarachnoid Haemorrhage

- Common in young adults. 5-10% stroke are due to subarachnoid haemorrhage.
- Cause—rupture of congenital berry aneurysm (most common cause, in 80% cases). Other causes—head injury, leaking from arteriovenous malformation.
- Features—severe headache, usually in the occipital region, like struck by the hammer or thunderclap. There may be vomiting, convulsion, rapid loss of consciousness.
- Neck rigidity and Kernig's sign are present.
- Fundoscopy shows subhyaloid haemorrhage with upward concavity (boot-shaped).
- Lumbar puncture and CSF study shows raised CSF pressure, which is frankly haemorrhagic. If CSF is kept for hours, xanthochromia may occur. CT scan is diagnostic. CT angiogram may be done.
- Treatment—control of hypertension, nimodipine, surgical treatment.

COMA OR UNCONSCIOUSNESS

Causes (remember the formula—**'AEIOU—DAMH'**):

- **A**poplexy—cerebral haemorrhage, subarachnoid haemorrhage.
- **E**pilepsy.
- **I**nfection (e.g. encephalitis, meningitis, cerebral malaria, severe septicaemia).
- **O**pium poisoning.
- **U**raemia (renal failure).
- **D**iabetes mellitus (ketoacidosis, hypoglycaemia, lactic acidosis, HONC).
- **A**lcohol.
- **M**etabolic—metabolic acidosis.
- **H**ypoglycaemia, hypoxaemia, hypertensive encephalopathy, hepatic coma, hypothyroidism (myxoedema coma), hyponatraemia, hypothermia, hyperpyrexia, head injury.

Investigations

- CBC, ESR.
- Blood sugar.
- Serum urea, creatinine, electrolytes.
- Arterial blood gas analysis.
- Chest X-ray.
- ECG.
- Thyroid function test.
- Liver function test.
- CT scan or MRI.
- Others according to suspicion of cause, e.g. malarial parasite (MP), lumbar puncture and CSF study, etc.

Management: A, B, C measures

- Airway should be kept clear.
- Breathing maintenance—O_2 inhalation, suction may be needed.
- Circulation should be maintained, IV channel.
- Nutrition should be maintained—NG tube feeding and correction of water and electrolytes.
- Care of bowel, bladder, mouth and eyes.
- Change posture 2 hourly to prevent bed sores.
- Parenteral antibiotic to prevent infection.
- Treatment of primary cause.

MYASTHENIA GRAVIS

Definition

It is an autoimmune disease of skeletal muscle characterised by weakness or fatigue specially ocular, facial, neck and bulbar muscles following activity.

Muscle groups involved in order are—extraocular, bulbar (swallowing or chewing), face, neck, limb girdle and trunk. Cardiac muscle is not affected.

Cause

Due to autoantibody (IgG) against postsynaptic nicotinic acetylcholine receptor (AchR).

Usually associated with other autoimmune disease (e.g. type 1 diabetes, Graves' disease, pernicious anaemia) and thymic hyperplasia in 70%.

Clinical Features

Common in women, age 15–50 years. Over 50 years, it is common in men and associated with thymic atrophy or thymic tumour 10–15%.

Symptoms

- Muscular weakness or fatigue after activity, usually at the end of the day.
- Ocular—drooping of upper eyelid and double vision.
- Bulbar—difficulty in chewing, swallowing, speaking.

Signs

Following bed side test can be done—

- Ptosis, usually bilateral, may be unilateral, frontalis over acitivity.
- Counting test—when the patient is asked to count 1–50, voice becomes gradually indistinct.
- Ceiling test—patient is asked to look at the ceiling for some time—ptosis will occur.
- Muscle power is initially normal, but with activity becomes weak.
- Peek sign—if the patient is asked to close the eyes tightly, after some time eye lids separate (peek) showing white sclera.
- Reflexes—normal.

Investigations

- CBC and ESR.
- Chest X-ray (to exclude bronchial carcinoma, thymoma).
- CT scan of chest (to exclude thymoma).
- Edrophonium (Tensilon) test.
- Vital capacity.
- Serum acetylcholine receptor antibody.
- Serum anti-MuSK.
- Single fibre EMG—shows progressive decremental response.
- Repetitive nerve stimulation test (RNS).
- To see other associations—thyroid function test, anti-skeletal muscle antibody (suggest presence of thymoma), ANA, rheumatoid factor, serum CPK, antibody against intrinsic factor.

Tensilon Test

2 mg edrophonium is injected initially to see any side effect. If no, another 8 mg is given after half a minute. Improvement in muscle power occurs within 30 seconds and persists for 2-3 minutes. Sensitivity is 80%. Occasionally, there may be bronchospasm and syncope. Resuscitation facilities must be available. Atropine should be kept ready.

Treatment

1. Anticholinesterase drug, e.g. pyridostigmine 60 mg tablet (4–16 tablets in divided doses up to five times a day).
2. Others—
   - Thymectomy—In all patients with thymoma and thymic hyperplasia.
   - Plasmapheresis—in severe myasthenia or myasthenic crisis or preoperative preparation.
   - IV immunoglobulin—it is an alternative to plasma exchange in short-term treatment of severe myasthenia.
   - Steroid—to minimize the side effect, low-dose prednisolone initially 5 mg/day, increase 5 mg/week up to 1 mg/kg. Continued for 1-3 months, then gradually modified to an alternate day regimen over the course of additional 1-3 months. On remission, reduce the dose (may take months). Azathioprine may be added (2.5 mg/kg daily) or weekly methotrexate may be given. Sometimes, I/V methylprednisolone may be tried.
   - Other immunosuppressive drugs—azathioprine, mycophenolate mofetil may be used.

Drugs to be avoided in MG

- Aminoglycoside.
- Penicillamine.
- Ciprofloxacin.
- Quinine.
- Antiarrhythmic drugs.

Myasthenic Crisis

It is the exacerbation of symptoms of myasthenia gravis. May be severe and require artificial ventilation in 10% cases. Precipitating factors are exertion, extremes of temperature, respiratory infection and surgery. The patient should be closely monitored for pulmonary function and should be treated in ICU.

Treatment

- Respiratory assistance and pulmonary physiotherapy.
- Stop all cholinesterase inhibitors.
- Plasmapheresis or I/V immunoglobulin.
- Antibiotic, if there is infection.

Cholinergic Crisis

Overdose of anticholinesterase drugs may cause cholinergic crisis, which is due to depolarization block of motor end plates. Features of cholinergic crisis are muscle fasciculation, paralysis, pallor, sweating, excessive salivation, lacrimation, bronchial secretion, small pupil (meiosis), abdominal colic, diarrhoea, urinary incontinence, respiratory insufficiency, confusion and collapse. Infection, diarrhoea, aminoglycoside, penicillamine, steroid may precipitate the crisis. Edrophonium should be avoided in these patients.

Difference between Myasthenic Crisis and Cholinergic Crisis

The clinical features are as above. In both cases, patient complains of weakness.

- Muscarinic features are present only in cholinergic crisis, but absent in myasthenic crisis.
- Pupil in constricted or small in cholinergic crisis, but normal in myasthenic crisis.
- In myasthenic crisis—edrophonium causes quick improvement.

EATON–LAMBERT SYNDROME

It is a paraneoplastic syndrome characterised by proximal muscle weakness, wasting and easy fatigability. It commonly involves the lower limbs, but may involve any muscle. Bulbar symptoms are rare (unlike MG).

Cause

There is defect in acetylcholine release at the neuromuscular junction, thought to be due to an autoantibody against P/Q type voltage gated calcium channel (VGCC, present in 90% cases) on the motor nerve terminal. It is commonly due to small cell carcinoma of lung. May be associated with or may precede 1–2 years before the manifestations of carcinoma.

Clinical Features

- Features like myasthenia gravis.
- Other features are—diminished or absent tendon reflexes (cardinal sign), appears immediately after sustained contraction of relevant muscle.
- There is transient improvement in muscle strength and deep tendon reflexes following brief exercise. Muscle power increases after repeated activity (reverse of myasthenia gravis).

Investigations

EMG is diagnostic—there is progressive incremental response following repeated stimulation (reverse of myasthenia gravis, where there is progressive decremental response).

Treatment

- Prednisolone plus azathioprine may be helpful.
- Occasionally plasmapheresis.
- 3, 4 diaminopyridine (DAP) is given.
- Guanidine hydrochloride may help.
- I/V immunoglobulin.
- No response to anticholinesterase drug. However anticholinesterase (pyridostigmine or neostigmine) either alone or in combination with guanidine hydrochloride shows variable response.
- Treatment of primary cause (e.g. bronchial carcinoma).

TRANSVERSE MYELITIS

Definition

Transverse myelitis (TM) is the acute inflammatory, demyelinating disorder of the spinal cord causing paraparesis or paraplegia or sometimes quadriplegia. Commonly due to postinfectious or postvaccinal inflammation. It is the common cause of noncompressive spinal cord syndrome.

Causes

1. Postinfectious or postvaccinal inflammation
   - Viral—coxsackie, polio, EBV, herpes virus, HIV.
   - Bacterial—pyogenic, tuberculous, syphilitic (rare).
   - Others—parasitic, fungal, schistosomiasis.
2. Traumatic.
3. Vascular—arteritis, anterior spinal artery occlusion.
4. Nutritional myelopathy.
5. Collagen vascular disease—SLE, Sjogren syndrome, MCTD.
6. Miscellaneous—ADEM, multiple sclerosis, sarcoidosis, neuromyelitis optica.
7. Idiopathic.

Common Site

Mid thoracic region.

Clinical Features

Usually follows viral illness or vaccination.

Symptoms

- Fever may be present, acute or subacute onset of paralysis or paraparesis associated with back pain.
- At the level of lesion—girdle constriction with hyperaesthesia just above the lesion may be present.
- Usually no root pain, spinal tenderness or spinal deformity.
- Urinary problem like retention, incontinence as bladder involvement is early.

Signs

Motor system:

- Muscle tone—may be increased.
- Muscle power—may be diminished.
- Reflexes—may be normal or exaggerated.
- Coordination—may be normal.

Sensory

Partial or complete sensory loss with a definite upper level.

Investigations

- CBC (leucocytosis in systemic infection).
- X-ray of dorsolumbar spine (to exclude other cause).
- CSF study (high protein and lymphocyte).
- CT scan and MRI of brain and spinal cord.

Treatment

1. General measures
   - Reassurance and psychological support.
   - Care of bowel, bladder (catheterisation), eyes, skin.
   - Passive physiotherapy.
   - For spasticity—baclofen, diazepam, tinazidine.
   - Rehabilitation.
2. Treatment of specific cause, if any.
3. In patient with severe and rapidly progressive disease—high-dose IV methylprednisolone and IV acyclovir.
4. Plasmapheresis.

CEREBELLAR LESION

Cerebellum consists of two hemisphere connected by vermis.

Function of Cerebellum

- Hemisphere cordinates movement of ipsilateral limb.
- Vermis controls axial functions—eye movement, head and trunk posture, stance and gait.

Signs of Cerebellar Lesions

- Titubation of head.
- Tilting of head towards the site of lesion.
- Nystagmus (horizontal).
- Scanning speech.
- Intention tremor.
- Incoordination.
- Dysdiadochokinesis.
- Past pointing (dysmetria).
- Ataxia.
- Hypotonia.
- Diminished tendon reflex (knee jerk may be pendular).

Causes of Cerebellar Lesion

1. Vascular—haemorrhage, infarction, arteriovenous malformation and brain stem vascular lesion.
2. Demyelinating—multiple sclerosis.
3. Drugs—phenytoin, carbamazepine, lithium.
4. Alcohol.
5. Neoplasm—haemangioblastoma, medulloblastoma, acoustic neuroma, secondary deposit.
6. Infection—cerebellar abscess, HIV infection.
7. Inherited—Friedreich's ataxia, ataxia telengiectesia and other hereditary ataxias.
8. Cerebellar syndrome of malignancy (paraneoplastic syndrome), which may be due to carcinoma of ovary, uterus, breast, small cell carcinoma of the lung.
9. Cerebellar syndrome—Shy-Drager syndrome, Steele- Richardson-Olszeweski syndrome, Creutzfeldt-Jakob disease, Wilson's disease.
10. Others—hypothyroidism, Arnold-Chiari lesion, trauma (punch-drunk syndrome).

Investigation

MRI.

FRIEDREICH'S ATAXIA

Definition

It is the most common type of hereditary ataxia, inherited as autosomal recessive trait and in some cases, autosomal dominant.

Sites of Lesion

- Cerebellum.
- Spinocerebellar tract.
- Posterior column lesion and dorsal root ganglia.
- Degeneration of peripheral sensory fibers.
- Corticospinal tract (lateral column lesion).
- Eye (primary optic atrophy).

There is progressive degeneration.

Clinical Features

Usual onset at 8–16 years.

Symptoms

- Difficulty in walking due to weakness of lower limbs and
- Hearing loss.
- Dysarthria.

Signs

- Cerebellar signs (dysarthria, nystagmus, intention tremor, ataxic gait).
- Posterior column lesion—absent vibration and position sense, positive Rhomberg sign.
- Corticospinal tract sign lesion—extensor plantar response, weakness.
- Peripheral nerve—absent reflexes in lower limb, wasting of muscles.

Others

- Diabetes mellitus (common).
- Kyphoscoliosis, pes cavus, cocking of toes, optic atrophy, spina bifida and hypertrophic cardiomyopathy.
- Normal mentation (may have mild dementia).

Investigations

Diagnosis is clinical.

- CBC, ESR.
- Blood sugar—high.
- Chest X-ray (cardiomegaly).
- ECG (arrhythmia).
- MRI of brain and spinal cord (shows atrophy of cerebellum and spinal cord).
- Nerve conduction study.

Treatment

Symptomatic and supportive.

Prognosis

Usually progresses slowly, death occurs before 40 years of age (usually 20 years after the onset of symptoms due to cardiac and respiratory complications).

RAISED INTRACRANIAL PRESSURE

Causes

1. Intracranial space occupying lesion—
   - Tumour (mainly posterior fossa lesion, high-grade glioma).
   - Abscess.
   - Secondary deposit.
   - Hydatid cyst.
   - Tuberculoma.
2. Intracranial haemorrhage—for example intracerebral haemorrhage, subdural haematoma, extradural haematoma.
3. Meningitis.
4. Encephalitis.
5. Benign (idiopathic) intracranial hypertension.
6. Intracranial venous sinus thrombosis.
7. Hydrocephalus.
8. Hypertensive encephalopathy.

Features of Raised ICP

- Headache, which is diffuse, dull in nature, more on waking from sleep, improves throughout the day, worse on bending forward, cough and straining.
- Morning vomiting without nausea.
- Deterioration of consciousness and mental function.
- Pulse—bradycardia.
- BP—may be high.
- Diplopia due to 6th nerve involvement (false localising sign).
- Fundoscopy shows papilloedema.

Investigations

CT scan or MRI.

Treatment

- Mannitol 200–300 cc IV in half an hour. May be repeated.
- Frusemide 40–80 mg IV.
- Inj. dexamethasone IV 6–8 hourly may be given.
- Treatment of primary cause.

INTRACRANIAL SPACE OCCUPYING LESION (ICSOL)

Mass lesion produces symptoms or signs by direct pressure to the brain tissue raised intracranial pressure or provoking seizure.

Clinical Features

1. Local effects on adjacent brain tissue, e.g. focal signs (depends upon the localisation of the tumour, whether frontal, temporal, etc. or parital, or cerebellum).
2. Features due to raised ICP—Headache, vomiting, papilloedema, depressed level of consciousness.
3. False localising signs—unilateral or bilateral 6th nerve palsy, ipsilateral hemiparesis, bilateral extensor plantar responses.
4. Others—seizure, mental changes, depression, fatigability.

BENIGN (IDIOPATHIC) INTRACRANIAL HYPERTENSION

Definition

Benign intracranial hypertension (BIH), also called idiopathic intracranial hypertension is defined as symptoms of raised intracranial pressure without space occupying lesion or ventricular dilatation or focal neurological sign.

Actual cause of BIH is unknown, it is due to reduced or defect of CSF reabsorption by arachnoid villi.

Clinical Features

It is common in young females, 18–40 years, obese, rarely familial. Benign intracranial hypertension may be associated with—

- Pregnancy.
- Obesity.
- Oral contraceptive pill.
- Hypo- or hyperthyroidism.
- Adrenal insufficiency.
- Steroid use or withdrawal.
- Drugs (sulfur, nitrofurantoin, nalidixic acid, tetracycline), hypervitaminosis A.

Clinical Features

The patient usually presents with—

- Frequent headache.
- Visual disturbance—transient obscurations of vision mainly with change in posture.
- 6th nerve palsy (false localizing sign).
- Usually no epileptic attack.
- Fundoscopy—shows papilloedema.
- Visual loss may occur due to optic atrophy.

Investigations

- CT scan or MRI of brain—normal with no ventricular dilatation (sometimes, ventricle is small and appear slit like).
- Lumbar puncture shows high CSF pressure (>30cm CSF), but normal CSF constituents.
- MR angiography or cerebral venography may be done to exclude cerebral venous sinus thrombosis.

Treatment

- Weight reduction.
- Avoid offending drugs.
- Loop diuretic or acetazolamide may be given.
- Repeated lumbar puncture.
- Occasionally, steroid may be used (it reduces intracranial pressure).
- Surgical treatment—ventriculoperitoneal or lumbo-peritoneal shunt, especially if there is progressive visual loss. Optic nerve fenestration may be done.

BRAIN TUMOURS

Primary brain tumours are rare, about 1% in adult, but higher in children. Metastatic tumours are common. Primary brain tumour does not metastasize to the other part due to absence of lymphatic drainage in the brain.

Classification

Malignant

- Glioma (astrocytoma)—common, glioblastoma multiforme is the most aggressive.
- Oligodendroglioma.
- Medulloblastoma.
- Ependymoma.
- Cerebral lymphoma.

Benign

- Meningioma—common
- Neurofibroma
- Craniopharyngioma
- Pituitary adenoma
- Colloid cyst
- Pineal tumours

Common Tumors of the Posterior Fossa or Cerebellopontine Angle

- Vestibular schwannoma (acoustic neuroma).
- Meningioma
- Epidermoid or dermoid cyst

Tumors of the Pituitary Region

- Pituitary adenoma—Microadenoma (<1 cm) and macroadenoma.
- Craniopharyngioma.
- Optic nerve glioma.
- Suprasellar meningioma.

Investigations

- CT scan and MRI with contrast.
- Chest X-ray.
- CT scan of chest.
- USG of abdomen and pelvis—to see any primary lesion.
- Bone scan.
- Lumbar puncture and CSF study in some cases.
- Biopsy.

Treatment

- Surgery.
- Chemotherapy.
- Radiotherapy

WILSON'S DISEASE

Definition

It is an inborn error of copper metabolism, characterised by failure of biliary excretion of copper, excess deposition of copper in several organs with their damage. It is also called 'hepatolenticular degeneration.' Inherited as autosomal recessive.

Commonly affected organs are liver, basal ganglia of brain, cornea, kidney and skeleton. Caeruloplasmin production is less due to unknown mechanism. Total body copper is increased.

Symptoms

Age 5–30 years. Hepatitis is common in children and neurological features in adults. Features are:

- Liver—acute hepatitis, may be recurrent, fulminating hepatic failure, chronic persistent hepatitis, chronic active hepatitis or cirrhosis.
- Neurological—extrapyramidal (Parkinsonism, batwing tremor, dysarthria, chorea, athetosis, dystonia), cerebellar syndrome, dementia. No sensory abnormality. Three main movement disorders are—**D**ystonia, **I**ncoordination, **T**remor (**DIT**).
- Eye—Kayser-Fleischer ring, common in 10–12 o'clock position (upper periphery), due to deposition of copper in Descemet's membrane of cornea. It is greenish-brown pigmentation at the sclerocorneal junction seen by naked eye, may require slit lamp examination. Rarely, sunflower cataract due to deposition of copper in lens (does not impair vision).
- Psychiatric problem like personality change, suicidal tendency, manic-depressive psychosis.
- Other features—renal (renal tubular acidosis, nephrolithiasis), cholelithiasis, spontaneous abortion, amenorrhoea. Haemolytic anaemia, aminoaciduria or Fanconi syndrome, osteoporosis may occur.

NB: If young patient presents with prolonged jaundice or recurrent hepatitis or CLD or neurological features like involuntary movement or abnormal speech or psychiatric features, Wilson's disease should be excluded.

Investigations

- Serum caeruloplasmin—low.
- Serum free copper—high.
- 24 hour urinary copper—high (Normal <40 mg, in Wilson's disease—100–1000 mg or 0.6 mmol/24 hours). 24 hour urinary copper following penicillamine therapy >25 mmol is a confirmatory test.
- Liver biopsy with quantitative measurement of copper (high hepatic copper, usually not done).

Treatment

- Penicillamine (drug of choice)—1–4 g (usually 1.5 g daily). Dose may be reduced when the disease is remission, to be continued lifelong, even in pregnancy.
- Trientine dihydrochloride—1.2–2.4 g daily and zinc acetate—150 mg daily may be given as an alternative, usually helpful in maintenance therapy and in asymptomatic case.
- Liver transplantation in fulminating hepatic failure or in advanced cirrhosis.

Prognosis: Excellent, if treatment is started before irreversible damage:

NB: Sibling and children must be investigated and treatment should be given, even they are asymptomatic.

Follow-up

- Clinical improvement with regular measurement of urinary copper.
- Compliance to treatment
- Clinical deterioration and its management.
- Assessment of complications of treatment—CBC, LFT, RFT.

PARAPLEGIA

It may be spastic or flaccid.

Some common definitions:

- Paraplegia—complete paralysis of both lower limbs.
- Paraparesis—weakness of both lower limbs.
- Monoplegia—paralysis of one limb.
- Hemiplegia—paralysis of one half of the body.
- Hemiparesis—weakness of one half of the body.
- Quadriplegia—complete paralysis of all four limbs.
- Quadriparesis—weakness of four limbs.

Spastic Paraplegia

Definition

Paraplegia of upper motor neuron type.

Causes

- Spinal cord compression due to any cause (see below).
- Demyelinating disease (multiple sclerosis, ADEM).
- Motor neuron disease (amyotrophic lateral sclerosis, primary lateral sclerosis).
- Friedreich's ataxia (early age).
- Hereditary spastic paraplegia.
- Subacute combined degeneration (SCD).
- Acute transverse myelitis.
- Anterior spinal artery thrombosis or occlusion.
- Tropical spastic paraplegia.

Causes of Spinal Cord Compression According to the Site of Lesion

1. Vertebral lesion (extradural, 80%)—
   - Trauma.
   - Tuberculosis of spine (Pott's disease).
   - Lymphoma.
   - Secondary deposit (elderly).
   - Multiple myeloma (elderly).
   - Paravertebral abscess.
   - Extramedullary haematopoiesis in thalassaemia.
2. Meningeal lesion (intradural, extramedullary, 15%)—
   - Meningioma.
   - Neurofibroma.
   - Ependymoma.
   - Secondary deposit (elderly).
   - Lymphoma.
   - Leukaemia.
   - Epidural abscess.

3. Spinal cord lesion (intradural, intramedullary)—
   - Spinal cord tumour—glioma, ependymoma, metastasis.
   - Syringomyelia.
   - Haematomyelia.

NB: Commonest causes of spastic paraplegia—7 T's

- **T**rauma.
- **T**uberculosis (Pott's disease).
- **T**umour (meningioma, neurofibroma, lymphoma, leukaemia, myeloma, glioma).
- **T**ransverse myelitis.
- **T**abes dorsalis.
- **T**welve (B12 deficiency).
- **T**hrombosis.

Clinical Features

Symptoms

1. Pain—localised over the spine or in a root distribution, aggravated by coughing, sneezing or straining.
2. Sensory—paraesthesia, numbness or cold sensations, especially in the lower limbs, which spread proximally to a level on the trunk.
3. Motor—weakness, heaviness or stiffness of the limbs, most commonly the legs.
4. Sphincter—retention followed by urinary incontinence.

Signs

- UMN sign (spastic paraplegia) below the level of compression and LMN sign at the level of compression.
- Segmental sensory loss (sensory loss up to a particular segmental level).

Other features

- Sphincter disturbance—urinary retention and loss of bladder control.
- Root pain—frequent at the site of compression.
- Pain radiates in a band around the chest (thoracic compression).

Investigations

- X-ray of dorso-lumbar spine.
- MRI of dorsal lumbar spine.
- Lumbar puncture and CSF study.
- Other test according to cause (tuberculosis and myeloma).

Treatment

General measures

- Care of bowel, bladder, mouth, skin.
- Prevention of bed sore by changing of posture every 2–4 hours, using special bed (air cushion bed).
- Physiotherapy.

Specific—according to cause, as for example

- Anti-Koch's in Pott's disease.
- Surgical removal of tumour, drainage of abscess.

Causes of Spastic Paraplegia due to Cerebral Lesion

- Parasagittal meningioma (usually falx meningioma).
- Thrombosis of superior longitudinal sinus.
- Thrombosis of unpaired anterior cerebral artery.
- Multiple cerebral infarction.
- Hydrocephalus.
- Trauma.
- In children, cerebral palsy (cerebral diplegia).

Noncompressive Causes of Spastic Paraparesis or Paraplegia

- MND (e.g. amyotrophic lateral sclerosis).
- Subacute combined degeneration of spinal cord.
- Transverse myelitis.
- Multiple sclerosis.
- Friedreich's ataxia.
- Lathyrism.
- Syringomyelia.
- Vascular disease of the spinal cord.
- Hereditary spastic paraplegia.
- Tropical spastic paraplegia.
- Postvaccination.
- Syphilitic amyotrophy.
- Nonmetastatic manifestation of malignancy.
- Radiation myelopathy.
- Functional.

Causes of Paraplegia of Sudden Onset

- Trauma (to vertebral column).
- Collapse of vertebra due to any cause.
- Acute transverse myelitis.
- Multiple sclerosis.
- Anterior spinal artery thrombosis.
- Postvaccination myelitis.
- Dissecting aneurysm.
- Haematomyelia (due to arteriovenous malformation or angioma).

Flaccid Paraplegia

Definition

It is the paraplegia of lower motor neuron type.

Causes of Flaccid Paraplegia

1. With bowel and bladder involvement:
   - Spinal shock.
   - Cauda equina syndrome.

2. Without bowel and bladder involvement—
   - Guillain Barré syndrome (GBS).
   - Motor neuropathy due to any cause (such as acute intermittent porphyria, Charcot Marie Tooth disease, chronic lead poisoning, paraneoplastic syndrome).
   - Progressive muscular atrophy (MND).
   - Acute inflammatory demyelinating polyradiculopathy (AIDP).
   - Tabes dorsalis.
   - Friedreich's ataxia.
3. UMN lesion in shock stage.
4. Peripheral neuropathy involving both lower limbs.
5. Periodic paralysis
6. Hypo- or hyperkalaemia.

Common Causes of Flaccid Paraplegia

- Guillain-Barré syndrome.
- Motor neuropathy due to any cause.
- Tabes dorsalis.
- Friedreich's ataxia.
- Progressive muscular atrophy (one type of MND).
- Acute inflammatory demyelinating polyradiculopathy (AIDP).
- Hysterical conversion reaction HCR.

NB: Most common causes of flaccid paraplegia are GBS and peripheral neuropathy.

Difference between Rigidity and Spasticity

- Spasticity means increased resistance during the initial part of passive movement, followed by lessening of the resistance. It may be clasp-knife type, where the initial resistance is followed by sudden loss of resistance. It is due to pyramidal lesions.
- Rigidity means sustained resistance during passive movement. It may be lead pipe in which resistance is uniform throughout the passive movement (better seen in elbow and knee) or cog wheel in which continuous resistance is interrupted by tremor (better seen in the wrist joint). Rigidity is found in extrapyramidal lesion.

GUILLAIN–BARRÉ SYNDROME

Definition

Guillain–Barré syndrome (GBS) is a postinfective demyelinating neuropathy of unknown cause, characterised by demyelination of peripheral nerve or spinal root.

Causes

It occurs 1–3 weeks after respiratory infection, postvaccination, surgery or diarrhoea. Triggering factors are *Campylobacter jejuni*, cytomegalo virus, mycoplasma, herpes zoster, HIV, EB virus infection. May be immunologically mediated. It does not recur (monophasic).

There are two mechanisms—

1. Demyelinating (acute inflammatory demyelinating neuropathy, AIDP).
2. Axonal, may be—
   - Motor (acute motor axonal neuropathy, AMAN).
   - Sensorimotor (acute motor and sensory axonal neuropathy, AMSAN)

Symptoms

- Weakness, usually starts in lower limbs, ascends rapidly and affects upper limbs (called ascending paralysis), more marked proximally than distally.
- Facial and bulbar weakness, respiratory weakness. Even respiratory failure may develop within hours.
- Low back pain, distal paraesthesia and pain may precede weakness.

Signs

- Muscle tone and power—diminished.
- Loss of all reflexes.
- Sensory loss—minimum or absent.
- Bilateral facial palsy (in 50% cases, unilateral in 25% cases).
- Sphincter involvement (rare).

Investigations

- Lumbar puncture and CSF study—typical finding is 'albumino-cytological dissociation' (albumin may be very high, >1000 mg%, lymphocytes are slightly raised or normal, <20/mm^3).
- Repeated monitoring of respiratory function tests (FVC, FEV_1, PEFR).
- Arterial blood gas analysis (respiratory failure may occur).
- Nerve conduction study (shows slow conduction or conduction block, demyelinating neuropathy, found after 1 week).
- Serum electrolytes.

Treatment

- The patient should be treated in ICU, respiratory function should be monitored regularly (vital capacity and arterial blood gases). May require artificial ventilation.
- High-dose intravenous gamma globulin should be given to all patients. Dose is 400 mg/kg/day for 5 days, helpful if given within 14 days.

- Plasma exchange, if given within 14 days is equally effective.
- Physiotherapy.
- Symptomatic treatment.

NB: Steroid has no proven value (may worsen). Methylprednisolone with immunoglobulin has no proven benefit.

Prognosis of GBS

- 80% recovery, may take several months (3-6 months). If axons have been damaged, the regeneration may require 6–18 months or longer.
- 10% residual disability.
- Three to five percent die (in some study up to 10% death).

Complications of GBS (Cause of Death)

- Respiratory muscle paralysis. The patient may develop respiratory failure within hours.
- Bulbar palsy (dysphagia, nasal regurgitation).
- Cardiac conduction block.
- Cardiac arrhythmia.

Miller–Fisher Syndrome

Miller–Fisher syndrome is a variant of GBS characterised by triad of ophthalmoplegia, ataxia and areflexia. It is a rare disease.

CHRONIC INFLAMMATORY DEMYELINATING POLYNEUROPATHY (CIDP)

Definition

Chronic inflammatory demyelinating polyneuropathy (CIDP) is an autoimmune demyelinating disease of peripheral nerves characterised by weakness and sensory loss in limbs, peripheral nerve enlargement and high CSF protein.

Clinical Features

Common in young adult, males slightly more affected than females.

Symptoms

- Onset is usually gradual, but sometimes subacute.
- Features are like GBS.
- Relapsing and remitting or progressive generalised neuropathy.
- Sensory, motor or autonomic nerves can be involved, but the signs are predominantly motor. Some patients may present with pure sensory ataxia.

Signs

Like GBS.

Difference between CIDP and GBS

CIDP is clinically similar to GBS except that it has a relapsing or steadily progressive course over months or years, autonomic dysfunction is generally less common. It is less common than GBS. CIDP responds to steroid, while GBS does not.

Investigations

- CSF examination (high protein, acellular).
- NCV of peripheral nerves—GBS like feature (marked slowing of motor and sensory conduction, and focal conduction block).
- MRI (plaques resembling multiple sclerosis are found in brain and spinal cord in some cases).
- Nerve biopsy (shows segmental demyelination).

Treatment

Depends on severity of disease—

1. Mild—follow-up only, spontaneous recovery may occur.
2. Functionally significant—
   - Prednisolone 60-80 mg daily for 2-3 months, then taper slowly.
   - Intravenous immunoglobulin (0.4 g/kg/day for 5 days)—usually used as an initial treatment with steroid.
   - Plasma exchange—2-3 times per week for 6 weeks.
   - If above treatment fails—azathioprine, methotrexate, ciclosporin or cyclophosphamide may be given.
3. Severe disease, nonambulatory—plasma exchange 2-3/week for 6 weeks and prednisolone 60-80 mg/day.

EPILEPSY

Seizure

It means convulsion caused by abnormal, excessive or synchronous discharge of cerebral neurons.

Epilepsy

It is characterised by recurrent and paroxysmal attack of convulsion or seizure.

Causes of Epilepsy

1. Primary or idiopathic—common in early age, before 20.
2. Secondary—
   - Traumatic.
   - Vascular—CVD, A-V malformation.
   - Infection—meningitis, encephalitis, cerebral abscess, cerebral malaria, tuberculosis, HIV.
   - Intracranial space occupying lesion—tumour, secondaries, abscess, subdural haematoma.
   - Inflammatory—SLE, vasculitis, sarcoidosis.
   - Metabolic—hypoglycaemia, hepatic failure, renal failure.
   - Cerebral anoxia—asphyxia, carbon monoxide and nitrous oxide poisoning.
   - Congenital—tuberous sclerosis, cerebral palsy.

Classification

1. Generalised—
   - Generalised tonic-clonic seizure (grand mal).
   - Absence seizure (petit mal)—it may be—
     - Typical absence.
     - Atypical absence.
     - Absence with special features.
   - Myoclonic seizure—myoclonic atonic and myoclonic tonic.
   - Tonic and atonic seizure.
2. Partial or focal—
   - Simple partial—no impairment of consciousness (e.g. Jacksonian seizure).
   - Complex partial—impairment of consciousness (e.g. psychomotor epilepsy).
   - Partial seizure evolving to secondary generalized seizure.
3. Unclassifiable seizure—does not fit to any category above.

GENERALISED SEIZURES

There is diffuse involvement of both cerebral hemisphere, cellular, structural or biochemical abnormality that is widespread. Consciousness is usually impaired and motor abnormalities are bilateral.

Grandmal or Generalised Tonic Clonic Seizure (GTCS)

- Prodromal symptoms or aura—nonspecific symptoms like change of mood, irritability, insomnia, hallucination may warn the patient that an attack is impending.

- Tonic phase—tonic spasm of all muscles, loss of consciousness. Typical epileptic cry due to spasm of respiratory and laryngeal muscles followed by clonic phase. This phase lasts for 10–30 seconds.
- Clonic Phase—spasm is followed by jerky movement of one or more limbs. There may be tongue bite, frothing around the mouth, incontinence of urine. This phase lasts for 1–3 minutes.
- Postictal phase—the patient remains flaccid and unconscious, persists for some minutes, then gains consciousness, but is confused and disoriented for half an hour or more. After the seizure, patient feels severe headache and goes into sleep.

Typical Absence Seizure (Petit mal)

- It is common in childhood below 14 years of age.
- Main feature is transient loss of consciousness with or without falling.
- Staring look or eyes are tilted up.
- Attack may occur several times a day.

Myoclonic jerks

Simple twitching of single or multiple muscles or jerky movements predominantly in arms may be found.

Akinetic seizure

There is sudden fall on the ground without warning followed by gaining of consciousness immediately.

Partial seizures

Seizure activity is restricted to one part of the cerebral cortex. There is structural abnormality of the brain, such as tumour, A-V malformation.

Complex Partial (Psychomotor Type or Temporal Lobe Epilepsy)

Usually arises from temporal lobe.

- Emotional state either with fear, horror or outrage.
- Feeling of epigastric sensation.
- Hallucinations of smell, taste, vision, hearing associated with disorientation and confusion.
- Disturbances of memory or perception—undue familiarity (deja vu phenomenon) or unreality (jamais vu).
- In a dreamy state, patient carries out purposeful action without subsequent memory.

Simple Partial (Jacksonian epilepsy)

There may be an irritative focus that starts at any part of the cortex. Convulsion starts at part of the body, then spreads to the whole body. After the attack, there is paralysis of one half of body called Todd's palsy.

Focal fits

In focal fits, symptoms depend on location of lesion in the brain.

Investigations

- Routine—CBC, ESR, urea, creatinine, electrolytes, calcium, magnesium, blood sugar.
- Chest X-ray.
- CT scan or MRI of brain.
- Video EEG.

Treatment

Generalised seizures

1. Explanation and reassurance.
2. Drugs:
   - Sodium valproate 500–1500 mg or
   - Carbamazepine 200–1200 mg or
   - Phenytoin 200–400 mg.
   - Others—lemotrigine, topiramate, vigabatrin.

Petit mal—

- Ethosuximide 100–1500 mg or
- Sodium valproate.

Psychomotor—

- Carbamazepine.
- Others—phenytoin, lemotrigine.

Advice to the Patient

- Must take the drug regularly.
- Should not work near fire, machine.
- Avoid swimming, cycling and driving.
- Precipitating factors should be avoided.

Status Epilepticus

Definition

It is defined as persistent or prolonged seizure lasting for 30 minutes or longer or recurrent seizure with no recovery of consciousness in between.

Treatment

- Better to be treated in ICU.
- O_2 inhalation, airway should be kept clear.
- IV channel.
- Initially—injection diazepam—10 mg IV over 5 minutes (or rectally). Or injection lorazepam 4 mg IV. Repeat after 15 minutes, if attack recurs.
- If seizure continues after 30 minutes—injection phenytoin 15 mg/kg plus 10 m/mL in saline, at 50 mg/minutes or fosphenytoin 15 mg/kg with 10 mg/mL saline at 100 mg/min or phenobarbital 10 mg/kg with distilled water at 100 mg/min.
- If seizures persists over 90 minutes—intubation, ventilation and general anaesthesia (injection thiopentone).
- Once status is controlled—oral anticonvulsant should be continued.

DISEASE OF THE MUSCLES AND MYOPATHY

Some Definitions

- Myopathy means weakness of voluntary muscle.
- Myositis means inflammation of muscle.
- Muscular dystrophies are inherited disorders of muscle cells.
- Myasthenia means fatigue or weakness, worse on exercise.
- Myotonia is sustained contraction or slow relaxation.
- Channelopathis—ion channel disorders of muscles.

Clinical Features

Symptoms

- Weakness, difficulty in walking, combing, raising upper limb above the head.
- Cramping, muscle pain.
- Stiffness.

Signs

Depends on type.

Investigations

- Creatine phosphokinase (CPK)—high, up to 40 fold in Duchenne type.
- EMG—short duration, low-amplitude spiky polyphasic action potential.
- ECG (cardiomyopathy and dysrhythmia), echocardiography,
- Muscle biopsy—shows variation of muscle fibre size, degenerative changes, regeneration and replacement by fat.
- Blood sugar.
- Lactic acid (to exclude mitochondrial myopathy).
- Molecular genetic testing.

Differences between Neuropathy and Myopathy

- Myopathy usually involves proximal muscles (except myotonia dystrophica which involves distal muscles).
- Neuropathy usually involves distal muscles except diabetic amyotrophy, which involves proximal muscles.

Classification of Muscular Disease

1. Genetic
   - Muscular dystrophy.
   - Myotonic dystrophy.
2. Acquired
   - Inflammatory—polymyositis, dermatomyositis, viral, bacterial or parasitic, sarcoidosis.
   - Endocrine—Cushing's syndrome, thyroid disease.
   - Myasthenic disease—myasthenia gravis, Lambert-Eaton myasthenic myopathic syndrome.
   - Metabolic—myophosphorylase deficiency (McArdle's syndrome).
   - Chennelopathy—hypokalaemic and hyperkalaemic periodic paralysis.
   - Drugs and alcohol.

MUSCULAR DYSTROPHY

Definition

It is a group of hereditary muscular disorder characterised by progressive degeneration of groups of muscles without involvement of nervous system. The types are—

1. Hereditary muscular dystrophy—
   - Duchenne type (pseudohypertrophic).
   - Becker muscular dystrophy.
   - Limb girdle myopathy.
   - Fascioscapulohumeral dystrophy.
   - Myotonia dystrophica.
   - Myotonia congenita.
   - Others—oculopharyngeal or ocular myopathy and congenital muscular dystrophy.
2. Congenital myopathy (rare)—
   - Central core.
   - Nemaline myopathy.
   - Myotubular myopathy.

DUCHENNE MUSCULAR DYSTROPHY

Definition

It is inherited as X linked recessive disorder (30% spontaneous mutation). Duchenne gene is on the short arm of X chromosome, Xp21 and its product called dystrophin is absent.

Clinical Features

Affects only male, age of onset is 3–4 years.

- The child presents with difficulty in walking or getting up from sitting or lying position. There is history of frequent fall and delayed motor activity (e.g. walking).
- Gower's sign—positive (while the child gets up from lying position, he uses the hands to climb up).
- There is pseudohypertrophy in early stage involving calf and deltoid muscles. Later there is weakness, first involves the proximal muscles.
- Gait—waddling (duck like).
- Other features—dilated cardiomyopathy, kyphoscoliosis and mental retardation. There is early respiratory involvement.
- Prognosis is poor, chair bound by the age of 10 years and few survive up to 20 years.
- Causes of death—dilated cardiomyopathy and respiratory failure or inanition.

BECKER MUSCULAR DYSTROPHY

Definition

It is inherited as X-linked disorder, only males are affected and features are same as Duchenne type with the exception of the following:

- Onset is late (5–25 years).
- Less severe, less rapid progression and less cardiomyopathy.

- Mental retardation and kyphoscoliosis are uncommon.
- Respiratory involvement is a late feature.
- Chair bound at about 25 years after the onset.
- Survival up to fourth to fifth decade.

LIMB GIRDLE MYOPATHY

Definition

It is a type of muscular dystrophy, inherited as an autosomal dominant (type 1)—10% and autosomal recessive (type 2)—90%, characterised by involvement of shoulder and pelvic girdle muscles.

- Age of onset is 10–30 years, male and female are equally affected.
- May involve cardiac muscle (may cause conduction abnormality or heart failure).
- Intelligence is normal, face is normal, muscle enzymes are normal or slightly elevated.
- Prognosis is poor, chair bound at 20–25 years of age (10–20 years after the onset of disease).

FACIOSCAPULOHUMERAL DYSTROPHY

Definition

It is a type of muscular dystrophy, inherited as an autosomal dominant, characterised by the involvement of muscles of face and shoulder girdle.

- Onset is 10–40 years of age.
- Course is variable, but usually relatively benign.
- There is wasting of muscles of face, neck and shoulder girdle (lower trapezei, pectoralis, biceps, triceps). Hypertrophy of the deltoid.
- Winging of scapula (due to involvement of serratus anterior muscle).
- Pain in shoulder girdle is common.
- Face looks dull, expressionless, lips open and slack, inability to whistle and puff the cheek.
- Eyes—bilateral partial ptosis.
- There may be distal lower limb weakness.
- Intelligence is normal.
- Prognosis—normal life span, and slowly progressive.
- Muscle enzymes are usually normal or slightly elevated.

MYOTONIA

Definition

It is the continued contraction of the muscles after cessation of voluntary contraction. It is of two types—

- Myotonia dystrophica.
- Myotoni congenita (Thomsen's disease).

MYOTONIA DYSTROPHICA

Clinical Features

Inherited as autosomal dominant. Males are affected more than females. Age of onset is usually 20–50 years.

In face—

- Frontal baldness.
- Long, lean, triangular, sad and expressionless face.
- Wasting of temporalis and masseter.

In Eyes—

- Partial ptosis (usually bilateral, may be unilateral) with smooth forehead.
- Cataract (stellate cataract). May be subcapsular fine deposit.
- Difficulty in opening the eyes after firm closure.

In Neck—

- Wasting of sternomastoid and shoulder girdle muscles.

In Hands—

- If the hands are closed tightly, it relaxes slowly if asked to open.
- Inability to relax hands after handshake.
- Percussion on thenar eminence shows depressions, which fill slowly.

Others—

- Percussion over the tongue shows depression.
- Wasting of distal muscles of arms and legs.
- Testicular atrophy.
- Gynaecomastia.
- In heart—cardiomyopathy and conduction defect.
- Diabetes mellitus and impaired glucose tolerance (IGT) may occur.
- Intellect and personality—mild deterioration.
- Small pituitary fossa and hypogonadism may occur.
- Low serum IgG levels.
- Tolerate anaesthesia poorly.

Treatment

Only symptomatic. No specific treatment.

- Myotonia may be treated by phenytoin. Procainamide or quinidine may be used, but may worsen cardiac conduction.
- Genetic counselling.

Myotonia Congenita

It is an inherited as autosomal dominant, characterised by failure to relax the muscle after forceful contraction. Present at birth with feeding difficulty, inability to open the eyes and a peculiar cry. It is mild disease, improves with age.

Treatment of Myotonia

Procainamide, quinidine, mexiletine may be helpful.

Prognosis

Normal life expectancy.

Causes of Proximal Myopathy

- Dermatomyositis or polymyositis.
- Myasthenia gravis.
- Myasthenic myopathic syndrome (Eaton-Lambert syndrome).
- Myopathy (limb girdle, fascioscapulohumeral and mitochondrial), except myotonic dystrophy.
- Cushing's syndrome.
- Diabetic amyotrophy.
- Thyrotoxicosis (also hypothyroidism).
- Polymyalgia rheumatica.
- Osteomalacia.
- Hyperparathyroidism.
- Periodic paralysis.
- Alcohol and drugs (steroid, chloroquine, amiodarone, lithium and zidovudine).
- McArdle's syndrome (myophosphorylase deficiency, there is stiffness and cramps of muscle after exercise, which is hard and painful on movement).

Causes of High CPK

- Exercise.
- Intramuscular injection.
- Muscle trauma or road traffic accident.
- Convulsion.
- Alcoholism.
- Dermatomyositis or polymyositis.
- Acute myocardial infarction (CPK-MB).
- Myopathy (Duchenne type of muscular dystrophy).
- Rhabdomyolysis.
- Chronic liver disease (CLD).
- Drugs—statin, busulphan, narcotic, colchicine and chloroquine.

Isoenzymes of CPK

- MM (mainly in skeletal muscle).
- MB (mainly in cardiac muscle).
- BB (in brain).

ALZHEIMER'S DISEASE

Definition

It is a progressive, neurodegenerative disease characterised by memory loss, language deterioration, poor judgment, indifferent attitude and progressive dementia. However, motor function remains preserved.

Alzheimer disease appears first as memory decline and, over several years, it destroys cognition, personality and person's ability to function. Confusion and restlessness may also occur.

Pathology

1. Macroscopically—hallmarks are deposition of β amyloid in the cortex. There is diffuse atrophy of brain, particularly cerebral cortex and hippocampus with secondary enlargement of ventricular system.
2. Microscopically—
   - Neuritic senile plaque containing β amyloid.
   - Silver staining neurofibrillary tangles in neuronal cytoplasm of cerebral cortex.
   - Accumulation of Aβ amyloid in arterial wall of cerebral blood vessels.

Biochemical Abnormality

Impairment of acetylcholinesterase transmission. Other neurotransmitters, such as noradrenaline, 5HT, glutamate and substance P are also involved.

Clinical Features

It usually begins after age 65 years. But may occur as early as 40 years.

- Gradual decline in daily activities, ultimately profound disability and dependent on others.
- Disturbance in memory—progressive loss of ability to learn, retain and process new information and recall previously learnt information. Both short- and long-term memory are involved, commonly short-term.
- Decline in language function, difficulty with names, word finding and understanding what is being said.
- Apraxia—inability to perform skilled motor activity.
- Agnosia—failure to recognise objects, such as cloth, place, people.
- Frontal executive function—impairment of organising, planning and sequencing.
- Abnormality in behaviour—childish behaviour, agitation, aggression.
- Depression, paranoid delusion.
- In early stage, patient may complain of any physical problem, but in later stage, usually may be reluctant to seek medical attention (anosognosia).

Investigation

- Routine—CBC, blood sugar, electrolytes, serum calcium, B12, thyroid function, chest X-ray.
- CT scan or MRI of brain—shows focal cortical atrophy.
- EEG.
- Lumbar puncture and CSF study (also TPHA).

Treatment

- Usually, acetylcholinesterase inhibitor drugs are used (donepezil, galantamine, rivastigmine).
- Another drug—memantine (affects glutamine transmission) may be used.
- Antidepressant may be needed.

CREUTZFELDT-JAKOB DISEASE

Definition

Creutzfeldt-Jakob disease is a slow viral encephalopathy, which leads to rapidly progressive dementia with myoclonus, multifocal neurological signs including aphasia, cerebellar ataxia, cortical blindness, spasticity and extrapyramidal signs.

It is common in middle-aged and elderly. It is characterized by profound neuronal loss, astrocytosis and typical spongiform degeneration of the brain. EEG is typical, which shows repetitive slow wave complex.

Iatrogenic transmission to human may occur by surgical specimen, autopsy, corneal graft, depth EEG electrode, neurosurgery (cadaveric dura mater graft), pooled cadaveric growth hormone.

Treatment

No treatment is available. Quinacrine is in trial. The disease usually rapidly progresses, leading to death within 4-6 months.

PARANEOPLASTIC SYNDROME

Definition

Paraneoplastic syndrome is characterised by bizarre neurological presentation, multiple signs and symptoms associated with malignancy unrelated to metastasis especially in elderly.

Most are associated with carcinoma of lung (small cell), ovary, breast, pancreas, prostate, nasopharyngeal and lymphoma.

Actual mechanism is unknown, causes vary according to the type of malignancy. The probable causes are as follows:

- Secretion of tumour product usually polypeptide.
- Autoimmunity—cross reaction between tumour antigen and normal tissue antigen.
- Release of cytokines (e.g. TNF α).
- Myelitis—commonly in cervical cord.

Clinical Features

Varies with primary cause. Paraneoplastic syndrome may precede the clinical presentation of primary carcinoma in 50% cases. Usual features are as follows:

- Neurological—neuropathy, cerebellar degeneration, motor neuron disease, myasthenic myopathic syndrome (Lambert-Eaton syndrome), GBS.
- Musculoskeletal—polymyositis or dermatomyositis, clubbing, hypertrophic osteoarthropathy.
- Endocrine—SIADH, ectopic ACTH syndrome, hypercalcaemia.
- Cachexia.

Investigations

- X-ray chest or other organ.
- USG of abdomen.
- CT scan or MRI.
- EMG.
- CPK.
- Biopsy of muscle.
- Other investigation according to suspicion of cause.

Treatment

Primary cause should be treated.

NEUROFIBROMA

Definition

It is a benign tumour of peripheral nerves arising from neurilemmal sheath.

Neurofibromatosis

It is an autosomal dominant disease characterised by multiple neurofibroma with skin lesions like café-au-lait spots and axillary freckling.

Types of Neurofibromatosis

- Type 1 or von Recklinghausen disease or peripheral.
- Type 2 or central.

Features of Type 1 Neurofibromatosis

- Multiple cutaneous neurofibroma.
- Café-au-lait patches more than 6 (up to 5 may be found in normal person).
- Axillary freckling.
- Hamartoma of iris (Lisch nodules).
- Optic glioma.
- Others—scoliosis, pseudoarthrosis, pulmonary stenosis.

Features of Type 2 Neurofibromatosis

- Bilateral acoustic neuroma.
- Glioma (cerebral or optic nerve).
- Meningioma.
- Spinal neurofibroma.
- Schwannoma.
- Juvenile posterior subcapsular lenticular opacity.

Café-au-lait Spot

These are round to ovoid, pale yellow or brown macules, usually present on the trunk. May be 1–15 cm. Up to 5 may be present in a normal person.

Lisch Nodule

It is a melanocytic hamartoma of iris, clear to yellow or brown. It increases with age, present in patient older than 20 years.

Plexiform Neurofibroma

In this type, entire nerve trunk and its branches are involved in diffuse neurofibromatosis with overgrowth of overhanging tissues, leading to gross deformities in temporal and frontal scalp. The most common sites are temporal region in relation to trigeminal nerve, upper eyelid and back of the neck.

Associated findings or Complications of Neurofibroma

- Kyphoscoliosis.

- Lung cyst (honeycomb lung).
- Pseudoarthrosis and other orthopaedic abnormalities.
- Glioma, meningioma, medulloblastoma.
- Phaeochromocytoma (in MEN IIa).
- Posterior mediastinal tumour called dumbbell tumour.
- Rarely, sarcomatous change.

Phacomatosis

It is a group of diseases in which neurological abnormalities are associated with cutaneous disease. These are:
- Neurofibromatosis type 1.
- Tuberous sclerosis.
- Von Hippel-Lindau syndrome.
- Sturge-Weber syndrome.

TUBEROUS SCLEROSIS

Definition

It is an autosomal dominant disease characterised by classic triad of mental retardation (or learning disability), epilepsy and skin lesions. Family history, convulsion and mental retardation are present.
Skin lesions:
- Papules on the face called adenoma sebaceum.
- Subungual fibroma (nodule arising from the nail bed).
- Shagreen patches (firm, flesh coloured, patches of leathery thick skin over the lower back).
- Ash leaf patches (hypopigmented areas of skin).
- Café-au-lait spots present in 30% cases.

Other lesions may be associated
- CNS hamartomas—Cortical tubers and subependymal hamartomas. There may be cerebral glioma and calcification of basal ganglia.
- Retinal phacoma (glial mass).
- Hyperplastic gum.
- Benign rhabdomyoma of heart.
- Renal angiomyolipoma.
- Cysts in lung, liver, pancreas, kidneys and bones.

Investigations

- Skull X-ray shows tram-line calcification at the basal ganglia.
- CT scan or MRI of brain.

Treatment

- No specific treatment. Symptomatic treatment for seizure.
- Genetic counselling should be done.

Cause of Death

Usually from seizure, intercurrent illness or associated neoplasm.

HYDROCEPHALUS

Definition

It is the excessive accumulation of CSF within the brain caused either by increased CSF production, by reduced CSF absorption, or by obstruction of the circulation. As a result, there is ventricular dilatation.

Symptoms

Depends on amount of accumulation of CSF with its pressure:
- May be asymptomatic.
- Headache, cognitive impairment.
- Features of raised intracranial pressure.
- Ataxia.

Causes

1. Congenital malformations (Infantile hydrocephalus). Head is enlarged.
   - Stenosis of aqueduct of Sylvius.
   - Arnold—Chiari malformation.
   - Dandy-Walker syndrome (cerebellar hypoplasia and obstruction of 4th ventricular outflow foramen).
   - Benign intracranial cysts.
   - Congenital CNS infections.
   - Craniofacial anomalies.
2. Acquired causes (adult hydrocephalus):
   - Mass lesions (especially those in the posterior fossa)—tumour, colloid cyst of third ventricle, abscess, haematoma.
   - Absorption blockages due to—inflammation (e.g. meningitis, sarcoidosis), subarachnoid haemorrhage.
   - Idiopathic in many cases.

Treatment

- Frusemide and acetazolamide may be given (decrease CSF production).
- Serial lumbar puncture.
- Removal of tumour, if any.
- Ventriculoperitoneal shunting.
- Endoscopic third ventriculostomy.

Normal Pressure Hydrocephalus

It is a syndrome of enlarged ventricle with normal CSF pressure, characterised by triad of:
- Gait apraxia.
- Dementia.
- Urinary incontinence.

Common in elderly. It is idiopathic in many cases, may be secondary to meningitis or subarachnoid haemorrhage. CT scan shows dilatation of ventricles but no cortical atrophy.

Treatment

Shunt—ventriculoperitoneal or less commonly ventriculoatrial shunt.

MULTI-INFARCT DEMENTIA (MID)

Definition

When dementia is due to multiple infarction of brain secondary to atherosclerosis. It is also called vascular dimentia.

It is a common cause of dementia in the elderly, occurs when thrombus block small blood vessels in the brain and destroy brain tissue. Over time, as more small vessels are blocked, there is gradual mental decline.

Multi-infarct dementia, typically begins in 60–75 years, more in men. In the late stage, there is dementia, pseudobulbar palsy and a shuffling gait, the marche a petis pas (small step) called atherosclerotic parkinsonism.

Risk factors are advanced age, high blood pressure, smoking, diabetes mellitus, dyslipidaemia.

Symptoms of Multi-infarct Dementia

Symptoms often develop in a stepwise manner:

- Disturbance with recent memory.
- Confusion.
- Personality change and behavioural difficulty, aggressive, wandering or getting lost in familiar places.
- Loss of bladder or bowel control (incontinence).
- Emotional problems, such as laughing or crying inappropriately.
- Difficulty following instructions, and problems handling money.

Investigation

MRI of brain shows multiple infarction of brain.

Treatment

- No specific treatment for MID that can reverse the damage that has already occurred.
- Control of risk factors, e.g. high blood pressure, DM, dyslipidaemia.
- Symptomatic and supportive.

DIZINESS AND VERTIGO

Dizziness

It means feeling of various types of sensations, such as feeling of imbalance, light-headedness, faintness (a feeling of impending syncope), giddiness.

Vertigo

It is a sensation of movement of the body or the surroundings, perceived as feeling of rotation. It is due to disturbance in the vestibular system.

Both dizziness and vertigo may be accompanied by nausea and vomiting or difficulty with balance, gait or both. Vertigo can also present with nystagmus and blurring vision.

Causes of Dizziness and Vertigo

May be central (brainstem or cerebellar lesion) or peripheral (labyrinthine or vestibular lesion):

- Central—
  - Brain stem haemorrhage or infarction.
  - Cerebellar haemorrhage or infarction.
  - Multiple sclerosis.
  - Acoustic neuroma.
  - Vertebral artery dissection.
  - Vertebro-basilar insufficiency.
  - TIA.
  - Temporal lobe epilepsy.
  - Migraine.
- Peripheral—
  - Benign positional vertigo.
  - Meniere's disease.
  - Vestibular neuronitis.
  - Labyrinthitis.
  - Otitis media.
  - Trauma—tympanic membrane rupture, temporal bone fracture.
  - Ototoxic drugs (e.g. aminoglycoside).
  - Chronic motion sickness.
- Global disturbance of CNS function—
  - Anaemia.
  - Hypoglycemia.
  - Hypotension.
  - Hypoxaemia.
- Other causes—
  - Pregnancy.
  - Psychiatric (e.g. anxiety, depression, panic attack, hyperventilation syndrome).

Investisgations

- CBC.
- ECG, echocardiography.

- Chest X-ray.
- Blood sugar
- Serum electrolytes.
- Carotid Doppler study.
- MRI of brain.
- Audiometry.
- Others according to suspicion of cause (e.g. pregnancy test).

Treatment

- Treatment is directed at the cause of dizziness or vertigo.
- Drugs—cinarizine, betahistine may be given.

SYNCOPE

Definition

It is defined as transient loss of consciousness due to inadequate blood supply to the brain.

Near Syncope or Presyncope

It is light headedness and a sense of an impending faint without loss of consciousness.

Causes of Syncope

1. **Cardiac Causes—**
   - Cardiac arrhythmias—sick sinus syndrome, complete heart block, atrial fibrillation, ventricular tachycardia, ventricular fibrillation, asystole.
   - Cardiac outflow or inflow obstruction—aortic stenosis, tetralogy of Fallot. Hypertrophic cardiomyopathy. Cardiac tumours or thrombi (left atrial myxoma).
   - Ventricular dysfunction—Acute myocardial infarction, myocarditis.
2. **Vasovagal attack**—prolong standing, strong emotions (pain, fear).
3. **Orthostatic hypotension**—drugs (nitrate, ACE inhibitor, prazocin), autonomic neuropathy.
4. **Cerebrovascular causes**—TIA, stroke, migraine.
5. **Other causes—**
   - Cough syncope.
   - Micturition syncope.
   - Carotid sinus hypersensitivity syndrome.

Investigations

As in vertigo (see above).

Treatment

- The patient should lie in horizontal position with legs elevated.
- If pulseless—CPR should be initiated.
- Synchronized DC shock may be needed.
- Treatment of cause.

FUNNY TURN OR BLACKOUT

Definition

Blackout is a descriptive term, mentioned by the patient as altered consciousness, visual disturbance or falling. It is like dizziness.

Causes

- Epilepsy.
- Syncope due to any cause.
- Nonepileptic attacks (pseudoseizure).
- Panic attack.
- Hypoglycaemia.
- Drop attacks.
- Hydrocephalic attack.
- Basilar migraine.
- Severe vertigo.
- Cataplexy, narcolepsy, sleep paralysis.

MÉNIÈRE'S DISEASE

Definition

It is a vestibular disorder of unknown origin characterised by recurrent attack of vertigo and progressive deafness.

It is due to distension of endolymphatic system in the inner ear (endolymphatic hydrops).

Clinical Features

Equal in both sexes, age 40–50 years.

- Recurrent attacks of severe vertigo.
- Tinnitus—constant, increases during attack.
- Feeling of fullness in the ear.
- Severe nausea or vomiting.
- Imbalance.
- Progressive hearing loss—recovers between attack, but later permanent and progressive.

Diagnostic Tests

- Audiometry.
- Vestibular testing.
- Gadolinium-enhanced MRI to rule out other causes.

Treatment

1. Low-salt diet.
2. Potassium sparing diuretic (spironolactone).
3. For vertigo, nausea and vomiting—prochlorperazine or cinnarizine or cyclizine can be given.
4. Tab. diazepam 2–5 mg orally at 6 or 8 hours interval can also be given.
5. Betahistine to reduce the frequency and severity of attacks.
6. For tinnitus—sound therapy, cognitive behavioural therapy (CBT).
7. Vestibular rehabilitation to cope with balance problems.
8. Surgery.

LATERAL MEDULLARY SYNDROME (WALLENBERG SYNDROME)

Definition

This syndrome is produced by infarction of small wedge of lateral medulla posterior to inferior olivary nucleus, due to occlusion of posterior inferior cerebellar artery (PICA). Occlusion of any of the vessels may be responsible—(i) vertebral, (ii) posterior inferior cerebellar, (iii) superior, middle or inferior lateral medullary arteries.

In the majority of cases of lateral medullary syndrome, there is also occlusion of vertebral artery and pyramidal signs are present.

Clinical Features

Symptoms

- Headache, nausea, vomiting.
- Vertigo.
- Hiccough.

Signs

1. Ipsilateral—
   - Horner's syndrome (lesion in descending spinothalamic tract lesion).
   - Cerebellar signs (lesion in cerebellum and its connection).
   - Palatal palsy and diminished gag reflex (dysphagia and hoarseness due to IXth, Xth nerve involvement.
   - Decreased pain and temperature (Vth nerve nucleus and its descending tract lesion).
2. Contralateral decrease of pain and temperature (spinothalamic tract lesion).

Medial Medullary Syndrome

Occlusion of lower basilar artery, vertebral artery or one of its medial branches produce medial medullary syndrome, characterised by:

- Contralateral hemiplegia, which spares the face.
- Contralateral loss of vibration and joint position sense.
- Ipsilateral paralysis and wasting of tongue.

Investigation

MRI of brain.

Treatment

- Control of hypertension and DM.
- Antiplatelet drug—aspirin, clopidogrel.

CENTRAL PONTINE MYELINOLYSIS (CPM)

Rapid correction of hyponatraemia by hypertonic saline (3%) results in central pontine myelinolysis, which is a dangerous complication.

There may be various types of neurological deficits, from quadriparesis to coma and death. In CPM, there is demyelination of central basal pons or other areas of brain.

Rapid correction of hyponatraemia by hypertonic saline should be avoided. Correction with IV normal saline and oral salt may be sufficient.

MRI of brain is the investigation of choice. There is no definitive treatment, only symptomatic and supportive.

NYSTAGMUS

Definition

It is the involuntary, rhythmical, oscillatory movement of one or both eyes. It is due to inability to maintain the posture of eyes, owing to the lack of balance of the opposing ocular muscles.

It is defined by the direction of fast phase and is exaggerated on gaze to that side. Nystagmus must be sustained for more than a few beats to be significant. Nystagmus may be jerky or phasic, pendular or ataxic (internuclear ophthalmoplegia).

Types of Nystagmus

1. According to the direction—
   - Horizontal.
   - Vertical.
   - Rotatory.
2. According to the site of lesion—
   - Cerebellar nystagmus (towards the site of lesion).
   - Vestibular nystagmus (away from the site of lesion).
   - Brain stem lesion (usually vertical, may be in other direction).
3. Others—
   - Positional nystagmus (associated with benign positional vertigo).
   - Ocular or fixation nystagmus (usually pendular type).
   - Optokinetic.
   - See-saw nystagmus.

Causes of Horizontal Nystagmus

1. Cerebellar.
2. Vestibular nystagmus.
3. Brain stem lesion.
4. Others—
   - Ocular or fixation nystagmus (usually pendular type).
   - Optokinetic
   - In normal person, in extreme lateral gaze.

Causes of Vertical Nystagmus

- Brain stem lesion up-beating (midbrain lesion) and down-beating (medulla associated with foramen magnum lesion).
- Rarely, ocular nystagmus.

Causes of Vestibular Nystagmus

It is usually horizontal or rotatory, and not vertical. It is of two types—peripheral and central.

1. **Peripheral:** Lesion is in the labyrinth or vestibular nerve. Fast component of nystagmus is contralateral to the site of lesion, may be associated with cochlear lesion. Its causes are:
   - Labyrinthitis (may be viral).
   - Meniere's disease.
   - Acoustic neuroma.

  - Head injury.
  - Middle ear disease.
  - Vestibular neuronitis (presents with acute vertigo, tinnitus and deafness).
2. **Central:** Lesion is in vestibular nuclei. Its causes are:
  - Cerebrovascular accident.
  - Multiple sclerosis.
  - Neoplasm.
  - Alcohol.
  - Anticonvulsant drugs.

Jerky or Phasic Nystagmus

It is characterised by eye movement faster in one direction than other. Seen in horizontal direction, on lateral gaze in one or both directions. Causes are cerebellar lesion, vestibular lesion or lesions of their connection in the brain stem.

Pendular Nystagmus

In this type, oscillations are equal in speed and amplitude in both directions of eye movement, seen in central gaze.

Cause is poor visual acuity (in severe refractive error or macular disease), usually congenital and asymptomatic.

Ataxic Nystagmus

In this type, on looking to one side, nystagmus is present in the abducting eye and there is failure of adduction of the other eye. It is also called "dissociated nystagmus", and is present in internuclear ophthalmoplegia. The most common cause is multiple sclerosis.

However, on covering the abducting eye, the adduction of other eye is normal. The lesion is in the medial longitudinal bundle which connects the 6th nerve nucleus on one side to the 3rd nerve nucleus on the opposite side of brain stem.

Optokinetic Nystagmus

It occurs when the patient follows a rapidly moving scene (as during travelling in a train, eye remains fixed to a telegraph pole). It is a normal phenomenon.

See-saw Nystagmus

In this condition, one eye raises and turns in and the other eye falls and turns out. It is due to parasellar tumour.

CHAPTER

14 Poisoning

CHAPTER CONTENTS

COMMON CAUSES OF POISONING

- Paracetamol.
- Salicylate (aspirin).
- Tricyclic antidepressant.
- Benzodiazepines.
- Corrosives.
- Organophosphorus.
- Methanol.
- Ethanol.
- Ethylene glycol.
- Kerosene.
- Datura.
- Cannabis.
- Opioid.
- Snake bite.

General Management

1. A—Airway should be kept clear (suction, airway tube).
2. B—Breathing (O_2, ventilatory support, endotracheal tube if indicated).
3. C—Circulation (IV or CV line, IV fluid infusion).
4. Other treatment:
   - Gastric lavage except in corrosive poisoning.
   - Antidote, if available.
   - Maintenance of water, electrolytes and nutrition.

PARACETAMOL POISONING

Lethal Dose

Intake of 15 g of paracetamol is serious in most cases.

Mechanism

Toxic metabolite of paracetamol is NAPQI, which is normally conjugated with glutathione and is excreted. In paracetamol poisoning, there is the production of excess toxic metabolite and depletion of cellular glutathione. Toxic metabolite causes massive hepatic necrosis and hepatic failure (not by the drug itself).

No liver damage until 18 hours. If blood level of paracetamol is > 200 μg/mL in 4 hours, it indicates severe poisoning. Maximum liver damage occurs after 72–96 hours of ingestion.

There is increased prothrombin time and aminotransferase activity (AST or ALT). There may be hypo- and hyperglycemia, metabolic acidosis, arrhythmia, GIT bleeding, cerebral oedema, lactic acidosis and coma. Brainstem coning may occur after 96 hours.

Prognostic Factors

Three important risk or prognostic markers for severe hepatic injury are as follows:

- Prothrombin time is > 20 sec in 24 hours.
- pH < 7.3.
- Serum creatinine > 300 μmol/L.

Without treatment, few patients may develop fulminant hepatic failure. Renal failure may develop, due to acute tubular necrosis in 25% cases.

Investigations

- Serum paracetamol level.
- Blood glucose.
- LFT—AST, ALT, Prothrombin time.
- Serum creatinine and electrolytes.

Treatment

- Gastric lavage within 4 hours.
- N-Acetylcysteine (NAC) IV or
- Methionine orally. More effective, if given within 10 hours. Protective effects decline rapidly and ineffective after 15–16 hours.
- If PT is prolonged—fresh frozen plasma.
- Glucose may be given.
- Forced diuresis and dialysis have no role. Dialysis is done, if renal failure.
- Liver transplantation should be considered, in some cases of acute liver failure.
- Monitor—LFT (ALT and PT), electrolytes, glucose and creatinine.

Dose of N-acetylcysteine (NAC)

Three consecutive doses are given in 21 hours.

- 1st dose—150 mg/kg with 200 mL 5% dextrose over 1 hour, then

- 2nd dose—50 mg/kg with 500 mL 5% dextrose over 4 hours, then
- 3rd dose—100 mg/kg with 1000 mL 5% dextrose over 16 hours.

Dose of Oral Methionine

If NAC is not available, alternatively methionine 2.5 gm orally every 4 hours to a total of four doses can be given.

SALICYLATE (ASPIRIN)

Clinical Features

- Nausea, vomiting, epigastric pain, restlessness, sweating, tinnitus and deafness.
- Direct stimulation of respiratory centre causes hyperventilation.
- Neurological effects—agitation, confusion, tremor, delirium, stupor, convulsion and coma.
- Petechiae and subconjunctival haemorrhages can occur due to reduced platelet aggregation.
- If poisoning due to very high dose—respiratory paralysis and cardiovascular collapse.

Investigations

- Serum aspirin level—In adults, concentrations above 500 mg/L and 700 mg/L suggest serious and life-threatening poisoning, respectively.
- Serum electrolytes.
- ABG and pH (Low $PaCO_2$ indicates respiratory alkalosis).
- Serum glucose.
- Urine for ferric chloride test is positive.

Treatment

- Gastric lavage up to 24 hours (better within 12 hours).
- Correction of water and electrolyte balance (IV fluid).
- If severe metabolic acidosis—IV sodium bicarbonate (8.4%).
- Activated charcoal may be given.
- If serum salicylate > 750 mg/L or 500 mg/L with severe acidosis—forced alkaline diuresis may be done.
- If no response or neurological feature with blood level > 1000 mg/L or 750 mg/L with renal failure or acidosis—haemodialysis should be considered.

TRICYCLIC ANTIDEPRESSANT (TCA)

Clinical Features

- Drowsiness, confusion, delirium, hallucination, agitation, myoclonic fit, convulsion and coma.
- Pulse—tachycardia.
- Pupil—dilated, loss of accommodation.
- Divergent strabismus.
- Reflex—exaggerated, hypertonia or spasticity, plantar—extensor.
- Retention of urine may occur.
- ECG—sinus tachycardia, QRS is prolonged, P is small, arrhythmia (SVT, VT).
- Metabolic acidosis, cardiorespiratory failure in severe case.
- Most patients recover in 48 hours. However, in some cases, there may be persistent agitation, confusion, hallucination, rapid jerky movement which may persist for several days.

Investigations

- Blood for TCA level.
- Serum electrolytes.
- Arterial blood gas analysis.
- ECG monitoring.

Treatment

- Gastric lavage, if > 250 mg tablet is taken. TCA causes delayed gastric emptying, so lavage can be given up to 12 hours and activated charcoal may be given, if the patient presents within 1 hour.
- Protection of airway and oxygen.
- IV fluid.
- Cardiac monitor—if ECG shows prolong QRS (>0.16 sec), arrhythmia may develop.
- If epileptic seizure—IV lorazepam or diazepam should be given.
- For acidosis, sodium bicarbonate (50 cc of 8.4%) should be given.
- SVT and VT should be treated with sodium bicarbonate (50 cc of 8.4%) IV over 20 minutes (even without acidosis). If VT with compromising cardiac output, Inj. amiodarone 300 mg IV over 20–60 minutes.
- Lipid emulsion therapy in severe intractable poisoning may be tried.
- No role of forced diuresis or haemodialysis.

METHANOL (RECTIFIED SPIRIT)

Methanol or methyl alcohol is a component of varnishes, paint remover, windshield washer solution and copy machine fluid. Methanol is metabolised by alcohol dehydrogenase to formaldehyde and formic acid. It is mainly metabolised in the liver (90%), only 10% is excreted unchanged by lungs and kidneys.

Formic acid can cause retinal injury. Patient suffers from reduced visual acuity, due to optic nerve damage by formic acid resulting from increased concentrations of formic acid. Mydriasis, reduced visual reflexes to light and hyperaemia of optic disc are early features of methanol toxicity. If untreated, patient may develop blindness.

Clinical Features

- Early manifestations (by methanol)—nausea, vomiting, abdominal pain, headache, vertigo, dizziness, ataxia, drowsiness, dysarthria, nystagmus, convulsion, confusion, stupor and coma.
- Later on (by metabolite formic acid)—visual impairment, photophobia associated with optic disc and retinal oedema, impaired pupil reflexes. Retinal injury may cause blindness. Ocular toxicity occurs 15–19 hours after ingestion. Pancreatitis and abnormal liver function may also occur.
- In severe cases—metabolic acidosis, bradycardia, myocardial depression and shock.

Investigations

- Serum methanol level.
- Serum electrolytes and creatinine.
- ABG.
- Plasma osmolality—high.
- Others—blood sugar, serum calcium, magnesium.

Treatment

- Gastric lavage within first 4 hours.
- IV fluid, oxygen.
- Correction of acidosis—Sodium bicarbonate in large dose (250 mL of 1.26% solution, repeated as necessary). Alkalinisation enhances formic acid excretion.
- In early stage—antidote of methanol is ethanol or fomepizol (ethanol inhibits methanol oxidation by competing the inhibition of enzyme). Ethanol is given 10 mL/kg of 10% ethanol IV or 1 mL/kg of 95% ethanol orally.
- Thiamine (100 mg qid), pyridoxine (50 mg qid) and folate (50 mg qid).
- Folinic acid 30 mg IV every 6 hourly. It reduces ocular toxicity (accelerates metabolism of formic acid).
- Dialysis—it is indicated, if ingestion of methanol is > 30 g or metabolic acidosis or blood methanol is > 500 mg/L.

ETHANOL OR ETHYL ALCOHOL

Ethanol is commonly ingested in beverages and deliberately with other substances in overdose. It is also present in many cosmetic and antiseptic preparations. Ethanol is a CNS depressant. After absorption, ethanol is oxidised to acetaldehyde and then to acetate.

Clinical Features

Related to blood concentrations:

Blood [Ethanol] 500–1500 mg/L

- Emotional lability.
- Mild impairment of coordination.

Blood [Ethanol] 1500–2000 mg/L

- Visual impairment.
- Incoordination.
- Slowed reaction time.
- Slurred speech.

Blood [Ethanol] 2000–3000 mg/L

- Marked incoordination.
- Blurred or double vision.
- Stupor.
- Occasionally hypoglycaemia, hypothermia and convulsions.

Blood [Ethanol] 3000–5000 mg/L

- Depressed reflexes.
- Respiratory depression.
- Hypotension.
- Hypothermia.
- Death (from respiratory or circulatory failure or aspiration).

Treatment

- Gastric lavage.
- IV fluid, oxygen.
- Correction of acidosis—sodium bicarbonate in large dose (250 mL of 1.26% solution, repeated as necessary).
- Correction of hypoglycaemia.
- Haemodialysis—if the blood ethanol concentration exceeds 7500 mg/L severe metabolic acidosis is present.

ETHYLENE GLYCOL

Ethylene glycol is a common constituent of antifreeze fluid used in car radiators, brake fluids and in lower concentrations, windscreen washes.

Ethylene glycol, itself is nontoxic but is metabolised to toxic products.

Clinical Features

1. Features are same as methanol poisoning.
2. Other toxic effects of ethylene glycol are:
   - Neurological—ophthalmoplegia, cranial nerve palsy, hyporeflexia and myoclonus.
   - Renal pain and acute tubular necrosis occur because of precipitation of calcium oxalate in the kidneys.
   - Hypocalcaemia, hypomagnesaemia and hyperkalaemia are common.

Urinalysis under Wood's light in patient with ethylene glycol poisoning may reveal oxalate crystals in the urine, but its absence does not exclude the diagnosis.

Treatment

- Same like methanol.
- Correction of electrolytes (mainly hyperkalaemia), hypoglycaemia, hypocalcaemia, hypomagnesaemia.

ORGANOPHOSPHORUS COMPOUNDS (OPC)

Organophosphorus insecticides (e.g. malathion and parathion) are irreversible inhibitors of acetylcholinesterase, resulting in accumulation of acetylcholine at muscarinic and nicotinic synapses.

Clinical Features

Due to acute cholinergic syndrome, occur within minutes to hours.

Muscarinic Effects

- Constriction of pupil.
- Increased salivation, lacrimation.
- GIT—nausea, vomiting, abdominal pain, urinary and faecal incontinence.
- Respiratory—breathlessness, wheezing, excess bronchial secretion.
- In severe poisoning—bradycardia, hypotension, heart block and pulmonary oedema may occur.

Nicotinic Effects

- Twitching or fasciculation of muscles.
- Muscle weakness.

CNS Effects

Headache, dizziness, confusion, drowsiness, fit, coma.

Investigations

- Blood gas analysis.
- Serum electrolytes, urea and creatinine.
- Blood glucose.
- ECG.

Treatment

- Contaminated clothings should be removed.
- Airway should be cleared, high-flow oxygen, if needed.
- Gastric lavage may be done within an hour of intake, followed by activated charcoal.
- If convulsion—intravenous diazepam.
- Atropine 1.8–3 mg IV as a bolus dose, followed by double the dose every five minutes until there are signs of atropinization (such as dry and hot skin, dry tongue, clear lung, tachycardia, pupil dilated).
- Antidote like pralidoxime or obidoxime may be given.
- Monitoring of ECG, blood gases, temperature, urea and electrolytes, amylase and glucose.

Three types of illness may occur in OPC poisoning:

1. Acute cholinergic phase (as described above).
2. Intermediate syndrome (IMS).
3. Organophosphate induced delayed polyneuropathy (OPIDN).

Intermediate Syndrome (IMS)

Begins 48 hours after poisoning, may be after 72–96 hours. Occurs after resolution of acute phase.

- Muscle weakness causing respiratory distress and failure.
- Muscle weakness involves the ocular, neck and proximal limbs muscles, also respiratory muscles (intercostal muscles and diaphragm).
- Paralysis may continue for 2–18 days.
- Usually, recovery occurs with adequate ventilatory care.

Treatment

- Ventilator support.
- Diazepam or midazolam may be used for sedation during ventilation.
- Parenteral nutrition.

Organophosphate induced Delayed Polyneuropathy (OPIDN)

Occurs for about 1–3 weeks after acute exposure.

- Cramping muscle pain in the legs.
- Acute weakness of muscles of upper and lower limbs causing shuffling gait, foot and wrist drop. Muscle wasting and deformity causing claw hands.
- Sensory loss is variable and is mild. Tendon reflexes are reduced or lost, absent ankle reflexes being a constant feature.
- Recovery from OPIDN is incomplete. Functional recovery after 1–2 years may occur in younger patients.

Treatment

- No specific therapy.
- Regular physiotherapy.

BENZODIAZEPINES

Benzodiazepines have low toxicity when taken alone in overdose, but can enhance CNS depression when taken with other sedative agents or alcohol.

Clinical Features

- Dizziness, drowsiness, confusion, hallucination, slurred speech.
- Ataxia, reduced muscle tone.
- Hypothermia.
- Diplopia, strabismus, nystagmus, normal pupil size.
- In severe poisoning, respiratory depression and hypotension may occur, even coma.

Investigations

- Serum drug level.
- Serum electrolytes.
- Serum creatinine.

Treatment

- Airway should be clear, if needed oxygen.
- Gastric lavage can be given, if more than 30 tablets are taken.
- Activated charcoal may be given within 1 hour of ingestion of drugs.
- Water and electrolytes balance.
- Benzodiazepine antagonist flumazenil may be given (It is avoided in mixed TCA and benzodiazepine poisoning, also if there is history of epilepsy).

DATURA POISONING

Powder of datura seeds is used as a stupefying agent. Common places are railway station, launch or bus terminal and in hotels. Basic constituent of datura is atropine.

Clinical Features

The clinical features are due to excess anticholinergic activity.
- Patient is restless, confused with peculiar behaviour.
- There is pill rolling movement of hands, incoherent talk, staggering gait.
- Face is flushed, pupils widely dilated, diplopia or photophobia may develop. Light reflex is lost.
- Dryness of mouth, thirst and difficulty in speech.
- Skin is hot and dry with rise in temperature.
- Patient may progress to stupor and coma.
- Death from respiratory failure.

Treatment

- Clear the airway, ensure ventilation, maintain circulation.
- Maintain nutrition and hydration.
- Stomach wash.
- Antipyretic if required, tepid sponging for hyperpyrexia.
- Anticonvulsant—Diazepam 10 mg IM.
- Physostigmine—0.5 mg IV/IM at hourly interval.
- Pilocarpine—5 mg subcutaneously.

CANNABIS (MARIJUANA)

Cannabis is derived from dried leaves and flowers of cannabis sativa. Usually, it is smoked but may be ingested as 'cake', mixed with tea or injected intravenously. It is one of the misused compounds.

Clinical Features

- Initially there is euphoria, followed by perceptual alteration (distorted images, colours and sounds, altered tactile sensation), conjunctival congestion.
- Visual and auditory hallucinations and acute psychosis, confusion.
- High dose can cause anxiety, depression, slurred speech and ataxia. Regular users are at risk of psychological dependence. Withdrawal symptoms are unusual.
- Intravenous injection may cause watery diarrhoea, tachycardia, hypotension and arthralgia.
- Long-term use may cause schizophrenia in later life.

Treatment

- Reassurance.
- Psychotherapy.
- Sedation with IV diazepam 10–20 mg or chlorpromazine 50–100 mg IM in an adult is sometimes required.
- IV fluid for hypotension.

CORROSIVE POISONING

Common Corrosives

- Acid.
- Alkali.
- Bleaching powder.
- Household disinfectants (harpic, savlon, dettol, etc).

Clinical Features

- Burning and pain in mouth, throat and abdomen.
- Nausea, vomiting.
- Difficulty in swallowing.
- Cough may be due to chemical pneumonitis.

Treatment

- Gastric lavage is contraindicated.
- IV fluid to maintain water, electrolyte balance.
- Parenteral nutrition, if the patient is unable to take by mouth.
- IV antibiotic.
- Analgesic (tramadol, morphine or pethidine).

Complications

- Oesophageal stricture.
- Perforation of oesophagus or stomach.
- Aspiration pneumonia.

OPIATE POISONING

Usually, morphine poisoning occurs if taken intravenously.

Clinical Features

- Difficulty in respiration, confusion, hallucination, slurred speech, stupor or even coma.
- Ataxia, reduced muscle tone.
- Pin point pupil.
- Hypotension, relative bradycardia.
- Low respiratory rate.
- Abdomen—distended due to paralytic ileus.
- Death due to respiratory depression.

Treatment

- Maintenance of airway, breathing and circulation.
- Specific antidote—Naloxone 0.8–2 mg IV, may be repeated if needed.
- Continuous monitoring of respiratory function.

KEROSENE POISONING

It is common accidental poisoning in children. It is an irritant to GI tract and when absorbed, it depresses CNS. Aspiration in the respiratory tract causes pneumonitis.

Clinical Features

- Smell of kerosene in breath and vomitus.
- Pain and burning in throat.
- Dry irritating cough, breathlessness.
- Nausea, vomiting, abdominal pain.
- Drowsiness, impaired consciousness, convulsion.
- Death may occur due to respiratory failure or ventricular fibrillation.

Treatment

- Gastric lavage and induced vomiting should be avoided.
- Airway should be kept clear, maintenance of breathing and circulation.
- Oxygen inhalation may be given.
- Removal of contaminated clothing.
- Liquid paraffin orally to delay absorption.
- Antibiotic to prevent infection.
- Corticosteroid—if chemical or aspiration pneumonia.

SNAKE BITE

The features are due to different toxins by different snakes like haematotoxin, cardiotoxin, neurotoxin, myotoxin, nephrotoxin and allergic toxin.

Clinical Features

- Local features—there may be fang marks, pain, numbness, tingling, local oedema, redness, warmth, bleeding from site, blister, necrosis.
- General—nausea, vomiting, headache, dizziness, fever, urticaria.
- Neurological—cranial nerve paly, ptosis, squint, facial weakness, respiratory paralysis.
- Muscular—weakness and paralysis.
- Cardiac—tachycardia, hypotension, shock, cardiac failure, arrhythmias.
- Renal—oliguria, anuria or even renal failure.
- Haematological—bleeding, thrombosis, DVT, DIC.
- Cobra and krait causes constitutional symptoms more than local symptoms. Neurotoxicity is more.
- Russel and scaled vipers cause severe local symptoms and haemorrhagic tendency.

Treatment

1. General:
   - Maintenance of airway, breathing and circulation.
   - Immobilisation and pressure bandage above the bite.
   - Local care of wound.
   - IV fluid, maintenance of nutrition.
   - Antibiotic and analgesic, if needed.
   - Antihistamine in some cases.
   - Corticosteroid in severe shock and allergic reactions.
   - Management of complication, if any.
2. Specific:

Antidote—Polyvalent antisnake venom IV.

CHAPTER

15 Psychiatric Diseases

CHAPTER CONTENTS

- Classification of psychiatric disorders
- Delusion
- Illusion
- Hallucination
- Acute stress reaction
- Post-traumatic stress disorder
- Adjustment disorder
- Anxiety disorders (anxiety neurosis)
  - Phobic disorder
  - Panic disorder
  - Generalised anxiety disorder
- Obsessive compulsive disorder
- Depression
- Mania and hypomania
- Bipolar affective disorder (bipolar mood disorder)
- Schizophrenia
- Eating disorders
  - Anorexia nervosa
  - Bulimia nervosa
- Somatoform disorders
- Hysteria
- Puerperal disorders
- Dementia
- Delirium
- Substance abuse
- Factitious disorders
- Munchausen's syndrome

CLASSIFICATION OF PSYCHIATRIC DISORDERS

Psychiatric disorders are classified into two types:

1. Major
   - Schizophrenia.
   - Bipolar mood disorder (manic depressive psychosis).
   - Major depression.
   - Dementia.
   - Postpartum psychosis.
2. Minor
   - Anxiety disorder (anxiety neurosis).
   - Obsessive compulsive disorder (OCD).
   - Somatoform disorders (conversion disorder).
   - Stress-related disorders.
   - Behavioural and personality disorders.
   - Eating disorders.

Another classification:

1. Stress-related disorders—
   - Acute stress reaction.
   - Post-traumatic stress disorder.
   - Adjustment disorder.
2. Anxiety disorders—
   - Generalised anxiety disorder.
   - Phobic disorder.
   - Panic disorder.
   - Obsessive compulsive disorder
3. Affective (mood) disorders—
   - Depressive disorder.
   - Mania and bipolar disorder.
4. Schizophrenia and delusional disorders
5. Substance misuse—
   - Alcohol.
   - Drugs.
6. Organic—
   - Acute, e.g. delirium.
   - Chronic, e.g. dementia.
7. Disorders of adult personality and behaviour—
   - Personality disorder.
   - Factitious disorder.
8. Eating disorders—
   - Anorexia nervosa.
   - Bulimia nervosa.

9. Somatoform disorders—
   - Somatisation disorder.
   - Dissociative (conversion) disorder.
   - Pain disorder.
   - Hypochondriasis.
   - Body dismorphic disorder.
   - Somatoform autonomic dysfunction.
10. Neurasthenia.
11. Puerperal disorders.

DELUSION

Definition

It is a false belief which is not a fact and the falsity cannot be corrected even after clear demonstration.

Causes

- Schizophrenia.
- Manic depressive psychosis.
- Dementia.
- Alcohol and drug abuse.

Types

- Delusions of control or influence—patient believes that their thought and actions are controlled by outside force.
- Delusions of persecution—patient believes that attempts are being made to harm or poison him by their nearest relatives.
- Delusions of reference—patient believes that people refer to him in a special way, also believes that anyone is looking at him or talking about him.
- Delusion of broadcasting—patients believe that his thoughts are being broadcasted and everyone knows whatever he is thinking.
- Grandiose delusions—it is the delusion of having power, wealth, knowledge or special relationship with important persons (e.g. prime minister, president).
- Nihilistic—patient believes that he is dead or part or organ of his body is dead, the world and even time has been lost or destroyed. Commonly found in severe depression.
- Delusion of infidelity—patient believes his wife to be unfaithful while in fact she is chaste.
- Hypochondriac—patient believes that something is wrong in his body, he has some serious disease though he is actually healthy.

ILLUSION

Definition

It is the false interpretation of a real object. Patient imagines a rope to be a snake, voice of a bird to be voice of human. Do not have significant diagnostic importance. May be found in high fever, toxaemia or anxiety.

HALLUCINATION

Definition

It is the false sense of perception without any real object.

Types

- Auditory hallucination—hearing of voice when nothing is present. Commonly found in schizophrenia, severe depression, bipolar disorder.

- Visual hallucination—seeing something while there is nothing. Found in dissociation and conversion disorder, organic mental conditions, substance abuse, occasionally in schizophrenia and severe affective disorders.
- Tactile hallucination—sensation of being touched, insects moving under the skin, while there is nothing. Found in cocaine abuse and occasionally in schizophrenia.
- Gustatory hallucination—abnormal taste sensation though there is nothing in mouth. Occurs in schizophrenia and severe depressive disorders.
- Olfactory hallucination—abnormal sense of smell while nothing is present. Occurs in schizophrenia and severe depressive disorders, but may be in temporal lobe epilepsy or irritation of the olfactory bulb or pathways by tumour.
- Others—
  - Hypnagogic—vivid dream like hallucination at the onset of sleep.
  - Hypnopompic—vivid dream like hallucination on awakening.
  - Lilliputian hallucination—person thinks that people, animal or object seem to be smaller. May occur in substance use disorders.

ACUTE STRESS REACTION

Definition

After a stressful situation like major accident, physical or sexual assault, serious illness like AIDS or cancer, there may be characteristic pattern of symptoms, such as tension, anger, depression, increased activity or under activity and withdrawal.

These symptoms are transient, subsides within 3 days of their onset.

POST-TRAUMATIC STRESS DISORDER

Definition

Post-traumatic stress disorder (PTSD) is defined as severe response to a stressful condition which is threatening or catastrophic in nature, such as natural disaster, terrorist activity, serious accident and witnessing violent death or even distressing medical treatment.

Symptoms

- Recurrent thinking of the traumatic event, sleep disturbance, nightmares from which the patient awakes in a state of anxiety.
- Avoidance of situations, persons, activities or places similar to the traumatic event.
- Anxiety and depression.

Management

- Reassurance, counselling.
- Antidepressant drug.
- A novel therapy called eye movement desensitization and reprocessing (EMDR) is effective.

ADJUSTMENT DISORDER

Definition

Psychological response to adapting new situations which are distressing to the patient. It is less severe, but emotional reaction is more prolonged.

Situations may be—change in work, school, living, migration, divorce and separation, death of close relative, onset of chronic or terminal illness and long-term adjustment to sexual abuse.

These stresses can precipitate major depressive disorder, anxiety disorders and even schizophrenia. So other psychiatric disorders must be excluded before diagnosis of anxiety disorder.

Symptoms

- Develop within a month of the onset of stress, features depend on the underlying condition.
- Improves with the removal of stressful condition.
- There may also be anger, aggressive behaviour and excessive alcohol use, depression or anxiety.

Management

- Reassure, explanation and advice.
- Does not require psychotropic medication.
- Sometimes benzodiazepines may be used.
- Psychotherapy.
- Usually, resolves in time.

ANXIETY DISORDERS (ANXIETY NEUROSIS)

Definition

Anxiety disorder is a disorder characterised by lack of concentration, loss of interest, excessive worry, which are difficult to control and cause significant distress and impairment.

Types

It is of three types—phobic, panic and generalised anxiety disorder.

Phobic Disorder

Definition

It is an abnormal or excessive fear of an object or situation, which leads to avoidance of it, e.g. avoidance of journey by plane due to fear of crash.

Types of Phobia

- Simple phobia—fear of animal, height, closed or dark room etc.
- Social—fear of speech in a public gathering.
- Agoraphobia—fear of open space or street. Phobia outside home, so the patient remains home bound.

Panic Disorder

Definition

It is a disorder in which there is sudden and unpredictable attack of severe anxiety associated with physical symptoms such as chest pain, palpitation, breathlessness etc. Even when patient is well, he fears of another attack at any time.

Symptoms

- Chest pain.
- Palpitation.
- Fear of suffering from serious illness such as heart attack or stroke.
- Hyperventilation, difficulty in breathing.
- Fear of losing control, going 'crazy', passing out.
- Fear of dying.
- Anticipatory avoidance, reluctant to go outside.

Generalised Anxiety Disorder

Definition

This is characterized by chronic uncontrollable worry, tension and apprehension about everyday events and problems.

Symptoms

- Psychological—irritability, worry, fear, lack of concentration, depersonalization.
- Somatic—palpitation, fatigue, tremor, dizziness, sweating, diarrhoea, chest pain, insomnia, breathlessness.

Management of Anxiety Disorders

- Explanation and reassurance, psychotherapy including relaxation, graded exposure (desensitization).
- Drugs—benzodiazepines are useful. β blocker such as propranolol for palpitation.
- For long term treatment—SSRI (escitalopram, fluoxetine etc.)

OBSESSIVE COMPULSIVE DISORDER

Definition

Obsessive compulsive disorder (OCD) is characterised by unwanted thought, idea, impulse or image (obsession), which forces the person to do the act repeatedly to get rid of anxiety (compulsion).

Example—washing and rewashing of hands as if hands are not clear or contaminated.

Management

1. Explanation, reassurance, psychotherapy, behavioral therapy.
2. Drugs—
   - First line—SSRI (sertraline, fluoxetine).
   - Second line—TCA (imipramine, clomipramine, amytriptiline).
   - Third line—combination of SSRI and TCA or antipsychotic.

DEPRESSION

Definition

It is defined as persistent mood disturbance, such as loss of mood, interest, pleasure, retardation from physical and mental activities.

Cardinal Features

- Depressed mood.
- Lack of enjoyment.
- Negative thinking.
- Reduced energy.
- Slowness of thought.

Types

1. Primary—no underlying cause.
2. Secondary—due to some chronic illness, malignancy.
3. It may be unipolar or bipolar affective disorder.

Symptoms

- Psychological—lack of interest and concentration, guilty feeling, unworthiness. Sometimes severe depressive psychosis is associated with restlessness, agitation and suicidal tendency.
- Somatic—anorexia, weight loss, headache, backache, amenorrhea, loss of libido, insomnia, early waking from sleep, slowing of activity.

Management

1. Supportive—psychotherapy, reassurance.
2. Drugs—
   - SSRI (selective serotonin reuptake inhibitor)—fluoxetine, paroxetine, citalopram, escitalopram, sertraline.
   - TCA—amitriptyline, nortriptyline, imipramine.
   - For single episode, drug should be continued for at least 6-9 months and for multiple episodes, up to 2 years.
   - Drug should not be discontinued abruptly.

MANIA AND HYPOMANIA

Definition

It is a disorder characterised by marked elevation of mood such as euphoria, over activity and disinhibition.

Hypomania is the mild form of mania. It lasts a shorter time and is less severe with no psychotic features and less disability.

Clinical Features of Mania

- Mood—elevated or irritable, frequent swings from one mood to another, flights of ideas.
- Talk—excessive, fast, pressurised.

- Energy—excessive.
- Delusions of wealth, power, influence or of religious significance, sometimes persecutory.
- Hallucinations—fleeting auditory.
- Behaviour—disinhibition, excessive drinking, lost relationships (from promiscuity or irritability), social ostracism and lost employment (from reckless or disinhibited behaviour).
- Disturbance of memories.
- Insomnia, weight loss, increased libido.
- Over spending of money leading to significant debts.
- Mixed features of mania and depressive illness may be seen in the same episode.

Treatment

- Explanation and reassurance, psychotherapy.
- Drugs—haloperidol 10–30 mg with procyclidine or chlorpromazine 200–600 mg or thioridazine 200–600 mg.
- To prevent relapse—lithium 400–1200 mg single dose daily or carbamazepine or sodium valproate or clonazepam may be used.

BIPOLAR AFFECTIVE DISORDER (BIPOLAR MOOD DISORDER)

Definition

It is characterised by relapsing mood disturbance with periods of elevated mood known as mania and depressive mood.

Depressive episode may not always be present. It was previously called 'manic depressive psychosis.'

Clinical Features

- The patient may be cheerful, speaks fluently and over talkative.
- Inappropriate behaviour, social binding is completely lost.
- Delusion of grandiose type—he may claim to have special powers or to be an important personality.
- Sleep—less, claiming to have many tasks.
- Idea—flights of ideas, rapid change of topics or shifting of ideas.
- Over activity.
- In sight—impaired, hallucination may be present.

Treatment

- Patient and family members should be educated about relapsing nature and measures to prevent further episode (adequate sleep, reduced stress).
- Antipsychotics—dibenzodiazepines (Olanzepine), dibenzothiazepine (quetiapine), phenothiazine (chlorpromazine, trifluoperazine) or butyrophenones (haloperidol) or thioxanthines (flupentixol decanoate).
- Prophylaxis to prevent recurrent episodes is important. Lithium, carbamazepine and sodium valproate, lamotrigine, quetiapine may be used.

SCHIZOPHRENIA

Definition

Schizophrenia is a major psychiatric disorder characterised by disturbance of perception, thought, emotion, personality and social behaviour.

Types

1. Simple—there is gradual loss of interest to surroundings, withdrawal from reality, lack of caring himself but not violent. Delusion and hallucination are uncommon.
2. Hebephrenic—disorganised, disinhibited behaviour, violent, irrelevant talk. Hallucination and delusion are present.
3. Catatonic—patient maintains an odd posture for a prolong period, disturbance of behaviour, there is homicidal and suicidal tendency.
4. Paranoid—occurs at later age, persecutory delusions are main features. There is suspiciousness but personality is intact.

Clinical Features

1. Disturbance of thought—
   - Speech may be uninformative, meaningless with irrelevant words.
   - Thought insertion—patient thinks that thoughts are being inserted in his mind.
   - Thought withdrawal—patient thinks that thoughts are being taken away from mind.
   - Thought broadcasting—patient thinks that everybody knows whatever he thinks.
   - Delusion of control, grandiose, paranoid, hypochondriac are present.
2. Disorder of perception—hallucination, commonly auditory, may be visual.
3. Disturbance of mood or emotion—
   - Inappropriate emotional response (crying during laughing situation).
   - Blunt mood.
   - Rapid change of emotion.
   - Perplexed mood (fearful without any reason).
4. Disturbance of behavior and activity -
   - Violent, assaultive and destructive.
   - Withdrawal of activity (does not take care of himself, eat).
   - Purposeless activity (continuous walking without any destination).
5. Personality deterioration which affects family, work and personal relationship.

Features of Acute Schizophrenia

A—Auditory hallucination.
B—Broadcasting (insertion or withdrawal of thoughts).
C—Controlled feelings, impulse or act ('passivity' phenomenon—patient thinks that somebody is controlling him).
D—Delusional perception.

Above symptoms are often described as **'Schneider's first rank symptoms'.**

Treatment

Acute schizophrenia may require admission. In some cases, patient may be at risk of harming himself or others. Chronic schizophrenia can be treated at home.

General Measures

- Explanation and reassurance.
- Environmental and social factors to be looked for.
- Counselling by nurses, doctors or social workers.
- After control of schizophrenic attack, social and occupational rehabilitation is required.

Drug Treatment

- Antipsychotic agents (called neuroleptics or major tranquillizers) are effective against positive symptoms of schizophrenia in the majority of cases. Take 2–3 weeks to be maximally effective.
- Once symptoms are controlled, drugs are usually continued to prevent relapse.
- Patient with first episode of schizophrenia, improves in 1–2 years. However, with multiple psychotic episodes, treatment may be required for many years.

Antipsychotic Drugs

- Phenothiazine—chlorpromazine 100–1500 mg daily.
- Fluphenazine—20–100 mg fortnightly.
- Butyrophenone—haloperidol 5-30 mg daily.
- Thioxanthene—flupentixol 40-200 mg fortnightly.
- Newer drugs—risperidone 2–16 mg daily, olanzapine 5–20 mg daily, quetipiane 150–400 mg daily. pimozide 4–30 mg daily, sulpiride 600–1800 mg daily, clozapine 25–900 mg daily.

Side Effects of Antipsychotic Drugs

- Weight gain due to increased appetite.
- Metabolic (dyslipidaemia, impaired glucose tolerance), more common in newer (second generation) antipsychotics.
- Cardiac (e.g. Q-T prolongation). Baseline and follow-up ECG should be done.
- Extrapyramidal symptoms—Parkinsonism, akathisia (motor restlessness), acute dystonia, tardive dyskinesia. More common in older (first generation) antipsychotics.
- Effects due to antiadrenergic blockade—sedation, postural hypotension.
- Effects due to cholinergic blockade—dry mouth, blurred vision, constipation, urinary retention, impotence.
- Galactorrhoea.
- Hypersensitivity reactions—cholestatic jaundice, photosensitive dermatitis, blood dyscrasia (neutropenia with clozapine).
- Ocular complications—corneal and lens opacities.

EATING DISORDERS

Anorexia Nervosa

Definition

It is an eating disorder where body image is profoundly disturbed and despite emaciation, patient feels overweight and is afraid of weight gain. As a result, there is marked weight loss due to self-starvation.

Common in young teenage girls, rare after 30 years. More in higher social class, the patient is hard working, perfectionist and ambitious. Endocrine abnormality is present, which reverts to normal after improvement of the disease.

Diagnostic Criteria

- Weight loss, at least 15% of expected body weight.
- Avoidance of high calorie diet.
- Distortion of body image, so the patient regards herself fatty even when she is thin or grossly underweight.
- Amenorrhoea for at least 3 months (in male, loss of sexual interest).

Clinical Features

- Patient may hide his/her emaciation by using loosely fitting clothes.
- Physically overactive, performs excessive exercise, may use laxative or diuretic and sometimes vomit after meal.
- There may be downy, lanugo hair on trunk and limb. Hypotension, bradycardia, increased sensitivity to cold, constipation, peripheral cyanosis may be found.
- Anxiety, depressions are common.
- Psychosexual immaturity is present.
- Osteoporosis may occur due to less oestrogen.
- Bilateral parotid enlargement may be present.

Investigations

- Low LH, FSH, oestradiol. In male, low LH and testosterone.
- Low T3, but normal T4 and TSH.
- High cortisol and high GH are present. Dexamethasone suppression test may be abnormal. All revert to normal after therapy.
- Glucose intolerance may occur due to starvation.

Physical Effects of Anorexia Nervosa

1. Cardiac
   - ECG changes—T-inversion, ST-depression, prolonged Q-T interval.
   - Arrhythmia—sinus bradycardia, ventricular tachycardia.
2. Haematological—anaemia, thrombocytopenia and leucopenia.

3. Endocrine
   - Delayed puberty or arrest.
   - Growth retardation.
   - Amenorrhoea.
   - Sick euthyroid state.
4. Metabolic—renal failure, renal stone, osteoporosis.
5. Gastrointestinal—constipation, abnormal LFT.

Treatment

1. In mild case—treated in outdoor basis.
2. Moderate to severe case—
   - Hospitalisation.
   - Controlled diet to increase the weight, 1 kg weekly.
   - Psychotherapy and behavioural therapy.

Prognosis

50% full recovery, 30% partial recovery and 20% do not improve. 2–5% death from suicide or physical complication.

Bulimia Nervosa

Definition

It is an eating disorder characterised by uncontrolled, excessive eating (called binges), followed by self-induced vomiting.

Patient's weight is usually normal or near normal.

Clinical Features

Common in late adolescent female. Diagnostic criteria is as follows:
- Recurrent bouts of binge eating.
- Lack of self-control, overeating during binges.
- Self-induced vomiting, purgation or dieting after binges.
- Weight maintained within normal limits.

Physical Signs

- Pitted teeth (from gastric acid due to repeated vomiting),
- Calluses on knuckles ('Russell's sign').
- Parotid gland enlargement.

Complications

- Dental abnormality.
- Oesophageal tear due to excessive vomiting.
- Electrolyte abnormalities.
- Tetany due to hypokalaemic alkalosis.
- Cardiac arrhythmias and renal problems.

Treatment

- Cognitive behavioural therapy (CBT) achieves both short-term and long-term improvements.
- Guided self-help and interpersonal psychotherapy may be helpful.
- Drugs—SSRI (fluoxetine 60 mg daily).

Prognosis

Not associated with mortality like AN. 10% remain unwell, 20% remain subclinical and the remainder recover.

SOMATOFORM DISORDERS

Definition

It is a group of disorders characterised by multiple somatic symptoms, without any demonstrable medical illness. Physical symptoms are due to psychological factors.

Types

1. Somatization disorder (Briquet's syndrome)—multiple somatic symptoms, but no physical cause. Common in women. Usual complains are—pain, vomiting, nausea, headache, dizziness, menstrual irregularity, sexual dysfunction.
2. Hypochondriasis—in this disorder, patient has a fear or belief that he or she has a serious, fatal disease that persists despite normal investigation.
3. Body dysmorhpic disorder—in this disorder, there is feeling of disfigured appearance or body shape without reality. Patient even may request for cosmetic surgery.
4. Somatoform autonomic dysfunction—commonly related to autonomic nervous system. Complains are—
   - Cardiovascular (cardiac neurosis)—palpitation, chest pain.
   - Respiratory—hyperventilation, breathlessness.
   - GIT—vomiting and irritable bowel syndrome.
5. Somatoform pain disorder—there may be severe, persistent pain, which cannot be explained by a medical condition.
6. Neurasthenia (chronic fatigue syndrome)—characterised by excessive fatigue after minimal physical or mental exertion. Also, poor concentration, dizziness, muscular aches and sleep disturbance.
7. Dissociative (conversion) disorder—It is characterised by profound loss of awareness or cognitive ability without organic disease. The term dissociative (conversion) disorder has replaced 'hysteria.'
   - Conversion means unresolved conflict is converted into symbolic physical symptoms as a defence against it, e.g. paralysis, sensory loss, abnormal movements, aphonia, gait disturbance, blindness.
   - Dissociate means disintegration of different mental activity, e.g. amnesia, fugue, pseudoseizure.
   - Sometimes, in dissociative disorder, there is rigidity, which increases more and more during more manoeuvres.

General Management of Somatoform Disorders

- Reassurance, explanation, advice, psychotherapy, behavioural therapy.
- Encourage to return to normal functioning.
- Drugs—antidepressant (sertraline, fluoxetine, escitalopram).
- Rehabilitation.
- Shared care with GP.

HYSTERIA

Definition

It is a disorder in which patient develops symptoms of illness or mental symptoms for real or imagined gain without fully aware of the underlying motive. It is called conversion disorder.

Clinical Features (Table 1)

Common in young female, low socioeconomic group.

- Neurological—gait disturbance, paraplegia, rigidity, aphonia, pseudoseizure, visual loss, sensory loss.
- Cardiovascular—palpitation, chest pain.
- Respiratory—breathlessness, hyperventilation.
- GIT—nausea, vomiting, abdominal pain, feeling of lump in throat (globus hystericus), loss of appetite, abstinence from food.
- Sexual—decreased libido or impotence.
- Unexplained pain in different parts of the body.

Treatment

- Explanation and reassurance.
- Removal of stress factor.
- Drugs—SSRI, TCA, carbamazepine.

Table 1
Difference between hysteria and epilepsy

Points	*Hysteria (Pseudo-seizure)*	*Epilepsy (True seizure)*
Age and sex	More in female, young	Any sex, early onset
Fit during sleep	Never	May occur
Consciousness	No real loss	Loss of consciousness
Place of occurence	Never alone. Usually in presence of people or family members	Occur alone
Tongue biting, frothing of saliva, incontinence of urine and faeces	Never	Common
Duration	Longer	Short, brief
Recovery	May be sudden	Gradual
Post-ictal amnesia	No	Yes
EEG	Normal	Abnormal
CT scan	Normal	May be abnormal
Treatment	Psychotherapy	Anticonvulsant drugs

PUERPERAL DISORDERS

Three common psychiatric complications after childbirth.

1. Postpartum blues—characterised by irritability, labile mood and tearfulness. Symptoms begin soon after childbirth, peak on about the fourth day and then resolve. Psychological and social supports are necessary. No drug treatment is required.
2. Postpartum depression—occurs in 10–15% cases. Women with a previous history of depression are at risk. Explanation and reassurance is important. Psychotherapy and antidepressant may be given.
3. Puerperal psychosis—develops in the first 2 weeks after childbirth. Usually manic or depressive psychosis, however, schizophrenia can also occur.

Treatment

According to type of illness, e.g. depression, psychosis.

DEMENTIA

Definition

It is a disorder characterised by progressive deterioration of intellectual function, memory and personality due to progressive degeneration of brain. Consciousness is clear.

Causes

1. Degenerative and hereditary—
   - Alzheimer's disease.
   - Parkinson's disease.
   - Pick's disease.
   - Huntington's disease.
   - Wilson's disease.
2. Vascular causes—
   - Multi infarct dementia.
   - Diffuse white matter disease.
3. Infections—HIV, neurosyphilis, progressive multifocal leucoencephalopathy, Creutzfeldt-Jakob disease, prion disease (kuru).
4. Inflammatory—multiple sclerosis, sarcoidosis.
5. Connective tissue disease—SLE, Sjogren syndrome.
6. Drugs and toxins (sedative, heavy metal poisoning, carbon monoxide poisoning, alcohol).
7. Trauma—head injury, chronic subdural haematoma, punch drunk syndrome.
8. Neoplastic—primary brain tumour, secondary.
9. Endocrine causes—hypothyroidism, hypopituitarism, Addison's disease, Cushing's syndrome, hypo- and hyperparathyroidism.
10. Metabolic—renal failure, liver failure, respiratory failure.
11. Vitamin deficiencies—B1, B12, B3 (nicotinic acid).
12. Others—normal pressure hydrocephalous.

Clinical Features

Depends on the cause. Main features are as follows:

- Memory disturbance,
- Disturbance of intellect (judgment and problem solving).
- Personality problem and disinhibition (not keeping clothes, exposing genitalia, etc.)
- Impairment of performance of activities of daily living.
- Hallucination.
- Agitation.
- Insomnia.
- Micturition and defaecation at inappropriate place.
- Undue suspiciousness.

Investigations

- According to suspicion of cause.
- CT or MRI of brain to identify brain atrophy and structural lesions.

Treatment

Treatment of underlying cause, if any.

- Usually symptomatic. Institutionalisation may be required.
- Explanation to family members and care givers. Advise regarding exercise, structured activity, music therapy, bright light therapy, environmental cues and instructions.
- Cholinesterase inhibitor drugs for memory disturbances—rivastigmine, donepezil, galantamine, tecrine.
- Symptomatic management of behavioural problems—haloperidol, thioridazine.

DELIRIUM

Definition

It is an acute, reversible mental disorder characterised by mental confusion, disorientation of time and place associated with emotional lability, illusion, auditory and visual hallucination, violent behaviour.

Causes

Remember the formula—**'I WATCH DEATH'.**

- **I**nfection—meningitis, encephalitis, septicaemia.
- **W**ithdrawal of sedatives and alcohol.
- **A**cute metabolic conditions—electrolyte imbalance, hepatic and renal failure.
- **T**rauma, head injury, burn.
- **C**NS lesion—tumour, epilepsy, Wernicke's encephalopathy.
- **H**ypoxia.
- **D**eficiencies—Thiamine, B12.
- **E**ndocrine disorders—hypothyroidism, adrenal insufficiencies.
- **A**cute vascular event—TIA, stroke, shock.
- **T**oxins and drugs.
- **H**eavy metals—lead and mercury.

Investigations

- Routine—CBC, ESR, serum urea, creatinine, electrolytes, calcium, magnesium, glucose.
- Renal and liver function tests.
- Thyroid function tests.
- CT or MRI of brain.
- Others according to suspicion of cause.

Treatment

- Treatment of underlying illness.
- Maintenance adequate hydration and nutrition, correction of electrolyte imbalance.
- Psychotropic drugs—
  - Younger patients—haloperidol 5-10 mg orally every 12 hours.
  - Older patients—risperidone 2 mg orally, olanzapine, thioridazone.

Delirium Tremens

It is a disorder due to sudden withdrawal of alcohol in a chronic alcoholic person, occurs 1–3 days after alcohol cessation. It is commonly seen a day or two after admission to hospital.

Clinical Features

- Disorientation, agitation, aggression and marked tremor.
- Autonomic hyperactivity, such as tachycardia, diaphoresis (excessive sweating), fever, anxiety, insomnia, and hypertension.
- Hallucinations, most frequently visual or tactile.
- Features of dehydration.

Complications

- Dehydration.
- Secondary infection.
- Hepatic disease.
- Wernick-Korsakoff syndrome.

Treatment

- Hospitalisation.
- Benzodiazepines—lorazepam I/V 0.1 mg/kg at 2.0 mg/min or diazepam 10–20 mg or chlordiazepoxide 30–60 mg orally.
- Thiamine (vitamin B1) in high dose IV and other vitamin B complex.
- Correction of electrolytes imbalance.
- Antibiotic, if infection.
- Phenytoin or carbamazepine, if previous history of withdrawal fits.

SUBSTANCE ABUSE

Definition

It is the dependence on and misuse of both illegal and prescribed drugs. In addition to alcohol and nicotine, many psychotropic drugs that are taken for prolong period, resulting in dependency, affect mood and mental function, even occupational disturbance. Also, causes withdrawal symptoms on abrupt cessation.

Common Drugs and Substances which are Misused

1. Sedatives—
   - Benzodiazepines
   - Barbiturates
2. Narcotics—
   - Morphine
   - Heroin
   - Pethidine
3. Stimulants—
   - Cocaine
   - Amphetamine
   - Ecstasy (MDMA)
4. Hallucinogens—
   - Cannabis
   - Solvents
   - Lysergic acid diethylamide (LSD)

Clinical Features

Vary according to the drug taken.

Treatment

- Explanation, reassurance, patient's cooperation and will are the vital parts.
- Gradual reduction of dose.
- Substitute or antagonist should be considered.
- Preventive measure to stop selling of the drugs by the chemist.

FACTITIOUS DISORDER

There is repeated and deliberate production of signs or symptoms of a disease to get medical care. Common in young woman. Example—deliberate intake of thyroxin to reduce weight can cause factitious thyrotoxicosis.

MÜNCHAUSEN'S SYNDROME

This is a severe form of factitious disorder in which the patient makes signs and symptoms of disease for hospital admission repeatedly, sometimes visiting several hospitals in one day.

CHAPTER

16 Vitamins

CHAPTER CONTENTS

DEFINITION

Vitamins are organic substances required in small quantities for a variety of biochemical functions, usually not synthesized in the body and supplied in the diet.

Types

There are two types of vitamins:
- Fat-soluble vitamins—A, D, E, K.
- Water-soluble vitamins—B complex and vitamin C.

FAT-SOLUBLE VITAMINS

VITAMIN A (RETINOL)

Dietary Source

Milk, egg, butter, cheese, egg yolk, fish, liver oil. Also green leafy vegetables, carrot, mango (beta carotene).

Function of Vitamin A

- Essential for normal retinal function.
- Cell growth and differentiation, mainly epithelial cells.
- Necessary for normal wound healing.

Deficiency of Vitamin A

Deficiency of vitamin A may cause:
- Night blindness.
- Xerosis of conjunctiva (dryness).
- Xerophthalmia.
- Bitot's spots.
- Keratomalacia.
- Blindness.
- Dryness of skin (Toad's skin).

Treatment

Vitamin A 30,000–50,000 IU orally daily for 5 days.

Prevention

- Intake of food rich in vitamin A.
- Single prophylactic oral dose of 60 mg retinyl palmitate (providing 2,00,000 IU retinol) to all preschool children.
- Pregnant women and lactating mother should eat dark green, leafy vegetables and yellow fruits. Vitamin A 20,000 IU every week.

Toxicity

Prolonged use may cause toxicity called hypervitaminosis A.

VITAMIN D (CHOLECALCIFEROL)

Source

Sunlight, fish oil, egg yolk, milk, margarine, fortified cereals.

Natural form of vitamin D is cholecalciferol or vitamin D3 is formed by the action of UV light on 7-dehydrocholesterol in the skin. Vitamin D is converted in the liver to 25-hydroxycholecalciferol, which is further hydroxylated in the kidney to 1, 25-dihydroxycholecalciferol,which is the active form of vitamin D.

Function of Vitamin D

- Absorption of calcium from gut.
- Mineralisation of bone.

Cause of Vitamin D Deficiency

- Lack of exposure to sunlight.
- Malabsorption.
- Less intake in food.

Deficiency may cause: Rickets in child, osteomalacia in adult.

Rickets

Definition

It is a disease which affects children due to the deficiency of vitamin D.

Clinical Features

- Irritability, restlessness, sweating in forehead.
- Delayed development.
- Muscle hypotonia.
- Swelling of costochondral junctions of ribs called 'Rickety Rosary'.
- Craniotabes (small unossified areas in membranous bones of skull that yield to finger pressure with a cracking feeling).
- Bossing of frontal and parietal bones.
- Delayed anterior fontanelle closure.
- Enlargement of epiphyses at the lower end of radius.
- Harrison's sulcus—depression of lower ribs along the attachment of diaphragm.
- When the child begins to walk—may be knock knee or bowing legs.
- Kyphosis, lordosis, pelvic deformity may occur.
- Delayed dentition.
- Abdominal distention due to weak abdominal muscle called pot belly.
- Prone to respiratory infection.

Osteomalacia

Definition

It is the disease in adult due to vitamin D deficiency. It causes softening of bone due to defective mineralisation.

Causes of Osteomalacia

- Lack of exposure to sunlight.
- Less intake in diet.
- Malabsorbtion.
- Obstructive jaundice.
- Chronic kidney diseases.

Clinical Features

- May be asymptomatic.
- Muscle and bone pain. Increased bone fragility and fracture.
- Proximal muscle weakness and waddling gait.
- X-ray shows pseudofracture called Looser's zone.

Treatment

- Ergocalciferol (vit D) 250–1,000 μgm daily for 3–4 months.
- Maintenance—10–20 μgm daily for few months.
- Diet rich in vitamin D.
- Oral calcium gluconate may be given.

NB: Prolong and excessive use of vit D may cause hypervitaminosis D characterised by nausea, vomiting, polyuria and other features of hypercalcaemia.

Prevention

- Regular intake of food rich in calcium, e.g. milk.
- Adequate sunlight exposure.

VITAMIN E (TOCOPHEROL)

Source

Vegetable and seeds oil, soya oil, sunflower, nuts.

Function

It is an important antioxidant protecting cells and membranes from free radicals.

Illnesses Related to Deficiency of Vitamin E

The deficiency of vitamin E can cause:

- Mild haemolytic anaemia.
- Ataxia, areflexia.
- Visual scotoma.
- Infertility.

Treatment

Vitamin E 100–400 mg orally daily.

VITAMIN K

Source

- Vit. K I (phylloquinone)—Green vegetables, dairy product, liver, soya-bean oil.
- Vit. K II (menaquinone)—Intestinal bacterial flora.

Vitamin K dependents clotting factors: II, VII, IX, X, which are produced in the liver.

Function of Vit. K: It acts as cofactor in the production of gamma carboxyglutamic acid, which helps in the production of these coagulation factors.

Causes of Deficiency

- Less intake in food.
- Obstructive jaundice.
- Malabsorption syndrome.
- Prolonged use of antibiotic which destroys bacterial flora.

Deficiency: Delayed coagulation and bleeding tendencies.

Treatment: Vitamin K 10 mg IV for 3–5 days.

WATER-SOLUBLE VITAMINS

THIAMINE (VITAMIN B_1)

Source

Cereals, beans, peas, grains, yeast, pork, beaf, liver.

Function

It is an essential coenzyme for the decarboxylation of pyruvate to acetyl coenzyme A.

Causes of Deficiency

- Dietary deficiency.
- Chronic alcoholism.
- Prolong use of polished rice (causes beri-beri).

Illness Related to Deficiency of Vitamin B

- Beri-beri.
- Wernick's encephalopathy.

Beri-beri

It is a disease caused by deficiency of vitamin B1. There are two forms of the disease in adults—

Dry (or Neurological) Beri-beri

Its features are as follows
- Peripheral neuropathy—tingling, numbness, wasting of muscles, loss of reflexes, wrist, foot drop.
- Wernicke's encephalopathy.
- Korsakoff's psychosis.

Wet (or Cardiac) Beri-beri

Its features are as follows:
- Generalised oedema.
- Biventricular heart failure.
- Pulmonary oedema.

Treatment

- Injection B1 I/V 50–100 mg for 3–5 days, then oral therapy.
- Diet rich in vitamin B1 should be given.

Wernick's Encephalopathy

Definition

It is the acute cerebral manifestation of vitamin B1 deficiency, commonly due to long-standing heavy drinking of alcohol and inadequate diet. May also occur after repeated vomiting, prolonged starvation or diarrhoea.

Lesion may be in (i) brainstem causing ophthalmoplegia, nystagmus and ataxia, (ii) superior vermis of cerebellum causing ataxia, (iii) Dorsomedial nucleus in thalamus and adjacent area of grey matter, causing amnesia.

Clinical Features

1. Cognitive changes—Acute confusion, disorientation, drowsiness or altered consciousness.
2. Eye changes—bilateral symmetrical ophthalmoplegia, bilateral or unilateral paralysis of lateral conjugate gaze, horizontal or vertical nystagmus, abnormal pupillary reflex. Rarely, ptosis, meiosis and unreactive pupil.
3. Gait ataxia—broad based gait, cerebellar sign and vestibular paralysis.
4. When associated with memory disturbance and confabulation, it is called Korsakoff's psychosis. Loss of recent memory is common, but past memory may be normal. Confabulation means falsification of memory with clear consciousness. The patient makes new stories unrelated to truth.

Investigations

Diagnosis is clinical. CT scan is normal and CSF also normal, but slight rise in protein may occur.

Treatment

- Injection B1, 500 mg IV over 30 minutes TDS 2 days, then 500 mg IV or IM daily for 5 days.
- Then oral B1 100 mg TDS and other B complex vitamins.
- If promptly treated, it is reversible. If not treated promptly, lesion may be irreversible.

RIBOFLAVIN (VITAMIN B_2)

Source

Milk, cheese, eggs, liver, kidney, cereal, bread.

Illnesses Related to Deficiency of Vitamin B_2

The deficiency of vitamin B_2 affects lips and tongue and may cause:
- Glossitis.
- Angular stomatitis.
- Cheilosis.
- Seborrhoic dermatitis. The genitals and the skin areas rich in sebaceous glands may be affected.

Treatment

Riboflavin 10 mg daily orally.

NIACIN (VITAMIN B_3)

Source

Meat, cereals, liver, kidney, fish.

Illnesses Related to Deficiency of Vitamin B_3

The deficiency of vitamin B3 causes pellagra, characterised by dermatitis, diarrhoea, dementia (3 'D's).

- Dermatitis—Over the sun-exposed areas, mainly limbs and neck (necklace area) but not face. Skin lesions are erythema, vesiculation, cracking, pigmentation.
- Diarrhoea—Associated with anorexia, nausea, glossitia, dysphagia.
- Dementia.

Treatment

Nicotinic acid 100 mg 8 hourly daily orally or parenterally.

Toxicity

- Reversible hepatotoxicity.
- Dose above 200 mg a day gives rise to vasodilatory symptoms (flushing, hypotension).

PYRIDOXINE (VITAMIN B_6)

Source

Milk, egg, meat, wheat, corn, cabbage.

Illness Related to Deficiency of Vitamin B_6

- Peripheral neuropathy.
- Mouth sores and glossitis.

Drugs

INH and penicillamine may antagonise the action of pyridoxine and mimic pyridoxine deficiency.

Treatment

Oral pyridoxine 10–20 mg daily. (Very high doses of vitamin B6 taken for several months may cause sensory polyneuropathy).

BIOTIN (VITAMIN B_7)

Causes of Deficiency

The deficiency of vitamin B7 may occur due intake of large quantities of raw eggs taken over a period of months or years. The other causes are:

- Scaly dermatitis.
- Alopecia.
- Paraesthesia.

Treatment

Biotin 10 mg daily.

VITAMIN B_{12} (CYANOCOBALAMINE)

Source

Foods of animal origin—liver, meat, fish, egg. No plant source.

Functions

- Acts as coenzyme for methionine synthesis and L-methylmelonyl Co-A mutase.

Causes of Deficiency

- Inadequate dietary intake (strict vegetarians).
- Pernicious anaemia.
- Partial or total gastrectomy (intrinsic factor deficiency).
- Ileal disease—resection, Crohn's disease.

Illnesses Related to Deficiency of Vitamin B_{12}

- Macrocytic or megaloblastic anaemia.
- Glossitis.
- Subacute combined degeneration of the spinal cord.
- Peripheral neuropathy.
- Dementia.
- Optic atrophy.

Treatment

Inj. hydroxycobalamine 1000 μg IM for 5 days 2–3 days apart. Then maintenance dose 1000 μg every 3 months for life.

FOLATE

Source

Green vegetables, potato, peas, beans, meat, liver, kidney.

Function

- It acts as a coenzyme for one carbon transfer in neuclic acid and amino acid metabolism.

Cause of Deficiency

- Dietary deficiency mainly less vegetable intake.
- Malabsorption.
- More demand—pregnancy.
- Drug—methotrexate.

Illnesses Related to Deficiency

- Macrocytic or megaloblastic anaemia.
- Neural tube defects—spina bifida, anencephaly and encephalocele.

Treatment

- Folic acid 5 mg daily for 3 weeks, then 5 mg weekly as maintenance dose.
- In pregnancy—folic acid is given to prevent megaloblastic anaemia and also foetal neural tube defect.

VITAMIN C (ASCORBIC ACID)

Source

Fresh citrous fruits and vegetables.

Functions

It is a powerful reducing agent and is involved in the hydroxylation of proline to hydroxyproline, which is necessary for the formation of collagen.

Cause of Deficiency

Less intake of fresh fruits and vegetables.

Scurvy

It is disease due to deficiency of vitamin C. Scurvy is classified into two types—infantile and adult scurvy. The features are as follows:

- Swollen and spongy gums (particularly the papilla between teeth, called scurvy bud), which bleed easily.
- Teeth become loose and fall easily.
- Cutaneous bleeding—perifollicular haemorrhage, bruise, ecchymoses.
- Bleeding into the joints (haemarthrosis).
- Gastrointestinal bleeding.
- Anaemia.
- Poor wound healing.
- In infants—Subperiosteal haemorrhage leads to painful limbs, occurs at the end of long bones, usually seen after 2 weeks of onset of clinical symptoms. There may be enlargement of costochondral junction (scorbutic rosary). Infants become very irritable, don't let touch even.

Treatment

- Vitamin C 250 mg, three to four times daily orally.
- Dietary supplements especially fresh fruits (orange, mango, pineapple, guava, etc.) and liver extract.
- Bottle-fed infants should be given fruit juice. Nursing mother should take sufficient vitamin C, which is secreted in the breast milk.

Toxicity

Daily intake of more than 1 gm/day may cause diarrhoea and formation of renal oxalate stones.

ZINC

Source

Red meat, sea food, meat, dairy products, whole wheat bread

Illnesses Related to Deficiency

- Growth retardation—dwarfism.
- Hypogonadism.
- Constipation, diarrhoea.
- Acrodermatitis enteropathica—growth retardation, hair loss and diarrhea.
- In starvation, zinc deficiency causes thymic atrophy.

PROTEIN–ENERGY MALNUTRITION (PEM)

Definition

Protein-energy malnutrition is a syndrome due to deficiency of protein, energy or both.

Types

This syndrome is classified into three types:
- Marasmus—deficiency in calorie intake.
- Kwashiorkor—protein malnutrition is predominant.
- Marasmic Kwashiorkor—marked protein and calorie insufficiency, sometimes referred to as the most severe form of malnutrition.

Marasmus

Definition

It is defined as a malnutrition where both protein and energy deficiency occurs.

Clinical Features

- Emaciation—there is obvious muscle wasting and loss of body fat resulting in wrinkling and loosening of skin.
- Peculiar old man like facies called monkey facies.
- Weight loss. Muscles are flabby with hypotonia.
- Milestone of child development is delayed (standing, sitting, crawling, walking).
- No oedema.
- Hair is thin and dry. Eyes are sunken, anterior fontanelle is depressed.
- Diarrhoea.
- Signs of infection may be present.

Treatment

- Diet should contain protein, fat, carbohydrate.
- Minerals and vitamins should be added.
- Infection should be controlled and underlying cause should be treated.

Kwashiorkor

Definition

It is a form of malnutrition caused by the deficiency of protein. Occurs typically in a young child displaced from breastfeeding by a new baby. It is often precipitated by infections such as measles, malaria and diarrhoeal illnesses.

Clinical Features

- Child is apathetic, lethargic with severe anorexia.
- Generalised oedema.
- Skin—erythematous, pigmentated, thick and shiny, occasionally there may desquamation.
- Muscles are flabby.

- Hair is dry, sparse lusterless, may be reddish or yellow in colour.
- Abdomen is distended due to hepatomegaly and/or ascites.

Treatment

- Diet should contain milk, milk proteins, fish, egg, fruits.
- Vitamins and minerals should be added.

Complications of PEM

- Hypoglycaemia.
- Shock.
- Hypothermia.
- Severe infection.

Investigations for PEM

- CBC—anaemia due to folate, iron and copper deficiency.
- Serum electrolytes—it may show abnormalities.
- Serum total protein, A:G ratio.
- Stool R/M/E—it may show parasitic infestations.

Chest X-ray—tuberculosis may be found.

CHAPTER

17 Electrolyte and Acid-Base Imbalance

CHAPTER CONTENTS

NORMAL RANGE OF SERUM ELECTROLYTES

- Sodium—135-145 mmol/L.
- Potassium—3.5-5.2 mmol/L.
- Chloride—95-107 mmol/L.
- Bicarbonate—21-28 mmol/L.

HYPERNATRAEMIA

Definition

When serum sodium level is above the upper normal limit.

Causes

1. Pure or predominant water depletion due to the following:
   - Decreased intake.
   - Fever.
   - Hot environment.
2. Hyperosmolar nonketotic diabetic coma (HONC).
3. Diabetes insipidus.
4. Excessive normal saline infusion.

Clinical Features

- May be asymptomatic.
- Altered mental status (confusion, stupor, coma).

Treatment

- Water by mouth or nasogastric tube or dextrose in aqua or 1/2 strength normal saline IV.
- Treatment of underlying disorder.

HYPONATRAEMIA

Definition

When sodium is below the lower normal limit.

Causes

1. True hyponatremia (hypovolaemic)—There is real loss of sodium.
   - GIT causes vomiting, diarrhoea, pancreatitis.
   - Renal cause diuretic phase of ARF, CKD, tubulo-interstitial disorder, salt loosing nephropathy.
   - Endocrine cause Addison's disease.
   - Drugs—diuretic.

2. Hypervolaemic or dilutional—No sodium loss, water volume is relatively high. The causes are as follows:
   - CCF.
   - Nephrotic syndrome.
   - Cirrhosis of liver.
3. Euvolaemic—
   - SIADH (Syndrome of inappropriate ADH secretion).
   - Psychogenic polydipsia.
   - Postoperative hyponatraemia.
   - Iatrogenic—dextrose in aqua infusion.
4. Pseudohyponatraemia—Body sodium is normal, but serum sodium is low due to interference of laboratory tests by the following conditions:
   - Hyperglycaemia.
   - Paraproteinaemia.
   - Hyperlipidaemia.

Clinical Features

- May be asymptomatic.
- Weakness, lassitude, tiredness.
- Muscle cramp.
- Dizziness, giddiness, confusion, stupor or even coma.

Treatment

According to type and cause:

1. True hyponatraemia—
   - Sodium should be corrected. In mild case, oral salt is sufficient.
   - If serum sodium is <125 mmol/L—IV normal saline.
2. Hypervolaemic or dilutional—
   - Water restriction—600–1000 mL/day.
   - Diuretic.
   - Treatment of underlying cause.
3. Euvolaemic—
   - Water restriction and treatment of cause, e.g. SIADH.

NB: 3% saline may be required in selected cases. Should be used with caution, as rapid correction may cause central pontine myelinolysis (CPM).

HYPERKALAEMIA

Definition

When serum potassium is high above the normal limit.

Causes

1. High potassium intake (oral or IV fluid with potassium, food or drugs containing potassium).
2. Renal diseases—
   - Acute and chronic renal failure.
   - Impaired tubular secretion of K+ (renal lupus, amyloidosis, transplanted kidney).
3. Endocrine diseases—
   - Addison's disease.
   - Diabetic ketoacidosis.
   - Primary hypoaldosteronism.
4. Drugs—
   - Potassium sparing diuretics (spironolactone, amiloride, triamterine).
   - ACE inhibitor.
   - NSAIDs.
   - Ciclosporin.
5. Miscellaneous—
   - Metabolic acidosis.
   - Rhabdomyolysis.
   - Tumor lysis syndrome.
   - Digoxin poisoning.
   - Vigorous exercise.
   - Hyperkalaemic periodic paralysis.
   - Hyporeninaemic hypoaldosteronism (Type IV RTA).
   - Transfusion of stored blood.
6. Pseudohyperkalaemia—due to abnormal release of K+ from abnormal or damaged cells, also called spurious hyperkalaemia.
   - If blood is kept at room temperature for long time before analysis.
   - Acute leukaemia (due to very high WBC).
   - Haemolysis.
   - Thrombocytosis.
   - Infectious mononucleosis.

ECG Changes in Hyperkalaemia

- T—tall, peaked and tented (in chest leads).
- P—wide, small, ultimately absent.
- PR interval—prolonged.
- QRS—wide, slurred and bizarre.

Clinical Features

- May be asymptomatic.
- Muscular weakness, may be severe causing flaccid paralysis.

- Loss of tendon jerk.
- Paralytic ileus (abdomen is distended).
- Tingling around the lip or finger.
- Sudden death due to cardiac arrest or arrhythmia.

Treatment

- Withdrawal of potassium, potassium containing food and drug.
- Injection 10% calcium gluconate, 10–20 cc IV slowly over 10 minutes. May be repeated (it protects the myocardium, also reduces the risk of cardiac arrest).
- Injection 50 mL of 50% glucose IV plus Inj. insulin 10 units. This can be repeated, if necessary.
- Correction of acidosis by IV sodibicarb (1.26%), 500 mL 6-8 hourly (until serum HCO_3 is normal).
- Inj. Frusemide may be given.
- Treatment of primary cause.
- In some cases, exchange resins (calcium resonium 15–30 g orally).
- Nebulised salbutamol. It causes potassium entry into the cell.
- If all fails, haemodialysis or peritoneal dialysis.

NB: Hyperkalaemia is dangerous, if K+ is >7 mmol/L. May cause cardiac arrest in systole.

HYPOKALAEMIA

Definition

When serum potassium is below normal physiological limit.

Cause

- Diuretic (thiazide, frusemide)—most common cause.
- Gastrointestinal loss—diarrhoea, vomiting, purgative abuse, villous adenoma, ileostomy.
- Renal loss—renal tubular acidosis type I and II, renal tubular necrosis (diuretic phase), diuretic phase of ARF, relief of urinary tract obstruction, Bartter's syndrome, Liddle's syndrome, Gitelman's syndrome.
- Endocrine cause—Cushing's syndrome, Conn's syndrome (primary hyperaldosteronism).
- Others—heart failure, liver failure, nephrotic syndrome, drug (salbutamol, fenoterol), insulin therapy (in diabetic ketoacidosis), alkalosis, hypokalaemic periodic paralysis, interstitial renal disease.
- Intracellular shift—metabolic alkalosis, insulin therapy.

Clinical Features

1. May be asymptomatic (if serum potassium >2.5 mmol/ L).
2. If severe hypokalaemia (serum potassium <2.5 mmol/L)—
   - Muscular weakness, paralysis, loss of tendon reflex.
   - Abdominal distension with sluggish or absent bowel sound due to paralytic ileus, constipation.
   - Arrhythmia, increased digoxin toxicity.

Treatment

- If serum potassium is >2.5 mmol/L—oral potassium therapy.
- If severe or serum potassium is < 2.5 mmol/L— potassium is given in infusion (with normal saline).
- Treatment of primary cause.

NB: Potassium should never be given directly IV. Failure to correct hypokalaemia may be due to concurrent hypomagnesaemia. So, it should be measured and corrected.

ECG Changes in Hypokalaemia

- U wave—prominent in chest leads (most common).
- Others—ST-depression, T is small or inverted, prolonged PR interval.

HYPOMAGNESAEMIA

Normal value: 0.5–1 mmol/L.

Causes

1. Less intake—
   - Starvation.
   - Malnutrition.
   - Chronic alcoholism.
   - Prolong parenteral nutrition.
2. GIT loss—
   - Prolong vomiting.
   - Chronic diarrhoea.
   - Laxative abuse.
   - Nasogastric suction.
   - Small bowel by-pass surgery.
   - Gastrointestinal fistula.
3. Renal loss—
   - Diuretic.
   - Recovery phase of acute tubular necrosis.
   - Drugs—gentamicin, cisplatin.
   - Primary hyperaldosteronism.
   - Diabetic ketoacidosis.
   - Others—Bartter's syndrome, Gitelman's syndrome.
4. Miscellaneous—acute pancreatitis.

Clinical Features

Usually, associated with hypocalcaemia.

- Features of tetany.
- Cardiac arrhythmia (mainly torsades de pointes).
- CNS abnormality (irritability, dizziness, giddiness, seizure).

Treatment

- IV magnesium chloride—0.5 mL/kg in first 24 hours.
- Treatment of primary cause.

METABOLIC ACIDOSIS

Definition

It is a condition characterised by reduction in plasma bicarbonate and rise in H^+ concentration (low pH).

Causes

- Acute and chronic renal failure.
- Diabetic ketoacidosis.
- Lactic acidosis.
- Diarrhoea.
- Poisoning with methanol and ethanol.
- Aspirin poisoning.
- Starvation.

Clinical Features

- Confusion, drowsiness.
- Kussmaul's breathing (deep sighing respiration).
- Arrhythmia.

Treatment

- Treatment of primary cause.
- Inj. sodibicarb (1.26%).
- Correction of dehydration and other electrolyte imbalance.

METABOLIC ALKALOSIS

Definition

It is a condition characterised by rise in plasma bicarbonate and fall in H^+ concentration (increased pH).

Causes

- Vomiting.
- Aspiration of gastric contents.
- Ingestion of alkali or overuse of antacid.
- Diuretic.
- Intravenous bicarbonate, acetate or citrate.
- Hyperaldosteronism.
- Cushing's syndrome or excess use of steroid.

Clinical Features

- May be asymptomatic.
- Confusion, stupor or even coma.
- May cause tetany.

Treatment

- IV fluid, usually normal saline.
- Treatment of primary cause.
- Correction of potassium.

RESPIRATORY ACIDOSIS

Definition

It is a condition characterised by increased PCO_2 and low pH due to the inadequate ventilation.

Causes

1. Respiratory centre depression—
   - Head injury.
   - CVD.
   - Encephalitis.
   - Overdose of morhine, pethidine, sedative.
2. Lung disease—
   - Collapse.
   - Extensive fibrosis.
   - Massive pleural effusion.
   - Large pneumothorax.
3. Neomuscular—
   - Poliomyelitis.
   - Myopathy.
4. Miscellaneous—kyphoscoliosis, Pickwikian syndrome, morbid obesity.

Treatment

- Treatment of primary cause.
- Nebulised bronchodilator.
- O_2 inhalation.
- In severe case, ventilatory support.

RESPIRATORY ALKALOSIS

Definition

It is a condition characterised by low PCO_2 and high pH secondary to hyperventilation.

Causes

- Hysterical hyperventilation, anxiety.
- Pregnancy.
- Respiratory—pulmonary embolism, pneumonia.
- CNS—meningitis, encephalitis.
- Salicylate poisoning.
- Metabolic acidosis.
- Vigorous assisted ventilation.

Treatment

- Correction of cause.
- Rebreathing in a closed bag.

CHAPTER

18 Paediatrics

CHAPTER CONTENTS

Common disease in children like measles, mumps, whooping cough, rheumatic fever, infectious disease, cardiac, respiratory, protein energy malnutrition (kwashiorkor, marasmus), etc. are described in respective chapters. Only few are described here.

CEREBRAL PALSY

Definition

Cerebral palsy (CP) is a disorder of posture and movement resulting from permanent, nonprogressive insult to the developing brain.

It may improve gradually with increasing age because of plasticity of brain.

Causes

- Intrauterine hypoxia.
- Perinatal asphyxia and hypoxic ischaemic encephalopathy.
- Birth trauma.
- Infection—meningitis, encephalitis.
- Intracerebral haemorrhage.
- Neonatal sepsis.
- Low birth weight.
- Kernicterus.
- Hypoglycaemia or other metabolic abnormalities.
- Congenital brain malformation.

Types

1. Spastic (75%)—
   - Hemiplegic.
   - Diplegic (lower limbs more severely affected).
   - Quadriplegic.
   - Monoplegic (rare).
2. Ataxic (15%).
3. Dyskinetic (choreoathetosis, tremor, rigidity, dystonia).
4. Hypotonic (1%).
5. Mixed type.

Clinical Features

Symptoms

1. Not achieving or delay of milestones of development, i.e. neck control, sitting, standing, crawling, walking, holding things etc.
2. Involuntary movements (e.g. choreoathetosis).
3. Other symptoms—
   - Seizure.
   - Mental retardation.

- Speech disturbance (e.g. dysarthria, dysrhythmia).
- Visual disturbance (e.g. squint, refractive error, defect in choroid or retina and blindness).
- Defect in hearing, interaction.

Signs

Due to involvement of pyramidal, extrapyramidal and cerebellum. Usual findings are as follows:

- Spasticity (e.g. scissoring, tight tendoachiles).
- Reflex—exaggerated.
- Ataxia.
- Involuntary movements.
- Occasionally hypotonia.
- Other findings—microcephaly, squint, persistence of primitive reflexes (e.g. palmer reflex, Moro reflex).

Investigations: Mainly Clinical

- CT scan or MRI of brain may be done to exclude other neurological disorders.

Management

1. Counselling of the parents.
2. Symptomatic treatment—
   - For seizures—anticonvulsants (phenytoin, phenobarbitone).
   - For spasticity—baclofen, diazepam, clonazepam, tinazidine.
   - In some cases, botulinum toxin to reduce spasticity.
3. Other therapies—
   - Physiotherapy.
   - Speech therapy.
   - Psychotherapy.
   - Social and rehabilitation.
   - Educational therapy.
   - Orthopaedic measures.
4. Follow-up, to assess improvement of the disabilities.

FEBRILE CONVULSION OR FEBRILE SEIZURE

Definition

It is defined as seizure during fever between 6 months and 5 years of age in the absence of intracranial infection.

It is the most common seizure disorder of children less than 5 years, more common in male child. Occurs among developmentally normal children following viral infection (90%), pneumonia, otitis media, tonsillitis, dysentery, UTI, etc.

Diagnostic Criteria

- Age—6 months to 5 years with a peak age 14–18 months.
- Temperature >38.8°C or 101.8°F.
- Seizures—mostly generalised tonic clonic, usually once within 24 hours, last from few seconds to few minutes, but not exceeding 15 minutes. Usually, one seizure attack in one episode, rarely two.
- Absence of signs of meningitis (e.g. bulging fontanelle, stiff neck. stupor and irritability).
- No residual neurological deficit.

Investigations

- CBC.
- Blood C/S.
- Throat swab C/S.
- X-ray chest.
- Urine R/E and C/S.
- Lumbar puncture andCSF study.
- Others—blood sugar, serum electrolytes, calcium.

NB: EEG and neuroimaging are not required in simple febrile seizure.

Treatment of Febrile Seizure

Acute episode—

- Explanation and reassurance to the parents.
- Maintaining airway, breathing and circulation.
- For fever—tepid sponging, fanning, paracetamol. Excess clothing is removed (ice-cold water should be avoided).
- Control of convulsion—diazepam per rectally (0.5 mg/kg) or IV (0.2–0.3 mg/kg).
- For infection—antibiotic (e.g. amoxicillin, ceftriaxone, etc.).

Prevention of Recurrence

- Intermittent prophylaxis—oral diazepam (1 mg/kg/day 8 hourly) with paracetamol should be given at the onset of fever, usually for 2–3 days.
- Continuous prophylaxis—not recommended, but may be considered if occurrence of seizure after 6 years of age, despite intermittent prophylaxis.

Counselling to the Parents

About the natural history, treatment and prognosis.

Prognosis

- Generally good.
- Recurrence is high in one-third of cases—50% in under 1-year of age, 30% in other situation. Frequency decreases after 5 year of age.
- In about 2% cases, may turn to epilepsy in later childhood.

Atypical Febrile Convulsion

If convulsion associated with fever persists for >15 minutes, occurs more than once in 24 hours, focal or unilateral in nature, followed by Todd's paralysis, but no significant other cause or CNS infection, it is called atypical febrile convulsion.

EEG may be abnormal for 2 weeks or more following the attack.

Treatment

Continuous prophylaxis therapy may be given—sodium valproate 30-60 mg/kg/day in two divided dose. To be continued for at least 2 year fit free or until the child is 6 years old whichever comes earlier.

NEONATAL PNEUMONIA

Definition

It is the infection and inflammation of lung parenchyma.

Causes

1. Early onset neonatal pneumonia, in first 7 days—
   - *E. coli.*
   - Group *B Streptococcus.*
   - *Klebsiella.*
   - *S. aureus.*
   - *Streptococcus pneumoniae.*
   - *Pseudomonas.*
2. Late onset neonatal pneumonia, after 3 weeks—
   - *Streptococcus pneumoniae.*
   - *S. aureus.*
   - *Klebsiella.*
   - *Streptococcus.*
   - *Pseudomonas.*

Clinical Features

Symptoms

- Fever (moderate to high).
- Cough.
- Respiratory distress.
- Not able to drink or stop feeding.
- Convulsion.
- Stridor.

Signs

- Wheeze.
- Cyanosis.
- Fast breathing.
- Chest indrawing.
- In chest—bronchial breath sounds, rhonchi, few crepitations.

Investigations

- CBC.
- CRP.
- X-ray chest P/A view.
- Arterial blood gas analysis.
- Nasopharyngeal or tracheal aspirate for C/S.

Treatment

- Counselling to the mother.
- Breastfeeding to be continued.
- Airway should be kept clear.
- O_2 inhalation.
- Bronchodilator.
- Antibiotic—Inj. ampicillin 50–100 mg/kg/day in four divided doseplus. Injection gentamycin 2.5 mg/kg/day, 8–12 hourly orcefotaxime 150 mg/kg/day or Inj. ceftriaxone 75 mg/kg/day. Antibiotic can be changed according to C/S.

BRONCHIOLITIS

Definition

It is an acute viral infection of the bronchioles resulting in inflammatory obstruction.

Causes

- Respiratory Syncytial virus (RSV), most common.
- Other organism—influenzae virus, parainfluenzae viruses, adenovirus, metapneumovirus, rhinovirus, sometimes mycoplasma.

Risk Factors

- Prematurity.
- Low socioeconomic status.
- Non breastfeeding.
- Crowded environment.
- Passive smoking.
- Indoor air pollution, etc.

Clinical Features

Symptoms

Common in children <2 years of age, peak 2–6 months. It occurs in epidemics, particularly during winter and rainy season.

- Running nose.
- Fever, usually low-grade.
- Cough.
- Respiratory distress.
- Loss of appetite.
- Irritability and crying.

Signs

- Tachypnoea.
- Flaring alaenasi.
- Movement of accessory muscles of respiration.
- Suprasternal, intercostal and subcostal recession.
- Cyanosis.
- Multiple rhonchi.
- Crepitaions.
- Liver and spleen—palpate due to downward pushing of diaphragm by hyperinflated lung.

Investigations

- X-ray chest—shows hypertranslucency and hyperinflation, interstitial shadow.
- CBC—normal.
- Blood gas analysis—shows low oxygen.
- Virus isolation from nasopharyngeal secretion by PCR or culture.

Treatment

Counselling the parents about the diseases.

Mild Case

- May be treated at home—normal feeding, cleaning nose with normal saline drop, bathing with lukewarm water.

Severe Case

- Hospitalisation if central cyanosis, unable to take food, restlessness, severe respiratory distress or chest indrawing, grunting.
- Propped up position.
- Oxygen inhalation.
- Correction of dehydration, if needed IV fluid.
- Nebulized salbutamol, 0.03 mL/kg/dose.
- For fever—tepid sponging, paracetamol.
- Antiviral—ribavirin in nebulized form, specially in cyanotic congenital heart disease, bronchopulmonary dysplasia, immunodeficiency.
- Steroid—short course prednisolone, mainly if family history of atopy.

Prognosis

- Good, most case recover in 5–7 days.
- Thirty to fifty percent may develop bronchial asthma, specially if there is family history of asthma.

MENINGITIS

Definition

It is the inflammation of leptomeninges (pia and arachnoid mater) by invasion of micro-organism.

Causes

It may be bacterial, viral, tuberculous, others (parasitic, fungal).

Bacterial (or Pyogenic) Meningitis

Causative Organisms

- Neonatal period (under 2 months)—*E. coli,* Pseudomonas, group B Streptococcus, Proteus.
- Two months to six years—*H. influenzae, S. pneumoniae, N. meningitidis.*
- Above 6 years—*Streptococcus pneumoniae, N. meningitidis.*

Clinical Features

Symptoms

In children

- High fever.
- Nausea, vomiting.
- Headache.
- Photophobia.
- Impaired consciousness.
- Recurrent convulsion.

In neonates: Presentations are nonspecific.

- Reluctant to feed.
- High-pitched cry.
- Vacant look.
- Hypo- or hyperthermia.
- Jitteriness.
- Convulsion.
- Respiratory distress.
- Features of sepsis.

Signs

- Altered sensorium or altered consciousness or stupor.
- Bulging of anterior fontanelle (in neonates and infants).
- Signs of meningeal irritation, e.g. neck rigidity, Kernig's sign (may not present in children <18 months).
- In Meningococcal septicaemia typical skin rash in different parts of body and sometimes features of shock.

Investigations

1. CBC shows polymorphonuclear leukocytosis.
2. Blood C/S may reveal the organism in 80% cases.
3. Lumbar puncture and CSF study—
   - Pressure—high.
   - Colour—cloudy or purulent.
   - Cytology—300-2000 cell/cmm, high neutrophil.
   - Biochemistry—protein (increased), glucose (decreased), corresponding blood sugar should be done.
   - Gram staining may show the organism.
   - Bacterial antigens may be detected by latex agglutination test or PCR for DNA of causative agent.
   - Culture and sensitivity.

Treatment

1. General
   - Maintenance of nutrition, IV fluid, 10% dextrose (if hypoglycaemia).
   - For fever—tepid sponging, paracetamol.
   - For convulsion—diazepam, phenytoin, phenobarbitone.
2. Specific
   - Ampicillin 400 mg/kg/day pluschloramphenicol 100 mg/kg/day 6 hourly or Ceftriaxone (100 mg/kg/day) once daily.
   - Vancomycin, if pneumococcus is suspected.
   - Antibiotic may be changed according to C/S.
   - Inj. dexamethasone IV 0.15/kg/dose 6 hourly for 2 days.

Duration of Treatment

7 days (if meningococcus), 10 days (if *H. influenzae*), 14 days (if pneumococcus).

Complications

Acute complications

- Hydrocephalus.
- Subdural effusion, empyema.
- Ventriculitis.
- Cerebral abscess.
- Cerebral infarction.
- Cranial nerve palsy.

Long-term complications

- Cerebral palsy.
- Deafness.
- Mental retardation.
- Epilepsy.
- Visual impairment.
- Learning and language disability.

VIRAL MENINGITIS

Causes

- Enterovirus (most common)—coxsackie virus, echo virus, polio virus, human enterovirus.
- Other viruses—herpes simplex, varicella zoster, cytomegalovirus, measles virus, Epstein-Barr virus, etc.

Clinical Features

Same as bacterial meningitis.

Investigations

1. CBC—normal, may be leucopenia with lymphocytosis.
2. Lumbar puncture and CSF study.
   - Colour—clear.
   - Cytology—lymphocytosis.
   - Biochemical (protein and glucose)—normal.
3. Others—blood glucose, electrolytes, creatinine, etc.

Treatment

Usually benign disease.

- General measures as in bacterial meningitis.
- In HSV, acyclovir 10 mg/kg 8 hourly for 14–21 days.

TUBERCULOUS MENINGITIS (TBM)

Cause

Mycobacterium tuberculosis.

Clinical Features

- History of contact with TB patient.
- History of fever, loss of weight, night sweating.
- Nausea, vomiting, headache, irritability.
- Convulsion, drowsiness, dizziness or impaired consciousness.
- Signs of meningeal irritation (neck rigidity, Kernig's sign).
- Cranial nerve palsy (3rd and 6th nerve).

Investigations

- CBC—high ESR.
- CSF study—high pressure, straw colour, high lymphocyte, high protein, low sugar, high ADA (adenosine deaminase), AFB may be positive, PCR.
- MT—may be positive.
- X-ray chest—may show primary focus.
- CT or MRI of brain.

Complications

- Hydrocephalus.
- Cranial nerve palsy.
- Deafness.
- Blindness.
- Hemiplegia or paraplegia.
- Mental retardation.

Treatment

- General measures.
- Specific—anti-TB (rifampicin, INH, pyrazinamide) for 2 months then INH and rifampicin for 10 months.
- Prednisolone 1-2 mg/kg/day for 4-6 weeks, then taper over 2-4 weeks.
- Pyridoxine to prevent peripheral neuropathy.

NB: Ethambutol is avoided in children, as they cannot complain of the features of optic neuritis (may become blind).

DIARRHOEA

Definition

It means frequent passage of loose stools. It is one of the important causes of death of children under 5 years of age.

Causes

- Virus—Rota virus, enterovirus.
- Bacteria—*E. coli, Shigella, Salmonella, Campylobacter, V. cholerae.*
- Parasitic—*Giardia lamblia, Entamoeba histolytica.*

Pathological Consequence

During diarrhoea, 3 important clinical consequences occur—

- Loss of water and electrolytes (sodium chloride, potassium bicarbonate) in the liquid stools.
- Loss of greater quantity of zinc in stool, which delays recovery of patients and make the child vulnerable to suffer afterwards.
- Weight loss due to less intake of food, less absorption and increased nutrient requirements.

Acute Watery Diarrhoea

When diarrhoea persists for <14 days.

Symptoms

- Patient passes loose watery stool several times (>3 times) daily that do not contain blood.
- Sometimes may have associated vomiting and low-grade fever.

Signs

- Signs of dehydration.
- Abdominal distension.
- Sign of severe malnutrition.

Signs of Dehydration

- Lethargy.
- Tears absent.
- Sunken eyes.
- Pinched face.
- Dry tongue.
- Unable to drink or drink poorly.
- Skin pinch goes back very slowly.

Assessment of Patient with Diarrhoea

- Frequency of diarrhoea, presence of blood.
- History of vomiting, attacks of crying with pallor, urine out put
- History about foods and feeding.
- Local reports of cholera outbreaks.

Investigations

- Stool for R/M/E and C/S.
- CBC and PBF.
- Serumurea, creatinine and electrolytes.
- Blood sugar.
- Others—plain X-ray of abdomen, ultrasonography.

Treatment

Essential elements in the management of diarrhoea are as follows:

- Rehydration therapy.
- Zinc supplementation.
- Continued feeding.
- Antimicrobials in specific cases.

Rehydration

No signs of dehydration: Plan A (treatment at home)—Advice to the mother about the following:

- Child is given more fluid to prevent dehydration until diarrhoea stops.
- More food to prevent under nutrition.
- If no improvement or baby drinks poorly or unable to drink or breastfeed orbecome more sick or develops fever or blood appears in stool—child should be transferred to the hospital or health center.

Rehydration at home with ORS or home based fluids after each loose stool as follows:

- Less than 2 years—50-100 mL.
- Two to ten years—100-200 mL.
- Ten years and above—as much as possible.

Some dehydration: Plan B

- Rehydration with ORS solution—75 mL/kg given in 4 hours at OPD and the child is monitored.
- Encourage mother for breastfeeding.
- For infant < 6 months who are not breastfed—100- 200 mL clear water should be given.
- After 4 hours of oral rehydration, the child's hydration status should be reassessed. If no signs of dehydration, treatment like A.
- If signs of severe dehydration still present - treatment is like plan C.

Severe dehydration: Plan C

1. Rapid IV rehydration 100 mL/kg, best IV fluid is Ringer's lactate solution (also called Hartman's solution) or cholera fluid. If not available, then 5% dextrose in normal saline can be used.
   - Infant under 12 months—30 mL/kg in 1 hour, then 70 mL/kg in 5 hour.
   - Older children—30 mL/kg in 30 minutes, then 70 mg/mg in 2½ hour.
2. Monitoring
   - Reassess the child every 15-30 minutes until a strong radial pulse is present.
   - When full amount of IV fluid has been given, reassess the child's hydration status.
   - If sign of severe dehydration still present—repeat IV fluid.
   - If signs of some dehydration—discontinue IV fluid and give ORS for 4 hours.
   - If no signs of dehydration—advise mother to give ORS after each loose stool as plan A.

Zinc Supplementation

- Less than 6 months—10 mg/day for 10–14 days.
- More than 6 months—20 mg/day for 10–14 days.

Continued Feeding

- Less than 6 months—breastfeeding.
- More than 6 months—breastfeeding plus freshly prepared high energy complementary foods like mashed rice, mashed banana, fresh fruit juice, etc.

Antimicrobials for Specific Disease

- Cholera—tetracycline (above 8 years), cotrimoxazole, azithromycin or erythromycin.
- Amoebiasis—metronidazole, tinidazole, nitazoxanide.
- Giardiasis—metronidazole, tinidazole.
- *Shigella*—ciprofloxacin, pivmecillinam, nalidixic acid, cotrimoxazole.

NEONATAL JAUNDICE

Definition

It is the yellow colouration of skin and mucous membrane of a newborn baby.

In adult, jaundice is seen when the serum bilirubin is >3 mg/dL, but in new born, jaundice is seen when serum bilirubin is >5 mg/dL.

Causes

According to age—

Early jaundice (jaundice within 10 days of age)

1. Within first 2 days—
   - Haemolytic disease of newborn (HDN)—Rh incompatibility, ABO incompatibility.
   - G-6-PD deficiency.
   - Congenital spherocytosis.
   - Congenital infection—TORCH (toxoplasmosis, rubella, cytomegalovirus, herpes).
2. Within 3–10 days—
   - Physiological jaundice.
   - Prematurity.
   - Hypoglycaemia.
   - Sepsis.
   - Congenital haemolyticanaemia.
   - Congenital nonhaemolytic hyperbilirubinaemia (Gilbert's syndrome, Dubin-johnson syndrome, Crigler-Najjar syndrome, Rotor syndrome).

Prolonged Jaundice (Jaundice >10 Days)

1. Prolonged unconjugated hyperbilirubinaemia—
   - Breast milk jaundice.
   - Sepsis.
   - Hypothyroidism.
   - Galactosaemia.
   - Rh incompatibility.
   - G-6-PD deficiency.
   - Congenital hemolytic anaemia.
2. Prolonged conjugated hyperbilirubinaemia—
   - Intrahepatic cholestasis
     - Infections—septicaemia, UTI, hepatitis.
     - Galactosaemia.
     - Alpha-1antitrypsin deficiency.
     - Hypothyroidism.
     - Idiopathic neonatal hepatitis.
   - Extrahepatic cholestasis
     - Biliary atresia.
     - Choledochal cyst.

Investigations

- CBC with PBF shows leucocytosis in sepsis, PBF shows fragmented or nucleated RBC in haemolytic disease.
- Serum bilirubin—high.
- Blood grouping ABO (to see ABO incompatibility) and Rh typing of mother and baby (negative mother and positive baby, if Rh incompatibility).
- Coomb's test—positive (if Rh incompatibility).
- Reticulocyte count—high in haemolytic disease.
- Others—enzyme assay, TORCH screening, USG of hepatobiliary system, chest X-ray, blood C/S.

Treatment

1. Counselling to the parents.
2. Nutrition—breastfeeding to be continued.
3. I/V fluid may be needed.
4. Spontaneous recovery in physiological jaundice.
5. In other cases, to reduce bilirubin—
   - Sunlight exposure—In early morning for 10–20 minutes every day.
   - Phototherapy—
     - If serum bilirubin >15 mg/dL for term baby.
     - If serum bilirubin 10–12 mg/dL for preterm baby.
   - Exchange transfusion when bilirubin >20 mg/dL with anaemiain Rh incompatibility and ABO incompatibility.
6. IV immunoglobulin may be helpful.
7. Treatment of underlying cause.

ABO Incompatibility

This is an ABO blood group incompatibility. If the mother has O group and the baby has A or B group, this causes haemolysis of RBC of the baby.

Rh Incompatibility

Here baby is Rh positive and mother is Rh negative. Rh antibody enters into the foetal blood stream resulting in destruction of foetal RBC.

KERNICTERUS

Definition

It is a neurological syndrome that occurs as a result of excess bilirubin in blood and it's deposition within the brain, mainly in basal ganglia.

Also involves hippocampus, subthalamic nuclei, thalamus. Cerebral cortex is spared.

Causes

- Prematurity.
- Haemolytic disease of the newborn.
- Congenital familial nonhaemolytic jaundice.

- Neonatal hepatitis.
- Congenital spherocytosis.

Clinical Features

Usually occur if bilirubin is >20 mg/dL.

Early Signs

- Lethargy, poor feeding and loss of Moro reflex are common initial signs.

Acute Bilirubin Encephalopathy, 3 Phases

- Phase I—hypotonia, lethargy, poor suck and depressed sensorium.
- Phase II—hypertonia progressing to opisthotonus, rigidity, oculogyric crisis.
- Phase III—high-pitched cry, convulsion, hypotonia, death.

Chronic Bilirubin Encephalopathy

- In the first year of life—opisthotonus, extrapyramidal rigidity, irregular movements and convulsion.
- Later, in older children—mental retardation, deafness, athetosis, poor formation and discolouration of teeth usually of green colour.

Treatment

Once established, kernicterus is irreversible and management is only symptomatic and supportive.

LOW BIRTH WEIGHT

Definition

Low birth weight (LBW) means baby with birth weight <2.5 kg irrespective of the gestational age.

It includes preterm or prematurity and small for date (SFD) or small or gestational age (SGA), also called intrauterine growth retardation (IUGR).

- Preterm: When baby is born before 37 weeks of gestation.
- Term: When baby is born after 37 weeks of gestation.
- Post-term: When baby is born beyond 2 weeks of expected date of delivery.
- Very-low birth weight baby: When birth weight is <1500 g but >1000 g.
- Extremely low birth weight baby: When birth weight is 1000 gm or less.
- Small for date or gestational age: Gestation is full-term but the baby is malnourished, therefore, low birth weight.

Causes of Prematurity

1. Foetal
   - Foetal distress.
   - Multiple gestations.
   - Erythroblastosisfoetalis.
2. Placental
   - Placental dysfunction.
   - Placenta previa.
   - Abruptio placentae.
3. Uterine
   - Bicornuate uterus.
   - Incompetent cervix.
4. Maternal
   - Teenage mother.
   - Pre-eclampsia.
   - Polyhydramnios.
   - Premature rupture of membrane.
   - Chronic medical illness (cyanotic heart disease, renal disease).
   - Infections (UTI, chorioamnionitis).
5. Others
   - Diabetes mellitus.
   - Rh incompatibility.

Causes of IUGR

1. Fetal
   - Chromosomal disorders (Trisomy).
   - Chronic foetal infection.
   - Radiation.
   - Multiple gestations.
2. Placental
   - Decreased placental weight or cellularity or both.
   - Villous placentitis.

- Tumour (chorioangioma, hydatidiform mole).
- Placental separation, infarction.
- Twin-twin transfusion syndrome.

3. Maternal
   - Toxaemia of pregnancy.
   - Hypertension.
   - Renal disease.
   - Hypoxaemia (high-altitude, cyanotic cardiac or pulmonary disease).
   - Malnutrition.
   - Chronic illness or anaemia.
   - Drugs (narcotics, alcohol).

Complications of Preterm Baby

1. Respiratory—
   - Respiratory distress syndrome or hyaline membrane disease.
   - Pneumothorax.
2. CVS—PDA.
3. GIT and hepatic—necrotising enterocolitis, poor motility, hyperbilirubinaemia.
4. Haematologic—early anaemia, DIC.
5. Neurological—intraventricular haemorrhage, seizure, retrolental fibroplasia in eye.
6. Electrolyte imbalance—hyponatraemia, hypokalaemia, hypokalaemia.
7. Metabolic—hypothermia, hypocalcaemia, hypoglycaemia.
8. Others—infection, neonatal death, still birth.
9. Late complication—cerebral palsy, seizure.

Complications of IUGR

- Meconium aspiration syndrome.
- Transient hypoglycaemic episode.
- Transient hyperglycaemia.

NEONATAL CONVULSION

Definition

It is defined as paroxysmal alteration in neurological function, such as behaviour, motor, autonomic function, either one or all three within 28 days of birth.

Causes

- Hypoxic ischaemic encephalopathy (most common).
- Birth trauma especially during forceps delivery.
- Infection—meningitis, viral encephalitis, TORCH.
- Metabolic—hypoglycaemia, hypocalcaemia, hypomagnesaemia, hyponatraemia.
- Kernicterus.
- Intracranial haemorrhage—intraventricular, subdural or subarachnoid.
- Congenital anomaly of brain.
- Toxic—maternal narcotic addiction.
- Pyridoxine deficiency.

Investigations

- CBC with ESR.
- Blood sugar.
- Serum electrolytes, serum calcium, serum magnesium.
- Arterial blood gas analysis.
- If indicated—lumbar puncture and CSF study.
- USG of the head.

Treatment

- Maintenance of airway, circulation.
- To prevent tongue biting, mouth gag is placed between jaws.
- Reduction of body temperature by tepid sponging.
- IV 10% dextrose, 5 mL/kg over 2-5 minutes.
- IV calcium gluconate 10%, 1 mL/kg mixed with distilled water.
- Inj. pyridoxine 50-100 mg, followed by 15 mg/kg as maintenance.
- For convulsion—diazepam 0.3 mg/kg or lorazepam 0.5 mg/kg IV or phenobarbitone 10-20 mg/kg IV and may be repeated 5-10 mg/kg. For maintenance dose 5-6 mg/kg twice daily. Or phenytoin may be given—20 mg/kg IV, then 8 mg/kg twice daily.
- If the baby is neurologically normal, drug may be discontinued. If neurologically abnormal, drug should be continued.

PERINATAL MORTALITY

Definition

Foetal death after 28 weeks of gestation and death occurring immediately after birth is called perinatal mortality.

Causes of Perinatal Mortality

- Low birth weight.
- Perinatal hypoxia.
- Neonatal infections.
- Congenital malformations.
- ABO and Rh incompatibility.
- Neonatal haemorrhage.
- Neonatal jaundice.
- Birth injuries.

CHAPTER

19 Genetics

CHAPTER CONTENTS

AUTOSOMAL DOMINANT DISEASES

It has the following characters:

- Consecutive generations are affected.
- Half of the offsprings are affected.
- Both male and female are equally affected.
- Unaffected individual cannot transmit the disease.
- Age of onset of the disease is variable. Affected person may remain symptom free up to adult life.

Some autosomal dominant diseases are as follows:

- Neurofibromatosis.
- Tuberous sclerosis.
- Huntington's disease.
- Adult polycystic kidney disease.
- Marfan's syndrome.
- Familial adenomatous polyposis coli.
- Pseudoxanthoma elasticum.
- Peutz-Jegher's syndrome.

AUTOSOMAL RECESSIVE DISEASES

It has the following characters:

- Half the children of unaffected carriers will be carriers.
- It affects both male and female.
- If both parents are carriers, 1 in 4 of children of heterozygous parents will be affected and half will be carrier.
- Usually only one generation is affected.
- Consanguinity increases the risk of autosomal recessive disorders.

Some autosomal recessive diseases:

- Hereditary haemochromatosis.
- Cystic fibrosis.
- Wilson's disease.
- Albinism.
- Xeroderma pigmentosum.
- Ataxia telangiectasia.
- Phenylketonuria.
- Alkaptonuria.

X-LINKED RECESSIVE DISEASES

It has the following characters: (X chromosome gene)

- Only males are affected, females are carrier.
- Unaffected female carriers transmit the disease.
- A female carrier will transmit the disease to half of her sons and half of her daughters will be the carrier.
- Affected males cannot transmit the disease to their sons, but all the daughters will be carrier.

Some X-linked Recessive Disorders

- Haemophilia A and B.
- Glucose-6 phosphate dehydrogenase deficiency.
- Duchenne muscular dystrophy.
- Alport syndrome.
- Fragile-X syndrome.

X-LINKED DOMINANT DISEASES

It has the following characters:
- X-linked diseases are rarely dominant.
- Females who are heterozygous for the mutant gene and males who have only one copy of the mutant gene on their single X chromosome will manifest the disease.
- Half of the male or female offspring of an affected mother will have the disease.
- All the female offspring of an affected man will have the disease.
- Affected man will always have affected daughter, never son.
- Women are more affected than men, M:F = 1:2.
- Affected males tend to have the disease more severely than the heterozygous female.

Some of the X-linked dominant diseases:
- Vitamin-D resistant ricket or familial hypophosphataemic ricket.
- Oro-facio-genital syndrome.

Nongerm line cytoplasmic inheritance (e.g. gene on mitochondrial DNA): It has the following characters—
- Males and females are affected.
- No males transmit the disease.
- Variable proportion of offspring from female are affected.

DOWN'S SYNDROME

Definition

It is a chromosomal abnormality, trisomy 21 (47, XX/XY, +21), caused by the presence of all or part of an extra 21 chromosome.

Types

1. Trisomy 21(47, XX/XY, +21)—most common (95%).
2. Mosaic variant.
3. Translocation variant.

Clinical Features

- Face—flat with flat nasal bridge, low set small ears.
- Mouth—appears small and tends to remain open with high arched palate.
- Tongue—appears protruding with large, horizontal fissure.
- Eyes—epicanthic folds and slanting eyes, Brushfield's spots on iris (yellow speckles), conjunctivitis.
- Neck—short and wide.
- Hands—single palmar crease (simian) and short stubby finger. Hand looks small and round (short, broad hands) and has clinodactyly (short inward curving of little finger).
- Foot—gap between first and second toe.
- Cardiac—VSD is common, also ASD, PDA, tetralogy of Fallot and mitral regurgitation due to endocardial cushion defect.
- Others—short stature, hypotonia, joint hyperextensibility, straight pubic hair and low IQ (from mild to severe).
- The child is fond of music.

NB: Down's syndrome is related to maternal age during pregnancy (incidence is high with increase of maternal age).

Investigations

- Karyotyping.
- Frequent follow-up to see complications.

Complications

- High incidence of leukaemia (in neonates, acute myeloid leukaemia and in older children, acute lymphoid leukaemia).
- Duodenal atresia.
- Presenile dementia of Alzheimer's type.
- Autoimmune hypothyroidism may occur.
- Mental retardation (mild to severe).
- Lenticular opacity.

Prenatal Screening

1. First trimester—
   - Nuchal translucency.
   - Human chorionic gonadotropin (HCG).
   - Pregnancy-associated plasma protein-A (PAPP-A).
2. At 13 to 20 weeks—
   - Maternal serum for alpha-fetoprotein, HCG , unconjugated oestriol (uE_3).
   - Foetal USG.
   - Amniocentesis.

TURNER'S SYNDROME

Definition

It is a sex chromosomal abnormality characterized by absence of one of X chromosomes (45, XO). It only affects females and all or part of one X chromosome is deleted, leading to failure of ovarian development. Externally, patient appears female, but does not produce female sex hormones. Hence, the patient remains sexually immature.

Clinical Features

Usually presents with amenorrhoea, underdeveloped secondary sexual characters. Features are:
- Short stature.
- Short, webbed neck, low hairline, redundant skinfold on the back of neck.
- Face—small lower jaw (micrognathia), small, fish-like mouth, high-arched palate, low-set deformed ears.
- Chest—broad, wide apart nipples (shield-like chest).
- Hand—short fourth metacarpal (other metacarpals may be short), lymphoedema of hands (also feet) and hypoplastic nails.
- Elbow—increased carrying angles (cubitus valgus).

Noonan's Syndrome

Definition

It is also called male Turner. It may affect both male and female equally.
- Female patients have Turner phenotype, but with normal 46, XX. They have normal ovarian function and normal fertility.
- In male, there is 46, XY. Cardiac lesion is present, more on right side (e.g. pulmonary stenosis). In Turner syndrome, left-sided cardiac lesion is more.

Clinical Features

- Short stature.
- Mental retardation (common).
- Downward slanting and wide-spaced eyes.
- Low set ear.
- Webbing of the neck.
- Low posterior hairline.
- Pulmonary stenosis.

KLINEFELTER'S SYNDROME

Definition

It is a chromosomal abnormality in which there is an extra X chromosome associated with hypogonadism (due to small testis).

Common **karyotype** abnormality usually 47, XXY which results from nondysjunction during meiosis in one of the parents, may be 46, XY or 47, XXY mosaic.

Clinical Features

- Tall stature (arm span greater than height and leg is more long, lower extremity is greater than upper extremity). Tallness is due to androgen deficiency with lack of epiphyseal closure in puberty.
- Obese.
- Gynaecomastia (carcinoma of breast may develop in 20% cases).
- Eunuchoid body proportion—see below.
- Absence or rudimentary external genitalia—small penis and testis (volume <5 mL).
- Absence of secondary sexual characters (axillary, pubic hair and beard).
- In mosaic, there may be normal puberty. Diagnosis is done during routine investigation for infertility.

Usual presentations of Klinefelter's Syndrome

- Poor sexual development.
- Infertility.
- Gynaecomastia.
- Small or undescended testis.

Associations in Klinefelter's Syndrome

- DM type 2.
- Low T_4.
- Bronchial asthma.
- Carcinoma of breast in male is more in Klinefelter's syndrome.

Investigations

- Serum testosterone (low), gonadotrophic hormones (increased FSH and LH).
- Serum oestrogen (increased).
- Azoospermia is universal.
- Chromosomal analysis (two or more X-chromosome, one or more Y-chromosome).

Treatment

- No specific treatment.
- Androgen (testosterone may be used in oral, injection, patch, gel and pellet).
- Plastic surgery for gynaecomastia.
- Life span is usually normal.

Abnormality of the testis in Klinefelter's syndrome: Both testes are small and firm. These show seminiferous tubules dysgenesis. Hyalinisation and fibrosis are present within the seminiferous tubules. Leydig cell function is impaired, resulting in hypogonadism. Also, there is azoospermia and high gonadotrophin.

Features of eunuchoid body proportion: Features are apparent from childhood—

- Tall stature with long leg.
- Hairless face (also sparse body hair).
- High-pitched voice.
- Small and poorly developed external genitalia.

Immature personality.

CHAPTER

20 Miscellaneous

CHAPTER CONTENTS

- Shock
- Proximal myopathy
- Vasculitis
- Wegener's granulomatosis
- Takayasu's disease
- Giant cell arteritis or temporal arteritis
- Polymyalgia rheumatica
- Polyarteritis nodosa
- Microscopic polyangitis
- Churg Strauss syndrome (allergic angiitis or granulomatosis)
- Behcet's syndrome
- Goodpasture's syndrome
- Restless leg syndrome
- HELLP syndrome
- Hereditary hemorrhagic telangiectasia
- Drowning
- Heat-related illness
- Alcoholism
- Wernicke's encephalopathy
- Adult Still's disease
- Rhabdoyolysis
- Toxic shock syndrome
- Pickwickian syndrome
- Hereditary angioedema
- Familial periodic paralysis
- Carcinoid syndrome
- Pseudomembranous colitis
- Kallman's syndrome
- Tumour lysis syndrome
- Kikuchi's disease
- Cavernous sinus thrombosis
- Fluid retention syndrome
- Hiccough
- Cystic fibrosis
- Oxygen therapy
- Paget's disease
- Charcot-Marie-Tooth disease
- HIV infection (AIDS)
- *Pneumocystis carinii* (jirovecii) pneumonia

SHOCK

Definition

Shock is a clinical syndrome characterized by inappropriate and inadequate tissue perfusion resulting in widespread reduction of oxygen and metabolic requirements to the tissues, leading to tissue damage or organ failure and death.

Classification: 4 Types—

- **Hypovolaemic shock**—there is reduction of blood volume, so decreased stroke volume and cardiac output.
- **Cardiogenic shock**—it is due to failure of the heart to maintain effective pump.
- **Extracardiacobstructive shock**—there is compression of the heart, so mechanical impairment of forward flow of blood.
- **Distributive shock**—there is profound impairment of peripheral circulation.Cardiac output may be normal or even high, but still inadequate tissue perfusion.

Pathophysiology

Sympathetic and adrenergic response: Due to hypotension, there is increase sympathetic nervous activity, release of adrenaline and noradrenaline. These cause vasoconstriction, increased cardiac contraction to maintain cardiac output and try to maintain blood pressure. Also, reduction to renal flow causes activation of renin-angiotensin mechanism, production of angiotensin II which stimulates aldosterone secretion by adrenal cortex, causing sodium and water retention which restore circulating volume.

Neuroendocrine response: There is release of pituitary hormones, such as ACTH, vasopressin, ADH. There is release of cortisol which causes fluid retention. Also, release of glucagon that raises blood sugar.

Release of pro- and anti-inflammatory mediators: Severe infection or hypoxia or prolong hypoperfusion may trigger exaggerated inflammatory response, causing release of chemical mediators, which are responsible for further organ damage.

Activation of coagulation system: Inflammatory response to shock, tissue injury and infection may be associated with systemic activation of clotting system, leading to platelet aggregation, multiple microvascular thrombosis and inadequate tissue perfusion. DIC also develops.

Clinical features of different shock: Some features are common in any shock and some features are according to the cause.

Hypovolaemic Shock

In this type of shock, there is reduction of blood volume, so decreased stroke volume and cardiac output, low BP, compensatory sympathetic over activity, peripheral vasoconstriction, all of which try to maintain BP. If not properly treated, there is profound hypotension, collapse of capillary and venous beds, tissue hypoxia and damage to the vital organs.

Causes

- Blood loss—bleeding due to any cause (e.g. haematemesis, melaena, multiple injury).
- Fluid and electrolytes loss—vomiting, diarrhoea, heat stroke, aspiration of fluid, diabetic ketoacidosis, excessive sweating.
- Plasma loss—burns, exfoliative dermatitis.

Signs of Hypovolaemic Shock

- Pinched face, shunken eyes.
- Cold and clammy extremities.
- Low BP—systolic BP <100 mmHg, narrow pulse pressure.
- Pulse—tachycardia (>100/min), low volume.
- Respiration—rapid and shallow.
- Oliguria (urinary output <30 mL/hour).
- Drowsiness, dizziness, irritability, confusion, stupor, coma.
- Low CVP and low pulmonary artery occlusion pressure (PAOP).
- If persists for long time, multiple organ failure and death may occur.

Treatment

- A—Airway should be kept clear.
- B—Breathing should be maintained, oxygen inhalation.
- C—Circulation, IV channel or CV line.
- Position—supine or leg raised.
- Replacement with blood, plasma or I/V fluid (crystalloids, such as normal saline, Ringer's lactate or colloids, such as albumin, dextran, haemaccel).
- Treatment of primary cause (bleeding, diarrhoea, etc.).

Cardiogenic Shock

In this type, there is impairment of cardiac function, because of structural damage of the heart.

Causes

- Acute myocardial infarction (commonest).
- Acute myocarditis.
- Cardiac arrest.
- Prolong cardiac bypass surgery.
- Dilated cardiomyopathy.
- Dissecting aortic aneurysm affecting ascending aorta.
- Cardiac arrhythmias.
- Acute valvular dysfunction, e.g. Acute MR or AR, severe AS or MS.
- Rupture of ventricular septum or wall.
- Ventricular aneurysm.

Signs of Cardiogenic Shock

- Features of primary disease (e.g. myocardial infarction).
- Raised JVP.

- Pulsus alternans.
- Gallop rhythm (in LVF).
- Bilateral basal crepitations (in pulmonary oedema).
- CVP and PAOP—increased.

Treatment

1. Treatment of primary cause.
2. General measures of shock (as above).
3. Inotropic drugs (dopamine, dobutamine, dopexamine, enoxamine).
4. Other therapy—
   - Diuretic.
   - Vasodilator therapy to reduce afterload.
   - Mechanical support of myocardium—Intra-aortic balloon counterpulsation (IABCP)
   - Corticosteroid—role is doubtful.

Extracardiac Obstructive Shock

In this type, heart is unable to contract, because of mechanical obstruction compressing the heart.

Causes

- Cardiac tamponade.
- Massive pulmonary embolism.
- Tension pneumothorax.

Signs of Extracardiac Obstructive Shock

- Features of primary disease (e.g cardiac tamponade, tension pneumothorax).
- Raised JVP.
- Pulsus paradoxus and muffled heart sounds in cardiac tamponade.
- Kussmaul's sign.

Treatment

- General measures like other shock (as above).
- Treatment of primary cause (e.g. aspiration in cardiac tamponade).

Distributive Shock

In this type, there is profound peripheral vasodilation and increased capillary permeability, cardiac output may be normal or even high, but still inadequate perfusion.

Causes

- Septic shock.
- Anaphylactic shock.
- Neurogenic shock.
- Vasodilator drug toxicity.
- Endocrine—Addisonian crisis, thyrotoxic crisis, myxoedema coma, hypopituitarism.

Treatment

- General measures of shock.
- Treatment of primary cause.

Septic Shock

Definition

It is characterized by development of shock as a result of septicaemiaor endotoxin produced by different micro-organisms.

It is common in very young and very old patients. May be associated with diabetes mellitus, malignancy, immunosuppressive therapy, hepatobiliary, GIT, gynaecological and urinary abnormalities.

Causative Organisms

- Gram-negative septicaemia is the commonest cause (eg *E. coli*, Klebsiella, Proteus, Pseudomonus, Serratia). Also Gram-positive organisms.
- Bacteroids.

Mechanism of Septic Shock

- Initially, exposure to trigger factors (organism, toxin or both).
- Then host response (inflammatory response), acts on leucocytes, endothelium and other cells.
- Then there is synthesis and release of chemical mediators from monocytes, macrophages, neutrophils, endothelial cells.
- Chemical mediators are—cytokines (IL I, II, VI, VIII and TNF), platelet activating factor, arachidonic acid metabolites (prostaglandin, prostacycline, thromboxane A_2), leukotriens, lysosomal enzymes, endothelial derived vasoactive mediators (endothelin-1 and NO).
- There are multiple effects on microcirculation, heart and blood.

Effect on microcirculation: There is vasodilation and also vasoconstriction, resulting in maldistribution of blood flow, arteriovenous shunting, endothelial destruction and increased capillary permeability.

Effect on heart: There is myocardial depression, so decreased strokevolume, decreased cardiac output, leading to shock.

Effect on blood: Activation of clotting cascade, platelet aggregation, activation of plasminogen to plasmin, which breaks the clot with formation of FDP resulting in DIC. Also damage of capillary endothelium may occur.

Because of these changes, multiple organs are affected. If properly treated, there is full recovery. If no recovery, shock develops which is irreversible, resulting in organ failure, renal failure, hepatic failure, ARDS, DIC, impaired consciousness, coma and death.

Signs of Septic Shock

- History of high fever with chill and rigor.
- Warm periphery.

- Pulse—high volume, bounding.
- Evidence of DIC.
- Multiple organ failure.
- Other features of shock (as in hypovolaemic shock).

Treatment

1. General measures—
   - A—Airway should be kept clear.
   - B—Breathing should be maintained,oxygen inhalation.
   - C—Circulation, IV channel or CV line.
   - Position—supine or leg raised.
2. Antibiotic—broad spectrum **plus** metronidazole.
5. Others—
   - Correction of anaemia to raise Hb >10g/dL.
   - O_2 saturation >92%
   - Correction of electrolytes, calcium, magnesium, albumin.
   - Respiratory support.
   - Steroid—methylprednisolone1g with 200cc 5% DA IV daily for 5 days.

NB: In any case of shock, intubation may be necessary if—

- $PaCO_2$—>6.5 kPa.
- Respiratory rate >25/min.
- Impaired consciousness.

Anaphylactic Shock

Definition

Anaphylaxis is a serious allergic reaction arises as acute IgE mediated immune reaction involving antigen, mast cell and basophil.

Pathogenesis

Initially, there is sensitization to an antigen. Subsequent exposure to that antigen produces IgE induced degranulation of mast cells and basophils, resulting in liberation of multiple chemical mediators, such as histamine, leukotriens, prostaglandin activating factors, kinins causing shock.

Causes

- Drugs—penicillin, cephalosporins, vancomycin, insulin, snake venoms, radiographic contrast media.
- Blood transfusion.
- Foods—fish, egg, milk, peanut, strawberry, soya product.
- Insect bite—bee, wasp sting.
- Serum and vaccines—ATS, anti-rabies vaccine.
- Latex.

Clinical Features

- **General**—local tingling, warm, itching, urticaria, angio-oedema, flushing, warm periphery, oedema of face, pharynx and larynx.

- **Respiratory**—bronchospasm, dyspnoea, wheeze, laryngealoedema causing stridor.
- **Abdominal**—nausea, vomiting, abdominal pain, diarrrhoea.
- **Cardiovascular**—tachycardia, hypotension, arrhythmias or myocardial infarction leading to shock, collapse and death.

Treatment

- A—Airway should be kept clear.
- B—Breathing should be maintained, oxygen inhalation (100%).
- C—Circulation, IV channel or CV line.
- Position—supine or leg raised.
- IV fluid—normal saline or 5% DNS.
- Injection—adrenaline 0.5 mg IM.
- Injection—hydrocortisone 100–200 mg IV.
- Injection—antihistamine (chlorphenamine 10–20 mg IV).
- Intubation may be necessary, if hypoxia or hypotension is severe.

Prevention

- Avoidance of allergen (food, drugs).
- Patient's education regarding the use of drugs, such as adrenaline, hydrocortisone during emergency.
- To maintain a **MedicAlert bracelet** naming the culprit allergen.
- Desensitization in some case, where allergen is unavoidable.

Neurogenic Shock

It is caused by major brain or spinal cord injury, which disrupt brain stem and neurogenic vasomotor control. There is arteriolar dilatation, venodilatation which causes pooling of blood in the venous system, decreased venous return and cardiac output, resulting in shock.

Clinical Features

Same like other shock. There is hypotension due to vasodilatation with paradoxically slow heart rate. Extremities are warm.

Treatment

- General measures as in other shock.
- Excessive fluid are required to maintain normal circulation.
- Norepinephrine may be necessary to maintain increased vascular resistance.
- Treatment of primary cause.

PROXIMAL MYOPATHY

Definition

It means weakness of upper arm and thigh muscles. Patient complains of difficulty in raising the arm above the head, combing, standing from sitting.

Causes

- Dermatomyositis or polymyositis.
- Myasthenia gravis.
- Myasthenicmyopathic syndrome (Eaton Lambert syndrome).
- Myopathy (limb girdle, fascioscapulohumeral and mitochondrial) except myotonic dystrophy.
- Cushing's syndrome.
- Diabetic amyotrophy.
- Thyrotoxicosis (also hypothyroidism).
- Polymyalgia rheumatica.
- Osteomalacia.
- Hyperparathyroidism.
- Familial periodic paralysis.
- Alcohol and drugs (steroid, chloroquine, amiodarone, lithium and zidovudine).
- McArdle's syndrome (myophosphorylase deficiency, there is stiffness and cramps of muscle after exercise, which is hard and painful on movement).

Causes of Distal Muscle Weakness

- Myotonic dystrophy.
- Charcot Marie Tooth disease.
- Peripheral neuropathy (except diabetic amyotrophy).
- Distal myopathy.

VASCULITIS

Definition

It is the Inflammation of the vessel wall.

Classification

1. Cutaneous small vessel (postcapillary venule)—
   - Idiopathic cutaneous small vessel vasculitis.
   - Henoch Schonlein purpura.
   - Acute hemorrhagic oedema of infancy.
   - Urticarial vasculitis.
   - Cryoglobulinaemic vasculitis.
   - Others—drug induced, malignancy, connective tissue diseases, inflammatory bowel disease, HIV infection, Behcet's syndrome, Sweet syndrome, erythema nodosum leprosum.
2. Medium vessel—
   - Polyarteritis nodosa.
   - Kawasaki's disease.

3. Mixed (medium and small) vessel disease—
   - Connective tissue disease (e.g. rheumatoid vasculitis).
   - Septic vasculitis.
   - ANCA associated—Microscopic polyangiitis, Wegener's granulomatosis, allergic granulomatosis (Churg-Strauss syndrome).
   - Drug induced (most are postcapillary venule only).
4. Large vessel vasculitis—
   - Giant cell arteritis.
   - Takayasu's arteritis.

WEGENER'S GRANULOMATOSIS

Definition

It is a disorder of unknown aetiology characterized by necrotising granulomatous vasculitis of upper and lower respiratory tract with glomerulonephritis (focal, segmental, necrotising). It is called granulomatous polyangitis.

Clinical Features

This occurs in both male and female.

- **Nasal**: Discharge, epistaxis, nasal obstruction, nasal crust, rhinitis and sinusitis. If untreated, destruction of nasal bone and cartilage causes depressed nose, deafness due to inner ear involvement (serous otitis media).
- **Respiratory**: Cough, haemoptysis, chest pain and breathlessness.
- **Eye**: Conjunctivitis, episcleritis, iritis. There may be proptosis (due of inflammation of retro-orbital tissue). This causes diplopia due to entrapmentof extraocular muscles, or loss of vision due to optic nerve compression. Disturbance of colour vision is an early feature of optic nerve compression.
- **Renal:** Features of glomerulonephritis or renal failure.

Investigations

- CBC and ESR (leucocytosis with very-high ESR)
- CRP—high.
- Urine RME.
- Serum urea, creatinine and electrolytes.
- Serum complement—normal or slightly high.
- Chest X-ray—single or multiple nodules (migrating lung lesion in 50% cases).
- MRI of chest may be done.
- Biopsy—from nasal lesions or nasal crusts and also from kidney. It shows necrotising vasculitis with granuloma formation.
- C-ANCA—positive (helpful for diagnosis and to see the relapse).

Treatment

- Cyclophosphamide (2 mg/kg) plus prednisolone (1 mg/kg). Or
- Intravenous cyclophosphamide (15 mg/kg) plus IV methylprednisolone (10 mg/kg) every fortnight and then every month.
- Once remission occurs (takes 3–6 months)—maintenance therapy with low-dose prednisolone and azathioprine, methotrexate or mycophenolatemofetil (MMF).
- Rituximab with high-dose steroid is equally effective as oral cyclophosphamide.
- Oral cotrimoxazole (960 mg, three times weekly) is given to prevent pneumocystis pneumonia.
- There is tendency to relapse -so follow-up regularly should be done to check for recurrence. Measurements of ESR, CRP and ANCA should be done.

TAKAYASU'S DISEASE

Definition

It is a chronic, inflammatory, granulomatous panarteritis of unknown cause involving the elastic arteries commonly aorta and its major branches, carotid, ulnar, brachial, radial and axillary.

Occasionally, may involve pulmonary artery, rarely abdominal aorta, renal artery resulting in obstruction.

It is also called pulseless disease or aortic arch syndrome.

Pathological Changes

Panarteritis, intimal hyperplasia, thickening of media, thickening of adventitia and later on fibrosis.

Clinical Features

Common in young females, 25–30 years, more in Asians. F:M ratio is 8:1.

- In acute stage—may present with fever, malaise, weight loss, arthralgia, myalgia and high ESR.
- In chronic case—dizziness, giddiness, headache, blurring of vision, syncope, claudication in the upper limb.
- There may be aortic regurgitation, renal artery stenosis or anginal pain.
- Features of hypertension.

Signs

- All the pulses of upper limbs are absent, but present in lower limbs (so it is called **reverse coarctation syndrome**).
- BP is undetectable in upper limb and normal or high in lower limb
- Bruit may be present over the carotid, also renal bruit.
- Signs of aortic regurgitation may be present.
- There may be less development of upper part of the body.
- Fundoscopy—shows wreath like anastomosis around the optic disk.

Types: 4 Types—

1. Type 1—Involves aortic arch and its major branches.
2. Type 2—Involves descending aorta and abdominal aorta.
3. Type 3—Involves both type 1 and type 2. This may be complicated by aortic regurgitation.
4. Type 4—Involves the pulmonary arteries.

Investigations

- CBC (high ESR and normocytic normochromic anaemia).
- Chest X-ray shows cardiomegaly and widening of aorta.
- Aortography of aortic arch and its branches—shows narrowing, coarctation and aneurysmal dilatation.
- Serum immunoglobulin—high.

Treatment

- Prednisolone 40–60 mg daily or 1–2 mg/kg.
- If refractory to steroid or difficult to taper steroid—methotrexate up to 25 mg weekly.
- Cyclophosphamide may be used in resistant case.
- Reconstructive vascular surgery in selected case.
- Angioplasty, stenting or bypass surgery may be done, if there is vascular complication.
- Treatment of hypertension.

Complications

Heart failure, stroke.

Prognosis

Ninety five percent survive up to 15 years.

GIANT CELL ARTERITIS OR TEMPORAL ARTERITIS

Definition

Giant cell arteritis (GCA) or temporal arteritis is an inflammatory granulomatous arteritis of unknown cause involving the large arteries, predominantly affecting temporal and ophthalmic artery.

Clinical Features

Common in female (F:M = 4:1), 60–75 years of age, rare <50 years.May be associated with polymyalgia rheumatica.

- Headache, mostly on temporal and occipital region with local tenderness.
- Temporal artery is thick, hard, tortuous and tender.
- Jaw claudication, worse on eating.
- Pain in the face, jaw and mouth (due to involvement of facial, maxillary and trigeminal branch of external carotid artery).
- TIA, visual disturbance.
- Most dangerous feature is sudden painless temporary or permanent loss of vision in one eye, due to involvement of the ophthalmic artery (called acute ischaemic optic neuritis).
- Systemic features—severe malaise, tiredness, weakness, weight loss, arthralgia, mayalgia, fever.
- PUO may be the only feature, common in elderly.

Investigations

- CBC and ESR—normocytic normochromic anaemia, very-high ESR.
- CRP—high.
- ANA and ANCA—negative.
- Temporal artery biopsy—shows intimal hypertrophy, inflammation of intima and subintima, breaking up or fragmentation of internal elastic lamina, infiltration of lymphocyte, plasma cells and giant cells in internal elastic lamina with necrosis of arterial media. Biopsy from the affected site should be taken before starting or within 7 days of starting steroid.
- Fundoscopy—optic disc may appear pale and swollen with haemorrhage.

Treatment

- Prednisolone 60–100 mg/day for 1–2 months, then taper slowly (with the guide of ESR and CRP). To be continued for long time.
- Low-dose aspirin.
- Monitoring ESR and CRP, markers of disease activity.
- Relapse may occur in 30% cases. May be difficult to taper the dose, then methotrexate or azathioprine may be added.

NB: If any elderly patient presents with unilateral headache associated with unexplained fever, arthritis with very-high ESR, giant cell arteritis or temporal arteritis is the likely diagnosis.

POLYMYALGIA RHEUMATICA

Definition

Polymyalgia rheumatica (PMR) is characterized by severe pain and stiffness of the muscles of shoulders, neck, hips, lower back and thigh, in limb girdle pattern. It occurs isolated or associated with giant cell arteritis.

Clinical Features

Common in middle age above 50, more in women.

- Symptoms are worse in the morning, lasting from 30 minutes to several hours.
- Because of pain and stiffness—patients complains of difficulty in combing the hair, raising from sitting.
- General features—tiredness, fever, weight loss, depression and occasionally nocturnal sweating.
- On examination—stiffness and painful restriction of active shoulder movement, but passive movements are preserved.Muscles may be tender, but weakness and muscle wasting are absent.

Investigations: Diagnosis is Clinical

- CBC, ESR—shows anaemia (mild normochromic, normocytic). High ESR and CRP are hallmark.
- Serum alkaline phosphatase and gumma-glutamyltranspeptidase may be high in acute inflammation.
- Temporal artery biopsy shows giant cell arteritis in 10–30%.

Treatment

- Prednisolone—15–30 mg/day. Steroid dose should be tapered when symptoms improve, 10–15 mg for 8 weeks.Then maintenance of 5–7.5 mg daily and continued for 12–24 months.
- Steroid sparing agents—methotrexate or azathioprine may be given if requirement of prednisolone is >7.5 mg daily.
- Prophylaxis against osteoporosis should be given in patients with low BMD.

POLYARTERITIS NODOSA

Definition

Polyarteritis nodosa (PAN) is a multisystem necrotizing vasculitis involving medium and small vessels accompanied by severe systemic manifestations. It is occasionally associated with hepatitis B antigenaemia with secondary to deposition of immune complexes.

Pathology

There is fibrinoid necrosis of small and medium-sized muscular artery with microaneurysm formation, thrombosis and infarction. Lesion is segmental, involves the bifurcation and branching artery. May spread circumferentially to involve the adjacent venule. In kidney, there is arteritis but no glomerulonephritis. No pulmonary artery involvement. No granuloma, no eosinophilia and no allergic features (these occur in Wegener's granulomatosis).

Clinical Features

Usually in middle age, 40–50 years, more in males, M:F is 2:1.

- General features—fever, malaise, weakness,weight loss, headache and myalgia. These initial symptoms are followed by dramatic acute features that are due to organ infarction.
- Neurological—features of peripheral neuropathy, mononeuritis multiplex (due to arteritis of vasa nervorum). CVD, seizure may also occur.
- GIT—abdominal pain, nausea, vomiting, cholecystitis, pancreatitis or appendicitis. GI bleeding occurs due to mucosal laceration.
- Renal—severe hypertension, renal impairment due to multiple renal infarctions, but glomerulonephritis is rare (in contrast to microscopic polyangiitis). May be haematuria and proteinuria.
- Cardiac—coronary arteritis causes myocardial infarction and heart failure. Pericarditis also occurs.
- Skin—rash, palpable purpura, nodule, ulceration, infarction and livedoreticularis, subcutaneous haemorrhage and gangrene.
- Raynaud's phenomenon may be present.
- Musculoskeletal—arthritis, arthralgia, myalgia.
- Lung—involvement is rare.

Investigations

- CBC, ESR—shows anaemia, neutrophilic leukocytosis, high ESR.
- HbsAg—positive in 10–30% cases.
- Biopsy of muscle or sural nerve or from an affected organ—shows features of vasculitis.
- Angiography—to see microaneurysms in hepatic, intestinal or renal vessels, if necessary.
- Other investigations as appropriate—ECG, abdominal ultrasound, depending on the clinical problem.
- ANCA is usually negative (positive only rarely in classic PAN).

Treatment

- Prednisolone 1 mg/kg body weight with cyclophosphamide 2 mg/kg for 6–12 months.
- Maintenance with azathioprine or methotrexate.

MICROSCOPIC POLYANGIITIS

Definition

Microscopic polyangiitis (MPA) is a disorder characterized by necrotising vasculitis with few or no immune complex affecting small vessels, such as capillaries, arterioles and venules.

Pathology

There is necrotisingvasculitis that involves small and medium size arteries with capillaries and venules. Renal arteritis causes rapidly progressive glomerulonephritis, often in association with pulmonary capillary involvement which causes alveolar haemorrhage.

Clinical Feature

Common in elderly, above 57 years, more in females.

- General features—fever, weight loss, arthralgia, myalgia.
- Renal—RPGN causing renal failure.
- Pulmonary—haemoptysis, cough, breathlessness, pleural effusions (15%).
- Cutaneous—palpable purpura, skin rash, nodule, ulceration.
- Gastrointestinal—abdominal pain, nausea, vomiting, diarrhoea.
- Neurologigal—peripheral neuropathy, mononeuritis multiplex.

Investigations

- CBC, ESR—shows high ESR, anaemia, leukocytosis, thrombocytosis.
- P-ANCA (myeloperoxidase-MPO)—positive in 75%.
- Chest X-ray—may be normal, infiltration due to haemorrhage.
- Kidney biopsy—shows necrotizing arteritis.

Treatment

- Prednisolone 1 mg/kg plus cyclophophamide 2 mg/kg for 3–6 months, then maintenance with azathioprine or methotrexate.

CHURG-STRAUSS SYNDROME (ALLERGIC ANGIITIS OR GRANULOMATOSIS)

Definition

It is a small and medium vessel necrotizing granulomatous vasculitis characterized by cutaneous vasculitic lesions, respiratory involvement, asthmatic symptoms with eosinophilia (less in PAN).

Clinical Features

Common in males, in 4th decade.

- Nasal polyp, allergic rhinitis and adult-onset asthma usually occur before vasculitis by many years. Pulmonary infiltrate and eosinophilia are the main features.
- Fever, arthralgia, myalgia, weight loss.
- Skin rash, tender nodules.
- Mononeuritis or polyneuropathy.
- Gastrointestinal and cardiac involvement may occur.
- Hypertension.
- Glomerulonephritis (uncommon).

American College of Rheumatology (ACR): Presence of 4 or more is highly indicative of Churg Strauss syndrome—

1. Asthma.
2. Eosinophilia (10% on WBC differential).
3. Mononeuropathy or polyneuropathy.
4. Migratory or transient pulmonary infiltrates.
5. Systemic vasculitis (cardiac, renal, hepatic).
6. Extravascular eosinophils on biopsy of artery, arteriole or venule.

Differential Diagnosis

- Wegener's granulomatosis.
- Microscopic polyangiitis (also polyarteritis nodosa).

Investigation

Diagnosis is usually clinical.

- CBC with ESR (eosinophilia is common).
- Chest X-ray—shows transient patchy pneumonia-like shadow.
- P-ANCA—usually positive.
- C-ANCA—negative, done to exclude Wegener's granulomatosis.
- Kidney biopsy—shows necrotizing granulomatous vasculitis with extravascular eosinophilic infiltration (lung or calf muscle biopsy may be done).
- ANA and anti-ds DNA (to exclude SLE).

Treatment

- High-dose steroid and cyclophosphamide, then maintenance therapy with low-dose steroid and azathioprine, MTX, mycophenolatemofetil (MMF).
- Major lifethreatening organ involvement may require treatment with pulse doses of IV methylprednisolone.

NB: Triad of asthma, eosinophilia and positive p-ANCA strongly suggests Churg Strauss syndrome.

BEHCET'S SYNDROME

Definition

It is a vasculitis of unknown cause, characterized by recurrent oral, genital ulcer, ocular and skin lesion. There may be joint and neurological lesion. It mainly involves small arteries and venules.

Clinical Features

Common in males. Oral and genital ulcers are present in most patients.

- Recurrent oral ulceration, deep and multiple.
- Genital ulcers.
- Skin—erythema nodosum, diffuse pustular rash, erythema multiforme.
- Ocular—recurrent uveitis and iridocyclitis, retinal vascular lesions and optic atrophy, can lead to loss of vision in 50%.
- Recurrent thrombophlebitis may occur, leading to venous thrombosis. Less often, superior or inferior vena caval thrombosis, abdominal pain and bloody diarrhoea may occur.
- Seronegative arthritis, involving knees, ankles and wrists.
- Asymptomatic proteinuria is a recognized feature, but rarely may cause renal amyloidosis.
- Neurological complications occur in 5% cases. Organic confusional state, meningoencephalitis, transient or persistent brainstem syndromes.

NB: All manifestations are self-limiting except ocular attacks. Repeated attacks of uveitis can cause blindness.

Investigations

No specific investigations.

- Pathergy test is a useful diagnostic sign. It is demonstrated by pricking the skin by needle, there is pustule formation at venipuncture site within 24–48 hours.

Criteria for Diagnosis

It is a clinical diagnosis. No specific test.

- Recurrent oral ulcers, at least three times in 12 months

Plus 2 of the following—

- Recurrent genital ulceration.
- Eye lesion.
- Skin lesion.
- Positive pathergy test.

Treatment

- For oral ulcer and genital ulcer—topical steroid.
- Thalidomide 100–300 mg/day for 28 days is effective in resistant oral and genital ulcer.
- Colchicine is effective in erythema nodosum and arthralgia.
- Systemic steroid, immunosuppressive agent or ciclosporin are used for uveitis and neurological disease.
- Anti-TNF agent can be used in severe uveitis, neurological and gastrointestinal manifestations.

GOODPASTURE'S SYNDROME

Definition

It is a clinical syndrome of glomerulonephritis and pulmonary hemorrhage mediated by anti-GBM antibody. The antibody is usually IgG type which binds with glomerular or alveolar basement membrane.

Clinical Features

It is more in males, age 20–40 years, exclusively in smoker. Females are affected more, if it occurs after the age of 60 years.

- Initially upper respiratory tract infection—cough, recurrent hemoptysis, dyspnea.
- Followed by renal involvement—proteinuria, haematuria due to progressive, proliferative glomerulonephritis or features of renal failure.
- In one-third cases, no lung injury, only glomerulonephritis is present.
- Systemic features like fever, malaise, arthritis, headache, weight loss are not common, but may occur. Hypertension is usually not a feature. Chest pain and pleurisy are also rare.

Investigations

- CBC.
- Chest X-ray (shows blotchy opacities due to lung haemorrhage).
- USG of abdomen to see KUB.
- Anti-GBM antibody is positive (usually IgG).
- p-ANCA—positive in 30% cases.
- ANA—negative.
- Complements—normal.
- Lung function test—increased CO transfer due to pulmonary haemorrhage. Restrictive lung disease may occur in advanced stage.
- In sputum—haemosiderin-laden macrophage may be present.
- Kidney biopsy—shows proliferative or crescentic glomerulonephritis.

Treatment

- Plasmapheresis—to remove circulating antobodies.
- Methylprednisolone IV, 1–2 g/day for 3 days.
- Cyclophosphamide 2–3 mg/kg/day may be given.
- Occasionally, kidney transplantation may be considered.
- Recurrence may occur in transplanted kidney.

NB: In young patient with renal and lung involvement, causes are—

- Goodpasture's syndrome.
- Microscopic polyangitis.
- Wegener's granulomatosis.
- SLE.
- In elderly, bronchial carcinoma with metastasis in the kidney or membranous glomerulonephritis.

RESTLESS LEG SYNDROME

Definition

Restless leg syndrome (RLS) (also called Ekbom's syndrome) is a neuromuscular abnormality, characterized by discomfort or abnormal sensation in the calf or feet requiring irresistable and frequent movement of the affected limb.

Causes

It is a common complication in chronic renal failure. May also occur in iron deficiency anaemia.

Clinical Features

It is worse in the evening or at the onset of sleep at night, interfering with sleep. Commonly involves the lower limbs, may also involve upper limbs. Exaggerated by pregnancy, inactivity, caffeine, sleep disturbance, etc.

It is common in normal population, 1-5% (average 2%) cases, in middle age. But frequency increases up to 20-30%, if occurs after 60 years. May be familial in one-third cases, multiple members in the family may be affected, occasionally inherited as autosomal dominant. When RLS is associated with iron deficiency anaemia and CRF, it is called secondary RLS.

Treatment

- Clonazepam (0.5-2 mg), levodopa (100-200 mg), dopamine agonist (pramipexole or ropinirole).
- Narcotics, benzodiazepine and anticonvulsant may be helpful.
- Treatment of primary cause, e.g. CKD.

HELLP SYNDROME (HELP SYNDROME)

Definition

HELLP syndrome usually occurs in a patient with preeclampsia. It stands for—

- **H**—Haemolysis.
- **EL**—Elevated liver enzymes.
- **LP**—Low platelet.

HELLP syndrome is a variant of preeclampsia, affects 1 per 1000 pregnancies, common in multiparous women. Perinatal mortality is 10-60% and maternal mortality is 1.5-5%. In 15% cases, BP may be normal and proteinuria may be absent.

HELLP syndrome usually occurs in last trimester of pregnancy or within the first week of delivery. Liver disease is associated with hypertension, proteinuria and fluid retention. Serum transaminases are high and the condition can be complicated by hepatic infarction and rupture.

Differential diagnoses are HUS (hemolytic uremic syndrome), TTP (thrombotic thrombocytopenic purpura) and fatty liver. However, in TTP and HUS, no hypertension or no proteinuria. In fatty liver, transaminases are very high.

Investigations

- CBC—low platelet, increased reticulocyte count.
- LFT (SGPT, SGOT)—high.
- Urine RE—proteinuria in preeclampsia.

- USG of hepatobiliary system.
- Others—blood sugar, electrolytes, calcium, magnesium, prothrombin time.

Treatment

1. Prompt delivery is indicated in the following conditions—
   - Pregnancies ≥34 weeks of gestation.
   - Nonreassuring tests of fetal status (e.g. biophysical profile, fetal heart rate testing).
   - Maternal disease—multiorgan dysfunction, DIC, liver infarction or hemorrhage, renal failure, abruptio placentae.
2. In <34 weeks—IV dexamethasone may be given.
3. Other therapies—
   - Control of hypertension.
   - Platelet and blood transfusion may be necessary.
   - If convulsion—magnesium sulfate intravenously.
   - In severe renal failure—dialysis may be necessary.

Complications of HELLP Syndrome

Maternal—

- DIC.
- Abruptio placentae.
- Acute renal failure.
- Pulmonary oedema.
- Subcapsular liver hematoma.
- Retinal detachment.

Foetus/neonate—

- Prematurity.
- Intrauterine growth retardation.
- Sequele of abruptio placentae, perinatal mortality.

HEREDITARY HAEMORRHAGIC TELANGIECTASIA

Definition

It is inherited as autosomal dominant, characterized by multiple telangiectasia in the skin and mucous membrane in different parts of the body. It is also called Osler-Weber-Rendu disease.

Clinical Features

Symptoms

- Epistaxis (common), usually recurrent and sometimes the only site of bleeding.
- GIT bleeding (haematemesis, melaena).
- Pulmonary arteriovenous fistula may develop causing haemoptysis, cyanosis and clubbing.
- Bleeding from other sites.
- Anaemia (due to chronic blood loss, especially from GIT).
- Paradoxical embolism, stroke and cerebral abscess may occur.
- AV aneurysm may also occur in liver.
- In the eye—bloody tear (conjunctival telangiectasia), retinal haemorrhage and even detachment may occur.
- Neurological telangiectasia may cause haemorrhage and mycotic aneurysm.

Signs

- Telangiectasia (It is the localized collection of multiple noncontractile capillaries. It is found in lip, face, tongue under surface, buccal mucosa, nasal mucosa, nail bed, palm, feet, and gastrointestinal tract).

Treatment

- Continuous iron therapy.
- If epistaxis is frequent, oestrogen therapy is used. Anti-fibrinolytic agent aminocaproic acid may be given.
- Laser therapy may be used for cutaneous and mucosal lesions.

DROWNING

Definition

It is defined as death due to asphyxia following immersion in water. In some cases, no water enters into the lungs and death follows intense laryngospasm, which is called 'dry drowning'.

'Near drowning' is defined as survival for longer than 24 hours after suffocation by immersion. Following drowning, the victim becomes unconscious, doesn't breath unless there is rescue.

Pathogenesis

- Following drowning, there is rapid ventilation-perfusion imbalance with hypoxaemia and development of severe pulmonary oedema.
- As fresh water is hypotonic, it is rapidly absorbed across the alveolar membrane, impairs surfacatant function that leads to alveolar collapse. Absorption of large amount of hypotonic fluid results in haemolysis.
- In salt water drowning, there is alveolar oedema, as salt water is hypertonic.

Clinical Features

Following drowning there are—

- Hypoxaemia.
- Metabolic acidosis.
- Lung injury.
- Acute respiratory distress syndrome.

Complications

- Dehydration.
- Hypotension.
- Haemoptysis.
- Rhabdomyolysis.
- Renal failure.
- Cardiac arrhythmia.
- Death.

Management

Prehospital management—

- Person should be taken out from water. Mouth should be cleaned.
- For breathing—mouth to mouth breathing.
- If the person is not breathing—CPR should be started (2 breaths followed by 30 chest compressions should be given). This cycle is continued until the person starts breathing or emergency help arrives.
- If the person starts breathing—transfer to hospital.

Hospital Management

- Oxygen inhalation.
- Maintenance of water and electrolyte balance.
- Adequate nutrition and hydration.
- If no spontaneous breathing, endotracheal intubation should be done.
- Antibiotic, if infection.

HEAT-RELATED ILLNESS

Exposure to excessive heat may cause—
- Heat cramps.
- Heat syncope.
- Heat exhaustion.
- Heat stroke.

Heat Stroke

Definition

Heat stroke occurs when body temperature is >40°C on exposure to high atmospheric temperature. There is failure of thermoregulation.

Clinical Features

- High body temperature with no sweating and red, hot, dry skin.
- Nausea, vomiting and throbbing headache.
- Rapid, shallow breathing.
- Muscle weakness or cramps.
- Tachycardia.
- Dizziness, confusion, disorientation, seizure, unconsciousness.

Complications

- Hypovolaemic shock.
- Lactic acidosis.
- DIC.
- Rhabdomyolysis.
- Hepatic and renal failure.
- Pulmonary oedema.
- Cerebral oedema.

Investigations

Diagnosis is clinical. Investigations are done to see the effect—
- CBC.
- Blood sugar.
- Serum electrolytes.
- Liver function tests.
- Renal function tests.
- CPK—high.
- Coagulation screening (to see DIC).
- Chest X-ray.

Treatment

- The patient should be transferred to a cool environment.
- Clothing should be removed.
- Body should be cooled by spraying with cold water, fanning, if possible with air cooler or conditioner. Ice packs in axilla, neck and groin may be used.
- IV infusion to correct hypotension and dehydration.
- O_2 inhalation.
- Benzodiazepine can be administered to prevent shivering.
- If patient is unconscious—should be immediately transferred to hospital.

ALCOHOLISM

Alcohol becomes harmful when taken more than 21 units in men and 14 units in women weekly. There may be social, psychological and physical problems with excessive use of alcohol.

Features of Acute Alcohol Intoxication

- Emotional and behavioural disturbance.
- Hypoglycaemia.
- Aspiration of vomitus.
- Respiratory depression.
- Accidents, injuries.

Complications of Chronic Alcohol Misuse

1. Social problems—
   - Disturbance of work.
   - Unemployment.
   - Marital disharmony.
   - Child abuse.
   - Financial difficulties.
   - Problems with the law (e.g. violence and traffic offences).
2. Psychological—
   - Depression, anxiety especially during sudden withdrawal.
   - Attempted and completed suicide, auditory hallucination.
   - Alcohol withdrawal symptoms appear 2–3 days after the last drink and may cause seizures.
   - Delirium tremens—a form of delirium associated with severe alcohol withdrawal.
3. Physical—Involves multiple systems of the body.
   - Neurological—peripheral neuropathy, cerebellar degeneration, cerebral haemorrhage, dementia.
   - Hepatic—fatty liver, alcoholic hepatitis, cirrhosis, liver cancer.
   - GIT—oesophagitis, gastritis, pancreatitis, oesophageal cancer, Mallory-Weiss syndrome, malabsorption.
   - Respiratory—pulmonary tuberculosis, pneumonia and other chest infections.
   - Skin—spider naevi, palmar erythema, Dupuytren's contracture, telangiectasia.
   - Cardiac—cardiomyopathy, arrhythmia, hypertension.
   - Haematological—macrocytosis.
   - Musculoskeletal—myopathy, osteopenia and fracture.
   - Endocrine and metabolic—pseudo-Cushing's syndrome, hypoglycaemia, gout.
   - Reproductive—hypogonadism, foetal alcohol syndrome, infertility.
   - Wernicke's encephalopathy—nystagmus, ophthalmoplegia, ataxia, confusion.
   - Korsakoff's syndrome—short-term memory deficit, confabulation.

Clinical Features of Alcohol Withdrawal

- Restlessness, anxiety, panic attack.
- Tachycardia, sweating, pupil dilatation.
- Nausea, vomiting.

- Delirium tremens—agitation, hallucinations, illusions.
- Delusion.
- Convulsion.

Treatment of Chronic Alcoholic

- Counseling regarding the harmful effects and safe-level alcohol consumption.
- Psychotherapy.
- Maintenance of balanced diet with vitamins specially thiamine.
- Disulfiram.

Delirium Tremens

It is a type of delirium associated with severe alcohol withdrawal. Features usually occur 4–5 days after withdrawal. It is characterized by restlessness, agitation, insomnia, hallucination, illusion, delusion, tremor. Dehydration and tachycardia are also common.

Treatment

- Correction of water and electrolytes.
- High-dose B complex.
- Sedative—diazepam may be given.

WERNICKE'S ENCEPHALOPATHY

Definition

It is the acute cerebral manifestation of vitamin B1 deficiency, commonly in long-standing heavy drinking of alcohol and inadequate diet.

It occurs after repeated vomiting, alcoholism, prolonged starvation or diarrhoea.

Site of lesion: Lesion may be in—

- Brainstem causing ophthalmoplegia, nystagmus and ataxia.
- Superior vermis of cerebellum causing ataxia.
- Dorsomedial nucleus in thalamus and adjacent area of grey matter, causing amnesia.

Clinical Features

- Cognitive changes—acute confusion, disorientation, drowsiness or altered consciousness.
- Eye changes—bilateral symmetrical ophthalmoplegia, bilateral or unilateral paralysis of lateral conjugate gaze, horizontal or vertical nystagmus, abnormal pupillary reflex. Rarely, ptosis, meiosis and unreactive pupil.
- Gait ataxia—broad-based gait, cerebellar sign and vestibular paralysis.
- When associated with memory disturbance and confabulation, it is called Korsakoff's psychosis. Loss of recent memory is common, but past memory may be normal.

NB: Following points are important—

- Confabulation means falsification of memory with clear consciousness. The patient makes several new stories unrelated to the truth.
- In alcoholic, if repeated vomiting is associated with confusion, drowsiness with eye abnormality, Wernicke's encephalopathy should be suspected.

Diagnosis: Mainly Clinical

- CT scan—normal
- CSF is also normal, but slight rise of protein may occur.

Treatment of Wernick's Encephalopathy

- Injection vitamin B_1—500 mg IV over 30 minutes TDS for 2 days, then 500 mg IV or IM daily for 5 days. Then oral B_1 100 mg TDS and other B complex vitamins. If promptly treated, it is reversible.
- Correction of dehydration and electrolyte imbalance.

ADULT STILL'S DISEASE

Definition

It is a diseaseof unknown cause, characterized by high fever, seronegative arthritis, skin rash and polyserositis.

It is usually diagnosed by exclusion of other diseases.

Clinical Features

Common in young adult, 16–35 years of age, rare after 60 years.

Diagnostic Criteria of Adult Still's Disease

1. Each of the four—
   - Fever >39°C.
   - Arthralgia or arthritis lasting 2 weeks or longer.
   - RA—negative
   - ANA—negative.
2. Plus two of the following—
   - Leucocytosis >15,000/mm^3.
   - Evanescent macular or maculopapular skin rash, salmon coloured, nonpruritic.
   - Serositis (pleurisy, pericarditis).
   - Hepatomegaly.
   - Splenomegaly.
   - Lymphadenopathy, usually cervical, may be generalized.

Investigation

- CBC and ESR—shows leukocytosis (may be very high) and high ESR.
- Serum ferritin—very high.
- LFT—may be high SGPT, SGOT.
- X-ray chest—may be pleural effusion, cardiomegaly (due to pericardial effusion).
- USG of whole abdomen—may be ascites, hepatosplenomegaly, lymphadenopathy.

Treatment

- NSAID—in mild to moderate cases or arthritis.
- High-dose steroid—prednisolone 60–100 mg/day. When improve, taper the dose.
- Disease modifying drug (e.g. Methotrexate).
- If no response, biologic agent (e.g. TNF alpha, etanercept, infliximab).

RHABDOMYOLYSIS

Definition

It is defined as acute muscle destruction associated with high myoglobinaemia and myoglobinuria.

Causes

- Trauma (crush injury).
- Vigorous exercise.
- Convulsion or epilepsy.
- Electrocution.
- Hypothermia, heat stroke.
- Alcoholism.
- Polymyositis.
- Neuroleptic malignant syndrome.
- Burn.
- Septicaemia.
- Infection (influenzae, Legionnaire's disease).
- Ecstasy or amphetamine abuse.

Rhabdomyolysis is associated with high AST, CPK, creatinine, potassium, phosphate and uric acid. There is low calcium, because free calcium is bound by myoglobin.

Rhabdomyolysis and renal failure: Muscle injury due to any cause followed by acute renal failure is highly suggestive of rhabdomyolysis. Myoglobin is highly toxic to the renal tubules and precipitates renal failure. Urine is red, but no RBC.

Investigations

- Urine for ammonium sulfate test.
- Spectroscopic examination of urine to detect myoglobin.

NB: Myoglobinuria gives false positive dipstick for blood (haemoglobin), which can be distinguished by the ammonium sulfate test. This test gives a coloured precipitate in haemoglobinuria and coloured supernatant in myoglobinuria.

Treatment

- Supportive—adequate hydration, alkalinization of urine to reduce precipitation of myoglobin in the renal tubules.
- Dialysis, if renal failure.
- Nonsymptomatic hypocalcaemia does not require treatment.
- Loop diuretic should be avoided, as it may cause an acidic urinary pH, aggravating renal failure.

TOXIC SHOCK SYNDROME

Definition

It is a syndrome characterized by high fever, hypotension, diffuse macular rash, desquamation of palms and soles with widespread multiorgan involvement caused by toxic shock syndrome toxin-1 (TSST-1) by *Staph. aureus* or enterotoxin secreted by *Streptococcus pyogens.*

Cause

- Toxic shock syndrome toxin 1 (TSST-1) in menstruating women.
- Enterotoxin in nonmenstruating.

Source of Infection

- In *Staph. aureus* infection—usually from tampons used during menstruation, also infection in nasopharynx, rectum, wound, abscess.
- In streptococcus β hemolyticus—due to soft-tissue infection, such as necrotizing fasciitis, myositis or cellulitis or secondary to pneumonia, osteomyelitis or peritonitis.

Clinical Features

In menstruating women, onset begin 2–3 days after menstruation.

1. High fever >39°C.
2. Hypotension—BP systolic <90 mmHg or postural diastolic drop.
3. Widespread erythematous macular skin rash.
4. Multiple organ involvement—
   - GIT—vomiting or diarrhoea, abdominal pain.
   - Mucosal involvement—oropharyngeal, vaginal, conjunctival.
   - Muscular—myalgia (high CPK).
   - CNS—drowsiness, confusion, disorientation, alteration in consciousness, no focal neurological sign.
   - Skin—desquamation of palms and soles during recovery.
   - Hepatic—high bilirubin, SGPT, low albumin.
   - Hematological—thrombocytopenia <1,00,000/cmm, DIC.
   - Renal involvement—high urea, creatinine.

NB: In streptococcal TSS, features are same like Staphylococcus TSS but skin rash does not develop.

Investigations

- CBC, ESR—shows leucocytosis with thrombocytopenia.
- Blood for C/S—usually negative.
- High endocervical swab for C/S.
- DIC screening—PT, APTT, D-dimer, FDP.
- LFT—high bilirubin, SGPT, SGOT.
- Albumin—low.
- Renal—urea, creatinine (high).
- Others—serum electrolytes, blood sugar, chest X-ray, USG of whole abdomen.

Treatment

1. General measures—
   - IV fluid.
   - Correction of water and electrolyte balance.
   - Nutritional support.
   - Ionotropic support if needed.
2. Broad-spectrum antibiotic—
   - For *Staph. aurues*—flucoxacillin or vancomycin plus clindamycin. Linezolid may be given.
   - For *Streptococcus pyogens*—Penicillin G 2–4 g IV 4 hourly plus clindamycin 600–900 mg IV 8 hourly plus immunoglobulin 2 g/kg single dose.
3. Other therapy—Surgical debridement if needed.

PICKWICKIAN SYNDROME

Definition

It is also called obesity hypoventilation syndrome, characterized by gross obesity associated with failure to breath properly enough resulting in hypoxaemia and hypercapnia. Most of these patient suffer from obstructive sleep apnoea syndrome.

Clinical Features

- Gross obesity.
- Sleep disturbance or sleep apnoea, with daytime sleepiness.
- Airway obstruction may be present, more in smokers.
- Snoring is common.
- Features of polycythaemia.
- Respiratory failure—there is reduced respiratory drive. In most cases, $PaCO_2$ is normal, but may be high.
- Serum leptin is high.

Treatment

- Weight reduction.
- Smoking should be stopped.
- Respiratory stimulants may be helpful. Theophylline, acetazolamide, medroxyprogesterone may be given (which increases respiratory drive).
- C-PAP or Bi-PAP may be used for sleep apnoea.

Complications

- Pulmonary hypertension and corpulmonale
- Sleep apnea syndrome.
- Secondary polycythemia.
- Type II respiratory failure due to alveolar hypoventilation.

HEREDITARY ANGIOEDEMA

Definition

It is disorder inherited as autosomal dominant, due to deficiency or activity of C1 esterase inhibitor (C1-INH), a component of complement system. As a result, there is uncontrolled activation of C1 with increased local bradykinin concentration giving rise to pain and swelling.

Rarely, this condition may be acquired, associated with lymphoma or SLE. However, in such cases, there are low C1-INH and also low C1, C2. Acquired form usually occurs in older age.

Clinical Features

Common in late childhood or early adolescence.

- Angioedema in face, extremities, GIT, upper airways.
- Due to GIT involvement, there is recurrent acute abdomen.
- Laryngeal obstruction is dangerous.
- No urticarial, no allergy, no itching.

Attack may be spontaneous or triggered by trauma, infection, dental procedures or emotional stress. Also, there is increasing frequency and severity during puberty, menstruation and ovulation. Usually family history is present. Patient can present with any combination of cutaneous angioedema, abdominal pain or acute airway obstruction.

Investigations

- During acute attack—Serum C4 is low.
- Barium meal and follow-through show intestinal sacked coin appearance during attack.
- Confirmed by measurement of serum C1-INH.

Treatment

1. During acute attack—
   - Purified C1-INH infusion.
   - Two new drugs—bradykinin receptor antagonist (icatibant) or plasma kallikrein inhibitor (ecallantide) may be used.
   - Fresh frozen plasma may be used.
   - Steroid and adrenaline are ineffective.
2. For prevention—danazol or stanozolol may be given, which increase C1-INH, C2 and C4 by hepatic synthesis. However, these should be avoided in children.
3. Screening of the family members.

FAMILIAL PERIODIC PARALYSIS

Definition

It is a disorder inherited as autosomal dominant, characterized by episodic extreme weakness which progresses from proximal to distal due to low potassium.

There is membrane abnormality. Cranial and respiratory muscles are spared.

Types: 3 Types—

1. Hypokalaemic—lasts for days. It is the common type, called hypokalaemic periodic paralysis.
2. Hyperkalaemic—lasts for hours (in this type, myotonia of tongue and eye may occur, common in <10 years of age).
3. Normokalaemic—rare.

Cause

Unknown, there is shift of potassium from extracellular fluid to the intracellular fluid. Symptoms can be precipitated by intravenous glucose and insulin which would support the diagnosis of potassium shift theory.

NB: It may be confused with thyrotoxic periodic paralysis.

Clinical Features

- Patient feels weakness with activity, which usually occurs periodically after some precipitating factors.

Precipitating Factors

- Increased carbohydrate meal.
- Cold.
- Rest after exercise.
- Alcohol.
- Anxiety or tension.
- It usually occurs during rest after prolonged exercise, also while the patient is asleep.

Treatment

- During acute attack—potassium therapy in IV mixed with normal saline infusion (potassium is never given directly IV).
- Long-term treatment with potassium supplement.
- Potassium sparing diuretic (spironolactone) is given.
- Acetazolamide may be helpful—to prevent attack.

Hyperkalaemic Periodic Paralysis

It is a disorder inherited as autosomal dominant characterized by severe weakness, usually after exercise. Starts in childhood, remit after the age of 20. Attack persists for 30–120 minutes. Myotonia of tongue and eye may occur.

Treatment

IV calcium gluconate during acute attack. Acetazolamide or thiazide diuretic may be helpful.

Thyrotoxic Periodic Paralysis (TPP)

If a thyrotoxic patient develops sudden or periodic weakness, it is called thyrotoxic periodic paralysis. It is due to hypokalaemia (caused by entry of potassium into the cell), common in Asians. May occur following excess carbohydrate or glucose or heavy exercise. Persists up to 7–72 hours. Treatment of thyrotoxicosis improves the condition.

CARCINOID SYNDROME

Definition

It is a syndrome characterized by systemic symptoms that occurs when secretory products released from carcinoid tumour enter into the systemic circulation.

Secretory products are—serotonin or 5-hydroxytryptamin (5-HT), bradykinin, histamine, tachykinin, prostaglandin.

Sites

Carcinoid tumor is derived from enterochromaffin cells, 90% found in GIT (common in ileum, also appendix, rectum) and 10% in the lung. In appendix, it is usually benign, presents as appendicitis (10%).

Clinical Features

Carcinoid tumors are asymptomatic, until metastasis. Only 5% develop carcinoid syndrome, when there is metastasis to the liver. Features are—

- Recurrent attack of bluish-red flushing mainly on face and neck, wheezing. Flushing is the hallmark.
- Abdominal pain, recurrent diarrhoea, vomiting.
- Pellagra and photosensitive dermatitis may occur.
- There may be hypotension, bradycardia, facialoedema.
- Cardiac abnormalities are found in 50% cases, usually right sided. Tricuspid regurgitation, pulmonary stenosis. Left-sided cardiac valves are not affected, but bronchial carcinoid causes left-sided valvular lesion.
- Hepatomegaly, which is firm, irregular due to metastasis.

Investigations

- 24-hours urine for 5-HIAA (5-hydroxy-indole-acetic acid).
- USG of abdomen (to see hepatic metastasis). CT scan may be done.
- Colour doppler echocardiography to see cardiac lesion.
- Serum chromogranin A—high.

Treatment

- Surgery or embolization for solitary liver metastasis or bronchial carcinoid.
- Octreotide or lanreotide improves the syndrome in 90%. Long-acting octreotide sometimes inhibits tumor growth.
- Interferon and chemotherapy may be used which reduces tumor growth, but does not prolong survival.
- Nicotinamide is helpful for pellagra.
- Survival is 5–10 years.

PSEUDOMEMBRANOUS COLITIS

Definition

It is an inflammatory colitis characterized by bloody diarrhoea due to *Clostridium difficile* that occurs after antibiotic therapy.

May occur due to any oral antibiotic therapy, commonly clindamycin, cephalosporin, ampicillin and amoxicillin. 5% healthy adults and 20% elderly are healthy carrier of this organism.

Pathogenesis

Two types of toxins—A (enterotoxin) and B (cytotoxin) are responsible. It is common (80%) in elderly, above 65 years. Colonic mucosa may be ulcerated, occasionally covered by creamy white membrane like material, so it is called pseudomembranous colitis. It may be confused with ulcerative colitis.

Clinical Features

Common in the first few days of using antibiotic, even up to 6 weeks after stopping the drug.

- Bloody diarrhoea.
- Abdominal pain, cramp.

Investigations

- Detecting A or B toxin in stool by ELISA.
- Stool for RE and C/S, culture is positive in 90% cases.
- Colonoscopy—erythema, wide area of plaque, adherent pseudomembrane. Biopsy should be taken.

Treatment

- Offending drug should be stopped.
- Metronidazole 400 mg 8 hourly or vancomycin 125 mg qds for 7–10 days.
- Correction of dehydration by IV infusion.
- In severe case, IV immunoglobulin may be given.

Complications

Toxic dilatation, perforation, ileus may occur.

KALLMANN'S SYNDROME

Definition

Kallman's syndrome is due to isolated gonadotropin releasing hormone (GnRH) deficiency, characterized by hypogonadotropic hypogonadism with anosmia.

Pathogenesis

It results from disordered migration of gonadotropin releasing hormone (GnRH) producing neurons into the hypothalamus. This leads to failure of GnRH secretion and subsequent failure of luteinizing hormone (LH), follicle stimulating hormone (FSH) and testosterone production.

It is often familial, may be inherited as X-linked, autosomal dominant or autosomal recessive.

Clinical Features

It is common in males, rare in females (male to female ratio 4:1).

- Short stature.
- Absence of secondary sexual characters (sparse body hair, under developed penis and small testis).
- Anosmia.
- Associated with cleft lip and palate, high-arched palate, nystagmus and sensorineural deafness.
- Renal agenesis may occur.
- May be cryptorchidism, cerebellar dysfunction, cerebral abnormality, colour blindness.

Investigation

- Measurement of gonadotropin releasing hormone (GnRH).
- MRI of brain to exclude other abnormalities.

Treatment

- GnRH hormone therapy restores pituitary function.
- In females—cyclic oestrogen and progesterone therapy should be given. Fertility is possible.

TUMOUR LYSIS SYNDROME

Definition

Tumour lysis syndrome (TLS) is characterized by hyperuricaemia, hyperkalaemia, hyperphosphataemia and hypocalcaemia, caused by destruction of large number of neoplastic cells after chemotherapy.

Acidosis and acute renal failure may occur. TLS usually occurs during or shortly (1–5 days) after chemotherapy. Rarely, spontaneous necrosis of malignancy can cause TLS.

Tumour lysis syndrome is associated with treatment of Burkitt's lymphoma, acute lymphoblastic leukemia, high-grade non-Hodgkin's lymphoma, chronic leukaemia and rarely with solid tumour.

Mechanism of renal failure in TLS: Chemotherapy kills malignant cells and increase production of serum uric acid, which is precipitated in the tubules, medulla and collecting ducts of the kidney, leading to renal failure. Uric acid crystals in urine indicate uric acid nephropathy.

Investigation

- Serum uric acid and phosphate—high.
- Serum calcium—low.
- LDH—high (marker of bulky disease, with a risk of TLS).
- Serum urea and creatinine—high, if renal failure.
- Serum electrolytes—hyperkalaemia.

Treatment

- Identification of risk and prevention are the most important steps in the management of this syndrome.
- Preventive measures—allopurinol, urinary alkalinization, plenty of fluid.
- Symptomatic hypocalcaemia should be corrected.
- If renal failure—dialysis, haemodialysis is preferred.

KIKUCHI'S DISEASE

Definition

It is a rare, benign disorder of unknown etiology, characterized by lymphadenopathy with or without systemic features. It is also known as histiocytic necrotizing lymphadenitis.

Clinical Features

Common in females.

- Lymphadenopathy (common), usually localized, involving cervical lymph nodes (80%), mainly posterior chain. May be generalized affecting axillary, inguinal and mesenteric nodes.
- Fever, headache, nausea, vomiting, malaise, arthralgia, myalgia, night sweat, rash, abdominal or thoracic pain and weight loss.
- There may be maculopapular or morbilliform rash, nodules, urticaria and malar rash (resembling SLE).
- Hepatosplenomegaly.
- Involvement of bone marrow, thyroid, parotid gland and myocardium is rare.
- Neurological manifestation—aseptic meningitis, acute cerebellar ataxia and encephalitis.

Differential Diagnosis

May be confused with lymphoma, tubercular lymphadenitis and SLE. Other differential diagnoses include viral or bacterial lymphadenitis, metastatic carcinoma, rheumatoid arthritis, infectious mononucleosis, sarcoidosis, cat scratch disease, Still's disease, tuberculosis.

Investigations

- CBC—shows mild granulocytopenia or atypical lymphocytes. ESR and CRP may be high.
- LDH may be high, if liver is involved.
- ANA and anti-ds DNA may be done to exclude SLE.
- FNAC or biopsy of lymph node shows—necrotizing lymphadenitis.
- Others—chest X-ray, USG of whole abdomen.

Treatment

Usually supportive.

- Reassurance.
- Fever and pain may be treated with NSAID.
- Steroid is indicated in severe extranodal disease, involvement of liver (elevated LDH) or nervous system, severe lupus like syndrome or generalized KD. Prednisolone 50–60 mg daily orally with tapering as symptoms resolve.
- Immunosuppressive drugs are used with steroid in severe, life-threatening cases.
- Some patients respond to minocycline, ciprofloxacin, chloroquine and hydroxychloroquine.

Prognosis

Kikuchi's disease is generally benign and self-limiting with a good prognosis. It usually resolves over several weeks to 6 months. Recurrence is unusual (3%) and fatalities are rare.

CAVERNOUS SINUS THROMBOSIS

If any patient has infection in upper lip followed by headache, fever and proptosis, it is highly suggestive of cavernous sinus thrombosis.

Mechanism

Facial veins drain into the sinus. Most common source of infection is due to squeezing of nasal furuncle without antibiotic cover. Other sources of infection are otitis media, sinusitis and dental infection. Commonest organism is *Staphylococcus aureus*.

Causes or Predisposing Factors

1. Infections of the face, nose, ear, teeth and sinuses.
2. Thromboembolism due to—
   - Inherited thrombophilic disease (e.g. deficiency of antithrombin III, protein S and C).
   - Hyperviscosity syndrome.
   - Immobilization.
   - Pregnancy and puerperium.
   - Oral contraceptive pill.
   - Behcet's syndrome.

Clinical Features

- Severe periorbital headache, which also affects the areas innervated by the ophthalmic and maxillary branches of trigeminal nerve.
- Fever and periorbital oedema usually develop later.
- Bilateral proptosis with ophthalmoplegia.
- Fundoscopy shows papillodema.

Investigations

- High-resolution CT scan of the orbit with contrast or
- Gadolinium-enhanced MRI scan of the orbit.

Treatment

- Intravenous flucloxacillin 500 mg 6 hourly.
- Heparin.
- Corticosteroid may be used, which may improve inflammation around the cranial nerves.
- Others—symptomatic and supportive.

Complications

- Ocular swelling.
- Chemosis.
- Ophthalmoplegia due to compression of third, fourth and sixth cranial nerves.
- Drowsiness.

FLUID RETENTION SYNDROME (IDIOPATHIC OEDEMA)

Definition

This syndrome is characterized by periodic episodes of oedema frequently accompanied by abdominal distension, without any detectable cause. It exclusively occurs in women.

Clinical Features

- Oedema is intermittent and often worse in the premenstrual phase.
- The patient complains of swelling of the face, hands, breasts, thighs and feeling of being bloated.
- Also, there may be headache, blurring of vision, abdominal pain and diarrhoea.
- Sodium retention during the day causes an increase in body weight. This is followed by increased sodium excretion during recumbency which causes reduction of weight (usually at night). Diurnal variation of weight >1.5 kg over 12 hours.

Investigations

Done to exclude other diseases.

Treatment

General measures—
- Restriction of salt intake.
- Wearing of elastic stockings.
- Rest in supine position for several hours in each day.
- Regular exercise.

Drugs—
- Diuretic may help initially, but later lose their efficacy.
- ACE inhibitors may be given.
- Others—Progesterone, bromocriptine may be used.

HICCOUGH

Definition

It is a disorder due to sudden spasmodic involuntary contraction of the diaphragm with the glottis remaining closed.

Causes

Due to irritation of diaphragm or phrenic nerve.

Causes below the Diaphragm

1. Stomach—gastric distension (due to air swallowing, overeating, hasty ingestion of food and fluids), neoplasm.
2. Oesophagus—obstruction, reflux esophagitis.
3. Intestinal distension.
4. Hepatobiliary—hepatomegaly, hepatitis, hepatic failure, cholecystitis.
5. Pancreatic—pancreatitis, malignancy.
6. Subphrenic abscess.
7. Peritonitis.
8. Renal—CKD.

Causes above the Diaphragm

1. Respiratory—pneumonia, empyema, neoplasm, respiratory failure.
2. Cardiac—myocardial infarction, pericarditis, aneurysm.

Other Causes

1. Central nervous system—neoplasm, infection (encephalitis), CVD, trauma.
2. Metabolic—hypocapnoea (hyperventilation), diabetic ketoacidosis, electrolyte imbalance.
3. Alcohol ingestion.
4. Mechanical ventilation.
5. Surgery—general anaesthesia, postoperative.
6. Psychogenic—emotional excitement, stress, laughing.
7. Idiopathic.

Investigations

According to history and suspicion of causes.
- CBC.
- Liver and renal function test (Serum urea, creatinine, elctrolytes).
- Chest X-ray.
- USG of abdomen.
- Upper GI endoscopy.
- Echocardiography.
- Bronchoscopy.
- Chest fluoroscopy.
- CT of the head, chest and abdomen.

Treatment

1. Symptomatic treatment—
   - Breathing and rebreathing into a paper bag.
   - Breath holding.
   - Drinking cold water.
   - Valsalva manoeuver, sneezing, gasping (fright stimulus).
   - Stimulation of vagus by carotid sinus massage.
   - Relief of gastric distension by belching or antacid or insertion of nasogastric tube.
2. Drugs—
   - Chlorpromazine 25–50 mg or haloperidol 5 mg tds.
   - Domperidone 10 mg tds or metoclopramide 10 mg tds.
   - Benzodiazepines (lorazepam, diazepam).
   - Anticonvulsants (phenytoin, carbamazepine).
   - Baclofen or gabapentine.
   - Occasionally general anaesthesia.
3. Treatment of primary cause.

CYSTIC FIBROSIS

Definition

Cystic fibrosis is an autosomal recessive disease characterized by abnormal transport of chloride and sodium ions across the epithelium, causing thick and viscous secretions, leading to bronchopulmonary infection and pancreatic insufficiency.Prevalence is 1/2500.

Pathogenesis

CF is due to mutation of a gene on the long arm of chromosome 7, which codes for chloride channel known as cystic fibrosis transmembrane conductance regulator (CFTR), which regulates salt and water movement across the epithelium of nose, lungs, salivary glands, pancreas, intestine and bile ducts.

Clinical Features

Vary according to age.

Neonate: Failure to thrive, meconium ileus, rectal prolapse.

Children and Young Adult

1. Respiratory—
   - Recurrent infection (by *Staph. aureus, Pseudomonas aeruginosa* are the commonest).
   - Features of bronchiectasis—cough, wheeze, haemoptysis.
   - May be pneumothorax, lung collapse, respiratory failure, corpulmonale, asthma, otitis media, sinusitis, nasal polyps.
2. Abdominal—
   - Pancreatic insufficiency causing steatorrhoea, malabsorption.
   - Cholesterol gallstone.
   - Secondary biliary cirrhosis and portal hypertension.
   - Distal intestinal obstruction syndrome (meconium ileus equivalent syndrome).
   - Increased incidence of peptic ulceration and GI malignancy.
3. Others—
   - Diabetes mellitus, in 25% cases.
   - Male infertility (due to failure of development of vas deferens and epididymis). About 20% of females with cystic fibrosis are infertile.
   - Delayed puberty and skeletal maturity.
   - Arthritis, osteoporosis.
   - Vasculitis.
   - Clubbing with hypertrophic pulmonary osteoarthropathy.
   - Stress incontinence due to repeated forced cough.

Investigations

Routine—
- CBC.
- Blood sugar
- Liver function tests.

- Serum creatinine and electrolytes.
- Throat swab and sputum culture.
- X-ray chest (shows hyperinflation, bronchiectasis).
- USG of whole abdomen (fatty liver, cirrhosis, chronic pancreatitis).
- Spirometry (to see obstructive defect).
- Fecal fat analysis.

Specific—
- Sweat test—high sweat sodium and chloride > 60 mmol/L.

Diagnosis of cystic fibrosis: Done by history and investigations—
- Family history of cystic fibrosis.
- Sweat test.
- Blood DNA analysis (to see gene defect).
- Radiological features of bronchiectasis.
- Absent vas deferens and epididymis.
- Blood immune-reactive trypsin levels (for screening purpose).

Treatment

1. General care—
   - Nutritional support.
   - Fat-soluble vitamin supplement—A, D, E, K.
   - Strict glucose control.
   - Smoking must be stopped.
   - Vaccination—influenza and pneumococcal vaccines.
2. For respiratory problems—
   - Physiotherapy (postural drainage, active cycle techniques, forced expiratory technique).
   - Antibiotic, if infection (oral or IV) and prophylactically (oral flucloxacillin or nebulized colomycin or tobramycin).
   - For symptomatic relief—mucolytic, bronchodilators, inhaled corticosteroid. In some patients, inhalation of recombinant DNAse or hypertonic saline may give some relief.
   - Oxygen therapy, as needed.
   - Pulmonary rehabilitation.
   - In advanced lung disease—oxygen, diuretic (in cor pulmonale), noninvasive ventilation, lung or heart-lung transplantation.
3. For abdominal problems—
   - Pancreatic enzyme.
   - If acute abdomen due to intestinal obstruction—then nothing by mouth, IV fluid and nasogastric suction. Acetylcysteine IV or through nasogastric tube is useful in bowel obstruction.
   - Ursodeoxycholic acid for impaired liver function.
   - Liver transplantation may be needed in cirrhosis.
4. Other treatment—for osteoporosis, sinusitis, vasculitis, infertility.
5. Gene therapy—is a possibility in future.
6. Genetic counselling.

Distal intestinal obstruction syndrome (meconium ileus equivalent syndrome): It is a form of small intestinal obstruction occurring during infancy and onward in a patient with cystic fibrosis, resulting from a combination of steatorrhoea and viscid intestinal secretions, causing faecal impaction in ascending colon or in ileocaecal junction.

Treatment

See above.

NB: Following points are important—

- Cystic fibrosis should be suspected in any young patient who presents with repeated chronic respiratory and GI problems.
- Gastrointestinal problems, malabsorption and diabetes mellitus in patient with cystic fibrosis is due to pancreatic insufficiency.
- Faecal elastase is used as a screening test for exocrine pancreatic dysfunction.
- *Pseudomonas aeruginosa* is the commonest organism, causing recurrent respiratory infection.
- Prognosis—median survival is over 30 years.

OXYGEN THERAPY

It is the administration of oxygen to treat hypoxaemia and to ensure adequate arterial oxygen saturation (PO_2 >90%) to meet the demand of the tissues.

Methods of Oxygen Delivery

- Nasal cannulae, flow rate for 1L/min, delivers FiO_2 of 24%, then for additional 1 L increases flow rate by 4%.
- Facemak or venturi mask, it permits precise delivery of oxygen. It delivers oxygen by 35–55%.
- CPAP (continuous positive airway pressure). Useful in obstructive sleep apnea syndrome.
- Bi-PAP (bilevel positive airway pressure). This method is useful in neuromuscular disease, COPD and postoperative respiratory insufficiency.

Indications

In chronic condition—Low flow

- COPD.

In acute conditions- High flow. Indicated where the injury or illness causes hypoxaemia. Oxygen flow should be adjusted according to pulse oximetry.

- Acute severe asthma.
- Major trauma.
- Myocardial infarction.
- Left ventricular failure (acute pulmonary oedema).
- ARDS.
- Massive haemorrhage.
- Anaphylaxis and shock.
- During resuscitation.

Complications

- In COPD or chronic bronchitis, it aggaravates respiratory failure.
- In lung—pulmonary oedema, ARDS, progressive decrease in lung compliance.
- In premature infants and neonates—retrolental fibroplasia and blindness, bronchopulmonary dysplasia.

NB: In COPD or chronic respiratory failure, high flow or continuous oxygen therapy should be avoided. Because, in such case, respiratory centre is insensitive to high CO_2 retention and hypoxia is the only stimulant to the respiratory centre. So total correction of hypoxia may aggravate respiratory failure.

PAGET'S DISEASE

Definition

Paget's disease is characterized by excessive and disorganized resorption and formation of bone, resulting in deformity and fracture. Commonly involved bones are pelvis, femur, tibia, lumbar spines, skull and scapula.

Common above 55 years of age, rare below 40 years. More in temperate climate.

Cause

Unknown. Genetic factors are important. Some slow viruses like measles may be involved.

Pathogenesis

In Paget's disease, there is increased osteoclastic bone resorption and increased osteoblastic activity, followed by abnormal bone formation. Bone formation exceeds resorption, the new bone is bigger, but weaker and filled with new blood vessels. The disease may involve one bone (monostotic, 10–15%) or many bones (polyostotic).

Clinical Features

Common in females, M:F= 2:3.

- Many cases are asymptomatic (60–80%), detected on routine investigation like radiologically.
- May be bone pain, joint pain or stiffness, bowing of the legs, deformities (in weight-bearing bones, such as femur, tibia), pathological fracture, enlarged head and other bony swelling.
- Neurological features—deafness, cranial nerve defect, nerve root pain, spinal cord compression and spinal stenosis may occur due to enlargement of affected bone.
- Warm skin over the affected bone, high-output cardiac failure due to hyperdynamic circulation (due to increased vascularity of the bone).

Investigations

- Bone X-ray shows enlargement of bone with typical lytic and sclerotic lesion. X-ray skull shows lytic lesion osteoporosis circumscripta, also enlargement and sclerosis, thickening of trabeculae.
- Serum alkaline phosphates (high, normal in 10% cases due to monostotic involvement).
- Isotope bone scan (to see extent of bone involvement. It cannot differentiate between Paget's disease and osteoblastic metastatic carcinoma).
- Urinary hydroxyproline (high, it is a marker of bone breakdown).
- CT scan or MRI of bone may be done.
- Rarely bone biopsy.
- Calcium and phosphate—Normal (calcium may be high in prolonged immobilization or fracture).

Treatment

1. For pain—NSAIDs
2. To prevent further bone breakdown—
   - Bisphosphonates—Pamidronate, zoledronate, risedronate are more effective. Also etidronate and tiludronate. Hypocalcaemia may occur, so calcium and vitamin D should be taken

- Calcitonin—May be used subcutaneously 100–200 IU, three times weekly, for 2–3 months. It is less convenient and more expensive.

3. Orthopaedic surgery—Joint replacement or osteotomy may be needed. Neurosurgery may be needed in spinal cord compression.

Complications

- Bone fractures and deformities.
- Deafness due to otosclerosis of the ossicles, less due to compression of VIIIth cranial nerve.
- High-output heart failure.
- Secondary osteoarthrosis.
- Optic atrophy.
- Spinal cord compression causing paraplegia.
- Spinal stenosis.
- Basilar invagination (platybasia) causing brainstem sign.
- Osteosarcoma (Rare but serious).

CHARCOT-MARIE-TOOTH DISEASE

Definition

It is a group of heterogenous motor and sensory neuropathy.

May be inherited autosomal dominant or recessive or X linked. Affected family members may have forme fruste with only pescavus and absent ankle jerks.

Clinical Features

- The patient usually presents with foot deformities or gait disturbance in early childhood or early adult life.
- Bilateral pescavus and clawing of toes are present.
- Distal weakness and wasting that begins in the leg, progress slowly, involves both lower limbs up to the middle of legs, giving rise to inverted champagne bottle (stork or spindle legs) appearance.
- Dorsiflexion—weak in both feet.
- Ankle jerk—absent bilaterally.
- Plantar response—bilaterally equivocal.
- Sensory—mild impairment of both superficial and deep sensation up to mid thigh (even marked sensory loss with trophic ulcer may be found).
- Gait—steppage gait with foot drop.
- Later wasting and weakness in upper limbs may occur.

Types

1. Hereditary motor and sensory neuropathy type I—there is demyelinating neuropathy. It is the commonest type (70%), inherited as autosomal dominant.
2. Hereditary motor and sensory neuropathy type II—there is axonal neuropathy. There is prominent sensory involvement with pain and paraesthesia. Inherited as AD, recessive or X-linked dominant.

3. Hereditary motor and sensory neuropathy type III (also called distal spinal muscular atrophy). It is inherited as autosomal recessive.
4. Hereditary motor and sensory neuropathy type IV—CMT with optic atrophy, deafness, retinitis pigmentosa and spastic paraparesis. It is inherited as autosomal recessive.

Investigation

Nerve conduction study.

Treatment

Symptomatic and supportive. Physiotherapy and orthopedic measure may be given.

HIV INFECTION (AIDS)

HIV

Human immunodeficiency virus is a single stranded RNA virus, belongs to lentivirus group of retrovirus family. Two types—HIV-1 and HIV-2.

HIV Disease

Spectrum of disorders are—
- Primary infection with or without acute HIV syndrome.
- Asymptomatic infected state, even in advanced disease.
- AIDS.

AIDS (Acquired Immunodeficiency Syndrome)

- HIV infected individual with CD4 T cell count <200 cells/mm^3 regardless of the presence of symptoms or
- HIV infected individual with AIDS defining conditions (category C) regardless of CD4 count is called AIDS.

Modes of Transmission of HIV

- Sexual contact with an infected person—more in homosexuals, multiple sexual partners and noncircumcised persons.
- Transplacental, perinatal exposure and breastfeeding.
- Parenteral exposure to infected body fluid.
- Sharing of needles, including intravenous drug abusers.
- Blood and blood product transfusion.
- Occupational transmission.
- Organ transplantation including cornea.

Routes not involved in Transmission of HIV

- Close personal contact (sleeping, shaking hands, kissing).
- Social contact (at school, swimming pool, shopping mall).
- Sharing toilet.
- Staying in a common ward in hospital.
- Sharing utensils.
- Insect or animal bite.
- Respiratory droplets, sputum.
- Through health workers like doctors, nurses.

Natural History of HIV or AIDS

Primary infection: It is symptomatic in 70–80% cases, usually occurs 2–6 weeks after exposure. Features are—
- Fever with rash.
- Pharyngitis with cervical lymphadenopathy.
- Myalgia, arthralgia.
- Headache.
- Mucosal ulceration.

Asymptomatic infection: The patient remains asymptomatic but potentially infectious to others. This stage may persist for 5–10 years. Laboratory investigations may show anaemia, leucopenia, lymphopenia and reduced CD4 count. Also, there is cutaneous anergy.

Mildly symptomatic disease (HIV symptomatic or indicator diseases, category B)—

- Constitutional—low-grade fever, night sweat, weight loss.
- Oral hairy leucoplakia.
- Recurrent oropharyngeal candidiasis, recurrent vaginal candidiasis.
- Herpes zoster involving more than 1 dermatome.
- Idiopathic thrombocytopenic purpura.
- Chronic diarrhoea.
- Peripheral neuropathy.
- Cervical dysplasia, severe pelvic inflammatory disease.

Acquired immunodeficiency syndrome (AIDS): AIDS defining diseases are (category C)—

- Oesophageal candidiasis.
- Cryptococcal meningitis.
- Chronic cryptosporidial diarrhoea.
- Cerebral toxoplasmosis.
- CMV retinitis or colitis.
- Chronic mucocutaneous herpes simplex.
- Disseminated *Mycobacterium avium*-intracellulare (MAI).
- Pulmonary or extra-pulmonary tuberculosis.
- *Pneumocystis jirovecii* (carinii) pneumonia.
- Progressive multifocal leukoencephalopathy.
- Recurrent nontyphi Salmonella septicaemia.
- Extrapulmonary coccidioidomycosis.
- Invasive cervical cancer.
- Extrapulmonary histoplasmosis.
- Kaposi's sarcoma.
- Non-Hodgkin's lymphoma (including Burkitt's lymphoma).
- Primary cerebral lymphoma.
- HIV associated wasting.
- HIV associated dementia.

Table 1 shows clinical categories of HIV.

Table 1

Clinical category of HIV

CD 4 count (/cmm)	Category A: Asymptomatic or persistent generalised lymphadenopathy or acute seroconversion illness.	Category B: (see above)	Category C: (see above)
>500	A1	B1	C1
200–499	A2	B2	C2
<200	A3	B3	C3

NB: Category C, A3, B3 (shaded area) indicates AIDS.

Common Infections in AIDS

- *Pneumocystis jiroveci.*
- *Candida albicans.*
- *Cryptococcus neoformans.*
- *Toxoplasma gondii.*
- Mycobacterium (typical and atypical).
- CMV.
- Amoebiasis.
- *Cryptosporidium.*

HIV-related Cancer

- AIDS defining cancers—Kaposi's sarcoma and non-Hodgkin's lymphoma.
- Non-AIDS defining malignancies—Anal cancer and Hodgkin's disease.

Correlation between CD4 Count and HIV Associated Diseases

1. 500 cells/mm^3—
   - Acute primary infection.
   - Recurrent vaginal candidiasis.
   - Persistent generalized lymphadenopathy.
2. <500 cells/mm^3—
   - Pulmonary tuberculosis.
   - Herpes zoster.
   - Oropharyngeal candidiasis.
   - Oral hairy leukoplakia.
   - Kaposi's sarcoma.
   - HIV associated idiopathic thrombocytopenic purpura.
   - Cervical intraepithelial neoplasia II and III.
3. <200 cells/mm^3—
   - *Pneumocystis jirovecii* pneumonia.
   - Mucocutaneous herpes simplex.
   - Oesophageal candidiasis.
   - Miliary or extrapulmonary tuberculosis.
4. <100 cells/mm^3—
   - Cerebral toxoplasmosis.
   - Cryptococcal meningitis.
   - Non-Hodgkin's lymphoma.
   - Progressive multifocal leukoencephalopathy.
   - HIV-associated dementia.
5. <50 cells/mm^3—
   - CMV retinitis.
   - CMV gastrointestinal disease.
   - Primary CNS lymphoma.
   - Disseminated MAI.

Cutaneous Manifestations of HIV

- Early HIV—Herpes simplex, varicella zoster, human papilloma virus.
- Late HIV—Kaposi's sarcoma, molluscum contagiosum, chronic mucocutaneous herpes simplex.

Findings in Mouth Cavity in HIV Patient

- Hairy leukoplakia.
- Oropharyngeal candidiasis.
- Aphthous ulcer.
- Herpes simplex.
- Periodontal disease.

Causes of Diarrhoea or Enteropathy in HIV Patient: Organisms are—

- Cytomegalovirus (CMV).
- *Cryptosporidium* and *microsporidium*.
- *Mycobacterium avium*-intracellulare (MAI).
- Other infections—Isospora, *Giardia, Entamoeba histolytica, Salmonella, adenovirus* and bacterial overgrowth, etc.

The patient presents with dysphagia, retrosternal pain, watery diarrhoea accompanied by blood, colicky abdominal pain, weight loss and fever.

Major Causes of Pulmonary Disease in HIV

- *Pneumocystis jirovecii* pneumonia.
- Tuberculosis.
- Bacterial pneumonia.
- Fungal infection (e.g. Histoplasma).
- *Cryptococcus*.
- Malignancy—non-Hodgkin's lymphoma, Kaposi's sarcoma.

Neurological Manifestations in AIDS Patient

- Acute meningitis—during acute seroconversion. May be aseptic meningitis, multiple cranial nerve palsy.
- Encephalitis—herpes simplex, varicella zoster virus.
- *Toxoplasma gondii* causes encephalitis characterized by headache, confusion, convulsion and focal signs. MRI shows multiple ring-enhancing lesions in cortical grey-white matter interface, basal ganglia or brain stem with oedema and mass effect. Retinitis may coexist.
- Primary CNS lymphoma (5%).
- AIDS dementia complex (ADC)—may precede the diagnosis of AIDS in 25% cases.
- Progressive multifocal leukoencephalopathy (PML)—presents with hemiparesis, visual or speech defects, altered mental status, ataxia. Seizures are rare and fever is absent. MRI shows nonenhancing white mater lesions without oedema.
- Retinitis—CMV, toxoplasmosis.
- Autonomic neuropathy.

- Spinal cord, root and peripheral nerve disease includes—
  - HIV myelopathy—presents with spastic paraparesis and sensory ataxia. There is involvement of lateral and posterior column of spinal cord.
  - Peripheral neuropathy—by HIV or drugs.
  - Others—Guillain-Barré syndrome, transverse myelitis, brachial neuritis, polyradiculitis and peripheral neuropathy.

Ocular Diseases in AIDS

- CMV retinitis. Fundoscopy shows—retinal cotton wool spots, sometimes fluffy white retinal lesions with area of haemorrhage.
- *Toxoplasma gondii* retinitis.

Renal, Cardiac and Endocrine Complications of HIV

Renal—
- Acute renal failure due to acute infection, drug toxicity.
- Chronic renal failure due to HIV associated nephropathy (HIVAN).
- HIV immune complex kidney diseases.
- Thrombotic microangiopathy.

Cardiac—
- Dilated cardiomyopathy.
- Zidovudine induced cardiomyopathy.
- HIV patients are at higher risk of coronary artery disease. It may be due to HIV itself and change of lipid by antiretroviral drugs.

Endocrine—
- Hypoadrenalism, hypogonadism, hypopituitarism.

Hematological—
- Anaemia—usually mild, normocytic normochromic.
- Leucopenia (neutropenia is common, also lymphopenia).
- Thrombocytopenia, may occur early and may be the only manifestation in early case.
- Lymphoma.
- Pancytopenia.

Investigations for Newly Diagnosed (Asymptomatic) HIV Infected Patient

Routine tests—
- CBC, PBF, LFT, renal function test, lipid profile, blood glucose, urinalysis, chest X-ray.

Related to HIV—
- HIV antibody (confirmatory).
- HIV rapid antibody test (result found in 10-20 minutes). Should be confirmed with ELISA and Western blot.
- CD4 count.
- Viral load.
- HIV genotype.

For other infections—

- Hepatitis serology (A, B, C), HCV RNA.
- Cytomegalovirus serology, PCR.
- Toxoplasma serology.
- Syphilis serology.
- Screening other for sexually transmitted disease.
- Cryptococcal antigen.

Others—

- Cervical cytology in women.
- Lymphocyte subsets.
- HLA-B*5701 screen for hypersensitivity to abacavir.
- Fundoscopy.

Diagnosis of HIV or AIDS

Screening by ELISA (positive 3–12 weeks after infection), confirmation by Western blot.

Pretest and Post-test Counselling for Suspected HIV or AIDS Patient

Pretest counselling—

- Purpose of the test should be discussed.
- Assessment of the risk factors.
- Explanation of the natural history of HIV to the patient.
- Discussion about mode of transmission and reduction of risk.
- Coping strategy.
- Explanation of the test procedure.
- Informed consent.

Post-test counselling—

1. If the test result is negative—
   - Discussion regarding behaviour modification including safer sex and needle exchange.
   - A second test should be carried out 3 months after last exposure.
2. If the test result is positive—
   - Explanation of significance and implications of result.
   - Urgent medical follow-up.
   - Strategy regarding fear of disclosure and social rejection.
   - Verbal and written information.
   - Emotional and practical support by providing phone number and name.

Aims of Treatment

- To reduce viral load to an undetectable level.
- To improve CD4 count to >200 cells/mL, so that severe HIV related disease becomes less.
- To improve quantity and quality of life without unacceptable drug related side effects or lifestyle alteration.
- To reduce transmission.

Indications of Antiretroviral Therapy in Patients with HIV Infection

1. Acute infection syndrome.
2. Chronic infection—
   - Symptomatic disease (including HIV associated nephropathy).
   - Asymptomatic diseases—
     - CD4+ T cell count <350/cmm.
     - Pregnancy.
     - Postexposure prophylaxis.

Treatment of AIDS

General Management

- Dietary and nutritional advice.
- Advice on smoking, alcohol, drug misuse and exercise.
- Proper advice on reducing the risk of HIV transmission including sexual practice.
- Psychological support for the patient, family, friends and caregivers.
- Information about childbearing.

Drug Treatment

Depends on clinical assessment, laboratory investigations including viral load and CD4 counts, also individual circumstances.

Drugs used in HIV-infected Patients

1. Reverse transcriptase inhibitors (RTI)—
   - Nucleoside reverse transcriptase inhibitors (NRTI)—zidovudine, didanosine, lamivudine, stavudine, abacavir, emtricitabine.
   - Nonnucleoside reverse transcriptase inhibitors (NNRTI)—nevirapine, efavirenz and etravirine.
2. Protease inhibitors (PIs)—indinavir, ritonavir, lopinavir, tipranavir, atazanavir, fosamprenavir and darunavir.
3. Entry inhibitors—
   - Fusion inhibitors—enfurvitide.
   - Co-receptor blockers—maraviroc.
   - Integrase inhibitors—raltegravir.

Treatment of CMV Retinitis in HIV

Gancyclovir. Adult dose is—

- Induction therapy—5 mg/kg IV, 12 hourly for 14–21 days.
- Maintenance therapy—5 mg/kg IV daily, 7 days/week. Or, 6 mg/kg IV daily, 5 days/week.
- Oral—1000 mg 3 times a day. Or, 500 mg 6 times a day (every 3 hours while awake) with food.
- If progression of CMV retinitis during maintenance treatment—reinduction should be given.

Prevention of HIV Infection

- Safe sexual practice.
- Effective treatment of STI.

- Screening of blood and blood products.
- Use of clean needles and syringes for IVDU.
- Antiretroviral drugs to reduce mother to child transmission.

Treatment of a Person Exposed to HIV Infection

When risk is significant, in both occupational and nonoccupational settings, lopinavir, tenofovir and emtricitabin are given. First dose is given as soon as possible, preferably within 6–8 hours, 4 weeks of therapy is recommended. Protection is not absolute and seroconversion may occur.

Treatment of HIV Positive Pregnant Woman

Antepartum

- Ritonavir-boosted PI (e.g. lopinavir) with zidovudine and lamivudine from 20 weeks given to all mothers. Or
- Oral zidovudine monotherapy for those with viral loads <10,000 copies/mL and wild type virus who are willing to have caesarean section.

During Delivery

- ZDV IV infusion at the onset of labour given to those on ZDV alone or those on HAART but with detectable virus, undergoing normal vaginal delivery.
- Delivery by caesarean section reduces the risk of transmission but if the patient is on HAART it is unnecessary.

After Delivery

- The neonate should get oral zidovudine for 6 weeks.
- Breastfeeding should be avoided.

PNEUMOCYSTIS CARINII (JIROVECII) PNEUMONIA (PCP)

Pneumocystis jirovecii (previously called *Pneumocystis carinii*) is an opportunistic fungus that causes pneumonia in HIV or AIDS patient, when CD4 is <200/mm^3. PCP may also occur in patients who are immunosuppressed due to cancer, corticosteroid or other immunosuppressive drugs, organ or bone marrow transplantation, etc.

The organism damages alveolar epithelium causing interstitial plasma cell pneumonia with foamy exudate in the alveoli that impedes gas exchange and reduces lung compliance.

Clinical Features

Develop slowly over weeks, may take months.

- Initially there is shortness of breath on exertion.
- Cough (usually dry).
- Fever, malaise, weight loss and night sweat.
- Tachypnoea, tachycardia, cyanosis.
- Fine crepitations may be present.

Investigations

- Chest X-ray—shows bilateral perihilar interstitial infiltrates.
- HRCT of chest—shows ground glass appearance.
- Sputum for cytology or PCR—organism may be found in 50–90% cases (by silver or Giemsa staining or immunofluorescent technique. Organism cannot be cultured).
- Bronchoscopy and bronchoalveolar lavage (shows organisms in 90–95% cases).
- Blood gas analysis (PO_2 is low, <90% on exercise).
- PCR amplification of the fungal DNA in blood.
- Lung function tests—restrictive pattern with reduced diffusion capacity.
- Lung biopsy.
- LDH—high.

Complications

- Respiratory failure.
- Pneumothorax.
- Pleural effusion (rare).
- Bacterial infection.

Treatment

- IV co-trimoxazole (120 mg/kg daily in divided doses for 21 days) is the first line treatment.
- If sensitive to co-trimoxazole—IV pentamidine (4 mg/kg/day) or dapsone and trimethoprim are given for the same duration.
- Atovaquone or combination of clindamycin and primaquine may be given.
- Prednisolone—40 mg bid for 5 days, then 40 mg daily for 5 days and 20 mg daily for 11 days.
- Systemic corticosteroid may be used in severe cases.
- CPAP or mechanical ventilation (if patient remains severely hypoxic or becomes too tired).

Prophylaxis

- Secondary prophylaxis is indicated in patient who recovered from PCP and CD4 remain <200/cmm. Usual regimen is co-trimoxazole 960 mg three times a week. Patient sensitive to sulphonamide are given dapsone, pyrimethamine or nebulized pentamidine.
- Primary prophylaxis therapy is recommended in—AIDS and CD4 counts <200/mm^3.

Bibliography

1. Burns T, Breathnach S, Cox N, Griffiths C. Rook's textbook of dermatology. 7th edn. Philadelphia: WB Saunder. 2011.
2. Dooley JS, Lok A, Burroughs A, Heathcote J. Sherlock's diseases of the liver and biliary system (Sherlock diseases of the liver). 12th edn, Oxford; Blackwell Scientific Publications: 2011.
3. Firkin F, Chesterman C, Rush B. de Gruchy's clinical haematology in medical practice, 6th edn. Oxford: Blackwell Scientific. 2012.
4. Glynn, Drake. Hutchison's clinical methods. 23rd ed. WB Saunders. 2012.
5. Houghton AR, Gray D. Chamberlain's symptoms and signs in clinical medicine. 13th edn. Hodder Arnold. 2010.
6. James WD, Berger T, Elston D. Andrew's diseases of the skin clinical dermatology. 11th edn. Philadelphia: WB Saunder. 2011.
7. Kumar P, Clark ML. Kumar & Clark's Clinical Medicine. 8th edn. London: Saunders Elsevier. 2012.
8. Longo DL, Fauci AS, Kasper DL, Hauser SL, Jameson JL, Loscalzo J. Harrison's principles of internal medicine. 19th edn. New York: McGraw Hill. 2015.
9. Macleod J, Douglas G, Nicol EF, Robertson CE. Macleod's clinical examination. 11th edn. Churchill Livingstone; Elsevier. 2009.
10. Ryder REJ, Mir MA, Freeman EA. An Aid to the MRCP PACES. 3rd edn; Oxford: Blackwell Publishing. 2003.
11. Seaton A, Seaton D, Leitch AG. Crofton and Douglas's: Respiratory disease. 5th edn, 2012.
12. SN Chugh. Bedside medicine without tears. 2nd edn. New Delhi; Jaypee Brothers Medical Publishers (P) Ltd. 2011.
13. SN Chugh. Clinical methods in medicine. 1st edn. New Delhi; Jaypee Brothers Medical Publishers (P) Ltd. 2008.
14. Talley NJ, O'Connor S. Clinical Examination: A systematic guide to physical examination. 7th edn, Elsevier Australia. 2014.
15. Tierney LM, McPhee SJ, Papadakis MA (Eds). Current medical diagnosis and treatment. 55th edn. New York: McGraw Hill. 2016.
16. Walker BR, Colledge NR, Ralston SH, Penman I. Davidson's principles and practice of medicine. 22th edn. Edinburgh: Churchill Livingstone; An imprint of Elsevier. 2014.
17. Warrell DA, Cox TM, John D. Oxford Textbook of Medicine. 5th edn. Oxford: Oxford University Press. 2012.

Index

Page numbers followed by *t* refer to table.

H

I

J

K

L

M

O

P

Q

R

S

U

W

X

Y

Z